MEDICAL TERMINOLOGY
WITH HUMAN ANATOMY

MEDICAL TERMINOLOGY
WITH HUMAN ANATOMY

Third Edition

Jane Rice, RN, CMA-C
Medical Assistant Program Director
Coosa Valley Technical Institute
Rome, Georgia

Spanish Language Consultant
Adie DeLaGuardia, A.S., CMA-C
Broward Community College

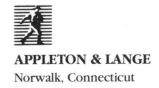

APPLETON & LANGE
Norwalk, Connecticut

95 96 97 98 99 / 10 9 8 7 6 5 4 3 2 1

Prentice Hall International (UK) Limited, *London*
Prentice Hall of Australia Pty. Limited, *Sydney*
Prentice Hall Canada, Inc., *Toronto*
Prentice Hall Hispanoamericana, S.A., *Mexico*
Prentice Hall of India Private Limited, *New Delhi*
Prentice Hall of Japan, Inc., *Tokyo*
Simon and Schuster Asia Pte. Ltd., *Singapore*
Editora Prentice Hall do Brasil Ltda., *Rio de Janeiro*
Prentice Hall, *Englewood Cliffs, New Jersey*

Library of Congress Cataloging–in–Publication Data

Rice, Jane.
    Medical terminology with human anatomy / Jane Rice. — 3rd ed.
        p.   cm.
    Includes index.
    ISBN 0-8385-6268-X
    1. Medicine—Terminology.   2. Human anatomy—Terminology.
  I. Title.
    [DNLM: 1. Nomenclature.   W 15 R496m 1994]
    R123.R523 1994
    610′.14—dc20
    DNLM/DLC   94-15792
    for Library of Congress   CIP

Figures and tables on the following pages were used with permission from Martini F, *Fundamentals of Anatomy and Physiology*, 2nd ed. Englewood Cliffs, NJ: Prentice Hall, 1992: 24, 48, 74, 106, 134, 162, 196, 224, 252, 282, 283, 312, 400, & 432.

Acquisitions Editor: Cheryl L. Mehalik
Production Editor: Elizabeth C. Ryan
Designer: Janice Barsevich Bielawa

ISBN 0-8385-6268-X

90000

9 780838 562680

Dedicated with love and appreciation to Larry Rice,
Melissa Rice-Noble, Doug Noble, and Zachary and Benjamin Noble.
You are the flowers in my life.

In special memory of my parents, Warren Galileo and Elizabeth Styles Justice.

CONTENTS IN BRIEF

CONTENTS

PREFACE

Medical Terminology with Human Anatomy, Third Edition, is a comprehensive, self-paced, text with a built-in dictionary. Written for the person in the fields of allied health, nursing, and business office technology, it is arranged by body systems and speciality areas. By using the body systems approach one may master the component parts of medical words as they are directly related to the topic of the chapter.

THREE-DIMENSIONAL TEXT

This text may be used in a traditional classroom setting, as a programmed text, or as a self-paced individualized instructional workbook.

WORD-BUILDING TECHNIQUE

To build a medical vocabulary, all you have to do is recall the word parts that you have learned and link them with the new component parts presented in the chapter. **Prefixes** and **suffixes** are repeated throughout the text, while **word roots** and **combining forms** are presented according to the system or specialty area to which they relate. Once the material in Chapters 1 and 2 has been mastered, you should know 30 prefixes, 45 suffixes, and 39 roots/combining forms. This word-building technique, while not complicated, is different from other terminology texts that have students learn prefixes, roots, combining forms, and suffixes as separate entities, generally not related to the terminology of a body system. It is much easier to learn component parts directly associated with a body system or specialty area and this is the key to the classic design of *Medical Terminology with Human Anatomy.*

ORGANIZATION AND CLASSIC DESIGN

The Third Edition has been redesigned, and throughout the text vibrant use of red, with its various shades, strengthens the presentation. The Anatomy and Physiology Overviews have been moved to the beginning of the chapters so that you may acquire an appreciation of the basic structure and function of the body before proceeding to the Terminology, Vocabulary, and other sections of the chapter. Each chapter is organized in the same manner, thereby allowing you to participate in a systematic learning experience in which medical terminology becomes a new, easily learned, and interesting part of your vocabulary.

Key Features

- 24 pages of full color illustrations for anatomy and physiology placed at the beginning of the text. This is a perfect complement to the discussion of the Anatomy and Physiology Overviews in Chapters 2 through 16.
- **Chapter Opening with Appropriate Art Work:** The chapter opening gives a brief

synopsis of the subject of the chapter and the art work enhances the presentation. Included in the chapter opening side bars are interesting facts and statistics about health.

- **Anatomy and Physiology Overview** (Chapters 2 through 16): Comprehensive coverage of the structure and function of the body with new art and tables. Many chapters have been updated and expanded.
- **Insights:** A *new feature* that presents a current finding in medicine or an interesting topic that relates to the subject of the chapter.
- **Drug Highlights**: A *new feature* that presents essential drug information that relates to the subject of the chapter.
- **Terminology with Surgical Procedures and Pathology:** Each term has a pronunciation guide directly under it, word parts are identified and defined, and the definition of the term is provided. Each term is presented in alphabetical order for easy reference, acting as a built-in dictionary.
- **Vocabulary Words:** Common words or specialized terms associated with the subject of the chapter. These words are provided to enhance your medical vocabulary. Each word is presented in alphabetical order, with a pronunciation guide and definitions.
- **Abbreviations:** Selected abbreviations with their meanings are included in each chapter. These abbreviations are in current use and directly associated with the subject of the chapter.
- **Communication Enrichment (English/Spanish):** This *new feature* provides you with the opportunity to learn Spanish for selected general and medical terms associated with the subject of the chapter.
- **Diagnostic and Laboratory Tests:** Describes currently used tests and procedures that are used in the physical assessment and diagnosis of certain conditions and diseases that are related to the subject of the chapter.
- **Learning Exercises:** Provides you with the opportunity to write in the correct answers for questions that relate to the anatomy and physiology. The Word Parts section is arranged in alphabetical order, and includes all of the word parts presented in the chapter. This is an excellent method for learning the component parts that are used to build medical words. Identifying Medical Terms allows you to build medical words and the Spelling Section allows you to test your spelling skills.
- **Review Questions:** The Review Questions include matching and fill-in-the-blank. These questions are based on the vocabulary words, abbreviations, and diagnostic and laboratory tests.
- **Appendix I:** Answer Key for the learning exercises and review questions. All answers are provided so that you may easily check your work.
- **Appendix II:** Includes common medical abbreviations, and medication and prescription abbreviations.
- **Appendix III:** Glossary of Component Parts includes 89 Prefixes, 640 Roots and Combining Forms, and 160 Suffixes with their meanings. It also includes 10 suffixes that mean "pertaining to" and 7 suffixes that mean "condition of." When you have completed *Medical Terminology with Human Anatomy,* you will know 889 component parts and be able to use these component parts to understand the technical language of medicine.
- **Index:** Includes over 3000 words plus a Spanish index of 700 words.
- **Flashcards:** The most commonly used prefixes, roots and combining forms, and suffixes are provided in a perforated format for you to use while studying medical terminology.

ANCILLARIES FOR THE INSTRUCTOR

- *Instructor's Guide/Test Bank:* Contains: A course Syllabus, Progress Sheet, Test Schedule, Answer Sheet for post test A and post test B, two tests for each chapter. Form A and Form B, two final exams, over 2000 questions and all answers are provided.
- Upon adoption, a **Computerized Test Generator** (IBM compatible) is available by contacting your local Appleton & Lange representative. A menu-driven computer program designed to create examinations, it consists of *the same* test items included in the Instructor's Guide/Test Bank, but provides the instructor with maximum flexibility due to the computerization of the material. The instructor can use the Computerized Test Generator to quickly create tests either by choosing specific items or by having the program randomly select test items. Any test items in the pool may be previewed, and test items from one or more chapters may be included in the exam. Once selected, test items can be scrambled or left in order. If more than one chapter is chosen, test items may be shuffled or left grouped by chapter. Test items may be edited, deleted or added to the test item pool by the instructor with a special, easy-to-use text editor incorporated into the program.

STUDY AIDS FOR THE STUDENT

- **Computerized Student Self-Assessment:** Over 1000 questions are provided in a multiple choice, true/false, fill-in-the-blank format. The learner is tested on material in a given chapter with the correct answer explained, as well as referenced by page number. A study plan is then generated from questions that were answered incorrectly. Study plans may be viewed directly on the computer screen or printed. Computerized Student Self-Assessment Guides are available for purchase from Educational Software Concepts, Inc., 660 S. 4th Street, Edwardsville, Kansas, 66113, 1-800-748-7734.
- A Three Tape Set (45 minutes each side) of all the terms listed in the terminology sections is available as an aid to pronunciation and understanding of the terms. Each term is pronounced, broken into its component parts, the definition of the part is given and then the term is pronounced again. By learning the component parts that are used to build medical words, one may easily acquire a working knowledge of medical terminology. These tapes are available for student purchase from Appleton & Lange at 1-800-423-1359 or by filling out the coupon found in Jane Rice's Medical Terminology with Human Anatomy, Third Edition.
- Free to both the student and the instructor upon request is a single Student Tape, which will contain two sides (thirty minutes each). The first side will focus on difficult terminology from three chapters: Integumentary System (Chapter 3), Endocrine System (Chapter 11) and Nervous System (Chapter 12). The "Tough Terms" will be pronounced and then defined. Side 2 will focus on key Spanish terms and short phrases. The term or phrase will be pronounced in Spanish, then defined in English. This offer is available through Appleton & Lange by filling out the coupon found in Jane Rice's MEDICAL TERMINOLOGY WITH HUMAN ANATOMY, THIRD EDITION. No telephone requests will be honored. Limit one per customer.

ACKNOWLEDGMENTS

I extend my warmest gratitude to the individuals who accepted *Medical Terminology with Human Anatomy* as their text and to the Allied Health, Nursing, and business office technology students that I have had the privilege to teach. I especially want to thank Betty Coffman, friend and colleague, who planted the seed for adding Spanish to this edition.

During this Autumn of my life, there is a person who has brought Springtime to me, and that is my editor at Appleton & Lange, Cheryl Mehalik. Through her guidance and hard work, this third edition of my "dream" has reached a new dimension. Cheryl, you have made it happen, and I thank you! I would also like to thank Janice Barsevich Bielawa for the classic new design of the text, Tracey Schelmetic, Elizabeth Ryan, John Williams, Kathy Mayer, Fred Velardi, Greg Vis, Norberto Escobales, Fran Levine, and all those at Appleton & Lange who worked on my text.

A special thank you to David Kendric Brake, Editor at Prentice-Hall, who worked with Cheryl Mehalik and allowed us to use selected art from *Fundamentals of Anatomy and Physiology,* Second Edition, by Frederic Martini, and Adie DeLaGuardia, who assisted me with the Spanish Communication Enrichment sections.

I would like to express my appreciation to the reviewers who provided me with feedback, based upon their experience with the book. They include:

Belinda Escamilla, MA, RT (R)
Department of Health Related Studies
Division of Radiologic Health Sciences
The University of Texas Medical Branch
  at Galveston
School of Allied Health Sciences
Galveston, Texas

Bonnie Deister, BSN, RN, CMA-C
Broome Community College
Department of Medical Assisting
Binghampton, New York

Patricia A. Suminski, RN
Milwaukee Area Technical College
Medical Assisting Program
Milwaukee, Wisconsin

Leslie Taylor, MS, PT
Department of Physical Therapy
Georgia State University
College of Health Sciences
Atlanta, Georgia

Betty L. Warrenfeltz, RN
Consultant
Hagerstown Business College
Hagerstown, Maryland

Ruben Gutierrez
Instructor
International Career Schools
Houston, Texas

I could never have completed this edition without the help of my best friend, partner-in-life, and husband, Charles Larry Rice. You are the Best!

Jane Rice

NOTE TO THE STUDENT

Don't be afraid of the long, strange-looking and sounding medical terms included in this text. Medical terms are made up of prefixes, roots, combining forms, and suffixes. By learning the various word parts included in each chapter, you will soon know the component parts used to build medical words. Next, you will be able to relate their definitions to the meanings of the terms, and be able to analyze almost any medical word that you encounter in your studies.

To assist you in learning to speak the language of medicine, a pronunciation guide is provided for each medical term, vocabulary word, and the diagnostic and laboratory tests. With this edition audiotapes are again available, so that you may listen to the word and then pronounce the word.

Enhance your medical vocabulary by learning the words included in the vocabulary section. This section has been expanded to include the most current words used in the field of medicine.

Further expand your knowledge of medicine by studying the abbreviations included in each chapter. Abbreviations are usually capitalized and periods are not generally used. Exceptions to this general rule are the abbreviations used for medications and prescriptions. Many of these are in lower case and do use periods. Since most abbreviations have more than one meaning, you will need to be careful with their use.

This text is not just about words and their meanings. Integrated within each chapter is information on diagnostic and laboratory tests, and the amazing human body. By studying these sections, you will be amazed at how much they can help you.

You can test yourself by using the learning exercises and review questions at the end of each chapter. An answer key, located in Appendix I at the back of the text, is provided for use in checking your progress. Further suggestions for studying medical terminology are:

1. Use a building process to learn medical terminology. Take the first ten terms in the chapter and learn their word parts and definitions. Then, relate this information to the meanings of the terms. Take the next ten terms and do the same thing. Review what you have learned and then continue with this same process.

2. You may wish to make additional flash cards with the word part on one side and the definition and an example term on the other side. This can be a helpful technique as you begin to learn word parts. Finally, check with your instructor to see if the accompanying audiotapes are available at your school. These audiotapes will help you correctly pronounce the words that are included in the Medical Terminology sections.

Thank you for choosing this text, and may you gain a "world of knowledge" that will help you in all that you do.

Jane Rice

MEDICAL TERMINOLOGY
WITH HUMAN ANATOMY

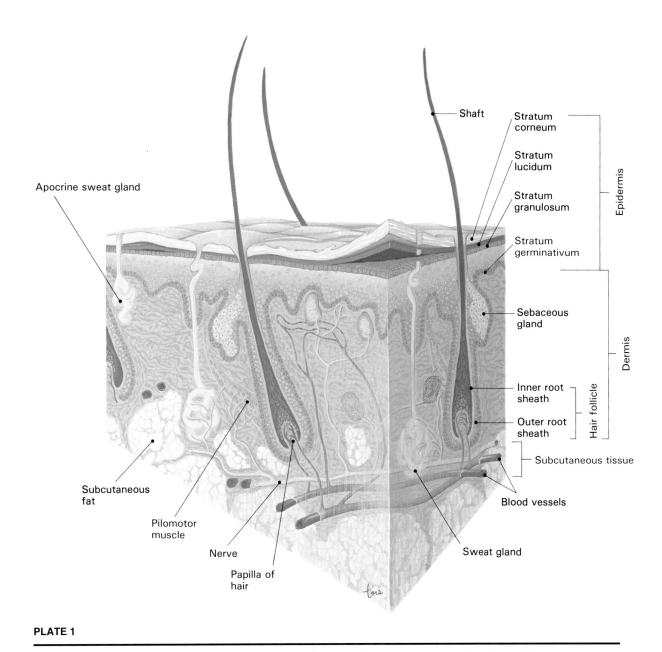

PLATE 1

The integument: epidermis, dermis, subcutaneous tissue, and associated structures. (*Adapted from Evans WF. Anatomy and Physiology, 3rd ed. Englewood Cliffs, NJ: Prentice-Hall, 1983, with permission.*)

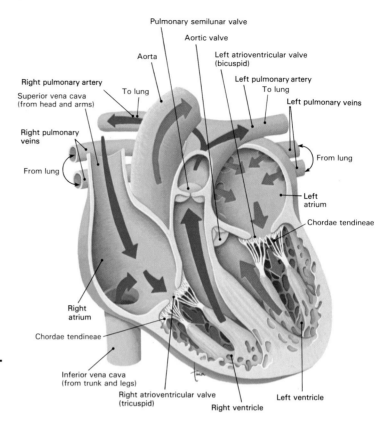

PLATE 2

Structure of the heart showing blood flow. (*Adapted from Evans WF.* Anatomy and Physiology, *3rd ed. Englewood Cliffs, NJ: Prentice-Hall, 1983, with permission.*)

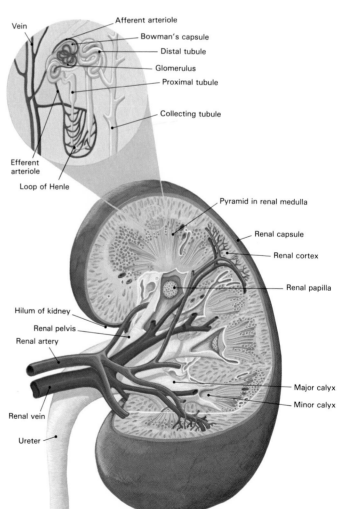

PLATE 3

The kidney with an exploded view of a nephron. (*Adapted from Evans WF.* Anatomy and Physiology, *3rd ed. Englewood Cliffs, NJ: Prentice-Hall, 1983, with permission.*)

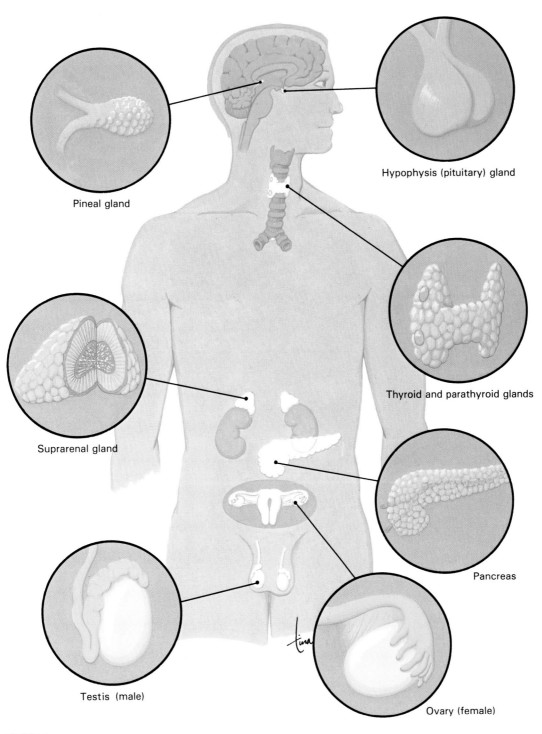

PLATE 4

The endocrine glands and their locations in the body. (*Adapted from Evans WF. Anatomy and Physiology, 3rd ed. Englewood Cliffs, NJ: Prentice-Hall, 1983, with permission.*)

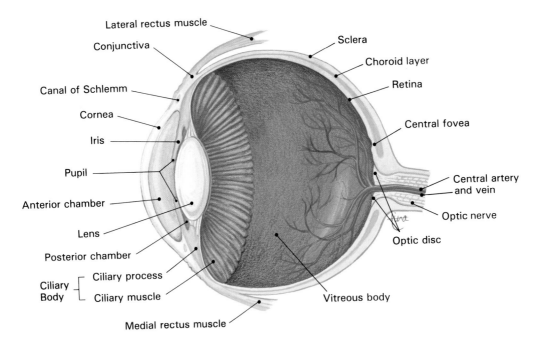

PLATE 5

The structure of the eyeball. (*Adapted from Evans WF. Anatomy and Physiology, 3rd ed. Englewood Cliffs, NJ: Prentice-Hall, 1983, with permission.*)

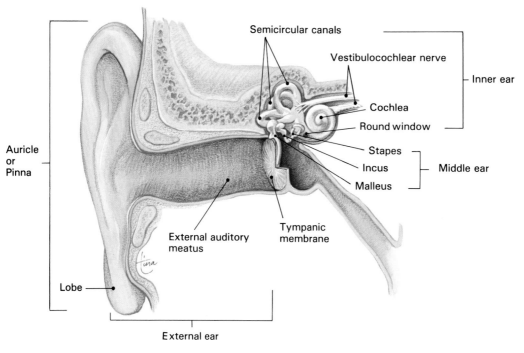

PLATE 6

The auditory apparatus and its anatomical relations. (*Adapted from Evans WF. Anatomy and Physiology, 3rd ed. Englewood Cliffs, NJ: Prentice-Hall, 1983, with permission.*)

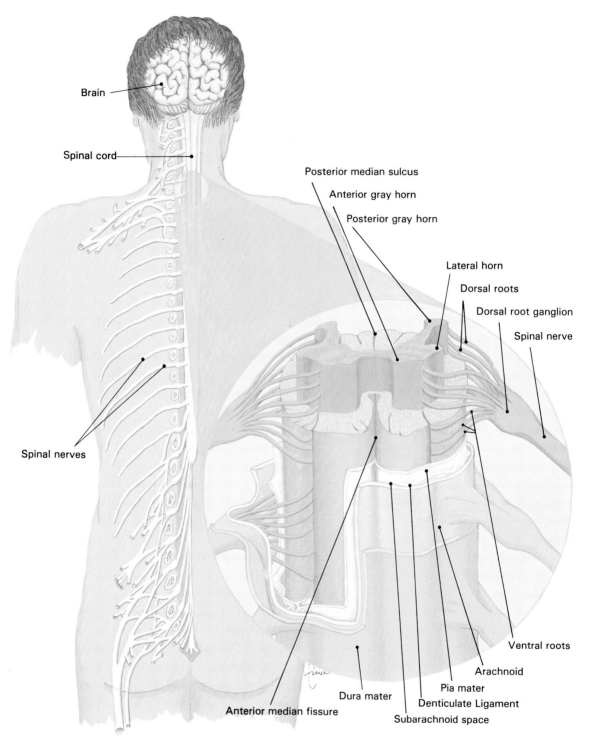

PLATE 7

The brain, spinal cord, and spinal nerves with an exploded view of a spinal nerve. (*Adapted from Evans WF.* Anatomy and Physiology, *3rd ed. Englewood Cliffs, NJ: Prentice-Hall, 1983, with permission.*)

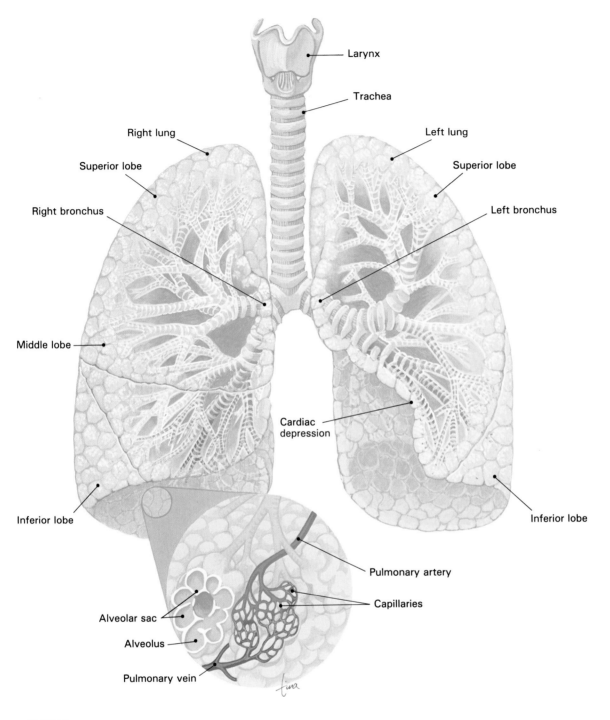

PLATE 8

The larynx, trachea, bronchi, and lungs with an exploded view of clusters of alveoli showing the pulmonary blood vessels. (*Adapted from Evans WF.* Anatomy and Physiology, *3rd ed. Englewood Cliffs, NJ: Prentice-Hall, 1983, with permission.*)

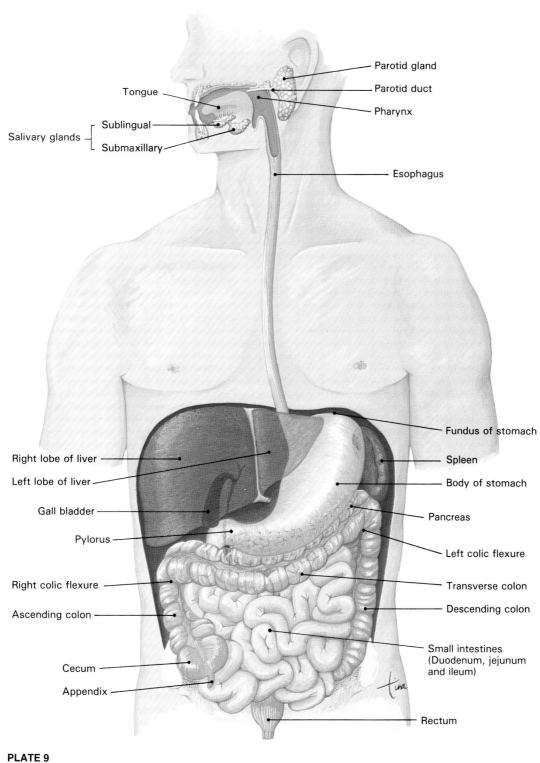

PLATE 9

The digestive system. (*Adapted from Evans WF. Anatomy and Physiology, 3rd ed. Englewood Cliffs, NJ: Prentice-Hall, 1983, with permission.*)

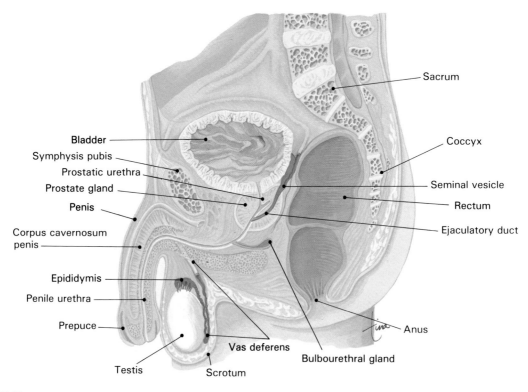

PLATE 10

Sagittal section through the male pelvis, showing organs of the reproductive system. (*Adapted from Evans WF. Anatomy and Physiology, 3rd ed. Englewood Cliffs, NJ: Prentice-Hall, 1983, with permission.*)

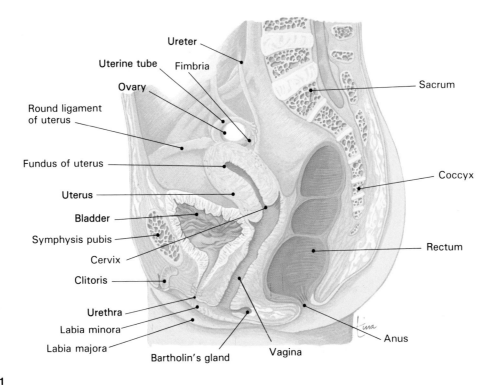

PLATE 11

Sagittal section through the female pelvis, showing organs of the reproductive system. (*Adapted from Evans WF. Anatomy and Physiology, 3rd ed. Englewood Cliffs, NJ: Prentice-Hall, 1983, with permission.*)

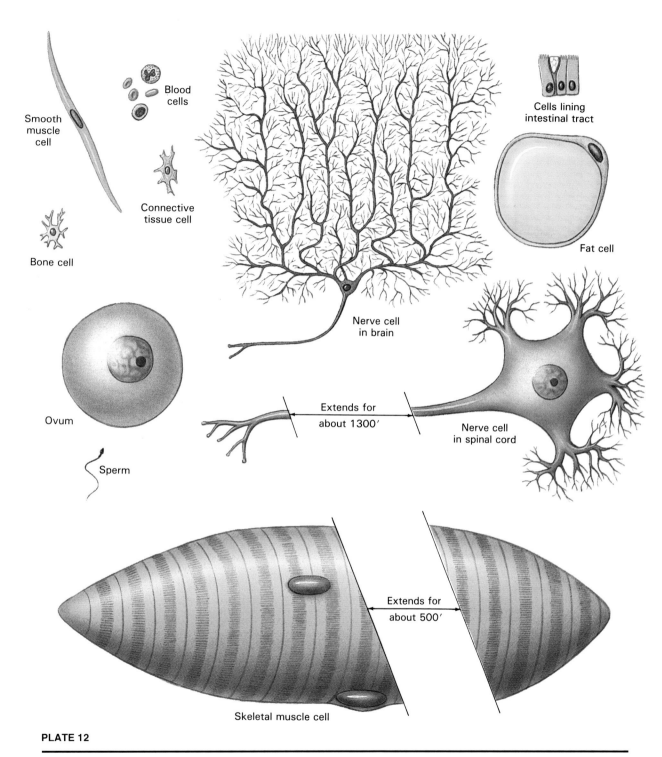

PLATE 12

The diversity of cells in the human body. The cells of the body have many different shapes and a variety of special functions. These examples give an indication of the range of forms and sizes; all of the cells are shown with the dimensions they would have if magnified approximately 500 times. (*From Martini F. Fundamentals of Anatomy and Physiology, 2nd ed. Englewood Cliffs, NJ: Prentice-Hall, 1992, with permission.*)

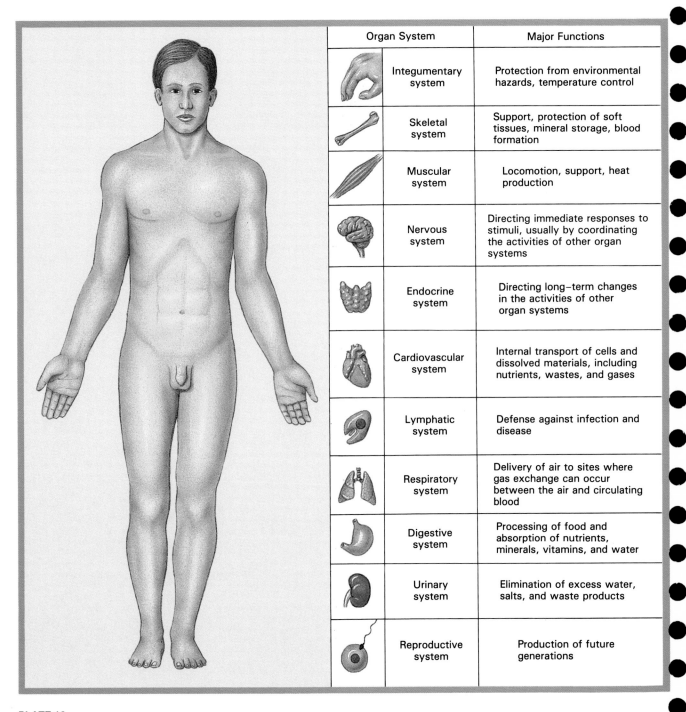

Organ System	Major Functions
Integumentary system	Protection from environmental hazards, temperature control
Skeletal system	Support, protection of soft tissues, mineral storage, blood formation
Muscular system	Locomotion, support, heat production
Nervous system	Directing immediate responses to stimuli, usually by coordinating the activities of other organ systems
Endocrine system	Directing long-term changes in the activities of other organ systems
Cardiovascular system	Internal transport of cells and dissolved materials, including nutrients, wastes, and gases
Lymphatic system	Defense against infection and disease
Respiratory system	Delivery of air to sites where gas exchange can occur between the air and circulating blood
Digestive system	Processing of food and absorption of nutrients, minerals, vitamins, and water
Urinary system	Elimination of excess water, salts, and waste products
Reproductive system	Production of future generations

PLATE 13

An introduction to organ systems. (*From Martini F. Fundamentals of Anatomy and Physiology, 2nd ed. Englewood Cliffs, NJ: Prentice-Hall, 1992, with permission.*)

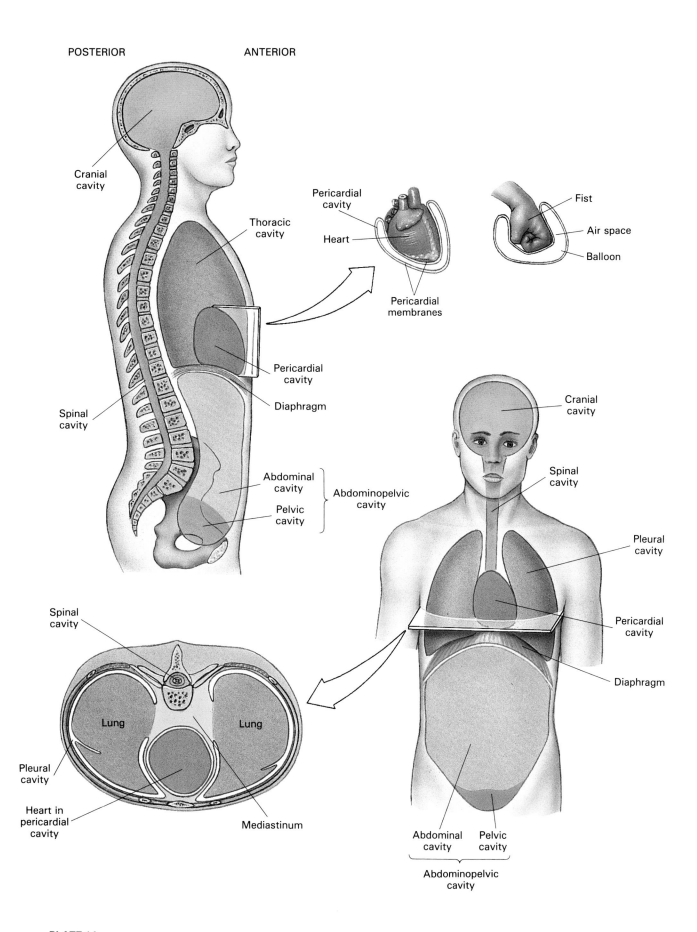

PLATE 14

Body cavities. (*From Martini F. Fundamentals of Anatomy and Physiology, 2nd ed. Englewood Cliffs, NJ: Prentice-Hall, 1992, with permission.*)

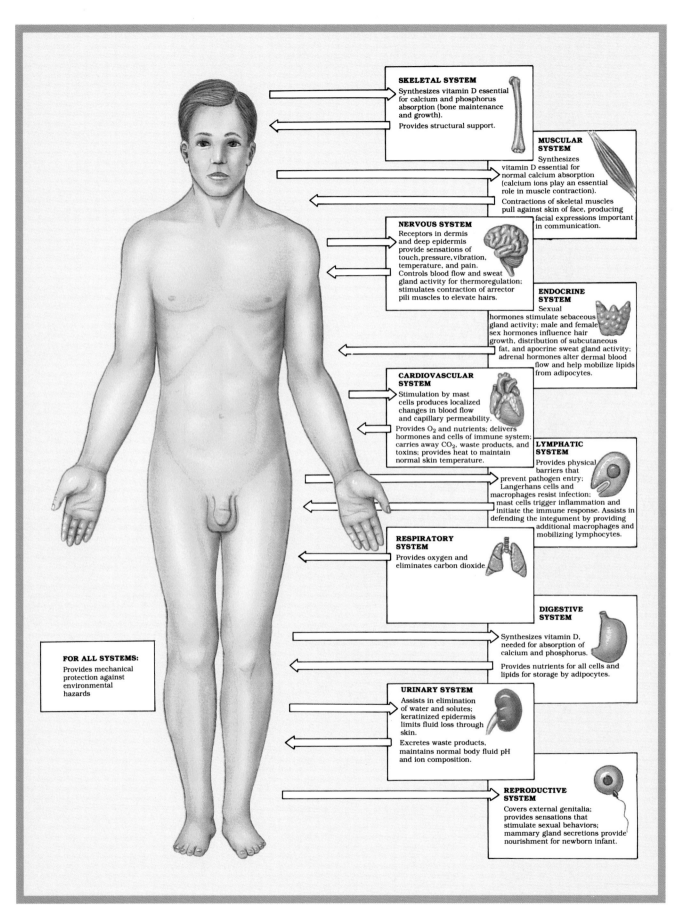

SKELETAL SYSTEM

Synthesizes vitamin D essential for calcium and phosphorus absorption (bone maintenance and growth).

Provides structural support.

MUSCULAR SYSTEM

Synthesizes vitamin D essential for normal calcium absorption (calcium ions play an essential role in muscle contraction).

Contractions of skeletal muscles pull against skin of face, producing facial expressions important in communication.

NERVOUS SYSTEM

Receptors in dermis and deep epidermis provide sensations of touch, pressure, vibration, temperature, and pain. Controls blood flow and sweat gland activity for thermoregulation; stimulates contraction of arrector pili muscles to elevate hairs.

ENDOCRINE SYSTEM

Sexual hormones stimulate sebaceous gland activity; male and female sex hormones influence hair growth, distribution of subcutaneous fat, and apocrine sweat gland activity; adrenal hormones alter dermal blood flow and help mobilize lipids from adipocytes.

CARDIOVASCULAR SYSTEM

Stimulation by mast cells produces localized changes in blood flow and capillary permeability.

Provides O₂ and nutrients; delivers hormones and cells of immune system; carries away CO₂, waste products, and toxins; provides heat to maintain normal skin temperature.

LYMPHATIC SYSTEM

Provides physical barriers that prevent pathogen entry; Langerhans cells and macrophages resist infection; mast cells trigger inflammation and initiate the immune response. Assists in defending the integument by providing additional macrophages and mobilizing lymphocytes.

RESPIRATORY SYSTEM

Provides oxygen and eliminates carbon dioxide.

DIGESTIVE SYSTEM

Synthesizes vitamin D, needed for absorption of calcium and phosphorus.

Provides nutrients for all cells and lipids for storage by adipocytes.

FOR ALL SYSTEMS:

Provides mechanical protection against environmental hazards

URINARY SYSTEM

Assists in elimination of water and solutes; keratinized epidermis limits fluid loss through skin.

Excretes waste products, maintains normal body fluid pH and ion composition.

REPRODUCTIVE SYSTEM

Covers external genitalia; provides sensations that stimulate sexual behaviors; mammary gland secretions provide nourishment for newborn infant.

PLATE 15

Functional relationships between the integumentary system and other systems. (*From Martini F.* Fundamentals of Anatomy and Physiology, *2nd ed. Englewood Cliffs, NJ: Prentice-Hall, 1992, with permission.*)

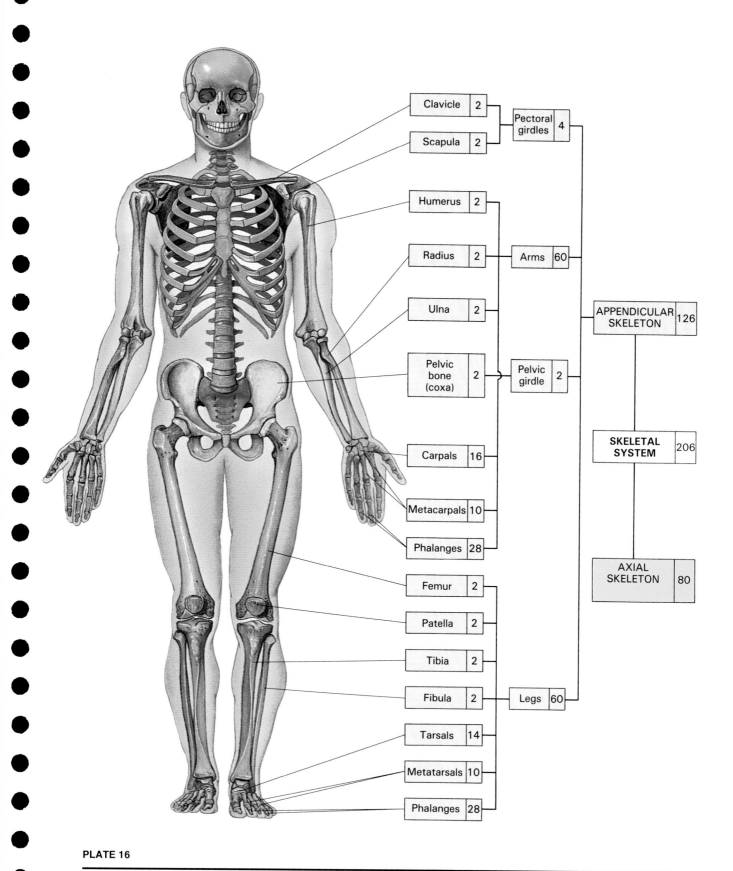

PLATE 16

The appendicular skeleton. (*From Martini F.* Fundamentals of Anatomy and Physiology, *2nd ed. Englewood Cliffs, NJ: Prentice-Hall, 1992, with permission.*)

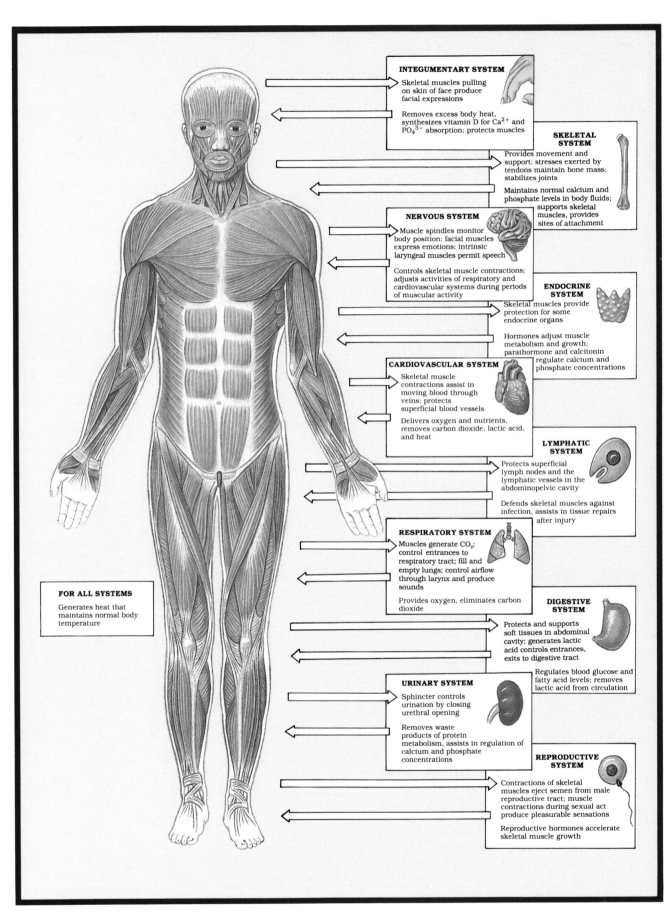

INTEGUMENTARY SYSTEM

Skeletal muscles pulling on skin of face produce facial expressions

Removes excess body heat, synthesizes vitamin D for Ca^{2+} and PO_4^{3-} absorption; protects muscles

SKELETAL SYSTEM

Provides movement and support; stresses exerted by tendons maintain bone mass; stabilizes joints

Maintains normal calcium and phosphate levels in body fluids; supports skeletal muscles, provides sites of attachment

NERVOUS SYSTEM

Muscle spindles monitor body position; facial muscles express emotions; intrinsic laryngeal muscles permit speech

Controls skeletal muscle contractions; adjusts activities of respiratory and cardiovascular systems during periods of muscular activity

ENDOCRINE SYSTEM

Skeletal muscles provide protection for some endocrine organs

Hormones adjust muscle metabolism and growth; parathormone and calcitonin regulate calcium and phosphate concentrations

CARDIOVASCULAR SYSTEM

Skeletal muscle contractions assist in moving blood through veins; protects superficial blood vessels

Delivers oxygen and nutrients, removes carbon dioxide, lactic acid, and heat

LYMPHATIC SYSTEM

Protects superficial lymph nodes and the lymphatic vessels in the abdominopelvic cavity

Defends skeletal muscles against infection, assists in tissue repairs after injury

RESPIRATORY SYSTEM

Muscles generate CO_2; control entrances to respiratory tract; fill and empty lungs; control airflow through larynx and produce sounds

Provides oxygen, eliminates carbon dioxide

DIGESTIVE SYSTEM

Protects and supports soft tissues in abdominal cavity; generates lactic acid controls entrances, exits to digestive tract

Regulates blood glucose and fatty acid levels; removes lactic acid from circulation

FOR ALL SYSTEMS

Generates heat that maintains normal body temperature

URINARY SYSTEM

Sphincter controls urination by closing urethral opening

Removes waste products of protein metabolism, assists in regulation of calcium and phosphate concentrations

REPRODUCTIVE SYSTEM

Contractions of skeletal muscles eject semen from male reproductive tract; muscle contractions during sexual act produce pleasurable sensations

Reproductive hormones accelerate skeletal muscle growth

PLATE 17

Functional relationships between the muscular system and other systems. (*From Martini F.* Fundamentals of Anatomy and Physiology, *2nd ed. Englewood Cliffs, NJ: Prentice-Hall, 1992, with permission.*)

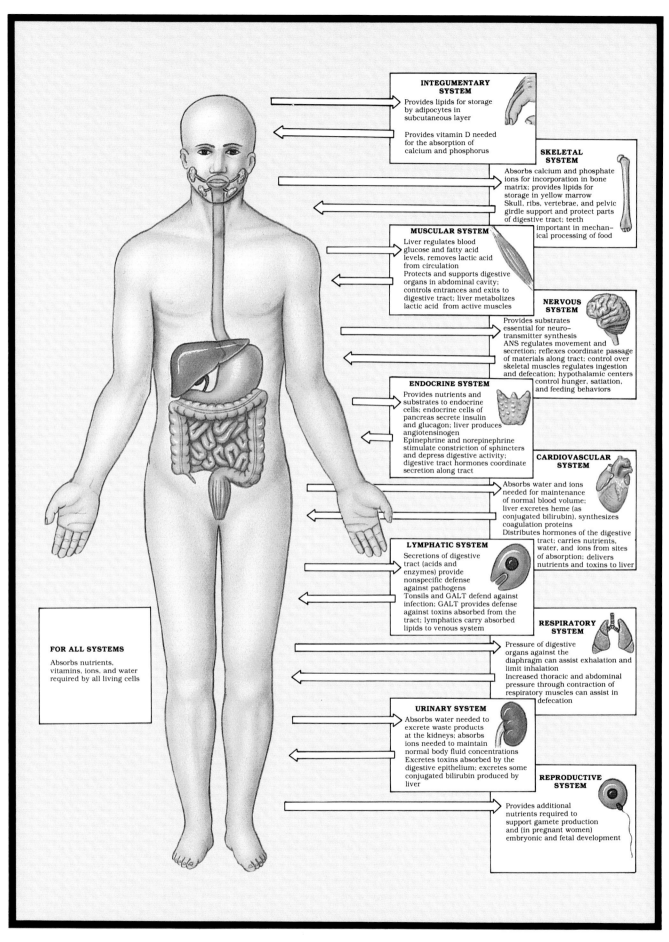

PLATE 18

Functional relationships between the digestive system and other systems. (*From Martini F.* Fundamentals of Anatomy and Physiology, *2nd ed. Englewood Cliffs, NJ: Prentice-Hall, 1992, with permission.*)

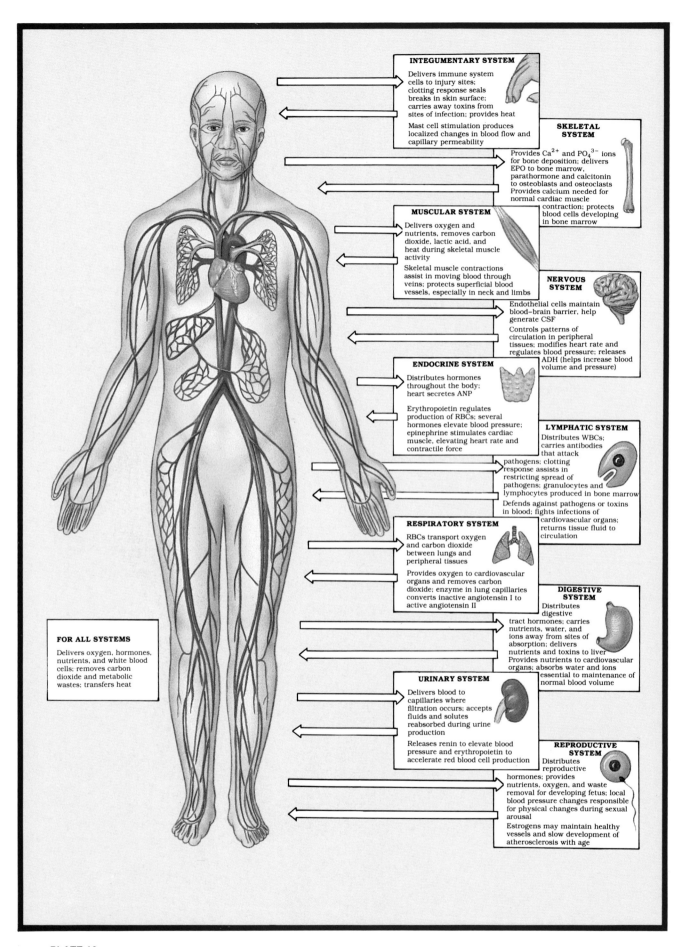

INTEGUMENTARY SYSTEM

Delivers immune system cells to injury sites; clotting response seals breaks in skin surface; carries away toxins from sites of infection; provides heat

Mast cell stimulation produces localized changes in blood flow and capillary permeability

SKELETAL SYSTEM

Provides Ca^{2+} and PO_4^{3-} ions for bone deposition; delivers EPO to bone marrow, parathormone and calcitonin to osteoblasts and osteoclasts
Provides calcium needed for normal cardiac muscle contraction; protects blood cells developing in bone marrow

MUSCULAR SYSTEM

Delivers oxygen and nutrients, removes carbon dioxide, lactic acid, and heat during skeletal muscle activity

Skeletal muscle contractions assist in moving blood through veins; protects superficial blood vessels, especially in neck and limbs

NERVOUS SYSTEM

Endothelial cells maintain blood–brain barrier, help generate CSF

Controls patterns of circulation in peripheral tissues; modifies heart rate and regulates blood pressure; releases ADH (helps increase blood volume and pressure)

ENDOCRINE SYSTEM

Distributes hormones throughout the body; heart secretes ANP

Erythropoietin regulates production of RBCs; several hormones elevate blood pressure; epinephrine stimulates cardiac muscle, elevating heart rate and contractile force

LYMPHATIC SYSTEM

Distributes WBCs; carries antibodies that attack pathogens; clotting response assists in restricting spread of pathogens; granulocytes and lymphocytes produced in bone marrow

Defends against pathogens or toxins in blood; fights infections of cardiovascular organs; returns tissue fluid to circulation

RESPIRATORY SYSTEM

RBCs transport oxygen and carbon dioxide between lungs and peripheral tissues

Provides oxygen to cardiovascular organs and removes carbon dioxide; enzyme in lung capillaries converts inactive angiotensin I to active angiotensin II

DIGESTIVE SYSTEM

Distributes digestive tract hormones; carries nutrients, water, and ions away from sites of absorption; delivers nutrients and toxins to liver
Provides nutrients to cardiovascular organs; absorbs water and ions essential to maintenance of normal blood volume

FOR ALL SYSTEMS

Delivers oxygen, hormones, nutrients, and white blood cells; removes carbon dioxide and metabolic wastes; transfers heat

URINARY SYSTEM

Delivers blood to capillaries where filtration occurs; accepts fluids and solutes reabsorbed during urine production

Releases renin to elevate blood pressure and erythropoietin to accelerate red blood cell production

REPRODUCTIVE SYSTEM

Distributes reproductive hormones; provides nutrients, oxygen, and waste removal for developing fetus; local blood pressure changes responsible for physical changes during sexual arousal

Estrogens may maintain healthy vessels and slow development of atherosclerosis with age

PLATE 19

Functional relationships between the cardiovascular system and other systems. (*From Martini F.* Fundamentals of Anatomy and Physiology, *2nd ed. Englewood Cliffs, NJ: Prentice-Hall, 1992, with permission.*)

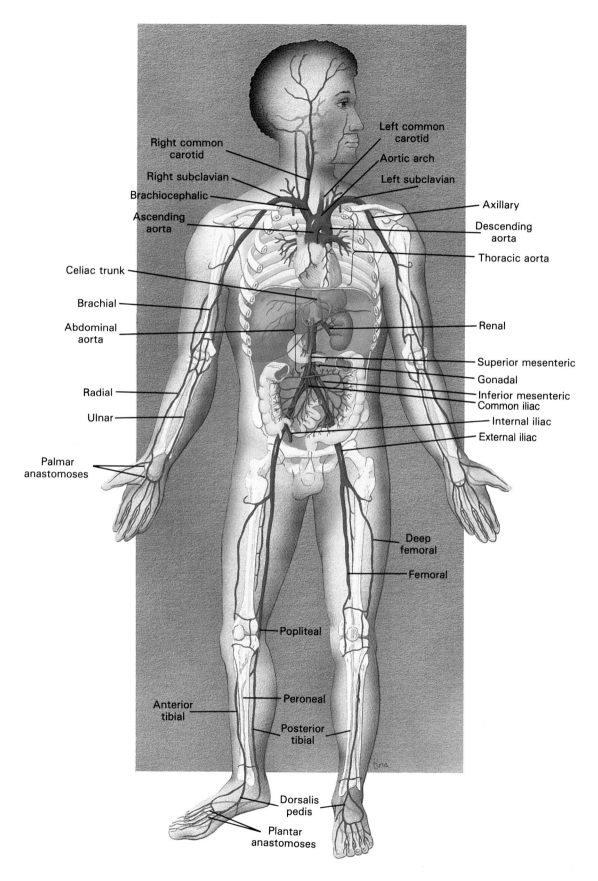

PLATE 20

An overview of the arterial system. (*From Martini F. Fundamentals of Anatomy and Physiology, 2nd ed. Englewood Cliffs, NJ: Prentice-Hall, 1992, with permission.*)

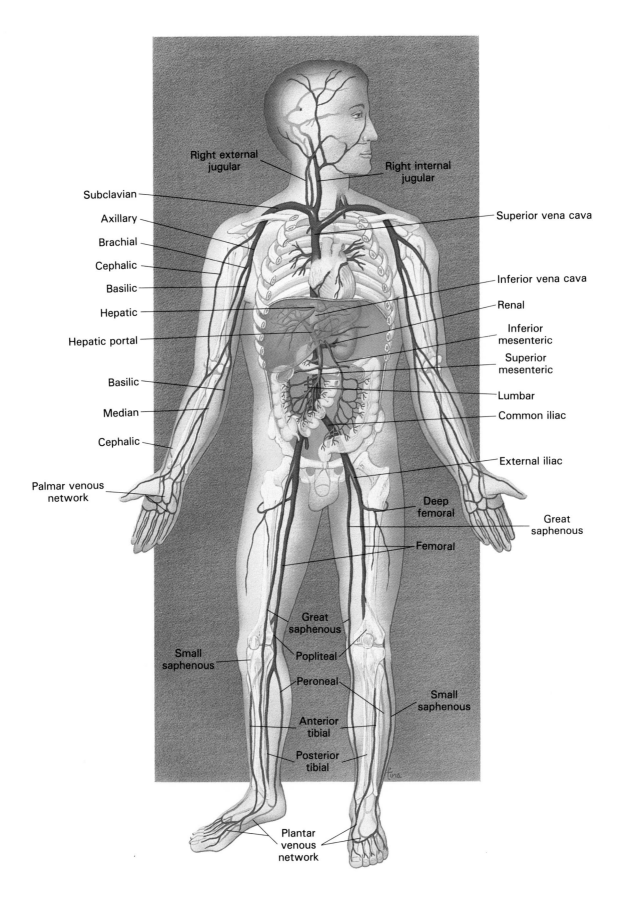

PLATE 21

An overview of the venous system. (*From Martini F.* Fundamentals of Anatomy and Physiology, *2nd ed. Englewood Cliffs, NJ: Prentice-Hall, 1992, with permission.*)

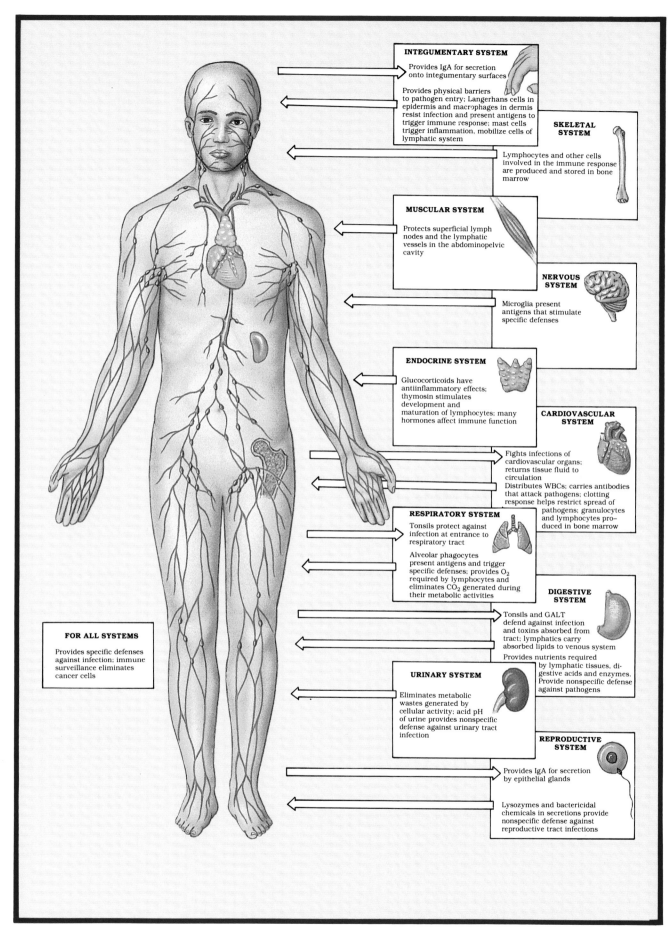

INTEGUMENTARY SYSTEM

Provides IgA for secretion onto integumentary surfaces

Provides physical barriers to pathogen entry; Langerhans cells in epidermis and macrophages in dermis resist infection and present antigens to trigger immune response; mast cells trigger inflammation, mobilize cells of lymphatic system

SKELETAL SYSTEM

Lymphocytes and other cells involved in the immune response are produced and stored in bone marrow

MUSCULAR SYSTEM

Protects superficial lymph nodes and the lymphatic vessels in the abdominopelvic cavity

NERVOUS SYSTEM

Microglia present antigens that stimulate specific defenses

ENDOCRINE SYSTEM

Glucocorticoids have antiinflammatory effects; thymosin stimulates development and maturation of lymphocytes; many hormones affect immune function

CARDIOVASCULAR SYSTEM

Fights infections of cardiovascular organs; returns tissue fluid to circulation

Distributes WBCs; carries antibodies that attack pathogens; clotting response helps restrict spread of pathogens; granulocytes and lymphocytes pro–duced in bone marrow

RESPIRATORY SYSTEM

Tonsils protect against infection at entrance to respiratory tract

Alveolar phagocytes present antigens and trigger specific defenses; provides O_2 required by lymphocytes and eliminates CO_2 generated during their metabolic activities

DIGESTIVE SYSTEM

Tonsils and GALT defend against infection and toxins absorbed from tract; lymphatics carry absorbed lipids to venous system

Provides nutrients required by lymphatic tissues, digestive acids and enzymes. Provide nonspecific defense against pathogens

FOR ALL SYSTEMS

Provides specific defenses against infection; immune surveillance eliminates cancer cells

URINARY SYSTEM

Eliminates metabolic wastes generated by cellular activity; acid pH of urine provides nonspecific defense against urinary tract infection

REPRODUCTIVE SYSTEM

Provides IgA for secretion by epithelial glands

Lysozymes and bactericidal chemicals in secretions provide nonspecific defense against reproductive tract infections

PLATE 22

Functional relationships between the lymphatic system and other systems. (*From Martini F.* Fundamentals of Anatomy and Physiology, *2nd ed. Englewood Cliffs, NJ: Prentice-Hall, 1992, with permission.*)

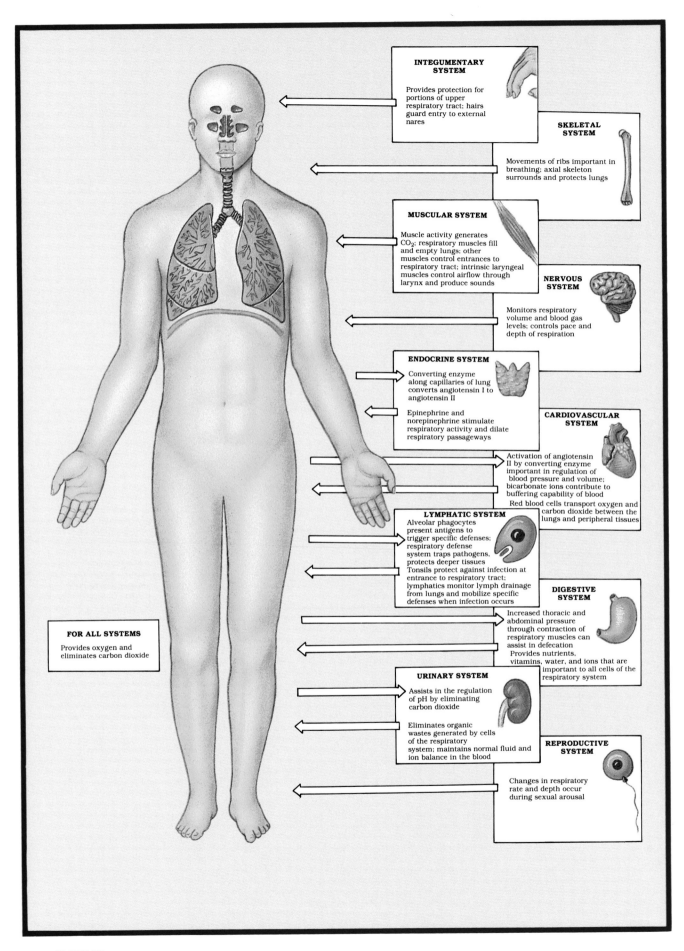

INTEGUMENTARY SYSTEM

Provides protection for portions of upper respiratory tract; hairs guard entry to external nares

SKELETAL SYSTEM

Movements of ribs important in breathing; axial skeleton surrounds and protects lungs

MUSCULAR SYSTEM

Muscle activity generates CO_2; respiratory muscles fill and empty lungs; other muscles control entrances to respiratory tract; intrinsic laryngeal muscles control airflow through larynx and produce sounds

NERVOUS SYSTEM

Monitors respiratory volume and blood gas levels; controls pace and depth of respiration

ENDOCRINE SYSTEM

Converting enzyme along capillaries of lung converts angiotensin I to angiotensin II

Epinephrine and norepinephrine stimulate respiratory activity and dilate respiratory passageways

CARDIOVASCULAR SYSTEM

Activation of angiotensin II by converting enzyme important in regulation of blood pressure and volume; bicarbonate ions contribute to buffering capability of blood

Red blood cells transport oxygen and carbon dioxide between the lungs and peripheral tissues

LYMPHATIC SYSTEM

Alveolar phagocytes present antigens to trigger specific defenses; respiratory defense system traps pathogens, protects deeper tissues

Tonsils protect against infection at entrance to respiratory tract; lymphatics monitor lymph drainage from lungs and mobilize specific defenses when infection occurs

DIGESTIVE SYSTEM

Increased thoracic and abdominal pressure through contraction of respiratory muscles can assist in defecation

Provides nutrients, vitamins, water, and ions that are important to all cells of the respiratory system

URINARY SYSTEM

Assists in the regulation of pH by eliminating carbon dioxide

Eliminates organic wastes generated by cells of the respiratory system; maintains normal fluid and ion balance in the blood

REPRODUCTIVE SYSTEM

Changes in respiratory rate and depth occur during sexual arousal

FOR ALL SYSTEMS

Provides oxygen and eliminates carbon dioxide

PLATE 23

Functional relationships between the respiratory system and other systems. (*From Martini F. Fundamentals of Anatomy and Physiology, 2nd ed. Englewood Cliffs, NJ: Prentice-Hall, 1992, with permission.*)

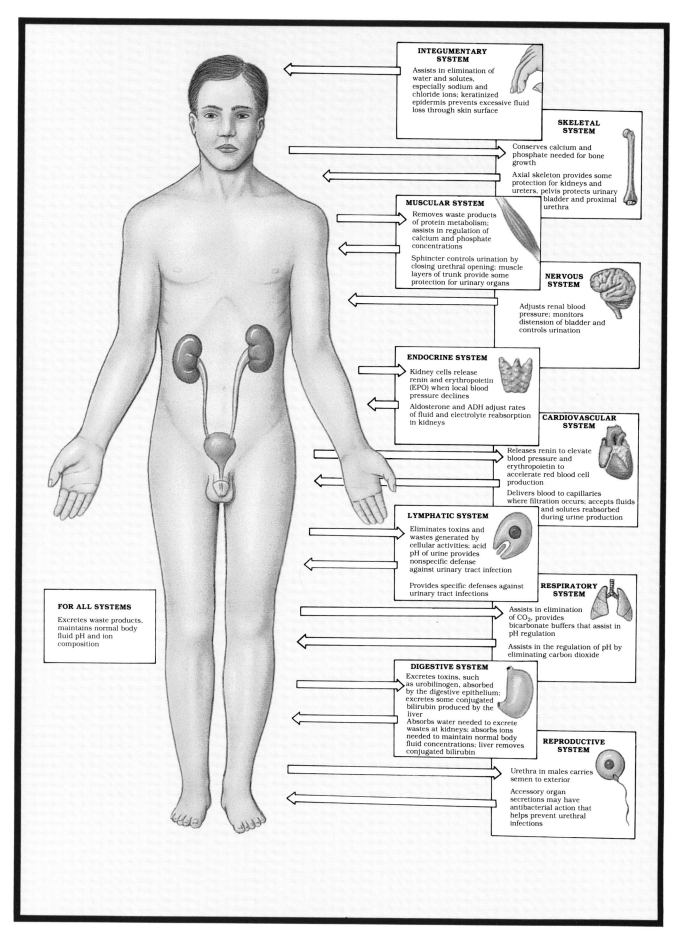

INTEGUMENTARY SYSTEM
Assists in elimination of water and solutes, especially sodium and chloride ions; keratinized epidermis prevents excessive fluid loss through skin surface

SKELETAL SYSTEM
Conserves calcium and phosphate needed for bone growth

Axial skeleton provides some protection for kidneys and ureters, pelvis protects urinary bladder and proximal urethra

MUSCULAR SYSTEM
Removes waste products of protein metabolism; assists in regulation of calcium and phosphate concentrations

Sphincter controls urination by closing urethral opening; muscle layers of trunk provide some protection for urinary organs

NERVOUS SYSTEM
Adjusts renal blood pressure; monitors distension of bladder and controls urination

ENDOCRINE SYSTEM
Kidney cells release renin and erythropoietin (EPO) when local blood pressure declines

Aldosterone and ADH adjust rates of fluid and electrolyte reabsorption in kidneys

CARDIOVASCULAR SYSTEM
Releases renin to elevate blood pressure and erythropoietin to accelerate red blood cell production

Delivers blood to capillaries where filtration occurs; accepts fluids and solutes reabsorbed during urine production

LYMPHATIC SYSTEM
Eliminates toxins and wastes generated by cellular activities; acid pH of urine provides nonspecific defense against urinary tract infection

Provides specific defenses against urinary tract infections

RESPIRATORY SYSTEM
Assists in elimination of CO_2, provides bicarbonate buffers that assist in pH regulation

Assists in the regulation of pH by eliminating carbon dioxide

FOR ALL SYSTEMS
Excretes waste products, maintains normal body fluid pH and ion composition

DIGESTIVE SYSTEM
Excretes toxins, such as urobilinogen, absorbed by the digestive epithelium; excretes some conjugated bilirubin produced by the liver

Absorbs water needed to excrete wastes at kidneys; absorbs ions needed to maintain normal body fluid concentrations; liver removes conjugated bilirubin

REPRODUCTIVE SYSTEM
Urethra in males carries semen to exterior

Accessory organ secretions may have antibacterial action that helps prevent urethral infections

PLATE 24

Functional relationships between the urinary system and other systems. (*From Martini F.* Fundamentals of Anatomy and Physiology, *2nd ed. Englewood Cliffs, NJ: Prentice-Hall, 1992, with permission.*)

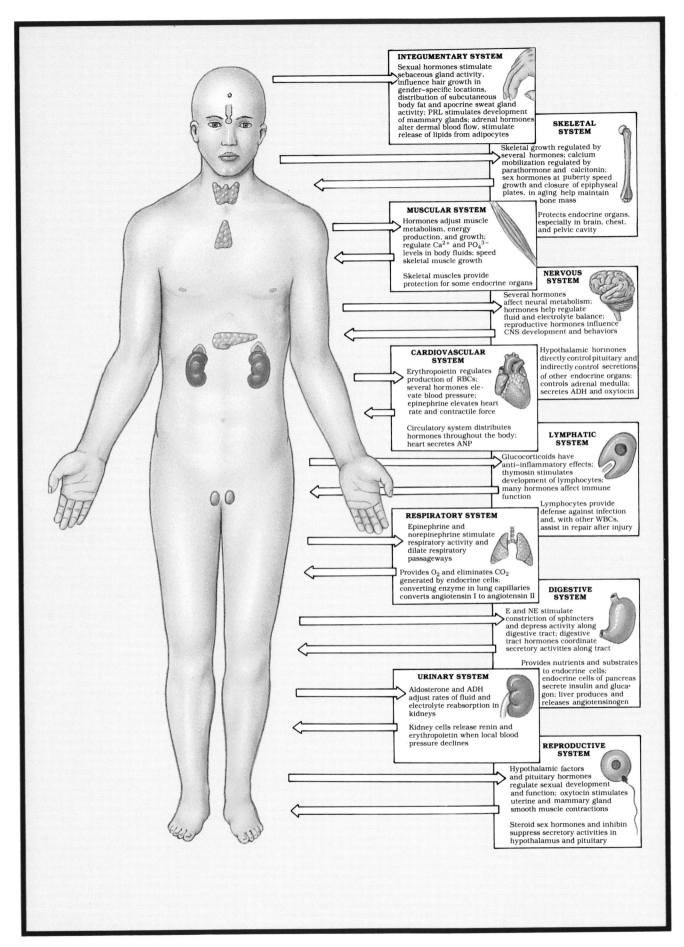

INTEGUMENTARY SYSTEM
Sexual hormones stimulate sebaceous gland activity, influence hair growth in gender–specific locations, distribution of subcutaneous body fat and apocrine sweat gland activity; PRL stimulates development of mammary glands; adrenal hormones alter dermal blood flow, stimulate release of lipids from adipocytes

SKELETAL SYSTEM
Skeletal growth regulated by several hormones; calcium mobilization regulated by parathormone and calcitonin; sex hormones at puberty speed growth and closure of epiphyseal plates, in aging help maintain bone mass

Protects endocrine organs, especially in brain, chest, and pelvic cavity

MUSCULAR SYSTEM
Hormones adjust muscle metabolism, energy production, and growth; regulate Ca^{2+} and PO_4^{3-} levels in body fluids; speed skeletal muscle growth

Skeletal muscles provide protection for some endocrine organs

NERVOUS SYSTEM
Several hormones affect neural metabolism; hormones help regulate fluid and electrolyte balance; reproductive hormones influence CNS development and behaviors

Hypothalamic hormones directly control pituitary and indirectly control secretions of other endocrine organs; controls adrenal medulla; secretes ADH and oxytocin

CARDIOVASCULAR SYSTEM
Erythropoietin regulates production of RBCs; several hormones elevate blood pressure; epinephrine elevates heart rate and contractile force

Circulatory system distributes hormones throughout the body; heart secretes ANP

LYMPHATIC SYSTEM
Glucocorticoids have anti–inflammatory effects; thymosin stimulates development of lymphocytes; many hormones affect immune function

Lymphocytes provide defense against infection and, with other WBCs, assist in repair after injury

RESPIRATORY SYSTEM
Epinephrine and norepinephrine stimulate respiratory activity and dilate respiratory passageways

Provides O_2 and eliminates CO_2 generated by endocrine cells; converting enzyme in lung capillaries converts angiotensin I to angiotensin II

DIGESTIVE SYSTEM
E and NE stimulate constriction of sphincters and depress activity along digestive tract; digestive tract hormones coordinate secretory activities along tract

Provides nutrients and substrates to endocrine cells; endocrine cells of pancreas secrete insulin and glucagon; liver produces and releases angiotensinogen

URINARY SYSTEM
Aldosterone and ADH adjust rates of fluid and electrolyte reabsorption in kidneys

Kidney cells release renin and erythropoietin when local blood pressure declines

REPRODUCTIVE SYSTEM
Hypothalamic factors and pituitary hormones regulate sexual development and function; oxytocin stimulates uterine and mammary gland smooth muscle contractions

Steroid sex hormones and inhibin suppress secretory activities in hypothalamus and pituitary

PLATE 25

Functional relationships between the endocrine system and other systems. (*From Martini F.* Fundamentals of Anatomy and Physiology, *2nd ed. Englewood Cliffs, NJ: Prentice-Hall, 1992, with permission.*)

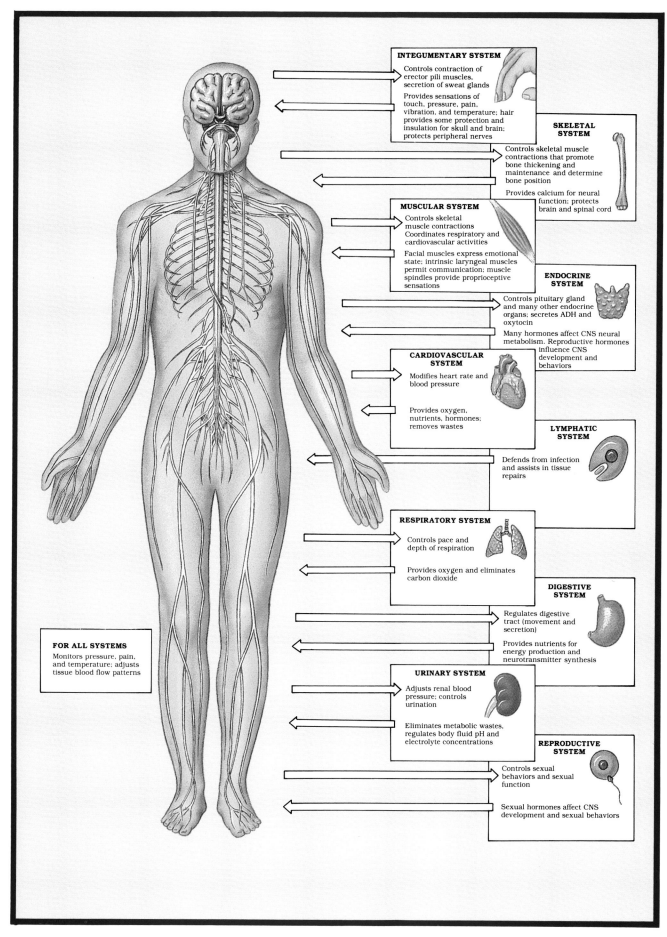

INTEGUMENTARY SYSTEM
Controls contraction of erector pili muscles, secretion of sweat glands

Provides sensations of touch, pressure, pain, vibration, and temperature; hair provides some protection and insulation for skull and brain; protects peripheral nerves

SKELETAL SYSTEM
Controls skeletal muscle contractions that promote bone thickening and maintenance and determine bone position

Provides calcium for neural function; protects brain and spinal cord

MUSCULAR SYSTEM
Controls skeletal muscle contractions
Coordinates respiratory and cardiovascular activities

Facial muscles express emotional state; intrinsic laryngeal muscles permit communication; muscle spindles provide proprioceptive sensations

ENDOCRINE SYSTEM
Controls pituitary gland and many other endocrine organs; secretes ADH and oxytocin

Many hormones affect CNS neural metabolism. Reproductive hormones influence CNS development and behaviors

CARDIOVASCULAR SYSTEM
Modifies heart rate and blood pressure

Provides oxygen, nutrients, hormones; removes wastes

LYMPHATIC SYSTEM
Defends from infection and assists in tissue repairs

RESPIRATORY SYSTEM
Controls pace and depth of respiration

Provides oxygen and eliminates carbon dioxide

DIGESTIVE SYSTEM
Regulates digestive tract (movement and secretion)

Provides nutrients for energy production and neurotransmitter synthesis

FOR ALL SYSTEMS
Monitors pressure, pain, and temperature; adjusts tissue blood flow patterns

URINARY SYSTEM
Adjusts renal blood pressure; controls urination

Eliminates metabolic wastes, regulates body fluid pH and electrolyte concentrations

REPRODUCTIVE SYSTEM
Controls sexual behaviors and sexual function

Sexual hormones affect CNS development and sexual behaviors

PLATE 26

Functional relationships between the nervous system and other systems. (*From Martini F.* Fundamentals of Anatomy and Physiology, *2nd ed. Englewood Cliffs, NJ: Prentice-Hall, 1992, with permission.*)

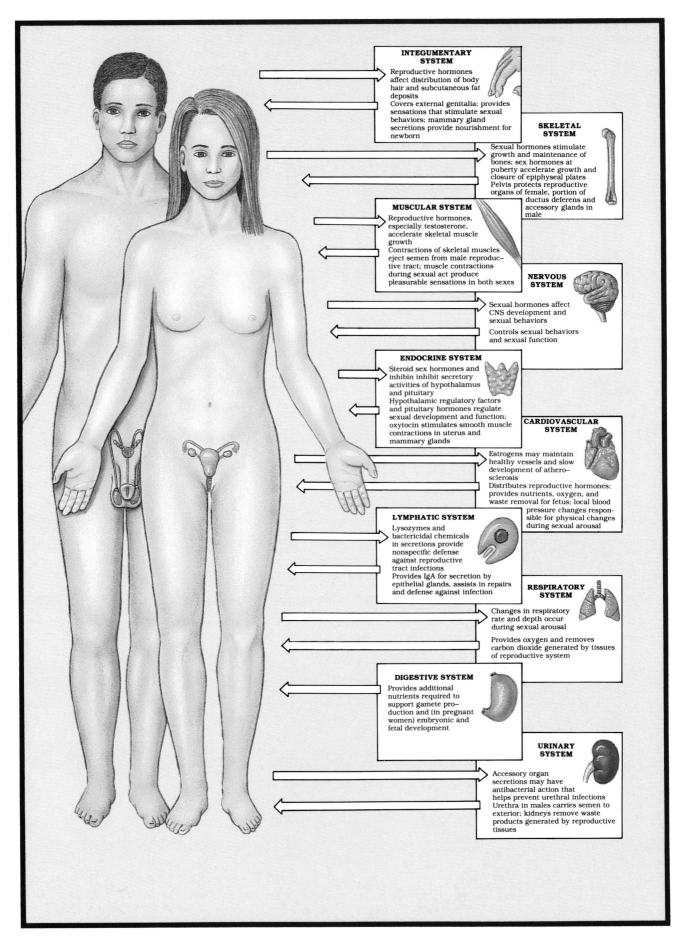

INTEGUMENTARY SYSTEM
Reproductive hormones affect distribution of body hair and subcutaneous fat deposits
Covers external genitalia; provides sensations that stimulate sexual behaviors; mammary gland secretions provide nourishment for newborn

SKELETAL SYSTEM
Sexual hormones stimulate growth and maintenance of bones; sex hormones at puberty accelerate growth and closure of epiphyseal plates
Pelvis protects reproductive organs of female, portion of ductus deferens and accessory glands in male

MUSCULAR SYSTEM
Reproductive hormones, especially testosterone, accelerate skeletal muscle growth
Contractions of skeletal muscles eject semen from male reproductive tract; muscle contractions during sexual act produce pleasurable sensations in both sexes

NERVOUS SYSTEM
Sexual hormones affect CNS development and sexual behaviors
Controls sexual behaviors and sexual function

ENDOCRINE SYSTEM
Steroid sex hormones and inhibin inhibit secretory activities of hypothalamus and pituitary
Hypothalamic regulatory factors and pituitary hormones regulate sexual development and function; oxytocin stimulates smooth muscle contractions in uterus and mammary glands

CARDIOVASCULAR SYSTEM
Estrogens may maintain healthy vessels and slow development of athero-sclerosis
Distributes reproductive hormones; provides nutrients, oxygen, and waste removal for fetus; local blood pressure changes responsible for physical changes during sexual arousal

LYMPHATIC SYSTEM
Lysozymes and bactericidal chemicals in secretions provide nonspecific defense against reproductive tract infections
Provides IgA for secretion by epithelial glands, assists in repairs and defense against infection

RESPIRATORY SYSTEM
Changes in respiratory rate and depth occur during sexual arousal
Provides oxygen and removes carbon dioxide generated by tissues of reproductive system

DIGESTIVE SYSTEM
Provides additional nutrients required to support gamete production and (in pregnant women) embryonic and fetal development

URINARY SYSTEM
Accessory organ secretions may have antibacterial action that helps prevent urethral infections
Urethra in males carries semen to exterior; kidneys remove waste products generated by reproductive tissues

PLATE 27

Functional relationships between the reproductive system and other systems. (*From Martini F.* Fundamentals of Anatomy and Physiology, *2nd ed. Englewood Cliffs, NJ: Prentice-Hall, 1992, with permission.*)

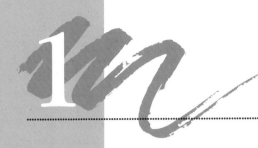

Fundamental Word Structure

This is the beginning of a new experience in learning for most students. Chapter 1 provides the basic **building blocks** necessary to the understanding of medical word structure. Also, some students may choose to benefit from a new feature, called *Communication Enrichment,* in which we have included the Spanish translation of key words used for communication in a medical setting.

1

UNDERSTANDING FUNDAMENTAL WORD STRUCTURE

Medical terminology is the study of terms that are used in the art and science of medicine. It is a specialized language with its origin arising from the Greek influence on medicine. Hippocrates was a Greek physician who lived from 460 to 377 BC and whose vital role in medicine is still recognized today. He is called "The Father of Medicine" and is credited with establishing early ethical standards for physicians. Because of advances in scientific computerized technology, many new terms are coined daily; however, most of these terms are composed of word parts that have their origins in ancient Greek or Latin. Because of this foreign origin, it is necessary to learn the English translation of terms when learning the fundamentals of word structure.

Fundamentals of Word Structure

The fundamental elements in medical terminology are the component parts used to build medical words. The terms for component parts used in this text are P = prefix, R = root, CF = combining form, and S = suffix. Each of these component parts is described in detail below.

PREFIX

The term **prefix** means to fix before or to fix to the beginning of a word. A prefix may be a syllable or a group of syllables united with or placed at the beginning of a word to alter or modify the meaning of the word or to create a new word.

For example: the word **abnormal** means pertaining to away from the normal. Note its component parts below:

ab	P or prefix meaning	away from
norm	R or root meaning	rule
al	S or suffix meaning	pertaining to

WORD ROOT

A root is a word or word element from which other words are formed. It is the foundation of the word. The root conveys the central meaning of the word and forms the base to which prefixes and suffixes are attached for word modification.

For example: the word **autonomy** means condition of being self-governed. Note its component parts below:

auto	P or prefix meaning	self
nom	R or root meaning	law
y	S or suffix meaning	condition

COMBINING FORM

A combining form is a word root to which a vowel has been added to join the root to a second root or to a suffix. The vowel "o" is used more often than any other to make combining forms. Combining forms may be found at the beginning of a word or within the word.

For example: the word **chemotherapy** means treatment of disease by using chemical agents. Note the relation of its component parts:

chemo	CF or combining form meaning	chemical
therapy	S or suffix meaning	treatment

SUFFIX

The term **suffix** means to fasten on beneath or under. A suffix or pseudo suffix may be a syllable or group of syllables united with or placed at the end of a word to alter or modify the meaning of the word or to create a new word.

For example: the word **centigrade** means having 100 steps or degrees and the word **centimeter** means one-hundredth of a meter:

centi	P or prefix meaning	a hundred
grade	S or suffix meaning	a step
centi	P or prefix meaning	a hundred
meter	S or suffix meaning	measure

In many medical terminology textbooks, all the prefixes, suffixes, and pseudo suffixes used throughout the text are grouped into one or two beginning chapters. Under this arrangement, you are forced to refer repeatedly back to these chapters to identify or define these word elements. In this book, however, prefixes, suffixes, and pseudo suffixes, along with their definitions, are integrated into each chapter throughout the text and provide a ready reference. Naturally, many of these same prefixes, suffixes, and pseudo suffixes will be used in each chapter. This repetition serves to reinforce the learning of the terms and their definitions and makes this text an improved learning tool.

Word roots and combining forms, together with their definitions, are included in each chapter according to the cell, tissue, organ, system, or element they describe. This arrangement makes it possible for you to form associations between medical terms and the various body systems. To reinforce this relation, this text provides you with a general anatomy and physiology overview for each of the body systems that it includes.

Principles of Component Parts

As you learn definitions for prefixes, roots, combining forms, and suffixes, you will discover that some component parts have the same meanings as others. This occurs most often with words that relate to the organs of the body and the diseases that affect them. The existence of more than one component part for a particular meaning can be traced to differences in the Greek or Latin words from which they originated. Most of the terms for the body's organs originated from Latin words, whereas terms describing diseases that affect these organs have their origins in Greek.

For example:

- **uterus**—a Latin word for one of the organs of the female reproductive system
- **hyster**—a Greek R (root) for womb
- **hysterectomy**—surgical excision of the womb from hyster R (root) meaning womb + ectomy S (suffix) meaning surgical excision
- **metri**—a Greek CF (combining form) for uterus
- **myometrium**—muscular tissue of the uterus from myo CF meaning muscle + metri CF meaning uterus + um S meaning tissue

Many prefixes and suffixes have more than a single definition. When learning medical terminology, you must learn to use the definition that best describes the term. The following are commonly used prefixes that have more than a single definition:

Prefix	Meanings	Prefix	Meanings
a-, an-	no, not, without, lack of, apart	extra-	outside, beyond
ad-	toward, near, to	hyper-	above, beyond, excessive
bi-	two, double	hypo-	below, under, deficient
de-	down, away from	in-	in, into, not
di-	two, double	mega-	large, great
dia-	through, between	meta-	beyond, over, between, change
dif-, dis-	apart, free from, separate	para-	beside, alongside, abnormal
dys-	bad, difficult, painful	poly-	many, much, excessive
ec-, ecto-	out, outside, outer	post-	after, behind
end-, endo-	within, inner	pre-	before, in front of
ep-, epi-	upon, over, above	pro-	before, in front of
eu-	good, normal	super-	above, beyond
ex-, exo-	out, away from	supra-	above, beyond

The following are commonly used suffixes that have more than a single definition:

Suffix	Meanings	Suffix	Meanings
-ate	use, action	-penia	lack of, deficiency
-blast	immature cell, germ cell	-plasm	a thing formed, plasma
-ectasis	dilatation, dilation, distention	-plegia	stroke, paralysis
-gen	formation, produce	-ptosis	prolapse, drooping
-genesis	formation, produce	-rrhea	flow, discharge
-genic	formation, produce	-scopy	to view, examine
-gram	weight, mark, record	-spasm	tension, spasm
-ic	pertaining to, chemical	-stasis	control, stopping
-ive	nature of, quality of	-staxia	dripping, trickling
-lymph	serum, clear fluid	-trophy	nourishment, development
-lysis	destruction, to separate	-y	process, condition, pertaining to
-megaly	enlargement, large		

Dictionaries, medical terminology texts, and other resources often differ in labeling component parts as prefixes, roots, and combining forms. For example, one source will list **hemato** as a prefix whereas another source will refer to it as a combining form. Occasionally, the same source will label a word part as a prefix in one instance and as a combining form in another. Throughout this book every effort has been made to provide consistency with respect to labeling component parts according to the more acceptable usage of the part.

Identifying Medical Terms

When identifying medical terms you will learn to distinguish between and select the appropriate component parts for the meaning of the term. It is most important that you learn the terms as they are listed, for the slightest change in the arrangement of a medical word's component parts can change its meaning.

For example: the word **microscope** means an instrument used to view small objects. Compare the following:

micro + scope	Proper placement of component parts (P + S) although the definitions translate micro = small and scope = instrument.
scope + micro	Improper placement of component parts (S + P). Although incorrect, this arrangement of word parts seems to correspond to the term's definition.

Spelling

Medical terms of Greek origin are often difficult to spell because many of them begin with a silent letter or have a silent letter within the word. The following are examples of words that begin with silent letters:

Silent Beginning	Pronounced	Medical Term	Pronunciation Guide
cn	n	**c**nemial	(nē′ mĭ-al)
gn	n	**g**nathic	(năth′ ĭ k)
kn	n	**k**nuckle	(nŭk′ ĕ l)
mn	n	**m**nemic	(nē′ mĭ k)
pn	n	**p**neumonia	(nū′-mō′ nĭ-ă)
ps	s	**p**sychiatrist	(sī-kī′ ă-trĭst)
pt	t	**p**tosis	(tō′ sĭ s)

The following are examples of medical terms that contain silent letters within the word:

Silent Letter	Medical Term	Pronunciation Guide
g	phle**g**m	(flĕm)
p	ble**p**haro**p**tosis	(blĕf′ ′ ă-rō-tō′ sis)

Correct spelling is extremely important in medical terminology as the addition or omission of a single letter may change the meaning of a term to something entirely different. The following examples illustrate this point:

Term/Letter Change	Meaning of Term	Term/Letter Change	Meaning of Term
a**b**duct	To lead **away** from the middle	art**er**itis	Inflammation of an **artery**
a**d**duct	To lead **toward** the middle	art**hr**itis	Inflammation of a **joint**

Listed below are some of the component parts that often contribute to spelling errors:

Prefix	Meaning	Suffix	Meaning
ante-	before	-poiesis	formation
anti-	against	-ptosis	prolapse, drooping
		-ptysis	spitting
ecto-	outside		
endo-	within	-rrhagia	bursting forth
		-rrhage	bursting forth
hyper-	above, beyond, excessive		
hypo-	below, under, deficient	-rrhaphy	suture
		-rrhea	flow
inter-	between	-rrhexis	rupture
intra-	within		
		-scope	instrument
para-	beside	-scopy	to view
peri-	around		
		-tome	instrument to cut
per-	through	-tomy	incision
pre-	before		
		-tripsy	crushing
pro-	before	-trophy	nourishment
super-	above, beyond		
supra-	above, beyond		

The following guidelines are provided to help with the identification and spelling of medical terms:

1. If the suffix begins with a vowel, drop the combining vowel from the combining form and add the suffix.

    For example: hemato + oma becomes hematoma when we drop the "o" from hemato.

2. If the suffix begins with a consonant, keep the combining vowel and add the suffix to the combining form.

    For example, kilo + gram becomes kilogram and we keep the "o" on the combining form kilo.

3. Keep the combining vowel between two or more roots in a term.

    For example: electro + cardio + gram becomes electrocardiogram and we keep the combining vowels.

Forming Plural Endings

To change the following singular endings to plural endings, substitute the plural endings as illustrated:

Singular Ending	Plural Ending	Singular Ending	Plural Ending
a as in burs**a**	to **ae** as in burs**ae**	**nx** as in phala**nx**	to **ges** as in phalan**ges**
ax as in thor**ax**	to **aces** as in thor**aces** or **es** as in thorax**es**	**on** as in spermatozo**on**	to **a** as in spermatozo**a**
		um as in ov**um**	to a as in ov**a**
en as in foram**en**	to **ina** as in foram**ina**		
is as in cris**is**	to es as in cris**es**	**us** as in nucle**us**	to i as in nucle**i**
is as in ir**is**	to **ides** as in ir**ides**	**y** as in arter**y**	to **i** and add **es** as in arter**ies**
is as in femor**is**	to a as in femor**a**		
ix as in append**ix**	to ices as in append**ices**		

Pronunciation

Pronunciation of medical words may seem difficult; however, it is very important to pronounce medical words with the same or very similar sounds to convey their correct meanings. As in spelling, one mispronounced syllable can change the meaning of a medical word. This text uses a phonetically spelled pronunciation guide adapted from *Taber's Cyclopedic Medical Dictionary*, and you should practice speaking each term aloud when working with the various lists of medical terms or vocabulary words. Accent marks are used to indicate stress on certain syllables. A single accent mark (′) is called a primary accent and is used with the syllable that has the strongest stress. A double accent (″) is called a secondary accent and is given to syllables that are stressed less than primary syllables.

Diacritics are marks placed over or under vowels to indicate the long or short sound of the vowel. In this text, the macron (-) shows the long sound of the vowel, the breve (˘) shows the short sound of the vowel, and the schwa (ə) indicates the uncolored, central vowel sound of most unstressed syllables [for example: antiseptic (an″ti - sep′ tik) or diathermy (di′ ə - thĕr″ mē)].

Learning Aids

Within each chapter you will find listings of terminology and vocabulary words along with pronunciation guides. The meaning for each term or vocabulary word has been provided, thereby reducing the need for a dictionary. These terms and words have been arranged in alphabetic order for easy use and reference.

Terminology with Surgical Procedures & Pathology

Term	Word Parts			Definition
abnormal (ăb-nōr′ măl)	ab norm al	P R S	away from rule pertaining to	Pertaining to away from the normal
adhesion (ăd′ hē–zhŭn)	adhes ion	R S	stuck to process	The process of being stuck together
antipyretic (ăn″ tĭ-pī-rĕt′ ĭk)	anti pyret ic	P R S	against fever pertaining to	Pertaining to an agent that works against fever
antiseptic (ăn″ tĭ-sĕp′ tĭk)	anti sept ic	P R S	against putrefaction pertaining to	Pertaining to an agent that works against sepsis; putrefaction
antitussive (ăn″ tĭ-tŭs′ ĭv)	anti tuss ive	P R S	against cough nature of, quality of	Pertaining to an agent that works against coughing
asepsis (ā-sĕp′ sĭs)	a sepsis	P S	without decay	Without decay; sterile, free from all living microorganisms
autoclave (ŏ′ tō-klāv)	auto clave	P S	self a key	An apparatus used to sterilize articles by steam under pressure
autonomy (ăw-tŏ′ nōm-ē) (ŏ-tŏ′ nōmē)	auto nom y	P R S	self law condition	The condition of being self-governed; to function independently
axillary (ăks′ ĭ-lār-ē)	axill ary	R S	armpit pertaining to	Pertaining to the armpit
cachexia (kă-kĕks′ ĭ-ă)	cac hexia	P S	bad condition	A condition of ill health, feeling bad
centigrade (sĕn′ tĭ-grād)	centi grade	P S	a hundred a step	Having 100 steps or degrees, as the Celsius temperature scale; boiling point = 100°C and freezing point = 0°C
centimeter (sĕn′ tĭ-mē-tĕr)	centi meter	P S	a hundred measure	Unit of measurement in the metric system; one-hundredth of a meter
centrifuge (sĕn′ trĭ-fūj)	centri fuge	CF S	center to flee	A device used in a laboratory to separate solids from liquids

(Terminology—continued)

Term	Word Parts			Definition
chemotherapy (kē″ mō-thĕr′ ă-pē)	chemo therapy	CF S	chemical treatment	Treatment using chemical agents
diagnosis (dī″ ăg-nō′ sĭs)	dia gnosis	P S	through knowledge	Determination of the cause and nature of a disease
diaphoresis (dī″ ă-fō-rē′ sĭs)	dia phoresis	P S	through to carry	To carry through sweat glands; profuse sweating
diathermy (dī′ ă-thĕr″ mē)	dia thermy	P S	through heat	Treatment using high-frequency current to produce heat within a part of the body
heterogeneous (hĕt″ ĕr-ō-jē′ nĭ-ŭs)	hetero gene ous	P R S	different formation, produce pertaining to	Pertaining to a different formation
kilogram (kĭl′ ō-grăm)	kilo gram	CF S	a thousand a weight	Unit of weight in the metric system; 1000 g
macroscopic (măk″ rō-skŏp′ ĭk)	macro scop ic	CF R S	large to examine pertaining to	Pertaining to objects large enough to be examined by the naked eye
malformation (măl″ fōr-mā′ shŭn)	mal format ion	P R S	bad a shaping process	The process of being badly shaped, deformed
microgram (mī″ krō-grăm)	micro gram	P S	small a weight	A unit of weight in the metric system; 0.001 mg
microorganism (mī″ krō-ōr′ găn-ĭzm)	micro organ ism	P R S	small organ condition	Small living organisms that are not visible to the naked eye
microscope (mī′ krō-skōp)	micro scope	P S	small instrument	An instrument used to view small objects
milligram (mĭl′ ĭ-grăm)	milli gram	P S	one-thousandth a weight	A unit of weight in the metric system; 0.001 g
milliliter (mĭl′ ĭ-lē″ tĕr)	milli liter	P S	one-thousandth liter	A unit of volume in the metric system; 0.001 L
multiform (mŭl′ tĭ-form)	multi form	P S	many, much shape	Occurring in or having many shapes
necrosis (nĕ-krō′ sĭs)	necr osis	R S	death condition of	A condition of death of tissue

(Terminology—continued)

Term	Word Parts			Definition
neopathy (nē-ŏp′ ă-thē)	neo pathy	P S	new disease	A new disease
oncology (ŏng-kŏl′ ō-jē)	onco logy	CF S	tumor study of	The study of tumors
paracentesis (păr″ ă-sĕn-tē′ sĭs)	para centesis	P S	beside surgical puncture	Surgical puncture of a body cavity for fluid removal
prognosis (prŏg-nō′ sĭs)	pro gnosis	P S	before knowledge	A condition of fore-knowledge; the prediction of the course of a disease and the recovery rate
pyrogenic (pī″ rō-jĕn′ ĭk)	pyro genic	CF S	heat, fire formation, produce	Pertaining to the production of heat, a fever
radiology (rā″ dē-ŏl′ ō-jē)	radio logy	CF S	ray study of	The study of radioactive substances
syndrome (sĭn′ drōm)	syn drome	P S	together, with a course	A combination of signs and symptoms occurring together that characterize a specific disease
thermometer (thĕr-mŏm′ ĕ-tĕr)	thermo meter	CF S	hot, heat instrument to measure	An instrument used to measure degree of heat
topography (tō-pŏg′ răh-fē)	topo graphy	CF S	place recording	A recording of a special place of the body
triage (trē-ahzh′)	tri age	P S	three related to	The sorting and classifying of injuries to determine priority of need and treatment

Vocabulary Words

Vocabulary words are terms that have not been divided into component parts. They are common words or specialized terms associated with the subject of this chapter. These words are provided to enhance your medical vocabulary.

Word	Definition
abate (ă-bāt ′)	To lessen, decrease, or cease
abscess (ăb′ sĕs)	A localized collection of pus, which may occur in any part of the body
acute (ă-cūt′)	Sudden, sharp, severe; a disease that has a sudden onset, severe symptoms, and a short course
afferent (ăf′ ĕr ĕnt)	Carrying impulses toward a center
ambulatory (ăm′ bŭ-lăh-tŏr″ ē)	The condition of being able to walk, not confined to bed
antidote (ăn′ tĭ-dōt)	A substance given to counteract poisons and their effects
apathy (ăp′ ă-thē)	A condition in which one lacks feelings and emotions and is indifferent
biopsy (bī ŏp-sē)	Surgical removal of a small piece of tissue for microscopic examination; used to determine a diagnosis of cancer or other disease processes in the body
chronic (krŏn′ ik)	Pertaining to time; a disease that continues over a long time, showing little change in symptoms or course
disease (dĭ-zēz′)	Lack of ease; an abnormal condition of the body that presents a series of symptoms that sets it apart from normal or other abnormal body states
disinfectant (dĭs″ĭn-fĕk′ tănt)	A chemical substance that destroys bacteria
efferent (ĕf ′ĕr ĕnt)	Carrying impulses away from a center
empathy (ĕm′ pă-thē)	A state of projecting one's own personality into the personality of another to understand the feelings, emotions, and behavior of the person
epidemic (ĕp″ i-dĕm′ ik)	Pertaining to among the people; the rapid, widespread occurrence of an infectious disease
etiology (ē″ tē-ŏl′ ō-jē)	The study of the cause(s) of disease
excision (ĕk-sī′ zhŭn)	The process of cutting out, surgical removal

(Vocabulary—continued)

Word	Definition
febrile (fē brĭl)	Pertaining to fever
gram (grăm)	A unit of weight in the metric system; a cubic centimeter or a milliliter of water is equal to the weight of a gram
illness (ĭl′ nĭs)	A state of being sick
incision (ĭn-sĭzh′ ŭn)	The process of cutting into
liter (lē′ tĕr)	A unit of volume in the metric system; equal to 33.8 fl oz or 1.0567 qt
malaise (mă-lāz′)	A bad feeling; a condition of discomfort, uneasiness; often felt by a patient with a chronic disease
malignant (mă-lĭg′ nănt)	A bad wandering; pertaining to the spreading process of cancer from one area of the body to another area
maximal (măks′ ĭ-măl)	Pertaining to the greatest possible quantity, number, or degree
minimal (mĭn′ ĭ-măl)	Pertaining to the least possible quantity, number, or degree
pallor (păl′ or)	Paleness, a lack of color
palmar (păl′ mar)	Pertaining to the palm of the hand
prognostication (prŏg-nŏs ′tĭ-că-shŭn)	The study of the likely course of a disease and the signs of a patient's failure to thrive
prophylactic (prō-fi-lăk′ tĭk)	Pertaining to preventing or protecting against disease
rapport (ră-pōr′)	A relationship of understanding between two individuals, especially between the patient and the physician

MEDICAL AND SURGICAL SPECIALTIES

The practice of medicine has evolved from the period in which the physician treated the patient as an entity to the present era of specialization. The specialties listed below have been identified as being within the field of medicine. A description of each specialty plus the physician's title is provided to familiarize you with these fields of medicine.

Allergy and Immunology. The branch of medicine concerned with diseases caused by the action of antibodies to antigens. The physician is an **allergist or immunologist.**

Anesthesiology. The branch of medicine that studies the partial or complete loss of sensation, pain, temperature, touch, etc. The physician is an **anesthesiologist.**

Cardiovascular Disease. The branch of medicine concerned with diseases of the heart, arteries, veins, and capillaries. The physician is a **cardiologist.**

Critical Care Medicine. The branch of medicine concerned with those who are dangerously ill or in a critical state.

Dermatology. The branch of medicine concerned with diseases of the skin. The physician is a **dermatologist.**

Emergency Care Medicine. The branch of medicine concerned with those who are acutely ill or suddenly injured. The physician is a board-certified emergency physician.

Endocrinology. The branch of medicine concerned with diseases of the endocrine system. The physician is an **endocrinologist.**

Epidemiology. The branch of medicine that studies the interrelationships of factors, causes, and probable causes of epidemic diseases. The physician is an **epidemiologist.**

Family Practice. The branch of medicine concerned with the care of all members of the family regardless of age and sex.

Gastroenterology. The branch of medicine concerned with diseases of the stomach and intestines. The physician is a **gastroenterologist.**

General Practice. The branch of medicine concerned with diseases of a general nature. No special title has been designated for this practitioner other than physician.

Geriatrics. The branch of medicine concerned with the aspects of aging. The physician is a **geriatrician.**

Gynecology. The branch of medicine that studies the diseases of the reproductive organs of the female. The physician is a **gynecologist.**

Hematology. The branch of medicine that studies the diseases of the blood and blood-forming tissues. The physician is a **hematologist.**

Infectious Disease. The branch of medicine concerned with diseases caused by the growth of pathogenic microorganisms within the body. The physician is an infectious disease specialist/internist.

Internal Medicine. The branch of medicine concerned with diseases of internal origin, those not usually treated surgically. The physician is an **internist.**

Neonatology. The branch of medicine concerned with the study and care of newborn infants (up to 6 weeks of age). The physician is a **neonatologist.**

Neoplastic Disease. The branch of medicine concerned with diseases of new, abnormal tissue formation.

Nephrology. The branch of medicine concerned with diseases of the kidney. The physician is a **nephrologist.**

Neurology. The branch of medicine that studies diseases of the nervous system. The physician is a **neurologist.**

Nuclear Medicine. The branch of medicine concerned with the diagnostic, therapeutic, and investigative use of atoms that disintegrate by emission of electromagnetic radiation.

Obstetrics. The branch of medicine concerned with treating the female during pregnancy, childbirth, and puerperium. The physician is an **obstetrician.**

Occupational Medicine. The branch of medicine concerned with the self-care, work, play, and task performance skills of well and disabled individuals. The physician is a specialist in occupational medicine.

Oncology. The branch of medicine that studies tumors. The physician is an **oncologist.**

Ophthalmology. The branch of medicine that studies the diseases of the eye. The physician is an **ophthalmologist.**

Orthopedics. The branch of medicine concerned with diseases and disorders involving the locomotor structures of the body. The physician is an **orthopedist.**

Otorhinolaryngology. The branch of medicine that studies the diseases of the ear, nose, and larynx. The physician is an **otorhinolaryngologist.**

Pathology. The branch of medicine that studies the structural and functional changes in tissues and organs caused by disease. The physician is a **pathologist.**

Pediatrics. The branch of medicine concerned with diseases of children. The physician is a **pediatrician.**

Physical Medicine. The branch of medicine concerned with the treatment of disease by physical agents such as heat, cold, light, electricity, manipulation, exercises, massage, or mechanical devices. The physician is a **physiatrist.**

Psychiatry. The branch of medicine concerned with diseases of the mind. The physician is a **psychiatrist.**

Pulmonary Disease. The branch of medicine concerned with diseases of the lungs. The physician is a **pulmonologist.**

Radiology. The branch of medicine that studies radioactive substances and their relation to prevention, diagnosis, and treatment of disease. The physician is a **radiologist.**

Rheumatology. The branch of medicine concerned with rheumatic diseases. The physician is a **rheumatologist.**

Space Medicine. The branch of medicine concerned with conditions, disorders, or diseases of astronauts and the effects of space travel on humans and animals.

Sports Medicine. The branch of medicine concerned with the prevention, diagnosis, and treatment of conditions that may occur because of an athletic endeavor.

Surgery. The branch of medicine concerned with the treatment of diseases by manual and operative procedures. Surgery may be classified as general, neurological, ophthalmologic, plastic, proctological, thoracic, urologic, and vascular. The physician is a **surgeon.**

Urology. The branch of medicine that studies diseases of the urinary system. The physician is a **urologist.**

ABBREVIATIONS

AB	abnormal	**FP**	family practice
ac	acute	**g, Gm**	gram
ax	axillary	**GP**	general practice
Bx	biopsy	**Gyn**	gynecology
C	centigrade, Celsius	**kg**	kilogram
cm	centimeter	**L**	liter
CT	computerized tomography	**mcg**	microgram
CVD	cardiovascular disease	**mg**	milligram
D/C	discontinue	**mL, ml**	milliliter
derm	dermatology	**Ob**	obstetrics
Dx	diagnosis	**Peds**	pediatrics
DRGs	diagnosis-related groups	**Psy**	psychiatry, psychology
ENT	otorhinolaryngology		

Communication Enrichment

This segment is provided for those who wish to enhance their ability to communicate in either English or Spanish.

WEIGHTS AND MEASURES

PESO Y MEDIDAS
(pĕ-sō ĭ mĕ-dǐ-dăs)

English	Spanish
length	longitud (lōn-hĭ-tūd)
width	anchura (ăn-chū-ră)
height	altura ăl-tū-ră
volume	volumen; tomo (vō-lū-mĕn; tō-mō)
weight	peso (pĕ-sō)
microgram	microgramo (mĭ-krō-gră-mō)
milligram	miligramo (mĭ-lĭ-gră-mō)
gram	gramo (gră-mō)
kilogram	kilogramo (kĭ-lō-gră-mō)
liter	litro (lĭ-trō)
millimeter	milímetro (mĭ-lĭ-mĕ-trō)
centimeter	centímetro (sĕn-tĭ-mĕ-trō)
cubic centimeter	centímetro cubico (sĕn-tĭ-mĕ-trō kŭ-bĭ-kō)
square	cuadrado (kū-ă-dră-dō)

DESCRIPTIVE WORDS

English	Spanish	English	Spanish
large	grande (grăn-dĕ)	weak	débil (dĕ-bĭl)
small	pequeño (pĕ-kĕ-ñō)	strong	fuerte (fū-ĕr-tĕ)
tall	alto (ăl-tō)	better	mejor (mĕ-hōr)

English	Spanish	English	Spanish
short	bajo (bă-hō)	worse	peor (pĕ-ōr)
fat	gordo (gōr-dō)	alive	vivo (vĭ-vō)
thin	flaco (flă-kō)	dead	muerto (mū-ĕr-tō)
dark	obscuro (ŏs-kŭ-rō)	healthy	sano (să-nō)
light	claro (clă-rō)	sick	enfermo (ĕn-fĕr-mō)
soft	blando (blăn-dō)	sweet	dulce (dūl-sĕ)
hard	duro (dŭ-rō)	sour	agrio (ăg-rĭ-ō)
hot	caliente (kă-lĭ-ĕn-tĕ)	bitter	amargo (ă-măr-gō)
wet	mojado (mō-hă-dō)	good	bueno (bway-no)
dry	seco (sĕ-kō)	bad	malo (mă-lō)
open	abierto (ă-bĭ-ĕr-tō)	pain	dolor (dō-lōr)
closed	cerrado (sĕ-ră-dō)	loud	fuerte (fŭ-ĕr-tĕ)

ESSENTIAL PHRASES

English	Spanish
Good day	Buenos días (bway-nōs dee-ahs)
What is your name?	¿Cómo se llama usted? (cō-mō sĕ yă-mă ūs-tĕd)
How old are you?	¿Cuántos años tiene? (kwan-tos ă-ñōs tĭ-ĕ-nĕ)
Do you understand me?	¿Me entiende? (me en-tē-en-dā)
Yes	Sí (sĭ)
No	No (nō)

CARDINAL NUMBERS

English	Spanish	English	Spanish
1	uno (*oo*-nō)	13	trece (*trĕ*-sĕ)
2	dos (dōs)	14	catorce (kă-*tōr*-sĕ)
3	tres (trĕs)	15	quince (*kĭn*-sĕ)
4	cuatro (*kwa*-trō)	20	veinte (*vĕn*-tĕ)
5	cinco (*sĭn*-kō)	30	treinta (*trĕn*-tă)
6	seis (sĕ-ĭs)	40	cuarenta (kŭ-ă-*rĕn*-tă)
7	siete (*sĭ*-ĕ-tĕ)	50	cincuenta (sĭn-*kwen*-tă)
8	ocho (ŏ-chō)	60	sesenta (sĕ-*sĕn*-tă)
9	nueve (*nŭ*-ĕ-vĕ)	70	setenta (sĕ-*tĕn*-tă)
10	diez (d'*yehs*)	80	ochenta (ō-*chĕn*-tă)
11	once (*ōn*-sĕ)	90	noventa (nō-*vĕn*-tă)
12	doce (*dō*-sĕ)	100	cien (sĭ-*ĕn*)

ORDINAL NUMBERS

English	Spanish	English	Spanish
first	primero (prĭ-*mĕ*-rō)	fourth	cuarto (*kwar*-tō)
second	segundo (sĕ-*gŭn*-dō)	fifth	quinto (*kĭn*-tō)
third	tercero (tĕr-*sĕ*-rō)	sixth	sexto (*sĕk*-tō)
seventh	séptimo (*sĕp*-tĭ-mō)	tenth	décimo (*dĕ*-sĭ-mō)
eighth	octavo (ōk-*tă*-vō)	eleventh	décimo primero (*dĕ*-sĭ-mō prĭ-*mĕ*-rō)
ninth	noveno (nō-*vĕn*-nō)	twelfth	décimo segundo (*dĕ*-sĭ-mō sĕ-*gŭn*-dō)

TIME

English	Spanish
hour	hora (ō-rǎ)
minute	minuto (mǐ-*nŭ*-tō)
second	segundo (sě-*gŭn*-dō)
at noon	al medio dia (ǎl *mě*-dǐ-ō *di*-ǎ)
at midnight	a la media noche (ǎ lǎ *mě*-dǐ-ǎ *nō*-chě)

MONTHS OF THE YEAR

English	Spanish	English	Spanish
January	enero (ě-*ně*-rō)	July	julio (*hŭ*-lǐ-ō)
February	febrero (fě-*brě*-rō)	August	agosto (a-*gōs*-tō)
March	marzo (*măr*-zō)	September	septiembre (sěp-*tǐ-ěm*-brě)
April	abril (ǎ-*brǐl*)	October	octubre (ōk-*tŭ*-brě)
May	mayo (*mǎ*-jō)	November	noviembre (no-*vǐ*-ěm-brě)
June	junio (*hŭ*-nǐ-ō)	December	diciembre (dǐ-*cǐ*-ěm-brě)

HOLIDAYS ———— (DIAS de FIESTA)

English	Spanish
Christmas	Navidad (Nǎ-vǐ-*dǎd*)
New Year	Año Nuevo (*A*-nō *Nŭ*-ě-vō)
Easter	Pascuas (*Păs*-qǔ-ǎs)
Holy Week	Semana Santa (Sě-*mǎ*-nǎ *săn*-tǎ)
Valentine's Day	Dia de los enamorados (*Dǐ*-ǎ dě lōs ě-nǎ-mō-*rǎ*-dōs)
July 4	Cuatro de julio (*Qǔ-ǎ*-trō dě *hŭ*-lǐ-ō)
Halloween	Dia de Todos los Santos (*Dǐ*-ǎ dě *tō*-dōs lōs *Săn*-tōs)

English	Spanish
birthday	cumpleaños (qŭm-plĕ-*ă*-ñōs)
anniversary	aniversario (ă-nĭ-vĕr-*să*-rĭ-ō)

DAYS OF THE WEEK

English	Spanish	English	Spanish
Monday	lunes (*lŭ*-nĕs)	Friday	viernes (*vĭĕr*-nĕs)
Tuesday	martes (*măr*-tĕs)	Saturday	sábado (*să*-bă-dōs)
Wednesday	miércoles (*mĭĕr*-qō-lĕs)	Sunday	domingo (dō-*mĭn*-gō)
Thursday	jueves (hŭ-*ĕ*-vĕs)		

Learning Exercises

Word Parts

1. In the spaces provided, write the definition of these prefixes, roots, combining forms, and suffixes. Do not refer to the listings of terminology words. Leave blank those terms you cannot define.
2. After completing as many as you can, refer back to the terminology word listings to check your work. For each word missed or left blank, write the term and its definition several times on the margins of these pages or on a separate sheet of paper.
3. To maximize the learning process, it is to your advantage to do the following exercises as directed. To refer to the terminology listings before completing these exercises invalidates the learning process.

PREFIXES

Give the definitions of the following prefixes:

1. a-	_____	2. ab-	_____
3. anti-	_____	4. auto-	_____
5. cac-	_____	6. centi-	_____
7. dia-	_____	8. hetero-	_____
9. mal-	_____	10. micro-	_____
11. milli-	_____	12. multi-	_____
13. neo-	_____	14. para-	_____
15. pro-	_____	16. syn-	_____
17. tri-	_____		

ROOTS AND COMBINING FORMS

Give the definitions of the following roots and combining forms:

1. adhes	_____	2. axill	_____
3. centri	_____	4. chemo	_____
5. format	_____	6. gene	_____
7. kilo	_____	8. macro	_____
9. necr	_____	10. nom	_____
11. norm	_____	12. onco	_____
13. organ	_____	14. pyret	_____
15. pyro	_____	16. radio	_____
17. scop	_____	18. sept	_____
19. thermo	_____	20. topo	_____
21. tuss	_____		

SUFFIXES

Give the definitions of the following suffixes:

1. -age _____
2. -al _____
3. -ary _____
4. -centesis _____
5. -clave _____
6. -drome _____
7. -form _____
8. -fuge _____
9. -genic _____
10. -gnosis _____
11. -grade _____
12. -gram _____
13. -graphy _____
14. -hexia _____
15. -ic _____
16. -ion _____
17. -ism _____
18. -ive _____
19. -liter _____
20. -logy _____
21. -meter _____
22. -osis _____
23. -ous _____
24. -pathy _____
25. -phoresis _____
26. -scope _____
27. -sepsis _____
28. -therapy _____
29. -thermy _____
30. -y _____

Identifying Medical Terms

In the spaces provided, write the medical terms for the following meanings:

1. _____ Process of being stuck together
2. _____ Without decay
3. _____ Pertaining to the armpit
4. _____ Treatment using chemical agents
5. _____ Pertaining to a different formation
6. _____ Process of being badly shaped, deformed
7. _____ An instrument used to view small objects
8. _____ Occurring in or having many shapes
9. _____ A new disease
10. _____ The study of tumors

Spelling

In the spaces provided, write the correct spelling of these misspelled terms:

1. antseptic _____
2. autnomy _____
3. centmeter _____
4. diphoresis _____
5. miligram _____
6. necosis _____
7. parcentesis _____
8. radilogy _____

Review Questions

Matching

Select the appropriate lettered meaning for each numbered line.

_____	1. abate	a. Lack of ease
_____	2. antipyretic	b. A state of being sick
_____	3. cachexia	c. The study of the likely course of a disease and the signs of a patient's failure to thrive
_____	4. diagnosis	
_____	5. disease	d. Pertaining to an agent that works against fever
_____	6. etiology	e. The sorting and classifying of injuries to determine priority of need and treatment
_____	7. illness	
_____	8. prognosis	f. To lessen, decrease, or cease
_____	9. prognostication	g. Determination of the cause and nature of a disease
_____	10. triage	h. A new disease
		i. The prediction of the course of a disease and the recovery rate
		j. A condition of ill health, feeling bad
		k. The study of the cause(s) of disease

Abbreviations

Place the correct word, phrase, or abbreviation in the space provided.

_____	1. AB
_____	2. ax
_____	3. biopsy
_____	4. CVD
_____	5. DRGs
_____	6. otorhinolaryngology
_____	7. family practice
_____	8. general practice
_____	9. Gyn
_____	10. Peds

The Organization of the Body

The human body is made up of atoms, molecules, cells, tissues, organs, and systems. As long as the body is in a state of balance known as *homeostasis* it is able to perform at its maximum potential. Chapter 2 provides basic information for understanding the organization of the human body. Also, some students may choose to benefit from learning the English and/or Spanish translation for body areas.

THE AMAZING HUMAN BODY

The body consists of :
30 trillion cells
206 bones
700 muscles
5 liters of blood
25,000 miles of blood vessels
70 miles of tubules in the kidney

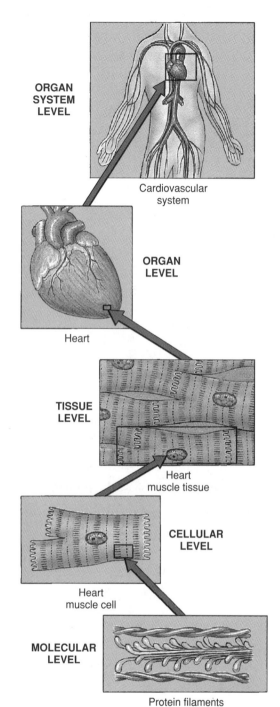

ORGAN SYSTEM LEVEL

Cardiovascular system

ORGAN LEVEL

Heart

TISSUE LEVEL

Heart muscle tissue

CELLULAR LEVEL

Heart muscle cell

MOLECULAR LEVEL

Protein filaments

ANATOMY AND PHYSIOLOGY OVERVIEW

This chapter introduces you to terms describing the body and its structural units. To aid you, these terms have been grouped into two major sections: the first offering an overview of the units that make up the human body, and the second covering terms used to describe anatomical positions and locations. The human body is made up of atoms, molecules, cells, tissues, organs, and systems. All of these parts normally function together in a unified and complex process. During homeostasis these processes allow the body to perform at its maximum potential.

The Human Body: Levels of Organization

ATOMS

An atom is the smallest chemical unit of matter. It consists of a nucleus that contains protons and neutrons and is surrounded by electrons. The nucleus is at the center of the atom and a proton is a positively charged particle, while a neutron is without an electrical charge. The electron is a negatively charged particle that revolves about the nucleus of an atom.

MOLECULES

A molecule is a chemical combination of two or more atoms that form a specific chemical compound. In a water molecule oxygen forms polar covalent bonds with two hydrogen atoms. Water is a tasteless, clear, odorless liquid that makes up 65% of a male's body weight and 55% of a female's body weight. Water is the most important constituent of all body fluids, secretions, and excretions. It is an ideal transportation medium for inorganic and organic compounds.

CELLS

The body consists of millions of cells working individually and with each other to sustain life. For the purposes of this book, cells are considered as the basic building blocks for the various structures that together make up the human being. There are several types of cells, each specialized to perform specific functions. The size and shape of a cell are generally related directly to its function. For example, cells forming the skin overlap each other to form a protective barrier, whereas nerve cells are usually elongated with branches connecting to other cells for the transmission of sensory impulses (see Plate 12). Despite these differences, however, cells can generally be said to have a number of common components. The common parts of the cell are the cell membrane and the protoplasm (Fig. 2–1). These parts are defined on the next page.

FIGURE 2–1

Major parts of the cell. (*Adapted from Evans, WF.* Anatomy and Physiology, *3rd ed. Englewood Cliffs, NJ: Prentice-Hall, 1983, with permission.*)

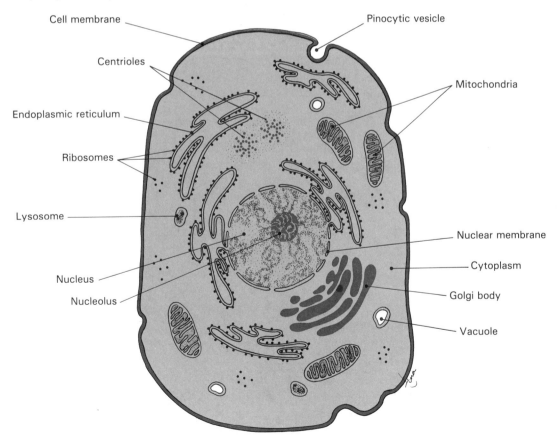

The Cell Membrane

The outer covering of the cell is called the cell membrane. Cell membranes have the capability of allowing some substances to pass into and out of the cell while denying passage to other substances. This selectivity allows cells to receive nutrition and dispose of waste just as the human being eats food and disposes of waste.

Protoplasm

The substance within the cell membrane is called protoplasm. Protoplasm is composed of cytoplasm and karyoplasm. These substances and their functions are described below.

Karyoplasm. Enclosed by its own membrane, karyoplasm is the substance of the cell's nucleus and contains the genetic matter necessary for cell reproduction as well as control over activity within the cell's cytoplasm.

Cytoplasm. All protoplasm outside the nucleus is called cytoplasm. The cytoplasm provides storage and work areas for the cell. Without mentioning their functions, the work and storage elements of the cell, called organelles, are the endoplasmic reticulum, ribosomes, Golgi apparatus, mitochondria, lysosomes, and centrioles.

TISSUES

A tissue is a grouping of similar cells that together perform specialized functions. There are four basic types of tissue in the body: epithelial, connective, muscle, and nerve. Each of the four basic tissues has several subtypes named for their shape, appearance, arrangement, or function. The four basic types of tissue are described below.

Epithelial Tissue

Epithelial tissue appears as sheet-like arrangements of cells, sometimes several layers thick, that form the outer layer of the skin, cover the surfaces of organs, line the walls of cavities, and form tubes, ducts, and portions of certain glands. The functions of epithelial tissues are protection, absorption, secretion, and excretion.

Connective Tissue

The most widespread and abundant of the body tissues, connective tissue forms the supporting network for the organs of the body, sheaths the muscles, and connects muscles to bones and bones to joints. Bone is a dense form of connective tissue.

Muscle Tissue

There are three types of muscle tissue: voluntary or striated, cardiac, and involuntary or smooth. Striated and smooth muscles are so described because of their appearance. Cardiac muscle is a specialized form of striated tissue under the control of the autonomic nervous system. Involuntary or smooth muscles are also controlled by this system. The striated or voluntary muscles are controlled by the person's will.

Nerve Tissue

Nerve tissue consists of nerve cells (neurons) and interstitial tissue. It has the properties of excitability and conductivity, and functions to control and coordinate the activities of the body.

ORGANS

Tissues serving a common purpose or function make up structures called organs. Organs are specialized components of the body such as the brain, skin, or the heart.

SYSTEMS

A group of organs functioning together for a common purpose is called a system. The various body systems function in support of the body as a whole. Listed in Figure 2–2 and Plate 13 are the organ systems of the body.

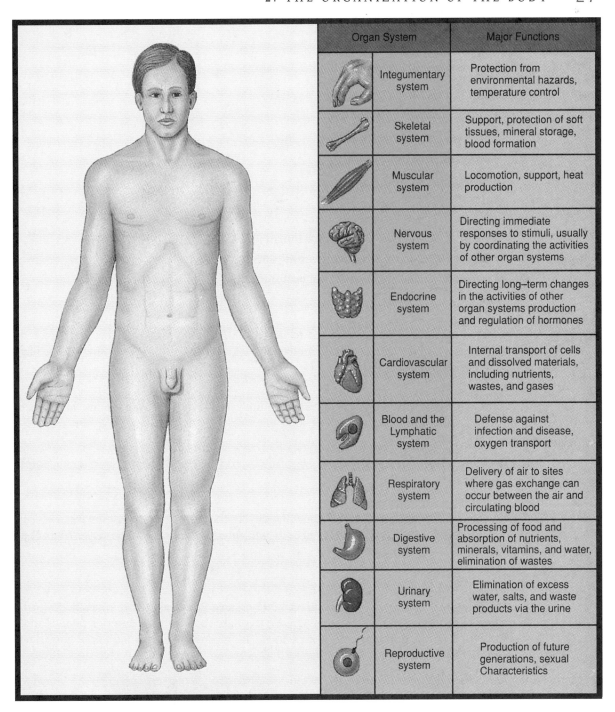

Organ System		Major Functions
	Integumentary system	Protection from environmental hazards, temperature control
	Skeletal system	Support, protection of soft tissues, mineral storage, blood formation
	Muscular system	Locomotion, support, heat production
	Nervous system	Directing immediate responses to stimuli, usually by coordinating the activities of other organ systems
	Endocrine system	Directing long–term changes in the activities of other organ systems production and regulation of hormones
	Cardiovascular system	Internal transport of cells and dissolved materials, including nutrients, wastes, and gases
	Blood and the Lymphatic system	Defense against infection and disease, oxygen transport
	Respiratory system	Delivery of air to sites where gas exchange can occur between the air and circulating blood
	Digestive system	Processing of food and absorption of nutrients, minerals, vitamins, and water, elimination of wastes
	Urinary system	Elimination of excess water, salts, and waste products via the urine
	Reproductive system	Production of future generations, sexual Characteristics

FIGURE 2–2

An introduction to organ systems. *(From Martini F. Fundamentals of Anatomy and Physiology, 2nd ed. Englewood Cliffs, NJ: Prentice-Hall, 1992, with permission.)*

Anatomical Locations and Positions

Four primary reference systems have been adopted to provide uniformity to the anatomical description of the body. These reference systems are direction, planes, cavities, and structural unit. The standard anatomical position for the body is erect, head facing forward, arms by the sides with palms to the front.

DIRECTION

The following terms are used to describe direction:

Superior. Above, in an upward direction

Anterior. In front of or before

Posterior. Toward the back

Cephalad. Toward the head

Medial. Nearest the midline

Lateral. To the side

Proximal. Nearest the point of attachment

Distal. Away from the point of attachment

Ventral. The same as anterior, the front side

Dorsal. The same as posterior, the backside

PLANES

The terms defined below are used to describe the imaginary planes that are depicted in Figure 2-3 as passing through the body and dividing it into various sections. These planes are discussed below.

Midsagittal Plane

The midsagittal plane vertically divides the body as it passes through the midline to form a right and left half.

Transverse or Horizontal Plane

A transverse or horizontal plane is any plane that divides the body into superior and inferior portions.

Coronal or Frontal Plane

A coronal or frontal plane is any plane that divides the body at right angles to the midsagittal plane. The coronal plane divides the body into anterior (ventral) and posterior (dorsal) portions.

CAVITIES

A cavity is a hollow space containing body organs. Body cavities are classified into two groups according to their location. On the front are the ventral or anterior cavities and on the back are the dorsal or posterior cavities. The various cavities found in the human body are depicted in Figure 2-4 and Plate 14.

The Ventral Cavity

The ventral cavity is the hollow portion of the human torso extending from the neck to the pelvis and containing the heart and the organs of respiration, digestion, reproduction, and elimination. The ventral cavity can be subdivided into three distinct areas: thoracic, abdominal, and pelvic.

The Thoracic Cavity. The thoracic cavity is the area of the chest containing the heart and the lungs. Within this cavity the space containing the heart is called the pericardial cavity and the spaces surrounding each lung are known as the pleural cavities. Other organs located in the thoracic cavity are the esophagus, trachea, thymus, and certain large blood and lymph vessels.

The Abdominal Cavity. The abdominal cavity is the space below the diaphragm, commonly referred to as the belly. It contains the kidneys, stomach, intestines, and other organs of digestion.

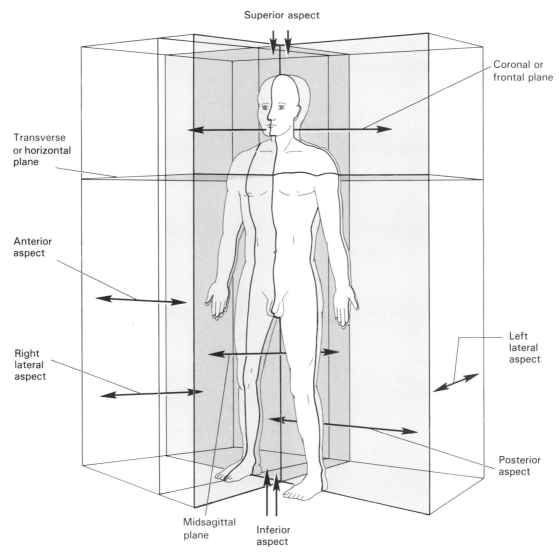

FIGURE 2–3

The body planes. *(Adapted from Evans WF. Anatomy and Physiology, 3rd ed. Englewood Cliffs, NJ: Prentice-Hall, 1983, with permission.)*

The Pelvic Cavity. The pelvic cavity is the space formed by the bones of the pelvic area and contains the organs of reproduction and elimination.

The Dorsal Cavity
Containing the structures of the nervous system, the dorsal cavity is subdivided into the cranial cavity and the spinal cavity.

The Cranial Cavity. The cranial cavity is the space in the skull containing the brain.

The Spinal Cavity. The spinal cavity is the space within the bony spinal column that contains the spinal cord and spinal fluid.

The Abdominopelvic Cavity
The abdominopelvic cavity is the combination of the abdominal and pelvic cavities. It is divided into nine regions.

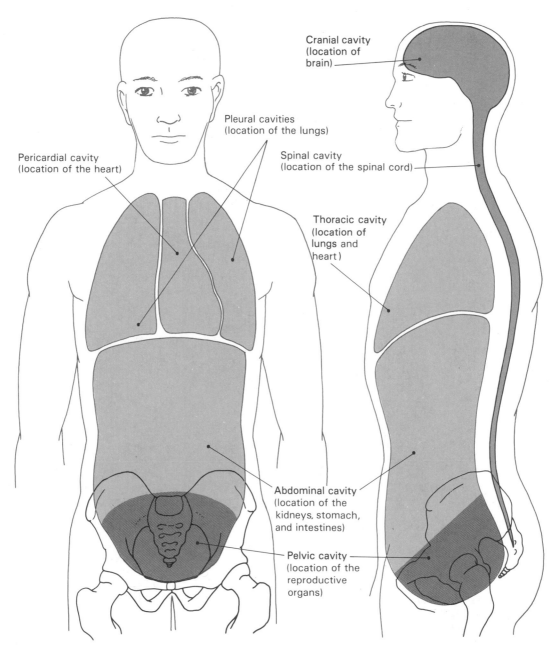

FIGURE 2–4

The body cavities: cranial, spinal, thoracic, abdominal, and pelvic. *(Adapted from Evans WF. Anatomy and Physiology, 3rd ed. Englewood Cliffs, NJ: Prentice-Hall, 1983, with permission.)*

NINE REGIONS OF THE ABDOMINOPELVIC CAVITY

As a ready reference for locating visceral organs, anatomists divided the abdominopelvic cavity into nine regions. Using a tic-tac-toe pattern drawn across the abdominopelvic cavity (Fig. 2–5) these regions are:

- **Right hypochondriac** - upper right region at the level of the ninth rib cartilage.
- **Left hypochondriac** - upper left region at the level of the ninth rib cartilage.
- **Epigastric** - region over the stomach.
- **Right lumbar** - right middle lateral region.

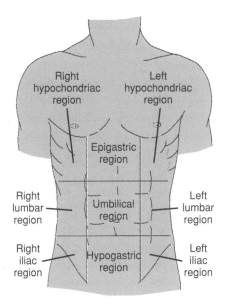

FIGURE 2–5

Nine regions of the abdominopelvic cavity. *(From Martini F.* Fundamentals of Anatomy and Physiology, *2nd ed. Englewood Cliffs, NJ: Prentice-Hall, 1992, with permission.)*

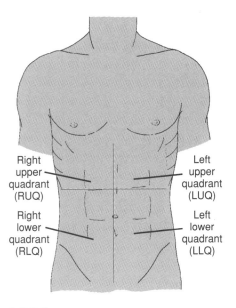

FIGURE 2–6

The four quadrants of the abdomen. *(From Martini F.* Fundamentals of Anatomy and Physiology, *2nd ed. Englewood Cliffs, NJ: Prentice-Hall, 1992, with permission.)*

- **Left lumbar** - left middle lateral region.
- **Umbilical** - in the center, between the right and left lumbar region. At the navel.
- **Right iliac (inguinal)** - right lower lateral region.
- **Left iliac (inguinal)** - left lower lateral region.
- **Hypogastric** - lower middle region below the navel.

ABDOMEN DIVIDED INTO QUADRANTS

The abdomen is divided into four corresponding regions that are used for descriptive and diagnostic purposes. By using these regions one may describe the exact location of pain, a skin lesion, surgical incision, and/or abdominal tumor. The four quadrants are (Fig. 2-6):

- right upper
- left upper
- right lower
- left lower

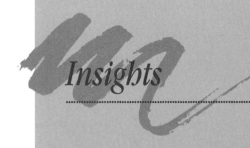

WATER—The Most Important Constituent of the Body

Water is the most important constituent of the human body and is essential to every body process. Bones depend on water intake to provide adequate blood for delivery and removal of calcium. The intestines and kidneys use water to remove waste. Muscles need water to remove acids that would otherwise build up, causing cramps and diminishing muscle action. Nerve function depends on the presence of certain minerals, which are kept in balance by water levels in the body. The immune system depends on sufficient water to ensure blood flow for delivery of immune cells and removal of diseased cells. Water in saliva and the stomach aids digestion and absorption of nutrients.

It is recommended that the average healthy adult drink eight 8-ounce glasses of water per day. To help meet a daily intake of adequate fluids you may choose to drink juices, milk, herbal teas, seltzer, and/or decaffeinated coffee.

- Regular coffee, tea, colas and alcohol contain diuretics that can trigger water loss. These beverages do not count towards the daily intake of ample fluids.
- Dehydration is the process whereby water loss exceeds intake. Symptoms may include thirst, headache, dry mouth, darkened urine, lethargy, fatigue, muscle cramps, and light-headedness.

Water Balance

Daily Input		Daily Output	
Moist foods	1000 mL	Urine	1000 mL
Ingested fluids	1000 mL	Skin (evaporation)	750 mL
Cell metabolism	300 mL	Lungs (evaporation)	400 mL
		Feces	150 mL
Total	2300 mL	Total	2300 mL

- You may need more than eight glasses of water per day before, during, and after exercise, in warm weather (especially, if you are doing any type of out-of-doors activity), during and after drinking alcohol or caffeine, when breast-feeding, during illness (especially diarrhea, fever, and/or prolonged vomiting), with certain medications (especially diuretics), after surgery, and/or severe burns or bleeding.

To maintain homeostasis it is essential that the body be supplied with adequate fluids. In the inserted box, you will find an average of input and output of fluids that can occur on a daily basis. Naturally, if one consumes more or less of these averages, the daily input and output will be affected.

Terminology with Surgical Procedures & Pathology

Term	Word Parts			Definition
adipose (ăd″ ĭ-pōs)	adip ose	R S	fat like	Fatty tissue throughout the body
ambilateral (ăm″ bĭ-lăt′ ĕr-ăl)	ambi later al	P R S	both side pertaining to	Pertaining to both sides
anatomy (ăn-ăt′ ō-mē)	ana tomy	P S	up incision	Literally means to cut up; the study of the structure of an organism such as humans
android (ăn′ droyd)	andr oid	R S	man resemble	To resemble man
bilateral (bī-lăt′ ĕr-ăl)	bi later al	P R S	two side pertaining to	Pertaining to two sides
biology (bi-ŏl′ ō-jē)	bio logy	CF S	life study of	The study of life
caudal (kŏd′ ăl)	caud al	R S	tail pertaining to	Pertaining to the tail
chromosome (krō-mō-sōm)	chromo some	P S	color body	Microscopic bodies that carry the genes that determine hereditary characteristics
cytology (sī-tŏl′ ō-jē)	cyto logy	CF S	cell study of	The study of cells
dehydrate (dē-hī′ drāt)	de hydr ate	P R S	down, away from water use, action	To remove water away from the body
diffusion (di-fū′ zhŭn)	dif fus ion	P R S	apart to pour process	A process in which parts of a substance move from areas of high concentration to areas of lower concentration
ectogenous (ĕk-tŏj′ ĕ-nŭs)	ecto gen ous	P R S	outside formation, produce pertaining to	Pertaining to formation outside the organism or body
ectomorph (ĕk′ tō-morf)	ecto morph	P S	outside form, shape	A slender physical body form
endomorph (ĕn″ dō-morf′)	endo morph	P S	within form, shape	A round physical body form

(Terminology—continued)

Term	Word Parts			Definition
histology (hĭs-tŏl′ ō-jē)	histo	CF	tissue	The study of tissue
	logy	S	study of	
homeostasis (hō″ mē-ō-stā′ sĭs)	homeo	P	similar, same	The state of equilibrium maintained in the body's internal environment
	stasis	S	control, stopping	
karyogenesis (kăr″ i-ō-jĕn′ ĕ-sĭs)	karyo	CF	cell's nucleus	Formation of a cell's nucleus
	genesis	S	formation, produce	
mesomorph (mĕs′ ō-morf)	meso	P	middle	A well-proportioned body form
	morph	S	form, shape	
pathology (pă-thŏl′ ō-jē)	patho	CF	disease	The study of disease
	logy	S	study of	
perfusion (pur-fū′ zhŭn)	per	P	through	The process of pouring through
	fus	R	to pour	
	ion	S	process	
physiology (fiz″ i-ŏl′ ō-jē)	physio	CF	nature	The study of the nature of living organisms
	logy	S	study of	
pinocytosis (pī″ nō-si-tō′ sis)	pino	CF	to drink	The condition whereby a cell absorbs or ingests nutrients and fluids
	cyt	R	cell	
	osis	S	condition of	
protoplasm (prō-tō-plăzm)	proto	P	first	The essential matter of a living cell
	plasm	S	a thing formed, plasma	
somatotrophic (sō″ mă-tō-trŏf′ ĭk)	somato	CF	body	Pertaining to stimulation of body growth
	troph	R	a turning	
	ic	S	pertaining to	
topical (tŏp′ ĭ-kăl)	topic	R	place	Pertaining to a place, definite locale
	al	S	pertaining to	
unilateral (ū″ nĭ-lăt′ ĕr-ăl)	uni	P	one	Pertaining to one side
	later	R	side	
	al	S	pertaining to	
visceral (vĭs′ ĕr-ăl)	viscer	R	body organs	Pertaining to body organs enclosed within a cavity, especially abdominal organs
	al	S	pertaining to	

Vocabulary Words

Vocabulary words are terms that have not been divided into component parts. They are common words or specialized terms associated with the subject of this chapter. These words are provided to enhance your medical vocabulary.

Word	Definition
anterior (an-tĕr′ ē-ōr)	In front of, before
anthropometry (ăn-thrō-pŏm′ ĕt-rē)	The measurement of the human body; includes measurement of the skull, bones, height, weight, and skin fold evaluation for subcutaneous fat estimation
apex (ā′ pĕks)	The pointed end of a cone-shaped structure
base (bās)	The lower part or foundation of a structure
center (sĕn′ tĕr)	The midpoint of a body or activity
cephalad (sĕf′ ă-lăd)	Toward the head
cilia (sĭl′ ē-ă)	Hairlike processes that project from epithelial cells; they help propel mucus, dust particles, and other foreign substances from the respiratory tract
deep (dēp)	Far down from the surface
distal (dĭs′ tăl)	Farthest from the center or point of origin
dorsal (dōr′ săl)	Pertaining to the backside of the body
filtration (fĭl-trā′ shŭn)	The process of filtering or straining particles from a solution
gene (jēn)	The hereditary unit that transmits and determines one's characteristics or hereditary traits
horizontal (hŏr′ă-zŏn′ tăl)	Pertaining to the horizon, of or near the horizon, lying flat, even, level
human genome (hū′ măn jē′ nōm)	The complete set of genes and chromosomes tucked inside each of the body's trillions of cells
inferior (ĭn-fē′ rē-or)	Located below or in a downward direction
inguinal (ĭng′ gwĭ-năl)	Pertaining to the groin, of or near the groin

(Vocabulary—continued)

Word	Definition
internal (ĭn-tĕr′nal)	Pertaining to within or the inside
lateral (lăt′ ĕr-ăl)	Pertaining to the side
medial (mē′ dē al)	Pertaining to the middle or midline
organic (or-găn′ĭk)	Pertaining to an organ
phenotype (fē′ nō-tīp)	The physical appearance or type of makeup of an individual
posterior (pŏs-tē′ rĭ-ōr)	Toward the back
proximal (prŏk′ sĭm-ăl)	Nearest the center or point of origin; nearest the point of attachment
superficial (sū″ pĕr-fĭsh′ ăl)	Pertaining to the surface, on or near the surface
superior (sū-pēr′ rĭ-ōr)	Located above or in an upward direction
systemic (sis-tĕm′ ĭk)	Pertaining to the body as a whole
ventral (vĕn′ trăl)	Pertaining to the front side of the body, abdomen, belly surface
vertex (vĕr′ tĕks)	The top or highest point; the top or crown of the head

ABBREVIATIONS

abd	abdomen, abdominal	**lat**	lateral
A&P	anatomy and physiology	**LLQ**	left lower quadrant
AP	anterior-posterior	**LUQ**	left upper quadrant
CNS	central nervous system	**PA**	posterior-anterior
CV	cardiovascular	**resp**	respiratory
ER	endoplasmic reticulum	**RLQ**	right lower quadrant
GI	gastrointestinal	**RUQ**	right upper quadrant

Drug Highlights

A drug is a medicinal substance that may alter or modify the functions of a living organism. There are thousands of drugs that are available as over-the-counter (OTC) medicines and do not need a prescription. A prescription is a written legal document that gives directions for compounding, dispensing, and administering a medication to a patient.

In general, there are five medical uses for drugs and these are: therapeutic, diagnostic, curative, replacement, and preventive or prophylactic.

- Therapeutic Use. Used in the treatment of a disease or condition, such as an allergy, to relieve the symptoms or to sustain the patient until other measures are instituted.
- Diagnostic Use. Certain drugs are used in conjunction with radiology to allow the physician to pinpoint the location of a disease process.
- Curative Use. Certain drugs, such as antibiotics, kill or remove the causative agent of a disease.
- Replacement Use. Certain drugs, such as hormones and vitamins, are used to replace substances normally found in the body.
- Preventive or Prophylactic Use. Certain drugs, such as immunizing agents, are used to ward off or lessen the severity of a disease.

Drug Names

Most drugs may be cited by their chemical, generic, and trade or brand (proprietary) name. The chemical name is usually the formula that denotes the composition of the drug. It is made up of letters and numbers that represent the drug's molecular structure. The generic name is the drug's official name, and is descriptive of its chemical structure. The generic name is written in lower case letters. A generic drug can be manufactured by more than one pharmaceutical company. When this is the case, each company markets the drug under its own unique trade or brand name. A trade or brand name is registered by the US Patent Office as well as approved by the US Food and Drug Administration (FDA). A trade or brand name is written with a capital.

Undesirable Actions of Drugs

Most drugs have the potential for causing an action other than their intended action. For example, antibiotics that are administered orally may disrupt the normal bacterial flora of the gastrointestinal tract and cause gastric discomfort. This type of reaction is known as a side effect. An adverse reaction is an unfavorable or harmful unintended action of a drug. For example, the adverse reaction of Demerol may be lightheadedness, dizziness, sedation, nausea, and sweating. A drug interaction may occur when one drug potentiates or diminishes the action of another drug. These actions may be desirable or undesirable. Drugs may also interact with foods, alcohol, tobacco, and other substances.

Medication Order and Dosage

The medication order is given for a specific patient and it denotes the name of the drug, the dosage, the form of the drug, the time for or frequency of administration, and the route by which the drug is to be given.

The dosage is the amount of medicine that is prescribed for administration. The form of the drug may be liquid, solid, semisolid, tablet, capsule, transdermal therapeutic patch, etc. The route of administration may be by mouth, by injection, into the eye(s), ear(s), nostril(s), rectum, vagina, etc.

It is important for the patient to know when and how to take a medication. The following are some hows, whens, and directions for taking medications. To assist you in communicating this information to a patient, both English and Spanish are provided for you to use.

English	Spanish
When	*Cuándo*
every hour	cada hora (*că*-dă ŏ-ră)
every two hours	cada dos horas (*că*-dă dōs ō-răs)
every three hours	cada tres horas (*că*-dă trĕs ō-răs)
every four hours	cada cuatro horas (*că*-dă *kū*-ă-trō ō-răs)
every six hours	cada seis horas (*că*-dă sĕ-ĭs ō-răs)
every eight hours	cada ocho horas (*că*-dă ō-chō ō-răs)
every twelve hours	cada doce horas (*că*-dă *dō*-sĕ ō-răs)
before meals	antes de comer (ăn-*tĕs* dĕ cō-*mĕr*)
after meals	después de comer (dĕs-*pū*-ĕs dĕ cō-*mĕr*)
before breakfast	antes de desayunar (*ăn*-tĕs dĕ dĕ-să-jū-*năr*)
after breakfast	después de desayunar (dĕs-*pū*-ĕs dĕ dĕ-să-jū-*năr*)
before lunch	antes de merendar (ăn-*tĕs* dĕ mĕ-rĕn-*dăr*)
after dinner	después de cenar (dĕs-pū-*ĕs* dĕ sĕ-*năr*)
at night	por la noche (pōr lă *nō*-chĕ)
in the morning	por la mañana (pōr lă mă-*ñă*-nă)
at bedtime	al acostarse (ăl ă-cōs-*tăr*-sĕ)
How	*Cómo*
with meals	con la comida (kōn lă *kō*-mĭ-dă)
with milk	con leche (kōn *lĕ*-chĕ)
with food	con alimento (kōn ă-lĭ-*mĕn*-tō)
with antacid	con anti-acido (kōn *ăn*-tĭ ă-*cĭ*-dō)

English	Spanish
in the right eye	en el ojo derecho (ĕn ĕl ō-hō dĕ-rĕ-chō)
in the left eye	en el ojo izquierdo (ĕn ĕl ō-hō ĭs-kĭ-ĕr-dō)
in both eyes	en los dos ojos (ĕn lōs dōs ō-hōs)
in the right ear	en el oido derecho (ĕn ĕl ō-ĭ-dō dĕ-rĕ-chō)
in the left ear	en el oido izquierdo (ĕn ĕl ō-ĭ-dō ĭs-kĭ-ĕr-dō)
in both ears	en los dos oidos (ĕn lōs dōs ō-ĭ-dōs)
into the nostrils	en la nariz (ĕn lă nă-rĭz)
into the rectum	en el recto (ĕn ĕl rĕc-tō)
into the vagina	en la vagina (ĕn lă vă-hĭ-nă)

Directions	*Dirección*
chew	mascar (măs-kăr)
do not chew	no mascar (nō măs-kăr)
avoid sunlight	evitar sol (ĕ-vĭ-tăr sōl)
avoid alcohol	evitar alcohol (ĕ-vĭ-tăr ăl-kōl)
shake well	agitar bien (ă-hĭ-tăr bĭ-ĕn)
for external use	para uso externo (pă-ră ū-sō ĕx-tĕr-nō)
keep refrigerated	mantener en el refrigerador (măn-tĕ-nĕr ĕn ĕl rĕ-frĭ-hĕ-ră-dōr)

Communication Enrichment

This segment is provided for those who wish to enhance their ability to communicate in either English or Spanish.

HEAD-TO-TOE ASSESSMENT

Body Area	Spanish	Component Part/Terminology
abdomen (belly)	vientre (vĭ-ĕn-trĕ)	abdomino (ăb-dō-mĭ-nō)
ankle	tobillo (tō-bĭ-jō)	ankylo (ăn-kĭ-lō)
arm	brazo (bră-zō)	brachi (bră-chĭ)
back	espalda (ĕs-pāl-dă)	posterior (pōs-tĕ-rĭ-ōr)
bones	huesos (wĕ-sos)	osteo (ōs-tē-ō)
chest	pecho (pĕ-chō)	thoraco (thō-ră-kō)
ear	oido (ō-ē-dōw)	oto (ō-tō)
elbow	codo (kō-dow)	cubital (cū-bĭ-tăl)
eye	ojo (ō-hō)	ophthalmo; oculo; opto (ōp-thăl-mō; ō-kū-lō; ōp-tō)
foot	pie (pĭĕ)	illus- (il-lus-)
gums	encías (ĕn-sĭ-ăs)	gingiv- (gĭn-gĭv-)
hand	mano (mă-nō)	manus (mă-nūs)
head	cabeza (că-bē-ză)	cephalo (sĕ-fã-lō)
heart	corazón (kō-ră-zōn)	cardio (kăr-dĭ-ō)
leg	pierna (pī-ĕr-nā)	crural; femoral (crū-răl; fĕ-mō-răl)
liver	higado (hĭ-gă-dow)	hepato (hĕ-pă-tō)
lungs	pulmones (pūl-mō-nĕs)	pulmo (pūl-mō)
mouth	boca (bō-kă)	oro (ō-rō)
muscles	músculos (mūs-kū-lōs)	musculo (mūs-cū-lō)

Body Area	Spanish	Component Part/Terminology
neck	cuello (*kŭe*-jō)	cervico (*sĕr*-vĭ-cō)
nerves	nervios (*ner*-vĭ-ōs)	neuro (*nū*-rō)
nose	nariz (*nă*-rĭz)	rhino; naso (*rĭ*-nō; *nă*-sō)
ribs	costillas (cōs-*tĭ*-jăs)	costo (*cōs*-tō)
side	costado (cōs-*tă*-dow)	lateral (lă-tĕ-*răl*)
skin	piel (pĕ-ĕl)	derma (*dĕr*-mă)
skull	cráneo (*krā*-nĕ-ō)	cranio (*krā*-nĭ-ō)
stomach	estómago (ĕs-tō-*mă*-gō)	gastro (*găs*-trō)
teeth	dientes (*dĭĕn*-tĕs)	denti (*dĕn*-tĭ)
temples	templo (*ti*-ĕm-plō)	tempora (tĕm-*pō*-ră)
thigh	muslo (*mŭs*-lō)	femoral; crural (fĕ-mō-răl; crŭ-răl)
throat	garganta (găr-*găn*-tă)	pharyngo (fă-*rĭn*-hō)
thumb	dedo pulgar (*dĕ*-dow *pŭl*-găr)	pollex (*pōl*-lĕx)
tongue	lengua (*lĕn*-gŭ-ă)	linguo; glosso (lĭn-gū-ō; glōs-sō)
wrist	muñeca (*mŭ*-ñĕ-kă)	carpo (*căr*-pō)

Learning Exercises

Anatomy and Physiology

Write your answers to the following questions. Do not refer back to the text.

1. The _____ consist of millions of _____ working individually and with each other to _____ life.

2. The outer covering of the cell is known as the _____ _____ which has the capability of allowing some substances to pass into and out of the cell.

3. The substance within the cell is known as _____ and is composed of _____ and _____ .

4. The cell's nucleus is composed of _____ , which contains its genetic material.

5. The two primary functions of the cell's nucleus are _____ and _____ .

6. List the four functions of epithelial tissue.

   a. _____   b. _____

   c. _____   d. _____

7. _____ tissue is the most widespread and abundant of the four body tissues.

8. Name the three types of muscle tissue.

   a. _____ b. _____ c. _____

9. Two properties of nerve tissue are _____ and _____ .

10. Define organ. _____

11. Define body system. _____
    _____ .

12. Name the organ systems listed in this text.

   a. _____   b. _____

   c. _____   d. _____

   e. _____   f. _____

   g. _____   h. _____

   i. _____   j. _____

   k. _____

13. Define the following directional terms:

   a. Superior _____   b. Anterior _____

   c. Posterior _____   d. Cephalad

   e. Medial _____   f. Lateral

   g. Proximal _____   h. Distal

   i. Ventral _____   j. Dorsal

14. The _____ _____ vertically divides the body. It passes through the midline to form a right and left half.

15. The _____ plane is any plane that divides the body into superior and inferior portions.

16. The _____ plane is any plane that divides the body at right angles to the plane described in question 14.

17. List the three distinct cavities that are located in the ventral cavity.

    a. _____ b. _____ c. _____

18. Name the two distinct cavities located in the dorsal cavity.

    a. _____ b. _____

Word Parts

1. In the spaces provided, write the definition of these prefixes, roots, combining forms, and suffixes. Do not refer to the listings of terminology words. Leave blank those terms you cannot define.
2. After completing as many as you can, refer back to the terminology word listings to check your work. For each word missed or left blank, write the term and its definition several times on the margins of these pages or on a separate sheet of paper.
3. To maximize the learning process, it is to your advantage to do the following exercises as directed. To refer to the terminology listings before completing these exercises invalidates the learning process.

PREFIXES

Give the definitions of the following prefixes:

1. ambi-	_____	2. ana-	_____
3. bi-	_____	4. chromo-	_____
5. de-	_____	6. dif-	_____
7. ecto-	_____	8. endo-	_____
9. homeo-	_____	10. meso-	_____
11. per-	_____	12. proto-	_____
13. uni-	_____		

ROOTS AND COMBINING FORMS

Give the definitions of the following roots and combining forms:

1. adip	_____	2. andr	_____
3. bio	_____	4. caud	_____
5. cyt	_____	6. cyto	_____
7. fus	_____	8. gen	_____
9. histo	_____	10. hydr	_____
11. karyo	_____	12. later	_____
13. patho	_____	14. physio	_____

15. pino _____   16. somato _____

17. topic _____   18. troph _____

19. viscer _____

SUFFIXES

Give the definitions for the following suffixes:

1. -al _____   2. -ate _____

3. -genesis _____   4. -ic _____

5. -ion _____   6. -logy _____

7. -morph _____   8. -oid _____

9. -ose _____   10. -osis _____

11. -ous _____   12. -plasm _____

13. -some _____   14. -stasis _____

15. -tomy _____

Identifying Medical Terms

In the spaces provided, write the medical terms for the following meanings:

1. _____ To resemble man

2. _____ Pertaining to two sides

3. _____ The study of cells

4. _____ A slender physical body form

5. _____ Formation of a cell's nucleus

6. _____ Pertaining to the stimulation of body growth

7. _____ Pertaining to one side

Spelling

In the spaces provided, write the correct spelling of these misspelled terms:

1. adpose _____   2. caual _____

3. cytlogy _____   4. difusion _____

5. histlogy _____   6. mesmorph _____

7. prefusion _____   8. pincytosis _____

9. somattrophic _____   10. unlateral _____

Review Questions

Matching

Select the appropriate lettered meaning for each numbered line.

_____ 1. ambilateral

_____ 2. anatomy

_____ 3. anthropometry

_____ 4. chromosome

_____ 5. cilia

_____ 6. homeostasis

_____ 7. human genome

_____ 8. phenotype

_____ 9. physiology

_____ 10. vertex

a. Hairlike processes that project from epithelial cells

b. The top or highest point

c. Pertaining to both sides

d. The study of the structure of an organism such as humans

e. The measurement of the human body

f. Microscopic bodies that carry the genes that determine hereditary characteristics

g. The complete set of genes and chromosomes

h. The physical appearance or type of makeup of an individual

i. The state of equilibrium maintained in the body's internal environment

j. The study of the nature of living organism

k. The study of disease

Abbreviations

Place the correct word, phrase, or abbreviation in the space provided.

_____ 1. abdomen

_____ 2. A&P

_____ 3. CNS

_____ 4. cardiovascular

_____ 5. gastrointestinal

_____ 6. lat

_____ 7. resp

_____ 8. ER

_____ 9. AP

_____ 10. PA

3

The Integumentary System

The integumentary system is composed of the skin and its accessory structures: the hair, nails, sebaceous glands, and sweat glands. The skin is the largest organ in the human body. In an average adult it covers more than 3000 square inches of surface area, and weighs more than 6 pounds.

47

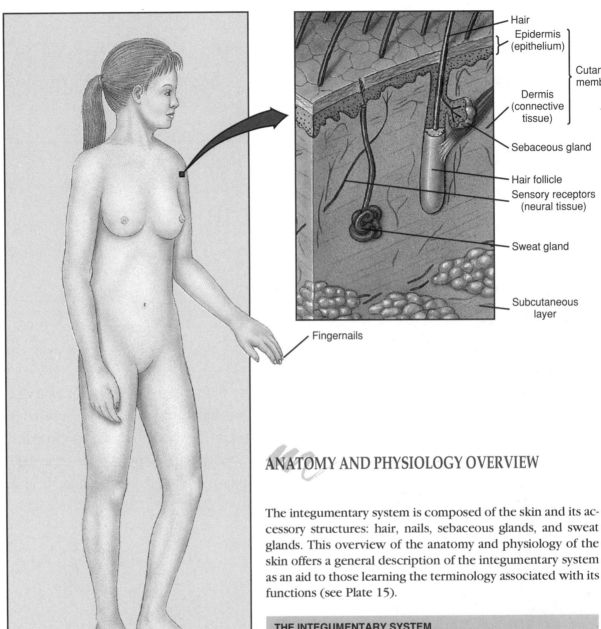

Hair
Epidermis (epithelium)
Cutaneous membrane
Dermis (connective tissue)
Sebaceous gland
Hair follicle
Sensory receptors (neural tissue)
Sweat gland
Subcutaneous layer
Fingernails

ANATOMY AND PHYSIOLOGY OVERVIEW

The integumentary system is composed of the skin and its accessory structures: hair, nails, sebaceous glands, and sweat glands. This overview of the anatomy and physiology of the skin offers a general description of the integumentary system as an aid to those learning the terminology associated with its functions (see Plate 15).

THE INTEGUMENTARY SYSTEM

Organ	Primary Functions
Cutaneous Membrane	
Epidermis	Protects underlying tissues
Dermis	Nourishes epidermis, provide strength
Hair Follicles	Produce hair
Hairs	Provide sensation, provide some protection for head
Sebaceous Glands	Secrete lipid coating that lubricates hair shaft
Sweat Glands	Produce perspiration for evaporative cooling
Nails	Protect and stiffen distal tips of digits
Sensory Receptors	Provide sensations of touch, pressure, temperature, pain
Subcutaneous Layer	Stores lipids, attaches skin to deeper structures

Functions of the Skin

The skin is the external covering of the body. In an average adult it covers more than 3000 square inches of surface area, weighs more than 6 pounds, and is the largest organ in the body. The skin is well supplied with blood vessels and nerves and has four main functions: protection, regulation, sensation, and secretion.

PROTECTION

The skin serves as a protective membrane against invasion by bacteria and other potentially harmful agents that might try to penetrate to deeper tissues. It also protects against mechanical injury of delicate cells located beneath its epidermis or outer covering. The skin also serves to inhibit excessive loss of water and electrolytes and provides a reservoir for food and water storage. The skin guards the body against excessive exposure to the sun's ultraviolet rays by producing a protective pigmentation, and it helps to produce the body's supply of vitamin D.

REGULATION

The skin serves to raise or lower body temperature as necessary. When the body needs to lose heat, the blood vessels in the skin dilate, bringing more blood to the surface for cooling by radiation. At the same time, the sweat glands are secreting more sweat for cooling by means of evaporation. Conversely, when the body needs to conserve heat, the reflex actions of the nervous system cause constriction of the skin's blood vessels, thereby allowing more heat-carrying blood to circulate to the muscles and vital organs.

SENSATION

The skin contains millions of microscopic nerve endings that act as sensory receptors for pain, touch, heat, cold, and pressure. When stimulation occurs, nerve impulses are sent to the cerebral cortex of the brain. The nerve endings in the skin are specialized according to the type of sensory information transmitted and, once this information reaches the brain, any necessary response is triggered. For example, touching a hot surface with the hand causes the brain to recognize the senses of touch, heat, and pain and results in the immediate removal of the hand from the hot surface.

SECRETION

The skin contains millions of sweat glands, which secrete perspiration or sweat, and sebaceous glands, which secrete oil for lubrication. Perspiration is largely water with a small amount of salt and other chemical compounds. This secretion, when left to accumulate, causes body odor, especially where it is trapped among hairs in the axillary region. Sebaceous glands produce sebum, which acts to protect the body from dehydration and possible absorption of harmful substances.

Layers of the Skin

The skin is essentially composed of two layers, the epidermis and the dermis.

THE EPIDERMIS

The epidermis can be divided into four strata: the stratum corneum, the stratum lucidum, the stratum granulosum, and the stratum germinativum. See Figure 3–1 and Plate 1 for the locations of these strata within the epidermis. A description of the four strata is given below and on the next pages.

The Stratum Corneum

The stratum corneum is the outermost, horny layer, consisting of dead cells filled with a protein substance called keratin. It forms the protective covering for the body, and its thick-

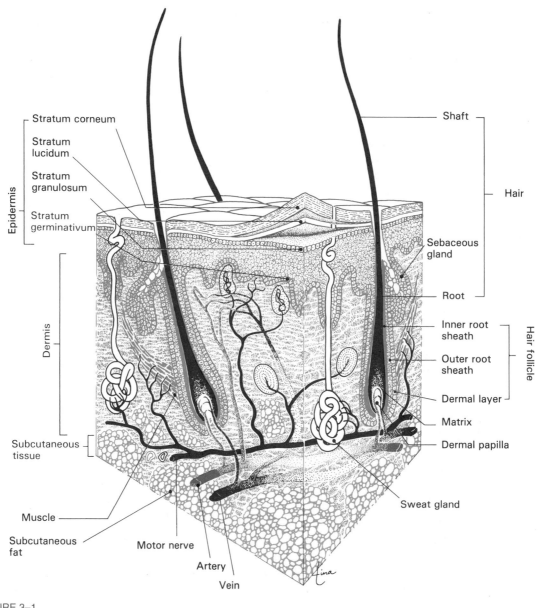

FIGURE 3–1

The integument: the epidermis, dermis, subcutaneous tissue, and associated structures. *(Adapted from Evans, WF. Anatomy and Physiology, 3rd ed. Englewood Cliffs, NJ: Prentice-Hall, 1983, with permission.)*

ness varies with the use made of the particular body part. Because of the pressure on their surfaces during use, the soles of the feet and palms of the hands have thicker layers of stratum corneum than do the eyelids or the forehead.

The Stratum Lucidum

The stratum lucidum is a translucent layer lying directly beneath the stratum corneum. It is frequently absent and is not seen in thinner skin. Cells in this layer are also dead or dying.

The Stratum Granulosum

The stratum granulosum consists of several layers of living cells that are in the process of becoming a part of the previously mentioned strata. Its cells are active in the keratinization process, during which they lose their nuclei and become hard or horny.

The Stratum Germinativum

The stratum germinativum is composed of several layers of living cells capable of mitosis or cell division. Sometimes called the mucosum or Malpighi, the stratum germinativum is the innermost layer and is responsible for the regeneration of the epidermis. Damage to this layer, as in severe burns, necessitates the use of skin grafts. Melanin, the pigment that gives color to the skin, is formed in this layer. The more abundant the melanin, the darker the color of the skin.

THE DERMIS

Sometimes called the corium or true skin, the dermis is composed of connective tissue containing lymphatics, nerves and nerve endings, blood vessels, sebaceous and sweat glands, elastic fibers, and hair follicles. It is divided into two layers: the upper or papillary layer and the lower or reticular layer. The papillary layer is arranged into parallel rows of microscopic structures called papillae. The papillae produce the ridges of the skin that are one's fingerprints or footprints. The reticular layer is composed of white fibrous tissue that supports the blood vessels. The dermis is attached to underlying structures by the subcutaneous tissue. The tissue supports, nourishes, insulates, and cushions the skin.

Accessory Structures of the Skin

The hair, nails, sebaceous glands, and sweat glands are the accessory structures of the skin. Each of these structures is described below.

HAIR

A hair is a thin, thread-like structure formed by a group of cells that develop within a hair follicle or socket. Each hair is composed of a shaft, which is the visible portion, and a root, which is embedded within the follicle. At the base of each follicle is a loop of capillaries enclosed within connective tissue called the hair papilla. The pilomotor muscle attaches to the side of each follicle. When the skin is cooled or the individual has an emotional reaction, the skin often forms "goose pimples" as a result of contraction by these muscles. Hair is distributed over the whole body with the exception of the palms of the hands and soles of the feet. It is thicker on the scalp and thinner on the other parts of the body. Hair around the eyes, in the nose, and in the ears serves to filter out foreign particles. The color of one's hair is a product of genetic background and is determined by the amount of pigmentation within the hair shaft. Hair grows at approximately 0.5 inch a month, and its growth is not affected by cutting.

NAILS

Finger- and toenails are horny cell structures of the epidermis and are composed of hard keratin. A nail consists of a body, a root, and a matrix or nailbed (Fig. 3–2). The crescent-shaped white area of the nail is the lunula. Nail growth may vary with age, disease, and hormone deficiency. Average growth is 1 mm per week, and a lost fingernail usually regenerates in $3\frac{1}{2}$ to $5\frac{1}{2}$ months. A lost toenail may require 6 to 8 months for regeneration.

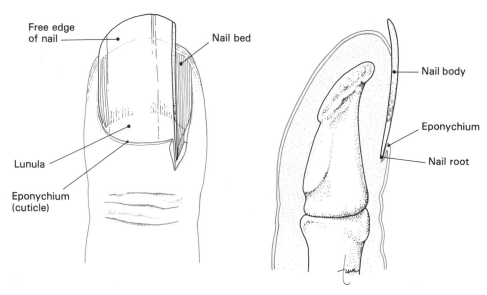

FIGURE 3–2

The nail, an appendage of the skin. *(Adapted from Evans WF. Anatomy and Physiology, 3rd ed. Englewood Cliffs, NJ: Prentice-Hall, 1983, with permission.)*

SEBACEOUS GLANDS

The oil-secreting glands of the skin are called sebaceous glands. They have tiny ducts that open into the hair follicles, and their secretion, sebum, lubricates the hair as well as the skin. The amount of secretion is controlled by the endocrine system and varies with age, puberty, pregnancy, and senility.

SWEAT (SUDORIFEROUS) GLANDS

There are approximately 2 million sweat glands. These coiled, tubular glands are distributed over the entire surface of the body with the exception of the margin of the lips, glans penis, and the inner surface of the prepuce. They are more numerous on the palms of the hands, soles of the feet, forehead, and axillae. Sweat glands secrete sweat or perspiration, which helps to cool the body by evaporation. Sweat also rids the body of waste through the pores of the skin. Left to accumulate, sweat becomes odorous by the action of bacteria. The body loses about 0.5 L of fluid per day through sweat.

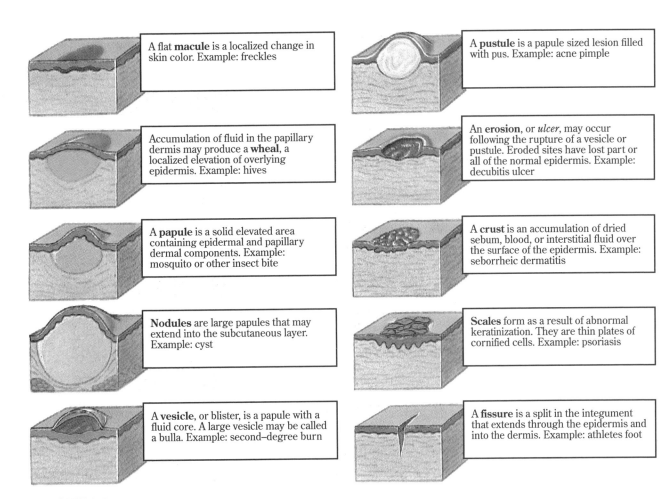

A flat **macule** is a localized change in skin color. Example: freckles

Accumulation of fluid in the papillary dermis may produce a **wheal**, a localized elevation of overlying epidermis. Example: hives

A **papule** is a solid elevated area containing epidermal and papillary dermal components. Example: mosquito or other insect bite

Nodules are large papules that may extend into the subcutaneous layer. Example: cyst

A **vesicle**, or blister, is a papule with a fluid core. A large vesicle may be called a bulla. Example: second–degree burn

A **pustule** is a papule sized lesion filled with pus. Example: acne pimple

An **erosion**, or *ulcer*, may occur following the rupture of a vesicle or pustule. Eroded sites have lost part or all of the normal epidermis. Example: decubitis ulcer

A **crust** is an accumulation of dried sebum, blood, or interstitial fluid over the surface of the epidermis. Example: seborrheic dermatitis

Scales form as a result of abnormal keratinization. They are thin plates of cornified cells. Example: psoriasis

A **fissure** is a split in the integument that extends through the epidermis and into the dermis. Example: athletes foot

FIGURE 3–3

Skin signs. *(From Martin F. Fundamentals of* Anatomy and Physiology, *2nd ed. Englewood Cliffs, NJ: Prentice-Hall, 1992, with permission.)*

Skin Signs

Skin signs are objective evidence of an illness or disorder. They can be seen, measured, or felt. They may be described as lesions that are circumscribed areas of pathologically altered tissue. Types of skin signs are shown and described in Figure 3-3.

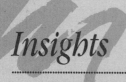
Insights

SKIN PATCH—A Transdermal System of Medication Delivery

Because of technological advances in medicine, there are new ways by which a drug can be prepared and delivered to a patient. Some of these preparations are known as "special delivery systems" that dispense the drug to a targeted area. Others are modified preparations of the conventional form of the drug.

- A transdermal system is a small adhesive patch or disc that may be applied to the skin near the treatment site.
- A transdermal system generally consists of four layers:

The Four Layers of a Typical Skin Patch

1. An impermeable back that keeps the drug from leaking out of the system.
2. A reservoir containing the drug.
3. A membrane with tiny holes in it that controls the rate of drug release.
4. An adhesive layer or gel that keeps the device in place.

The first patch on the medical scene was the scopolamine patch used for motion sickness. Worn behind the ear, the small patch is effective for up to 3 days. **Transderm-Nitro** is an example of a transdermal therapeutic system that provides controlled release of nitroglycerin through a semipermeable membrane continuously for 24 hours following application to intact skin. This type of patch is used to treat angina pectoris. **ESTRADERM** is an estrogen skin patch that relieves menopausal symptoms such as hot flashes, night sweats and vaginal dryness. **NICODERM** is a nicotine patch used to relieve the body's craving for nicotine. **CATAPRES-TTS-1** is a skin patch that is used to treat hypertension.

In the future we will see other transdermal systems, as researchers are working on developing other patches, possibly for Alzheimer's, osteoporosis, and birth control.

Terminology with Surgical Procedures & Pathology

Term	Word Parts			Definition
acanthosis (ăk″ ăn-thō′ sis)	acanth osis	R S	a thorn condition of	A condition of thickening of the prickle-cell layer of the skin
actinic dermatitis (ăk-tĭn′ ĭk dĕr″ mă-tī′ tĭs)	actin ic dermat itis	R S R S	ray pertaining to skin inflammation	Inflammation of the skin caused by exposure to actinic rays
albinism (ăl′ bĭn-ĭsm)	albin ism	R S	white condition of	Absence of pigment in the skin, hair, and eyes
anhidrosis (ăn″ hī-drō′ sĭs)	an hidr osis	P R S	without, lack of sweat condition of	A condition in which there is a lack or complete absence of sweating
autograft (ŏ-tō-grăft)	auto graft	P S	self pencil	A graft taken from one part of the patient's body and transferred to another part
causalgia (kŏ-săl′ jĭ-ă)	caus algia	R S	heat pain	Intense burning pain associated with trophic skin changes in the hand or foot after trauma to the part
cutaneous (kū-tā′ nē-ŭs)	cutane ous	R S	skin pertaining to	Pertaining to the skin
dermatitis (dĕr″ mă-tī′ tĭs)	dermat itis	R S	skin inflammation	Inflammation of the skin
dermatologist (dĕr″ mah-tol′ ŏ-jĭst)	dermato log ist	CF R S	skin study of one who specializes	One who specializes in the study of the skin
dermatology (dĕr″ mă-tol′ ŏ-jē)	dermato logy	CF S	skin study of	The study of the skin
dermatome (dĕr″ mah-tōm)	derma tome	CF S	skin instrument to cut	An instrument used to cut the skin for grafting
dermatopathy (dĕr″ mă-top′ ă-thē)	dermato pathy	CF S	skin disease	Skin disease
dermatoplasty (dĕr′ mă-tō-plăs″ tē)	dermato plasty	CF S	skin surgical repair	Surgical repair of the skin

(Terminology—continued)

Term	Word Parts			Definition
dermomycosis (děr′ mō-mī-kō′ sĭs)	dermo myc osis	CF R S	skin fungus condition of	A skin condition caused by a fungus
ecchymosis (ĕk-ĭ-mō′ sĭs)	ec chym osis	P R S	out juice condition of	A condition in which the blood seeps into the skin causing discolorations ranging from blue-black to greenish-yellow
eponychium (ĕp″ ō-nĭk′ ĭ-ŭm)	ep onychi um	P CF S	upon nail tissue	The horny embryonic tissue from which the nail develops
erysipelas (ĕr″ ĭ-sĭp′ ĕ-lăs)	erysi pelas	R S	red skin	Redness of the skin with inflammation caused by invasion by Group A hemolytic streptococci
erythroderma (ĕ-rĭth″ rō-dĕr′-mă)	erythro derma	CF S	red skin	Abnormal redness of the skin occurring over widespread areas of the body
excoriation (ĕks-kō″ rē-ā′ shŭn)	ex coriat ion	P R S	out corium process	Abrasion of the epidermis by scratching, trauma, chemicals, burns, etc.
hidradenitis (hī-drăd-ĕ-nī′ tĭs)	hidr aden itis	R R S	sweat gland inflammation	Inflammation of the sweat glands
hyperhidrosis (hī″ pĕr-hī-drō′ sĭs)	hyper hidr osis	P R S	excessive sweat condition of	A condition of excessive sweating
hypertrichosis (hī″ pĕr-trĭ-kō′ sĭs)	hyper trich osis	P R S	excessive hair condition of	A condition of excessive hair growth
hypodermic (hī″ pō-dĕr′ mĭk)	hypo derm ic	P R S	under skin pertaining to	Pertaining to under the skin
hypodermoclysis (hī″ pō-dĕr-mŏk′ lĭ-sĭs)	hypo dermo clysis	P CF S	under skin injection	Injection of fluids under the skin to supply the body with a rapid replacement of fluids
icteric (ik-tĕr′ ĭk)	icter ic	R S	jaundice pertaining to	Pertaining to jaundice

(Terminology—continued)

Term	Word Parts			Definition
intradermal (in″ trăh-děr′ măl)	intra derm al	P R S	within skin pertaining to	Pertaining to within the skin
keloid (kē′ lŏyd)	kel oid	R S	tumor resemble	Overgrowth of scar tissue caused by excessive collagen formation
leukoderma (lū″ kō-děr′ mă)	leuko derma	CF S	white skin	Localized loss of pigmentation of the skin
melanoblast (měl′ ăn-ō-blăst″)	melano blast	CF S	black immature cell, germ cell	A germ cell found in the basal layers of the epidermis that is capable of forming melanin
melanocarcinoma (měl″ ă-nō-kar″ sĭn-ō′ mă)	melano carcin oma	CF R S	black cancer tumor	A cancerous tumor that has black pigmentation
melanoma (měl″ ă-nō′ mă)	melan oma	R S	black tumor	A malignant black mole or tumor
melanonychia (měl″ ă-nō-nĭk′ i-ă)	melan onych ia	R R S	black nail condition	A condition in which the nails are blackened by melanin pigmentation
onychectomy (ŏn″ ĭ-kěk′ tō-mē)	onych ectomy	R S	nail excision	Surgical excision of a nail
onychitis (ŏn″ ĭ-kī′ tĭs)	onych itis	R S	nail inflammation	Inflammation of the nail
onychomalacia (ŏn″ ĭ-kō-mă-lā′ sĭ-ă)	onycho malacia	CF S	nail softening	Softening of the nail
onychophagia (ŏn″ ĭ-kŏf′ ă-jĭ-ă)	onycho phagia	CF S	nail to eat	Nail biting
pachyderma (păk-ē-der′ mă)	pachy derma	R S	thick skin	Thick skin
pachyonychia (păk″ ē-ō-nĭk′ ĭ-ă)	pachy onych ia	R R S	thick nail condition	A condition of thick nail or nails
paronychia (păr″ ō-nĭk′ ĭ-ă)	par onych ia	P R S	around nail condition	An infectious condition of the marginal structures around the nail
pediculosis (pĕ-dĭk″ ū-lō′ sĭs)	pedicul osis	R S	a louse condition of	A condition of infestation with lice

(Terminology—continued)

Term	Word Parts			Definition
rhytidectomy (rĭt″ ĭ-dĕk′ tō-mē)	rhytid	R	wrinkle	Surgical excision of wrinkles
	ectomy	S	excision	
rhytidoplasty (rĭt′ ĭ-dō-plăs″ tē)	rhytido	CF	wrinkle	Plastic surgery for the removal of wrinkles
	plasty	S	surgical repair	
scleroderma (skli rō-dĕr′ mă)	sclero	CF	hard	A chronic condition with hardening of the skin and other connective tissues of the body
	derma	S	skin	
seborrhea (sĕb″ or-ē′ ă)	sebo	CF	oil	Excessive flow of oil from the sebaceous glands
	rrhea	S	flow	
senile keratosis (sĕn′ ĭl kĕr″ ă-tō′ sĭs)	senile	R	old	A condition occurring in older people wherein there is dry skin and localized scaling caused by excessive exposure to the sun
	kerat	R	horn	
	osis	S	condition of	
subcutaneous (sŭb″ kū-tā′ nē-ŭs)	sub	P	below	Pertaining to below the skin
	cutane	R	skin	
	ous	S	pertaining to	
subungual (sŭb-ŭng′ gwăl)	sub	P	below	Pertaining to below the nail
	ungu	R	nail	
	al	S	pertaining to	
thermanesthesia (thĕrm″ ăn-ĕs-thē′ zē-ă)	therm	R	hot, heat	Inability to distinguish between the sensations of heat and cold
	an	P	without, lack of	
	esthesia	S	sensation	
trichomycosis (trĭk″ ō-mi-kō′ sĭs)	tricho	CF	hair	A fungus condition of the hair
	myc	R	fungus	
	osis	S	condition of	
xanthoderma (zăn″ thō-dĕr′ mă)	xantho	CF	yellow	Yellow skin
	derma	S	skin	
xeroderma (zē″ rō-dĕr′ mă)	xero	CF	dry	Dry skin
	derma	S	skin	

Vocabulary Words

Vocabulary words are terms that have not been divided into component parts. They are common words or specialized terms associated with the subject of this chapter. These words are provided to enhance your medical vocabulary.

Word	Definition
acne (ăk′ nē)	An inflammatory condition of the sebaceous glands and the hair follicles; pimples
acrochordon (ăk″ rō-kor′ dŏn)	A small outgrowth of epidermal and dermal tissue
alopecia (al″ ō-pē′ shĭ-ă)	Loss of hair, baldness
avulsion (ă-vŭl′ shŭn)	The process of forcibly tearing off a part or structure of the body, such as a finger or toe
boil (boil)	An acute, painful nodule formed in the subcutaneous layers of the skin, gland, or hair follicle; most often caused by the invasion of staphylococci; furuncle
bulla (bŭl′ lă)	A larger blister; a bleb
burn (burn) (bərn)	An injury to tissue caused by heat, fire, chemical agents, electricity, lightning, or radiation; burns are classified according to degree or depth of skin damage
callus (kăl′ ŭs)	Hardened skin
carbuncle (kăr′ bŭng″ kl)	An infection of the subcutaneous tissue, usually composed of a cluster of boils
cellulitis (sĕl-ū-lī′ tĭs)	Inflammation of cellular or connective tissue
cicatrix (sĭk′ ă-trĭks)	The scar left after the healing of a wound
comedo (kŏm′ ē-dō)	Blackhead
corn (korn) (ko(ə)rn)	A horny induration and thickening of the skin on the toes caused by ill-fitting shoes
cyst (sĭst)	A bladder or sac; a closed sac that contains fluid, semifluid, or solid material
decubitus (dē-kū′ bĭ-tŭs)	Literally means a lying down; a bedsore
dehiscence (dē-hĭs′ ĕns)	The separation or bursting open of a surgical wound

(Vocabulary—continued)

Word	Definition
eczema (ĕk′ zĕ-mă)	An inflammatory skin disease of the epidermis
erythema (ĕr″ ĭ-thē′ mă)	A redness of the skin; may be caused by capillary congestion, inflammation, heat, sunlight, or cold temperature
eschar (ĕs′ kăr)	A slough, scab
exudate (ĕks′ ū-dāt)	The production of pus or serum
folliculitis (fō-lĭk″ ū-lĭ′ tĭs)	Inflammation of a follicle or follicles
herpes simplex (hĕr′ pēz sĭm′ plĕks)	An inflammatory skin disease caused by a herpes virus (Type I); cold sore or fever blister
hives (hīvz)	Eruption of itching and burning swellings on the skin; urticaria
impetigo (ĭm″ pĕ-tī′ gō)	A skin infection marked by vesicles or bullae; usually caused by streptococci or staphylococci
integumentary (ĭn-tĕg″ ū-mĕn ′ tă-rē)	A covering; the skin, consisting of the dermis and the epidermis
intertrigo (ĭn″ tĕr-trī′ gō)	A superficial dermatitis that occurs in the folds of the skin
jaundice (jawn′ dĭs)	Yellow; a symptom of a disease in which there is excessive bile in the blood; the skin, whites of the eyes, and mucous membranes are yellow; icterus
lentigo (lĕn-tī′ gō)	A flat, brownish spot on the skin sometimes caused by exposure to the sun and weather; freckle
leukoplakia (loo″ kō-plā′ kē-ă)	White spots or patches formed on the mucous membrane of the tongue or cheek; the spots are smooth, hard, and irregular in shape and may become malignant
lupus (lū′ pŭs)	Originally used to describe a destructive type of skin lesion; current usage of the word is usually in combination with the words vulgaris or erythematosus: lupus vulgaris or lupus erythematosus
mole (mōl)	A pigmented, elevated spot above the surface of the skin; a nevus
petechiae (pē-tē′ kĭ-ē)	Small, pinpoint, purplish hemorrhagic spots on the skin

(Vocabulary—continued)

Word	Definition
pityriasis (pĭt″ ĭ-rī′ ă-sĭs)	A skin disease characterized by branny (like bran) scales
pruritus (proo-rī′ tŭs)	A severe itching
psoriasis (sō-rī′ ă-sĭs)	A chronic skin disease characterized by pink or dull-red lesions surmounted by silvery scaling
purpura (pur′ pū-ră)	A purplish discoloration of the skin caused by extravasation of blood into the tissues
rubella (roo-bĕl′ lă)	A systemic disease caused by a virus and characterized by a rash and fever; also called German measles and three-day measles
rubeola (roo-bē′ ō-lă)	A contagious disease characterized by fever, inflammation of the mucous membranes, and rose-colored spots on the skin; also called measles
scabies (skā′ bēz) or (skā′ bĭ-ēz)	A contagious skin disease characterized by papules, vesicles, pustules, burrows, and intense itching; it is caused by the itch mite and is also called "the itch" or the "seven-year itch"
scar (skahr)	The mark left by the healing process of a wound, sore, or injury
sebum (sē′ bŭm)	The fatty or oil secretion of sebaceous glands of the skin
striae (plural) (strī′ ē)	Streaks or lines on the breasts, thighs, abdomen, or buttocks caused by weakening of elastic tissue
taut (tot)	Tight, firm; to pull or draw tight a surface, such as the skin
telangiectasia (tĕl-ăn″ jē-ĕk-tā′ zē-ă)	Dilatation of small blood vessels that may appear as a "birthmark"
tinea (tĭn′ ē-ă)	Fungus infection of the skin; also call ringworm
ulcer (ŭl′ sĕr)	An open lesion or sore of the epidermis or mucous membrane
varicella (văr″ i-sĕl′ ă)	A contagious viral disease characterized by fever, headache, and a crop of red spots that become macules, papules, vesicles, and crusts; also called chickenpox
vitiligo (vĭt″ ĭl-ī′ gō)	A skin condition characterized by milk-white patches surrounded by areas of normal pigmentation

(Vocabulary—continued)

Word	Definition
wart (wōrt)	An elevation of viral origin on the epidermis; verruca
wen (wĕn)	A sebaceous cyst; steatoma
wound (woond)	An injury to soft tissue caused by trauma; generally classified as open or closed

ABBREVIATIONS

decub	decubitus	**SG**	skin graft
derm	dermatology	**SLE**	systemic lupus erythematosus
FB	foreign body	**STD**	skin test done
FUO	fever of unknown origin	**STSG**	split thickness skin graft
H	hypodermic	**subcu**	subcutaneous
Hx	history	**subq**	subcutaneous
ID	intradermal	**T**	temperature
I&D	incision & drainage	**TTS**	transdermal therapeutic system
PUVA	psoralen-ultraviolet-light	**ung**	ointment
		UV	ultraviolet

Drug Highlights

Drugs that are used for dermatological diseases or disorders include emollients, keratolytics, local anesthetic, antipruritic, antibiotic, antifungal, antiviral, anti-inflammatory, and antiseptic agents. Other drugs include Retin-A and Rogaine.

Emollients

Substances that are generally oily in nature. These substances are used for dry skin caused by aging, excessive bathing, and psoriasis.
Examples: Dermassage, Neutragena, and Destin.

Keratolytics

Agents that cause or promote loosening of horny (keratin) layers of the skin. These agents may be used for acne, warts, psoriasis, corns, calluses, and fungal infections.
Examples: Duofilm, Keralyt, and Saligel.

Local Anesthetic Agents

Agents that inhibit the conduction of nerve impulses from sensory nerves and thereby reduce pain and discomfort. These agents may be used topically to reduce discomfort associated with insect bites, burns, and poison ivy.
Examples: Solarcaine, Xylocaine, and Dyclone.

Antipruritic Agents

Agents that prevent or relieve itching.
Examples: Topical- PBZ (tripelennamine HCl); Oral-Benadryl (diphenhydramine HCl).

Antibiotic Agents

Agents that destroy or stop the growth of microorganisms. These agents are used to prevent infection associated with minor skin abrasions and to treat superficial skin infections, and acne. Several antibiotic agents are combined in a single product to take advantage of the different antimicrobial spectrum of each drug.
Examples: Neosporin, Polysporin, and Mycitracin.

Antifungal Agents

Agents that destroy or inhibit the growth of fungi and yeast. These agents are used to treat fungus and/or yeast infection of the skin, nails, and scalp.
Examples: Fungizone, Micatin, and Desenex.

Antiviral Agents

Agents that combat specific viral diseases. *Zovirax (acyclovir)* is used in the treatment of herpes simplex virus types 1 and 2, varicella-zoster, Epstein-Barr, and cytomegalovirus.

Anti-inflammatory Agents

Agents used to relieve the swelling, tenderness, redness, and pain of inflammation. Topically applied corticosteroids are used in the treatment of dermatitis and psoriasis.
Examples: Hydrocortisone and Decadron.

Antiseptic Agents   Agents that prevent or inhibit the growth of pathogens. Antiseptics are generally applied to the surface of living tissue.

Examples: Isopropyl alcohol and Zephrian (benzalkonium chloride)

Other Drugs   *Retin-A (tretinoin)* is available as a cream, gel or liquid. It is used in the treatment of acne vulgaris. *Rogaine (minoxidil)* is available as a topical solution to stimulate hair growth. It was first approved as a treatment of male pattern baldness.

Communication Enrichment

This segment is provided for those who wish to enhance their ability to communicate in either English or Spanish.

RELATED TERMS

English	Spanish	English	Spanish
skin	piel (pĭ-*ĕl*)	hair	pelo (*pĕ*-lō)
glands	glándulas (*glăn*-dŭ-lăs)	perspiration	perspiracion (pers-pir-a-*sion*)
bald	calvo (*căl*-vō)	rash	erupción (ĕ-*rŭp*-sĭ-ōn)
chickenpox	varicela (*vă*-rĭ-cĕ-lă)	redness	enrojecimiento (ĕn-rō-*hĕ*-sĭ-mĭ-ĕn-tō)
heat, warmth	calor (*că*-lōr)	sores	úlceros (ŭl-*sĕ*-răs)
itching	picazón (pĭ-*că*-zōn)	sweating	sudar (*sŭ*-dăr)
jaundice	ictericia (*ĭk*-tĕ-rĭ-sĭ-ă)	wound	herida (ĕ-*rĭ*-dă)
measles	sarampión (*să*-răm-pĭ-ōn)		

COLORS

English	Spanish (Colores)	Combining Form
red	rojo (*rō*-hō)	erytho; rubeo; rhodo (ĕ-*rĭ*-thō; *rŭ*-bĕ-ō; *rō*-dō)
white	blanco (*blăn*-cō)	leuko; albin (lĕ-ō-kō; *ăl*-bĭn)
green	verde (*vĕr*-dĕ)	chloro (*klō*-rō)

English	Spanish (Colores)	Combining Form
blue	azul (*ă*-zŭl)	cyano (sĭ-*ă*-nō)
black	negro (*nĕ*-grō)	melano (*mĕ*-lă-nō)
gray	gris (grĭs)	polio (*pō*-lĭ-ō)
yellow	amarillo (*ă*-mă-ri-jō)	xantho (*zăn*-thō)
purple	morado (mō-*ră*-dō)	purpura (pūr-*pū*-rā)
pink	rosado (rō-*să*-dō)	
rose	rosa (*rō*-să)	
orange-yellow	cirrho (*sĭr*-ō)	

DIAGNOSTIC AND LABORATORY TESTS

Test	Description
blastomycosis skin test (blăs″ tō-mī-kō′ sĭs)	An intradermal test performed on the inner aspect of the forearm to identify the presence of *Blastomyces* dermatitis. Antigen (0.5 mL) is injected and test results are read 48 hours later.
coccidioidomycosis skin test (kŏk-sĭd″ ĭ-oyd-ō-mī-kō′ sĭs)	An intradermal test performed on the inner aspect of the forearm to identify the presence of *Coccidioides immitis.* Antigen (0.5 mL) is injected and test results are read 48 hours later.
histoplasmosis skin test (hĭs″ tō-plăs-mō′ sĭs)	An intradermal test performed on the inner aspect of the forearm to identify the presence of *Histoplasma capsulatum.* Antigen (0.5 mL) is injected and test results are read 48 hours later.
toxoplasmosis skin test (tŏks-ō-plăs-mō′ sĭs)	An intradermal test performed on the inner aspect of the forearm to identify the presence of *Toxoplasma gondii.* Transmission of the organism to humans is by mammals and birds.
trichinosis skin test (trĭk″ ĭn-ō′ sĭs)	An intradermal test performed on the inner aspect of the forearm to identify the presence of *Trichinella spiralis.* This condition is caused by the eating of infected, poorly cooked pork.
tuberculosis skin test (tū-bĕr″ kū-lō′ sĭs)	A test performed to identify the presence of the *Tubercle bacilli.* The Tine, Mono-Vacc, patch, or Mantoux test may be used. The **Tine/Mono-Vacc** is an intradermal test performed using a sterile, disposable, multiple-puncture lancet. The tuberculin is on metal tines that are pressed into the skin. Test results are read in 48 hours.

Test	Description
	The **patch** test is performed by placing the tuberculin on a small square of gauze and applying it to the skin of the forearm. Test results are read in 48 hours.
	In the **Mantoux** test 0.5 mL of purified protein derivative tuberculin (PPD) is intradermally injected. Test results are read in 48 hours.
sweat test (chloride) (swĕt)	A test performed on **sweat** to determine the level of chloride concentration on the skin. In **cystic fibrosis,** there is an increase in skin chloride.
Tzank test (tsănk)	A microscopic examination of a small piece of tissue that has been surgically scraped from a pustule. The specimen is placed on a slide and stained, and the type of viral infection can be identified.
wound culture (woond)	A test done on wound exudate to determine the presence of microorganisms. An effective antibiotic can be prescribed for identified microbes.
biopsy (skin) (bī′ ŏp-sē)	Any skin lesion that exhibits signs or characteristics of malignancy may be excised and examined microscopically to establish a diagnosis. Usually only a small piece of living tissue is needed for examination.

Learning Exercises

Anatomy and Physiology

Write your answers to the following questions. Do not refer back to the text.

1. Name the primary organ of the integumentary system. _____

2. Name the four accessory structures of the integumentary system.

   a. _____   b. _____

   c. _____   d. _____

3. State the four main functions of the skin.

   a. _____   b. _____

   c. _____   d. _____

4. The skin is essentially composed of two layers, the _____ and the _____.

5. Name the four strata of the epidermis.

   a. _____   b. _____

   c. _____   d. _____

6. _____ is a protein substance found in the dead cells of the epidermis.

7. _____ is a pigment that gives color to the skin.

8. The _____ is known as the corium or true skin.

9. Name the two layers of the part of the skin described in question 8.

   a. _____   b. _____

10. The crescent-shaped white area of the nail is the _____.

Word Parts

1. In the spaces provided, write the definition of these prefixes, roots, combining forms, and suffixes. Do not refer to the listings of terminology words. Leave blank those terms you cannot define.
2. After completing as many as you can, refer back to the terminology word listenings to check your work. For each word missed or left blank, write the term and its definition several times on the margins of these pages or on a separate sheet of paper.
3. To maximize the learning process, it is to your advantage to do the following exercises as directed. To refer to the terminology listings before completing these exercises invalidates the learning process.

PREFIXES

Give the definitions of the following prefixes:

1. an-   _____   2. auto-   _____

3. ec-   _____   4. ep-   _____

5. ex-   _____   6. hyper-   _____

7. hypo- _____   8. intra- _____

9. par- _____   10. sub- _____

ROOTS AND COMBINING FORMS

Give the definitions of the following roots and combining forms:

1. acanth _____   2. actin _____

3. aden _____   4. albin _____

5. carcin _____   6. caus _____

7. chym _____   8. coriat _____

9. cutane _____   10. derm _____

11. derma _____   12. dermat _____

13. dermato _____   14. dermo _____

15. erysi _____   16. erythro _____

17. hidr _____   18. icter _____

19. kel _____   20. kerat _____

21. leuko _____   22. log _____

23. melan _____   24. melano _____

25. myc _____   26. onych _____

27. onychi _____   28. onycho _____

29. pachy _____   30. pedicul _____

31. rhytid _____   32. rhytido _____

33. sclero _____   34. sebo _____

35. senile _____   36. therm _____

37. trich _____   38. tricho _____

39. ungu _____   40. xantho _____

41. xero _____

SUFFIXES

Give the definitions of the following suffixes:

1. -al _____   2. -algia _____

3. -blast _____   4. -clysis _____

5. -derma _____   6. -ectomy _____

7. -esthesia _____   8. -graft _____

9. -ia _____   10. -ic _____

11. -ion _____   12. -ism _____

13. -ist _____   14. -itis _____

15. -logy _____   16. -malacia _____

17. -oid _____   18. -oma _____

19. -osis _____   20. -ous _____

21. -pathy _____   22. -pelas

23. -phagia _____   24. -plasty _____

25. -rrhea _____   26. -tome _____

27. -um _____

Identifying Medical Terms

In the spaces provided, write the medical terms for the following meanings:

1. _____ Inflammation of the skin caused by exposure to actinic rays

2. _____ Pertaining to the skin

3. _____ Inflammation of the skin

4. _____ The study of the skin

5. _____ Skin disease

6. _____ Condition of excessive sweating

7. _____ Pertaining to under the skin

8. _____ Pertaining to jaundice

9. _____ Surgical excision of a nail

10. _____ Thick skin

11. _____ Inability to distinguish between the sensations of heat and cold

12. _____ Yellow skin

Spelling

In the spaces provided, write the correct spelling of these misspelled terms.

1. caualgia _____   2. dermomcosis _____

3. echymosis _____   4. ersipelas _____

5. hypdermoclysis _____   6. melnoma _____

7. onchophagia _____   8. rhytiectomy _____

9. sleroderma _____   10. sebrrhea _____

Review Questions

Matching

Select the appropriate lettered meaning for each numbered line.

_____ 1. acne

_____ 2. alopecia

_____ 3. cicatrix

_____ 4. comedo

_____ 5. decubitus

_____ 6. dehiscence

_____ 7. exudate

_____ 8. leukoplakia

_____ 9. petechiae

_____ 10. pruritus

a. Small, pinpoint, purplish hemorrhagic spots on the skin

b. The production of pus or serum

c. A severe itching

d. An inflammatory condition of the sebaceous gland and the hair follicles

e. The scar left after the healing of a wound

f. Loss of hair, baldness

g. White spots or patches formed on the mucous membrane of the tongue or cheek

h. Blackhead

i. The separation or bursting open of a surgical wound

j. A bedsore

k. A slough, scab

Abbreviations

Place the correct word, phrase, or abbreviation in the space provided.

_____ 1. fever of unknown origin

_____ 2. transdermal therapeutic system

_____ 3. H

_____ 4. incision and drainage

_____ 5. skin graft

_____ 6. ID

_____ 7. temperature

_____ 8. ultraviolet

_____ 9. FB

_____ 10. PUVA

Diagnostic and Laboratory Tests

Select the best answer to each multiple choice question. Circle the letter of your choice.

1. The _____ _____ is an intradermal test performed using a sterile, disposable, multiple puncture lancet.

   a. patch test

   b. Mantoux test

   c. Tine/Mono-Vacc

   d. Tzank test

2. A test done on wound exudate to determine the presence of microorganisms is:

   a. sweat test

   b. biopsy

   c. Tzank test

   d. wound culture

3. A microscopic examination of a small piece of tissue that has been surgically scraped from a pustule is:

   a. Tzank test

   b. sweat test

   c. biopsy

   d. wound culture

4. _____ is transmitted to humans by mammals and birds.

   a. Trichinosis

   b. Toxoplasmosis

   c. Histoplasmosis

   d. Blastomycosis

5. _____ is caused by the eating of infected, poorly cooked pork.

   a. Trichinosis

   b. Toxoplasmosis

   c. Histoplasmosis

   d. Blastomycosis

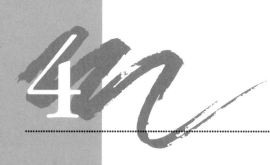

The Skeletal System

The skeletal system is composed of 206 bones that, together with cartilage and ligaments, make up the framework or skeleton of the human body. The skeleton can be divided into two main groups of bones, the axial and the appendicular skeleton.

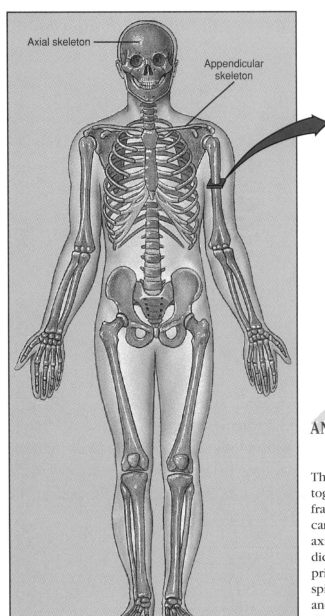

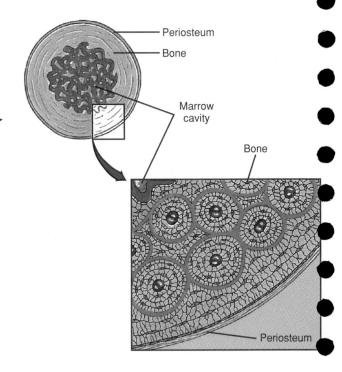

ANATOMY AND PHYSIOLOGY OVERVIEW

The skeletal system is composed of 206 bones that, together with cartilage and ligaments, make up the framework or skeleton of the body. The skeleton can be divided into two main groups of bones: the axial skeleton consisting of 80 bones and the appendicular skeleton with the remaining 126 bones. The principal bones of the axial skeleton are the skull, spine, ribs, and sternum. The shoulder girdle, arms, and hands and the pelvic girdle, legs, and feet are the primary bones of the appendicular skeleton (Fig. 4–1 and Plate 16).

THE SKELETAL SYSTEM	
Organ	**Primary Functions**
Bones (206), Cartilages, and Ligaments	Support, protect soft tissues, store minerals
Axial skeleton	Protects brain, spinal cord, sense organs, and soft tissues of chest cavity; supports the body weight over the legs
Appendicular skeleton	Internal support and positioning of arms and legs, supporting and moving axial skeleton

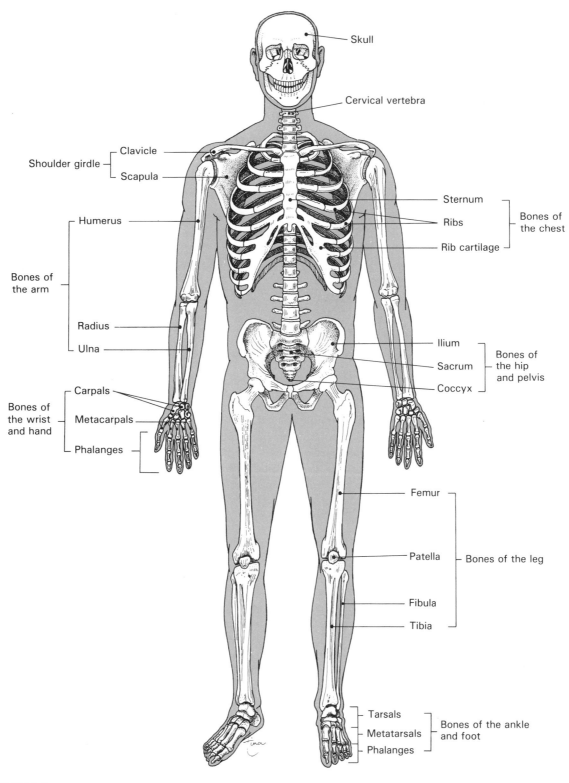

FIGURE 4–1

The axial and appendicular skeleton. (Adapted from Evans WF. Anatomy and Physiology, 3rd ed. Englewood Cliffs, NJ: Prentice-Hall, 1983, with permission.)

Bones

The bones are the primary organs of the skeletal system and are composed of about 50% water and 50% solid matter. The solid matter in bone is a calcified, rigid substance known as osseous tissue.

CLASSIFICATION OF BONES

Bones are classified according to their shapes. The following table classifies the bones and gives an example of each type:

Shape	Example of This Classification
Flat	Ribs, scapula, parts of the pelvic girdle, bones of the skull
Long	Tibia, femur, humerus, radius
Short	Carpal, tarsal
Irregular	Vertebrae, ossicles of the ear
Sesamoid	Patella

FUNCTIONS OF BONES

The following are the main functions of the skeletal system:

1. Bones provide shape and support and form the framework of the body.
2. Bones provide protection for internal organs.
3. Bones serve as a storage place for mineral salts, calcium, and phosphorus.
4. Bones play an important role in the formation of blood cells as hemopoiesis takes place in the bone marrow.
5. Bones provide areas for the attachment of skeletal muscles.
6. Bones help to make movement possible through articulation.

BONE DEVELOPMENT

Bone begins to develop during the second month of fetal life as cartilage cells enlarge, break down, disappear, and are replaced by bone-forming cells called osteoblasts. Most bones of the body are formed by this process known as endochondral ossification. In this process, the bone cells deposit organic substances in the spaces vacated by cartilage to form bone matrix. As this process proceeds, blood vessels form within the bone and deposit salts such as calcium and phosphorus that serve to harden the developing bone. Throughout a person's lifetime, osteoblasts continue to form new bone. To prevent overaccumulation of bone, large cells called osteocytes, located in depressions on the bone's surface, reabsorb the various components of bone. This material is then carried away for use by the body.

THE STRUCTURE OF A LONG BONE

Long bones, such as the tibia, femur, humerus, or radius, have most of the features found in all bones. These features, which are listed below, are shown in Figure 4–2.

Epiphysis. The ends of a developing bone

Diaphysis. The shaft of a long bone

Periosteum. The membrane that forms the covering of bones except at their articular surfaces

Compact bone. The dense, hard layer of bone tissue

Medullary canal. A narrow space or cavity throughout the length of the diaphysis

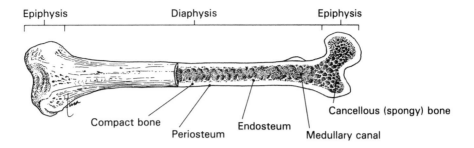

FIGURE 4-2

The gross structure of a long bone (tibia). *(Adapted from Evans WF. Anatomy and Physiology, 3rd ed. Englewood Cliffs, NJ: Prentice-Hall, 1983, with permission.)*

Endosteum. A tough, connective tissue membrane lining the medullary canal and containing the bone marrow

Cancellous or spongy bone. The reticular tissue that makes up most of the volume of bone

BONE MARKINGS

There are certain commonly used terms that describe the markings of bones. These markings are listed for your better understanding of their role in joining bones together, providing areas for muscle attachments, and serving as a passageway for blood vessels, ligaments, and nerves.

Marking	Description of the Bone Structure
Condyle	A rounded process that enters into the formation of a joint, articulation
Crest	A ridge on a bone
Fissure	A slit-like opening between two bones
Foramen	An opening in the bone for blood vessels, ligaments, and nerves
Fossa	A shallow depression in or on a bone
Head	The rounded end of a bone
Meatus	A tube-like passage or canal
Process	An enlargement or protrusion of a bone
Sinus	An air cavity within certain bones
Spine	A pointed, sharp, slender process
Sulcus	A groove, furrow, depression, or fissure
Trochanter	A very large process of the femur
Tubercle	A small, rounded process
Tuberosity	A large, rounded process

Joints and Movement

A joint is an articulation, a place where two or more bones connect. The manner in which bones connect determines the type of movement allowed at the joint. Joints are classified into the following three types:

Synarthrosis. Does not permit movement. The bones are in close contact with each other and there is no joint cavity. An example is the cranial sutures.

Amphiarthrosis. Permits very slight movement. An example of this type of joint is the vertebrae.

Diarthrosis. Allows free movement in a variety of directions. Examples of this type of joint are the knee, hip, elbow, wrist, and foot.

The following terms describe types of body movement that occur at the diarthrotic joints (Fig. 4–3):

Abduction. The process of moving a body part away from the middle.

Adduction. The process of moving a body part toward the middle.

Circumduction. The process of moving a body part in a circular motion.

Dorsiflexion. The process of bending a body part backward.

Eversion. The process of turning outward.

Extension. The process of straightening a flexed limb.

Flexion. The process of bending a limb.

Inversion. The process of turning inward.

Pronation. The process of lying prone or face downward; also the process of turning the hand so the palm faces downward.

Protraction. The process of moving a body part forward.

Retraction. The process of moving a body part backward.

FIGURE 4–3

Body movements. *(Adapted from Evans WF.* Anatomy and Physiology, *3rd ed. Englewood Cliffs, NJ: Prentice-Hall, 1983, with permission.)*

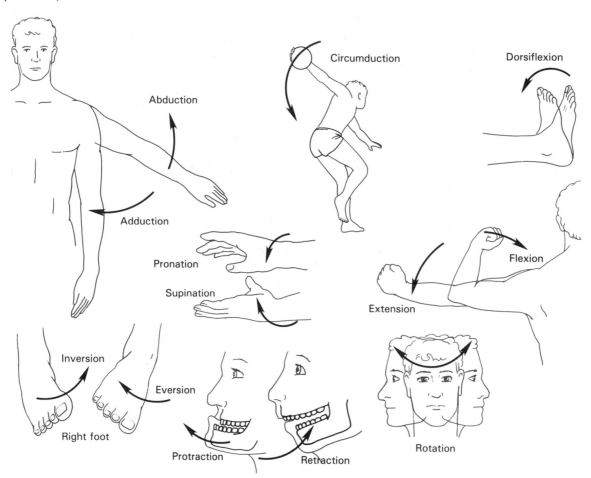

Rotation. The process of moving a body part around a central axis.

Supination. The process of lying supine or face upward; also the process of turning the palm or foot upward.

The Vertebral Column

The vertebral column is composed of a series of separate bones (vertebrae) connected in such a way as to form four spinal curves. These curves have been identified as the cervical, thoracic, lumbar, and sacral. The cervical curve consists of the first seven vertebrae, the thoracic curve consists of the next twelve vertebrae, the lumbar curve consists of the next five vertebrae, and the sacral curve consists of the sacrum and coccyx (tailbone) (Fig. 4–4).

It is known that a curved structure has more strength than a straight structure. The spinal curves of the human body are most important, as they help support the weight of the body and provide the balance that is necessary to walk on two feet.

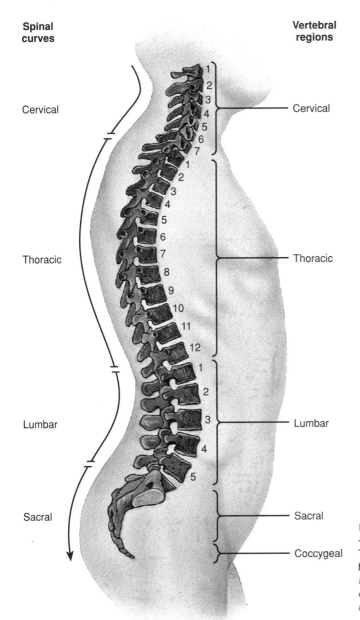

Spinal curves

Cervical

Thoracic

Lumbar

Sacral

Vertebral regions

Cervical

Thoracic

Lumbar

Sacral

Coccygeal

FIGURE 4–4

The vertebral column. The major divisions of the vertebral column, showing the four spinal curves. *(From Martini, F. Fundamentals of Anatomy and Physiology, 2nd ed. Englewood Cliffs, NJ: Prentice-Hall, 1992, with permission.)*

Abnormal Curvatures of the Spine

Scoliosis, Lordosis, and Kyphosis:

In **scoliosis,** there is an abnormal lateral curvature of the spine. This condition usually appears in adolescence, during periods of rapid growth. Treatment modalities may include the application of a cast, brace, traction, electrical stimulation, and/or surgery. See Figure 4-5A.

In **lordosis,** there is an abnormal anterior curvature of the spine. This condition may be referred to as "swayback" as the abdomen and buttocks protrude due to an exaggerated lumbar curvature. See Figure 4-5B.

In **kyphosis,** the normal thoracic curvature becomes exaggerated, producing a "humpback" appearance. This condition may be caused by a congenital defect, a disease process such as tuberculosis and/or syphilis, a malignancy, compression fracture, faulty posture, osteoarthritis, rheumatoid arthritis, rickets, osteoporosis, or other conditions. See Figure 4-5C.

The Male and Female Pelvis

The pelvis is the lower portion of the trunk of the body. It forms a basin bound anteriorly and laterally by the hip bones and posteriorly by the sacrum and coccyx.

The bony pelvis is formed by the sacrum, the coccyx, and the bones that form the hip and pubic arch, the ilium, pubis, and ischium. These bones are separate in the child, but become fused in adulthood.

THE MALE PELVIS

The male pelvis is shaped like a funnel forming a narrower outlet than the female. It is heavier, and stronger than the female pelvis, therefore it is more suited for lifting and running. See Figure 4-6A.

FIGURE 4–5
___

Abnormal curvature of the spine. **(A)** Scoliosis. **(B)** Lordosis. **(C)** Kyphosis. *(From Fong E, Scott AS, Ferris EB, Skelley EG.* Body Structures & Functions, *8th ed. Albany, NY: Delmar, 1993, with permission.)*

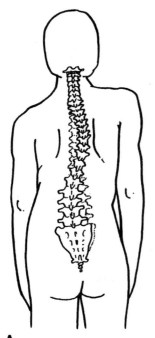
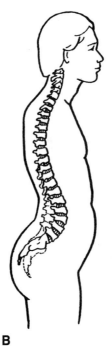
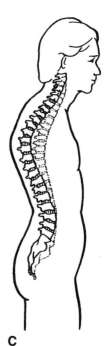

A　　　　　　　　　　　　B　　　　　　　　　　　　C

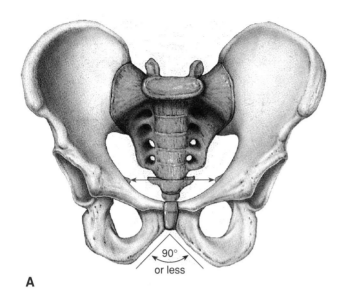

A

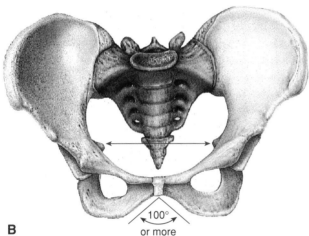

B

FIGURE 4–6

Differences in the male and female pelvis. Note the much sharper pubic angle in the pelvis of a male **(A)** than in that of a female **(B)** *(From Martini F. Fundamentals of Anatomy and Physiology, 2nd ed. Englewood Cliffs, NJ: Prentice-Hall, 1992, with permission.)*

THE FEMALE PELVIS

The female pelvis is shaped like a basin. It may be oval to round, and it is wider than the male pelvis. The female pelvis is constructed to accommodate the fetus during pregnancy and to facilitate its downward passage through the pelvic cavity in childbirth. In general the female pelvis is broader and lighter than the male pelvis. See Figure 4-6B.

FRACTURES

Fractures are classified according to their external appearance, the site of the fracture, and the nature of the crack or break in the bone. Important fracture types are indicated in Figure 4-7 and several have been paired with representative x-rays. Many fractures fall in more than one category. For example, Colles' fracture is a transverse fracture, but depending on the injury it may also be a comminuted fracture that can be either open or closed.

Fracture Type

Closed, or **simple,** fractures are completely internal; they do not involve a break in the skin

Open, or **compound,** fractures project through the skin; they are more dangerous because of the possibility of infection or uncontrolled bleeding

Comminuted fractures shatter the affected area into a multitude of bony fragments

Transverse fractures break a shaft bone across its long axis

In a **greenstick** fracture, only one side of the shaft is broken, and the other is bent; this usually occurs in children whose long bones have yet to fully ossify

Spiral fractures, produced by twisting stresses, spread along the length of the bone

A **Colles'** fracture is a break in the distal portion of the radius, the slender bone of the forearm; it is often the result of reaching out to cushion a fall

A **Pott's** fracture occurs at the ankle and affects both bones of the lower leg

Compression fractures occur in vertebrae subjected to extreme stresses, as when landing on your seat after a fall

Epiphyseal fractures usually occur where the matrix is undergoing calcification and chondrocytes are dying. A clean transverse fracture along this line usually heals well. Fractures between the epiphysis and the epiphyseal plate can permanently halt further longitudinal growth unless carefully treated; often surgery is required

Nondisplaced fractures retain the normal alignment of the bone elements or fragments

Displaced fractures produce new and abnormal arrangements of bony elements

Description

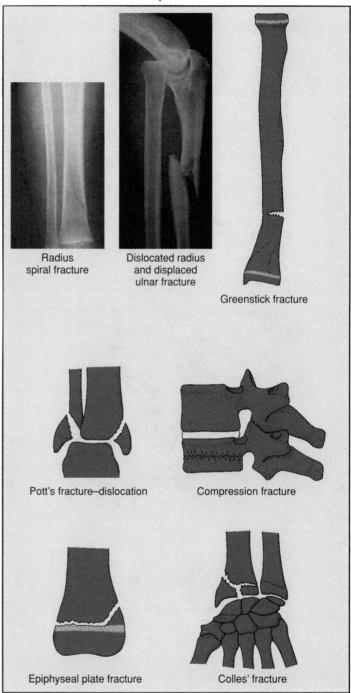

Radius spiral fracture

Dislocated radius and displaced ulnar fracture

Greenstick fracture

Pott's fracture–dislocation

Compression fracture

Epiphyseal plate fracture

Colles' fracture

FIGURE 4–7

A classification of fractures. *(From Martini F. Fundamentals of Anatomy and Physiology, 2nd ed. Englewood Cliffs, NJ: Prentice-Hall, 1992, with permission.)*

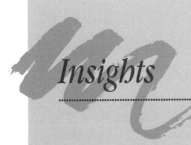
Insights

OSTEOPOROSIS

Osteoporosis, a condition in which there is a reduction in bone mass, affects more than 25 million Americans. Bone loss may occur during the aging process in the male and female, but proceeds at a faster rate in women. One-third to one-half of all postmenopausal women will be affected by osteoporosis, according to the National Osteoporosis Foundation. After menopause, changes in estrogen production may lead to weak, thin, or brittle bones. These changes are not generally felt by the patient, but signs of change may be noted as kyphosis, decrease in height, and dowager's hump (cervical lordosis with dorsal kyphosis due to loss of bone).

In America, approximately 250,000 hip fractures a year are caused by osteoporosis. Postmenopausal women are twice as likely to break their hip as men. Most hip fractures occur as a result of falling. It has been estimated that about 50% of all accidental deaths in persons over 65 are a result of falls.

Risk Factors

There are some risk factors involved in developing osteoporosis and these are:
- family history of osteoporosis
- thin, petite build
- early menopause (before 45 years of age)
- never been pregnant
- avoided dairy products as a child
- lack of exercise
- smoking, drinking alcoholic beverages
- diet high in salt, caffeine, or fat
- prone to fractures, and loss of height in the past few years

---

Prevention is a key concept in keeping the body functioning at its maximum potential. To help prevent osteoporosis, one should begin early in life. It is recommended that a prevention program include a regular exercise regimen, a diet rich in calcium, phosphorus, magnesium, and vitamins A, C, D, and the B-complex vitamins.

Vitamin A is important for the development of bones and teeth and good sources of this vitamin are dairy products, fish, liver oils, animal liver, green and yellow vegetables. Vitamin D aids in the proper use of calcium and phosphorus and good sources of this vitamin are ultraviolet rays, dairy products, and commercial foods that contain supplemental vitamin D (milk and cereals). Vitamin C is important for the maintenance of bones, teeth, and small blood vessels. Good sources of this vitamin are citrus fruits, tomatoes, melons, fresh berries, raw vegetables, and sweet potatoes.

The B-complex vitamins are essential for cellular oxidation, aid in metabolism of foods, and formation of red blood cells. Good sources of these vitamins are organ meats, dried beans, poultry, eggs, yeast, fish, whole grains, and dark-green vegetables.

Calcium, in combination with phosphorus, helps form strong bones and teeth. Good sources of calcium include dairy products, beans, cauliflower, egg yolk, molasses, leafy green vegetables, tofu, sardines, clams, and oysters. Good sources of phosphorus are dairy products, eggs, fish, poultry, meats, dried peas and beans, whole grain cereals, and nuts.

Magnesium aids in bone and tooth development. It is widely distributed in foods, especially whole grains, fruits, milk, nuts, vegetables, seafood, and meats.

Terminology with Surgical Procedures & Pathology

Term		Word Parts		Definition
acetabular (ăs″ ĕ-tăb′ ū-lăr)	acetabul	R	vinegar cup	The cup-shaped socket of the hipbone into which the thighbone fits
	ar	S	pertaining to	
achillobursitis (ă-kil″ ō-bŭr-sī′ tĭs)	achillo	CF	achilles, heel	Inflammation of the bursa lying over the Achilles' tendon
	burs	R	a pouch	
	itis	S	inflammation	
achondroplasia (ă-kŏn″ drō-plā′ sĭ-ă)	a	P	without	A defect in the formation of cartilage at the epiphyses of long bones
	chondro	CF	cartilage	
	plasia	S	formation	
acroarthritis (ăk″ rō-ăr-thrī′ tĭs)	acro	CF	extremity	Inflammation of the joints of the hands or feet
	arthr	R	joint	
	itis	S	inflammation	
acromion (ă-krō′ mĭ-ŏn)	acr	R	extremity, point	The projection of the spine of the scapula that forms the point of the shoulder and articulates with the clavicle
	omion	S	shoulder	
ankylosis (ăng″ kĭ-lō′ sĭs)	ankyl	R	stiffening, crooked	A condition of stiffening of a joint
	osis	S	condition of	
arthralgia (ăr-thrăl′ jĭ-ă)	arthr	R	joint	Pain in a joint
	algia	S	pain	
arthrectomy (ăr-thrĕk′ tō-mē)	arthr	R	joint	Surgical excision of a joint
	ectomy	S	excision	
arthredema (ăr″ thrĕ-dē′ mă)	arthr	R	joint	Swelling of a joint
	edema	S	swelling	
arthritis (ăr-thrī′ tĭs)	arthr	R	joint	Inflammation of a joint
	itis	S	inflammation	
arthrocentesis (ăr″ thrō-sĕn-tē′ sĭs)	arthro	CF	joint	Surgical puncture of a joint for removal of fluid
	centesis	S	surgical puncture	
arthrodesis (ăr″ thrō-dē′ sĭs)	arthro	CF	joint	The surgical binding of a joint for immobilization
	desis	S	binding	
arthropathy (ăr-thrŏp′ ă-thē)	arthro	CF	joint	Any joint disease
	pathy	S	disease	
arthroplasty (ăr″ thrō-plăs′ tē)	arthro	CF	joint	Surgical repair of a joint
	plasty	S	surgical repair	

(Terminology—continued)

Term	Word Parts			Definition
arthropyosis (ăr″ thrō-pī-ō′ sĭs)	arthro py osis	CF R S	joint pus condition of	A condition of pus at a joint
bursectomy (bŭr-sĕk′ tō-mē)	burs ectomy	R S	a pouch excision	Surgical excision of a bursa
bursitis (bŭr-sī′ tĭs)	burs itis	R S	a pouch inflammation	Inflammation of a bursa
calcaneal (kăl-kā′ nē-ăl)	calcane al	R S	heel bone pertaining to	Pertaining to the heel bone
calcaneodynia (kăl-kā″ nē-ō-dĭn′ ĭ-ă)	calcaneo dynia	CF S	heel bone pain	Pain in the heel bone
carpal (kăr′ păl)	carp al	R S	wrist pertaining to	Pertaining to the wristbone
carpopedal (kăr″ pō-pēd′ ăl)	carpo ped al	CF R S	wrist foot pertaining to	Pertaining to the wrist and the foot
carpoptosis (kăr″ pŏp-tō′ sĭs)	carpo ptosis	CF S	wrist drooping	Wrist drop
chondral (kŏn′ drăl)	chondr al	R S	cartilage pertaining to	Pertaining to cartilage
chondralgia (kŏn-drăl′ jĭ-ă)	chondr algia	R S	cartilage pain	Pain in or around cartilage
chondrectomy (kŏn-drĕk′ tō-mē)	chondr ectomy	R S	cartilage excision	Surgical excision of a cartilage
chondroblast (kŏn′ drō-blăst)	chondro blast	CF S	cartilage immature cell, germ cell	A cell that forms cartilage
chondrocostal (kŏn″ drō-kŏs′ tăl)	chondro cost al	CF R S	cartilage rib pertaining to	Pertaining to the rib cartilage
chondropathology (kŏn″ drō-pă-thŏl′ ō-jē)	chondro patho logy	CF CF S	cartilage disease study of	The study of the diseases of cartilage
clavicular (klă-vik′ ū-lăr)	clavicul ar	R S	little key pertaining to	Pertaining to the clavicle

(Terminology—continued)

Term	Word Parts			Definition
cleidorrhexis (klī″ dō-rĕks′ sĭs)	cleido rrhexis	CF S	clavicle rupture	Rupture of the clavicle of the fetus to facilitate delivery
coccygeal (kŏk-sĭj′ ĭ-ăl)	coccyge al	CF S	tailbone pertaining to	Pertaining to the coccyx
coccygodynia (kŏk-sĭ-gō-dĭn′ ĭ-ă)	coccygo dynia	CF S	tailbone pain	Pain in the coccyx
collagen (kŏl′ ă-jĕn)	colla gen	CF S	glue formation, produce	A fibrous insoluble protein found in the connective tissue, skin, ligaments, and cartilage
connective (kə′ nĕk′ tĭv)	connect ive	R S	to bind together nature of	That which connects or binds together
costal (kăst′ əl)	cost al	R S	rib pertaining to	Pertaining to the rib
costosternal (kŏs″ tō-stĕr′ năl)	costo stern al	CF R S	rib sternum pertaining to	Pertaining to a rib and the sternum
coxalgia (kŏk-săl′ jĭ-ă)	cox algia	R S	hip pain	Pain in the hip
coxofemoral (kŏk″ sō-fĕm′ ŏ-răl)	coxo femor al	CF R S	hip femur pertaining to	Pertaining to the hip and femur
craniectomy (krā″ nĭ-ĕk′ tŏ-mē)	crani ectomy	R S	skull excision	Surgical excision of a portion of the skull
cranioplasty (krā′ nĭ-ō-plăs″ tē)	cranio plasty	CF S	skull surgical repair	Surgical repair of the skull
craniotomy (krā″ nĭ-ŏt′ ō-mē)	cranio tomy	CF S	skull incision	Incision into the skull
dactylic (dăk′ tĭl′ ĭk)	dactyl ic	R S	finger or toe pertaining to	Pertaining to the finger or toe
dactylogram (dăk-til′ə grăm)	dactylo gram	CF S	finger or toe mark, record	A fingerprint
dactylogryposis (dăk″ tĭ-lō-grĭ-pō′ sĭs)	dactylo gryp osis	CF R S	finger or toe curve condition of	Permanent contraction of the fingers
dactylomegaly (dăk″ tĭ-lō-mĕg′ ă-lē)	dactylo megaly	CF S	finger or toe enlargement, large	Enlargement of the fingers and toes

(Terminology—continued)

Term	Word Parts			Definition
epicondyle (ĕp-ĭ-kŏn′ dīl)	epi condyle	P R	upon, above knuckle	A projection from a long bone near the articular extremity above or upon the condyle
femoral (fĕm′ ŏr-ăl)	femor al	R S	femur pertaining to	Pertaining to the femur; the thighbone
fibular (fĭb′ ū-lăr)	fibul ar	R S	fibula pertaining to	Pertaining to the fibula
humeral (hū′ mĕr-ăl)	humer al	R S	humerus pertaining to	Pertaining to the humerus
hydrarthrosis (hi″ drăr-thrō′ sĭs)	hydr arthr osis	P R S	water joint condition of	Condition of fluid in a joint
iliac (ĭl′ ē-ăk)	ili ac	R S	ilium pertaining to	Pertaining to the ilium
iliosacral (ĭl″ ĭ-ō-sā′ krăl)	ilio sacr al	CF R S	ilium sacrum pertaining to	Pertaining to the ilium and the sacrum
iliotibial (ĭl″ ĭ-ō-tĭb′ ĭ-ăl)	ilio tibi al	CF R S	ilium tibia pertaining to	Pertaining to the ilium and tibia
intercostal (ĭn″ tĕr-kŏs′ tăl)	inter cost al	R R S	between rib pertaining to	Pertaining to between the ribs
ischial (ĭs′ kĭ-al)	ischi al	R S	ischium, hip pertaining to	Pertaining to the ischium, hip
ischialgia (ĭs″ kĭ-ăl′ jĭ-ă)	ischi algia	R S	ischium, hip pain	Pain in the ischium, hip
kyphosis (kī-fō′ sĭs)	kyph osis	R S	a hump condition of	Humpback
laminectomy (lăm″ ĭ-nĕk′ tō-mē)	lamin ectomy	R S	lamina (thin plate) excision	Surgical excision of a vertebral posterior arch
lordosis (lŏr-dō′ sĭs)	lord osis	R S	bending condition of	Abnormal anterior curvature of the spine
lumbar (lŭm′ băr)	lumb ar	R S	loin pertaining to	Pertaining to the loins
lumbodynia (lŭm″ bō-dĭn′ ĭ-ă)	lumbo dynia	CF S	loin pain	Pain in the loins

(Terminology—continued)

Term	Word Parts			Definition
mandibular (măn-dĭb′ ū-lăr)	mandibul ar	R S	lower jawbone pertaining to	Pertaining to the lower jawbone
maxillary (măk′ sĭ-lĕr″ ē)	maxill ary	R S	jawbone pertaining to	Pertaining to the upper jawbone
metacarpal (mĕt″ ă-kär′ pəl)	meta carp al	P R S	beyond wrist pertaining to	Pertaining to the bones of the hand
metacarpectomy (mĕt″ ă-kär-pĕk′ tō-mē)	meta carp ectomy	P R S	beyond wrist excision	Surgical excision of one or more bones of the hand
myelitis (mī-ĕ-lī′ tĭs)	myel itis	R S	marrow inflammation	Inflammation of the bone marrow
myeloma (mī-ĕ-lō′ mă)	myel oma	R S	marrow tumor	A tumor of the bone marrow
myelopoiesis (mī′ ĕl-ō-poy-ē′ sĭs)	myelo poiesis	CF S	marrow formation	The formation of bone marrow
olecranal (ō-lĕk′ răn-ăl)	olecran al	R S	elbow pertaining to	Pertaining to the elbow
osteoarthritis (ŏs″ tē-ō-ăr-thrī′ tĭs)	osteo arthr itis	CF R S	bone joint inflammation	Inflammation of the bone and joint
osteoarthropathy (ŏs″ tē-ō-ăr-thrŏp′ ă-thē)	osteo arthro pathy	CF CF S	bone joint disease	Any disease of the bones and joints
osteoblast (ŏs′ tē-ō-blăst″)	osteo blast	CF S	bone immature cell, germ cell	A bone-forming cell
osteocarcinoma (ŏs″ tē-ō-kăr″ sĭn-ō-mă)	osteo carcin oma	CF R S	bone cancer tumor	A cancerous tumor of a bone; new growth of epithelial tissue
osteochondritis (ŏs″ tē-ō-kŏn-drī′ tĭs)	osteo chondr itis	CF R S	bone cartilage inflammation	Inflammation of the bone and cartilage
osteoclasia (ŏs″ tē-ō-klā′ zĭ-ă)	osteo clasia	CF S	bone a breaking	Surgical fracture of a bone to correct a deformity
osteodynia (ŏs″ tē-ō-dĭn′ ĭ-ă)	osteo dynia	CF S	bone pain	Pain in a bone

(Terminology—continued)

Term	Word Parts			Definition
osteofibroma (ŏs″ tē-ō-fĭ-brō′ mă)	osteo	CF	bone	A tumor of bone and fibrous tissues
	fibr	R	fibrous	
	oma	S	tumor	
osteogenesis (ŏs″ tē-ō-jĕn′ ĕ-sĭs)	osteo	CF	bone	The formation of bone
	genesis	S	formation, produce	
osteomalacia (ŏs″ tē-ō-măl-ā′ shĭ-ă)	osteo	CF	bone	Softening of the bones
	malacia	S	softening	
osteomyelitis (ŏs″ tē-ō-mī″ ĕl-ī′ tĭs)	osteo	CF	bone	Inflammation of the bone marrow
	myel	R	marrow	
	itis	S	inflammation	
osteonecrosis (ŏs″ tē-ō-nĕ-krō′ sĭs)	osteo	CF	bone	A condition in which there is death of bone tissue
	necr	R	death	
	osis	S	condition of	
osteopenia (ŏs″ tē-ō-pē′ nĭ-ă)	osteo	CF	bone	A lack of bone tissue
	penia	S	lack of	
osteoporosis (ŏs″ tē-ō-por-ō′ sĭs)	osteo	CF	bone	A condition that results in reduction of bone mass
	por	R	a passage	
	osis	S	condition of	
osteorrhagia (ŏs″ tē-ō-rā′ jĭ-ă)	osteo	CF	bone	Hemorrhage from a bone
	rrhagia	S	to burst forth	
osteorrhaphy (ŏs-tē-or′ ă-fē)	osteo	CF	bone	Suture of a bone
	rrhaphy	S	suture	
osteosarcoma (ŏs″ tē-ō-săr-kō′ mă)	osteo	CF	bone	A malignant tumor of the bone; cancer arising from connective tissue
	sarc	R	flesh	
	oma	S	tumor	
osteosclerosis (ŏs″ tē-ō-sklĕ-rō′ sĭs)	osteo	CF	bone	A condition of hardening of the bone
	scler	R	hardening	
	osis	S	condition of	
osteotome (ŏs′ tē-ō-tōm″)	osteo	CF	bone	An instrument used for cutting bone
	tome	S	instrument to cut	
patellapexy (pă-tĕl′ ă-pĕk″ sē)	patella	R	kneecap	Surgical fixation of the patella
	pexy	S	fixation	
patellar (pă-tĕl′ ăr)	patell	R	kneecap	Pertaining to the patella
	ar	S	pertaining to	
pedal (pĕd ′ĭ)	ped	R	foot	Pertaining to the foot
	al	S	pertaining to	

(Terminology—continued)

Term	Word Parts			Definition
perichondral (pĕr″ i-kŏn′ drăl)	peri chondr al	P R S	around cartilage pertaining to	Pertaining to the membrane that covers cartilage
periosteoedema (pĕr″ ĭ-ŏs″ tē-ō-ē-dē′ mă)	peri osteo edema	P CF S	around bone swelling	Swelling around a bone
phalangeal (fā-lăn′ jē-ăl)	phalange al	CF S	closely knit row pertaining to	Pertaining to the bones of the fingers and the toes
polyarthritis (pŏl″ ē-ăr-thrī′ tĭs)	poly arthr itis	P R S	many, much joint inflammation	Inflammation of more than one joint
rachialgia (rā″ kĭ-ăl′ jĭ-ă)	rachi algia	CF S	spine pain	Pain in the spine
rachigraph (rā′ kĭ-grăf)	rachi graph	CF S	spine to write	An instrument used to measure the curvature of the spine
rachiotomy (rā″ kĭ-ŏt′ ō-mē)	rachio tomy	CF S	spine incision	Surgical incision of the spine
radial (rā′ dĭ-ăl)	radi al	CF S	radius pertaining to	Pertaining to the radius
scapular (skăp′ ū-lăr)	scapul ar	R S	shoulder blade pertaining to	Pertaining to the shoulder blade
scoliosis (skō″ lĭ-ō′ sĭs)	scoli osis	R S	curvature condition of	A condition of lateral curvature of the spine
scoliotone (skō′ lĭ-ō-tōn)	scolio tone	CF S	curvature tension	A device for correcting the curve in scoliosis by stretching the spine
spinal (spī′ năl)	spin al	R S	spine pertaining to	Pertaining to the spine
spondylitis (spŏn-dĭl-ī′ tĭs)	spondyl itis	R S	vertebra inflammation	Inflammation of one or more vertebrae
sternal (stĕr′ năl)	stern al	R S	sternum pertaining to	Pertaining to the sternum
sternalgia (stĕr-năl′ jĭ-ă)	stern algia	R S	sternum pain	Pain in the sternum
sternotomy (stĕr-nŏt′ ō-mē)	sterno tomy	CF S	sternum incision	Surgical incision of the sternum

(Terminology—continued)

Term	Word Parts			Definition
subclavicular	sub	P	under, beneath	Pertaining to beneath the
(sŭb″ klă-vĭk′ ū-lăr)	clavicul	R	a little key	clavicle
	ar	S	pertaining to	
subcostal	sub	P	under, beneath	Pertaining to beneath the ribs
(sŭb-kŏs′ tăl)	cost	R	rib	
	al	S	pertaining to	
submaxilla	sub	P	under, beneath	The lower jaw or mandible
(sŭb″ măk-sĭl′ ă)	maxilla	R	jaw	
symphysis	sym	P	together	A growing together
(sĭm′ fĭ-sĭs)	physis	S	growth	
syndesis	syn	P	together	Binding together; surgical
(sĭn′ dē-sĭs)	desis	S	binding	fixation or ankylosis of a joint
tendoplasty	tendo	CF	tendon	Surgical repair of a tendon
(tĕn′ dō-plăs″ tē)	plasty	S	surgical repair	
tenonitis	tenon	R	tendon	Inflammation of a tendon
(tĕn″ ō-nī′ tĭs)	itis	S	inflammation	
tibial	tibi	R	tibia	Pertaining to the tibia
(tĭb′ ĭ-ăl)	al	S	pertaining to	
ulnar	uln	R	elbow	Pertaining to the elbow
(ŭl′ năr)	ar	S	pertaining to	
ulnocarpal	ulno	CF	elbow	Pertaining to the ulna side of
(ŭl″ nō-kăr′ păl)	carp	R	wrist	the wrist
	al	S	pertaining to	
ulnoradial	ulno	CF	elbow	Pertaining to the ulna and
(ŭl″ nō-rā′ dĭ-ăl)	radi	CF	radius	radius
	al	S	pertaining to	
vertebral	vertebr	R	vertebra	Pertaining to a vertebra
(vĕr′ tĕ-brăl)	al	S	pertaining to	
vertebrectomy	vertebr	R	vertebra	Surgical excision of a vertebra
(vĕr″ tĕ-brĕk′ tō-mē)	ectomy	S	excision	
vertebrosternal	vertebro	CF	vertebra	Pertaining to a vertebra and
(vĕr″ tĕ-brō-ster′ năl)	stern	R	sternum	the sternum
	al	S	pertaining to	
xiphoid	xiph	R	sword	Resembling a sword
(zĭf′ oyd)	oid	S	resemble	

Vocabulary Words

Vocabulary words are terms that have not been divided into component parts. They are common words or specialized terms associated with the subject of this chapter. These words are provided to enhance your medical vocabulary.

Word	Definition
arthroscope (ăr-thrŏs′ kōp)	An instrument used to examine the interior of a joint
bone marrow transplant (bōn măr′ ō trăns′ plànt)	The surgical process of transferring bone marrow from a donor to a patient
breakbone fever (brāk′ bōn fē′ vėr)	An acute febrile disease characterized by intense, arthritis-like pain; also known as dengue fever
bursa (bŭr′ sah)	A small space between muscles, tendons, and bones that is lined with synovial membrane and contains a fluid, synovia
calcium (kăl′ sĭ-ŭm)	A mineral that is essential for bone growth, teeth development, blood coagulation, and many other functions
carpal tunnel syndrome (kär′ pĕl tŭn′ ĕl sĭn′ drōm)	A condition caused by compression of the median nerve by the carpal ligament; symptoms: soreness, tenderness, weakness, pain, tingling, and numbness at the wrist
cartilage (kär′ tĭ-lĭj)	A specialized type of fibrous connective tissue present in adults, which forms the major portion of the embryonic skeleton
cast (kàst)	A type of material, usually made of plaster of Paris, used to immobilize a fractured bone, a dislocation, or a sprain
clawfoot (klō fùt)	A deformity of the foot characterized by an abnormally high arch; also known as pes cavus
dislocation (dĭs″ lō-kā′ shŭn)	The displacement of a bone from a joint
fixation (fĭks-ā′ shŭn)	The process of holding or fastening in a fixed position; making rigid, immobilizing
flatfoot (flăt fùt)	An abnormal flatness of the sole and arch of the foot; also known as pes planus
genu valgum (jē′ nū văl′ gŭm)	Knock-knee
genu varum (jē′ nū vā′ rŭm)	Bowleg
gout (gowt)	A hereditary metabolic disease that is a form of acute arthritis; usually begins in the knee or foot but can affect any joint

(Vocabulary—continued)

Word	Definition
hallux (hăl″ ŭks)	The big or great toe
hammertoe (hăm′ er-tō)	An acquired flexion deformity of the interphalangeal joint
ligament (lĭg′ ă-měnt)	A band of fibrous connective tissue that connects bones, cartilages, and other structures; also serves as a place for the attachment of fascia or muscle
phosphorus (fŏs′ fō-rŭs)	A mineral that is essential in bone formation, muscle contraction, and many other functions
radiograph (rā′ dĭ-ō-grăf)	An x-ray photograph of a body part
reduction (rē-dŭk′ shŭn)	The manipulative or surgical procedure used to correct a fracture or hernia
rheumatoid arthritis (roo′ mă-toyd ăr-thrī′ tĭs)	A chronic systemic disease characterized by inflammation of the joints, stiffness, pain, and swelling that results in crippling deformities
rickets (rĭk′ ĕts)	A deficiency condition in children primarily caused by a lack of vitamin D; may also result from inadequate intake or excessive loss of calcium
sequestrum (sē-kwĕs′ trŭm)	A fragment of a dead bone that has become separated from its parent bone
splint (splĭnt)	An appliance used for fixation, support, and rest of an injured body part
sprain (sprān)	Twisting of a joint that causes pain and disability
spur (spər)	A sharp or pointed projection, as on a bone
tennis elbow (těn′ ĭs ěl′ bō)	A chronic condition characterized by pain caused by excessive pronation and supination activities of the forearm; usually caused by strain, as in playing tennis
traction (trăk′ shŭn)	The process of drawing or pulling on bones or muscles to relieve displacement and facilitate healing

ABBREVIATIONS

AP	anteroposterior	**C-1**	cervical vertebra, first
CDH	congenital dislocation of hip	**C-2**	cervical vertebra, second
C-3	cervical vertebra, third	**ortho**	orthopedics, orthopaedics
Ca	calcium	**OA**	osteoarthritis
DJD	degenerative joint disease	**PEMFs**	pulsing electromagnetic fields
Fx	fracture	**PWB**	partial weight bearing
JRA	juvenile rheumatoid arthritis	**RA**	rheumatoid arthritis
jt	joint	**SAC**	short arm cast
KJ	knee jerk	**SLC**	short leg cast
L-1	lumbar vertebra, first	**SPECT**	single-photon emission
L-2	lumbar vertebra, second		computed tomography
L-3	lumbar vertebra, third	**T-1**	thoracic vertebra, first
LAC	long arm cast	**T-2**	thoracic vertebra, second
lig	ligament	**T-3**	thoracic vertebra, third
LLC	long leg cast	**TMJ**	temporomandibular joint
LLCC	long leg cylinder cast	**Tx**	traction

Drug Highlights

Drugs that are generally used for skeletal system diseases and disorders include anti-inflammatory drugs, antirheumatic drugs, and analgesics. Fractures, arthritis, rheumatoid arthritis, bursitis, carpal tunnel syndrome, dislocation, and pain are some of the conditions involving the skeletal system and the need for pharmacological therapy.

Anti-inflammatory Agents
Relieve the swelling, tenderness, redness, and pain of inflammation. These agents may be classified as steroidal (corticosteroids) and nonsteroidal.

Corticosteroids
Steroid substance with potent anti-inflammatory effects.

Examples: Depo-Medrol (methylprednisolone acetate), Aristocort (triamcinolone), Celestone (betamethasone), and Decadron (dexamethasone).

Nonsteroidal
Agents that are used in the treatment of arthritis and related disorders.

Examples: Bayer Aspirin (acetylsalicylic acid), Motrin (ibuprofen), Oxalid; Tanderaril (oxyphenbutazone), and Feldene (piroxicam).

Antirheumatic Drugs
Prevent or relieve rheumatism. Rheumatism is defined as an acute or chronic condition characterized by inflammation, soreness and stiffness of muscles, and pain in joints and associated structures. *Gold therapy* and *Rheumatrex* are used in the treatment of rheumatoid arthritis.

Gold therapy (chrysotherapy)
Used in the long-term treatment of rheumatoid arthritis. Gold preparations have shown to be effective in reducing the progression of the disease, as well as relieving inflammation, but its use is limited by the toxicity of the gold compound.

Examples: Ridaura (auranofin), Myochrysine (gold sodium thiomalate), and Solganal (aurothioglucose).

Rheumatrex

A low-dose form of *methotrexate* approved for adult rheumatoid arthritis. It is recommended for selected adults with severe, active, classical or definite rheumatoid arthritis who have had insufficient response to other forms of treatment. The patient may see improvement within 3 to 6 weeks.

Analgesics

Agents that relieve pain without causing loss of consciousness. They are classified as narcotic or non-narcotic.

Narcotic
Non-narcotic

Examples: Demerol (meperidine HCl) and morphine sulfate.
Examples: Tylenol (acetaminophen), aspirin, ibuprofen (Advil, Motrin, Nuprin), Naprosyn (naproxen), and Zomax (somepirac sodium).

Communication Enrichment

This segment is provided for those who wish to enhance their ability to communicate in either English or Spanish.

RELATED TERMS

English	Spanish
fracture	fractura (frăc-*tŭ*-ră)
sprain	torcer (*tōr*-sĕr)
bones	huesos (*wĕ*-sŏs)
shoulder	hombros (*ōm*-brōs)
elbow	codo (*kō*-dō)
wrist	muñeca (mŭ-*ñĕ*-kă)
fingers, toes	dedos (*dĕ*-dōs)
hip	cadera (kă-*dĕ*-ră)
knee	rodilla (rō-*dĭ*-jă)
ankle	tobillo (tō-*bĭ*-jō)
plaster	yeso (*jĕ*-sō)

English	Spanish
ray	rayo (*ră*-jō)
crutches	muletas (mŭ-*lĕ*-tăs)
foot	pie (*pĭ*-ĕ)
hands	manos (*mă*-nōs)
joint	cojuntura (kō-jŭn-*tŭ*-ră)
leg	pierna (pĭ-*ĕr*-nă)
neck	cuello (*kŭ*-ĕ-jŏ)
chest x-ray	radiografia del tórax (*ră*-dĭ-ō-gră-fĭ-ă dĕl *tō*-răx)
rib	costilla (kōs-*tĭ*-jă)
cartilage	cartilago (*kăr*-tĭ-lă-gō)
ligament	ligamento (*lĭ*-gă-mĭĕn-tō)
skeleton	esqueleto (ĕs-kĕ-lĕ-tō)
skull	craneo (*kră*-nĕ-ō)
spine	espinazo (ĕs-pĭ-*nă*-zō)
calcium	calcio (*kăl*-sĭ-ō)
phosphorus	fósforo (*fōs*-fō-rō)
water	agua (*ă*-gŭ-ă)
thigh	muslo (*mŭs*-lō)
pelvis	pelvis (*pĕl*-vĭs)
shape	forma (*fōr*-mă)
support	sustento (*sŭs*-tĕn-tō)
protection	protección (*prō*-tĕk-sĭ-ōn)
reduction	reducción (*rĕ*-dŭk-sĭ-ōn)

DIAGNOSTIC AND LABORATORY TESTS

Test	Description
arthrography (ăr-thrŏg' ră-fē)	A diagnostic examination of a joint (usually the knee) in which air and, then, a radiopaque contrast medium is injected into the joint space, x-rays are taken, and internal injuries of the meniscus, cartilage, and ligaments may be seen, if present
arthroscopy (ăr-thrŏs' kō-pē)	The process of examining internal structures of a joint via an arthroscope; usually done after an arthrography and before joint surgery
goniometry (gō" nē-ŏm' ĕt-rē)	The measurement of joint movements and angles via a goniometer
photon absorptiometry (fō' tŏn ăb-sorp' shē-ŏm' ĕt-rĕ)	A bone scan that uses a low beam of radiation to measure bone-mineral density and bone loss in the lumbar vertebrae; useful in monitoring osteoporosis
thermography (thĕr-mŏg' ră-fē)	The process of recording heat patterns of the body's surface; can be used to investigate the pathophysiology of rheumatoid arthritis
x-ray (ĕks' rā)	The examination of bones by use of an electromagnetic wave of high energy produced by the collision of a beam of electrons with a target in a vacuum tube; used to identify fractures and pathologic conditions of the bones and joints such as rheumatoid arthritis, spondylitis, and tumors
alkaline phosphatase blood test (ăl' kă-lĭn fŏs' fă-tās)	A blood test to determine the level of alkaline phosphatase; increased in osteoblastic bone tumors, rickets, osteomalacia, and during fracture healing
antinuclear antibodies (ANA) (ăn" tĭ-nū' klē-ăr ăn' tĭ-bŏd" ēs)	Present in a variety of immunologic diseases; positive result may indicate rheumatoid arthritis
calcium (Ca) blood test (kăl' sē-ŭm)	The calcium level of the blood may be increased in metastatic bone cancer, acute osteoporosis, prolonged immobilization, and during fracture healing; may be decreased in osteomalacia and rickets
C-Reactive protein blood test (sē-rē-ăk" tĭv prō' tē-in)	Positive result may indicate rheumatoid arthritis, acute inflammatory change, and widespread metastasis
phosphorus (P) blood test (fŏs' fō-rŭs)	Phosphorus level of the blood may be increased in osteoporosis and fracture healing
serum rheumatoid factor (RF) (sē' rŭm roo' mă-toyd făk' tōr)	An immunoglobulin present in the serum of 50 to 95% of adults with rheumatoid arthritis
uric acid blood test (ū' rĭk ăs' ĭd)	Uric acid is increased in gout, arthritis, multiple myeloma, and rheumatism

Learning Exercises

Anatomy and Physiology

Write your answers to the following questions. Do not refer back to the text.

1. The skeletal system is composed of _____ bones.

2. Name the two main divisions of the skeletal system.

    a. _____   b. _____

3. Name the five classifications of bone and give an example of each.

    a. _____   Example _____

    b. _____   Example _____

    c. _____   Example _____

    d. _____   Example _____

    e. _____   Example _____

4. State the six main functions of the skeletal system.

    a. _____   b. _____

    c. _____   d. _____

    e. _____   f. _____

5. Define the following features of a long bone:

    a. Epiphysis _____

    b. Diaphysis _____

    c. Periosteum _____

    d. Compact Bone _____

    e. Medullary Canal _____

    f. Endosteum _____

    g. Cancellous or Spongy Bone _____

4. THE SKELETAL SYSTEM   99

6. Match the term in column one with its definition from column two. Place the correct number from column two in the space provided in column one.

    _____ a. Meatus

    _____ b. Head

    _____ c. Tuberosity

    _____ d. Process

    _____ e. Condyle

    _____ f. Tubercle

    _____ g. Crest

    _____ h. Trochanter

    _____ i. Sinus

    _____ j. Fissure

    _____ k. Fossa

    _____ l. Spine

    _____ m. Foramen

    _____ n. Sulcus

1. An air cavity within certain bones
2. A shallow depression in or on a bone
3. A pointed, sharp, slender process
4. A large, rounded process
5. A groove, furrow, depression, or fissure
6. A tube-like passage or canal
7. An opening in the bone for blood vessels, ligaments, and nerves
8. A rounded process that enters into the formation of a joint, articulation
9. A ridge on a bone
10. A small, rounded process
11. The rounded end of a bone
12. A slit-like opening between two bones
13. An enlargement or protrusion of a bone
14. A very large process of the femur

7. Name the three classifications of joints.

a. _____   b. _____

c. _____

8. _____ is the process of moving a body part away from the middle.

9. Adduction is _____ .

10. _____ is the process of moving a body part in a circular motion.

11. Dorsiflexion is _____ .

12. _____ is the process of turning outward.

13. Extension is _____ .

14. _____ is the process of bending a limb.

15. Inversion is _____ .

16. _____ is the process of lying face downward.

17. Protraction is _____ .

18. _____ is the process of moving a body part backward.

19. Rotation is _____ .

20. _____ is the process of lying face upward.

Word Parts

1. In the spaces provided, write the definition of these prefixes, roots, combining forms, and suffixes. Do not refer to the listings of terminology words. Leave blank those terms you cannot define.
2. After completing as many as you can, refer back to the terminology word listings to check your work. For each word missed or left blank, write the term and its definition several times on the margins of these pages or on a separate sheet of paper.
3. To maximize the learning process, it is to your advantage to do the following exercises as directed. To refer to the terminology listings before completing these exercises invalidates the learning process.

PREFIXES

Give the definitions of the following prefixes:

1. a- _____   2. epi- _____
3. hydr- _____   4. inter- _____
5. meta- _____   6. peri- _____
7. poly- _____   8. sub- _____
9. sym- _____   10. syn- _____

ROOTS AND COMBINING FORMS

Give the definitions of the following roots and combining forms:

1. acetabul _____   2. achillo _____
3. acr _____   4. acro _____
5. ankyl _____   6. arthr _____
7. arthro _____   8. burs _____
9. calcane _____   10. calcaneo _____
11. carcin _____   12. carp _____
13. carpo _____   14. chondr _____
15. chondro _____   16. clavicul _____
17. cleido _____   18. coccyge _____
19. coccygo _____   20. colla _____
21. condyle _____   22. connect _____
23. cost _____   24. costo _____
25. cox _____   26. coxo _____
27. crani _____   28. cranio _____
29. dactyl _____   30. dactylo _____
31. femor _____   32. fibr _____
33. fibul _____   34. gryp _____
35. humer _____   36. ili _____
37. ilio _____   38. ischi _____
39. kyph _____   40. lamin _____

41. lord _____   42. lumb _____

43. lumbo _____   44. mandibul _____

45. maxill _____   46. maxilla _____

47. myel _____   48. myelo _____

49. necr _____   50. olecran _____

51. osteo _____   52. patell _____

53. patella _____   54. patho _____

55. ped _____   56. phalange _____

57. por _____   58. py _____

59. rachi _____   60. rachio _____

61. radi _____   62. sacr _____

63. sarc _____   64. scapul _____

65. scler _____   66. scoli _____

67. scolio _____   68. spin _____

69. spondyl _____   70. stern _____

71. sterno _____   72. tendo _____

73. tenon _____   74. tibi _____

75. uln _____   76. ulno _____

77. vertebr _____   78. vertebro _____

79. xiph _____

SUFFIXES

Give the definitions of the following suffixes:

1. -ac _____   2. -al _____

3. -algia _____   4. -ar _____

5. -ary _____   6. -blast _____

7. -centesis _____   8. -clasia _____

9. -desis _____   10. -dynia _____

11. -ectomy _____   12. -edema _____

13. -gen _____   14. -genesis _____

15. -gram _____   16. -graph _____

17. -ic _____   18. -itis _____

19. -ive _____   20. -logy _____

21. -malacia _____   22. -megaly _____

23. -oid _____   24. -oma _____

25. -omion _____   26. -osis _____

27. -pathy _____   28. -penia _____

29. -pexy _____   30. -physis _____

31. -plasia _____   32. -plasty _____

33. -poiesis _____   34. -ptosis _____

35. -rrhagia _____   36. -rrhaphy _____

37. -rrhexis _____   38. -tome _____

39. -tomy _____   40. -tone _____

Identifying Medical Terms

In the spaces provided, write the medical term for the following meanings:

1. _____ Inflammation of the joints of the hands or feet

2. _____ The condition of stiffening of a joint

3. _____ Surgical excision of a joint

4. _____ Inflammation of a joint

5. _____ Any joint disease

6. _____ Pertaining to the heel bone

7. _____ Wrist drop

8. _____ Pertaining to cartilage

9. _____ Study of the diseases of cartilage

10. _____ Pain in the coccyx

11. _____ Pertaining to the rib

12. _____ Surgical excision of a portion of the skull

13. _____ Pertaining to the finger or toe

14. _____ Condition of fluid in a joint

15. _____ Pertaining to between the ribs

16. _____ Pain in the hip

17. _____ Pertaining to the loins

18. _____ A tumor of the bone marrow

19. _____ Inflammation of the joint and bone

20. _____ Pain in a bone

21. _____ Inflammation of the bone marrow

22. _____ A lack of bone tissue

23. _____ Pertaining to the foot

24. _____ Pain in the sternum

25. _____ Resembling a sword

Spelling

In the spaces provided, write the correct spelling of these misspelled terms:

1. acrmoin _____   2. arthedema _____

3. buritis _____   4. chondblast _____

5. conective   _____   6. cranplasty   _____

7. dactlomegaly   _____   8. ischal   _____

9. melyitis   _____   10. ostchonditis   _____

11. ostnecrosis   _____   12. patelar   _____

13. phalangal   _____   14. rachgraph   _____

15. scolosis   _____   16. spondlitis   _____

17. symphsis   _____   18. tennitis   _____

19. ulncarpal   _____   20. vertbral   _____

Review Questions

Matching

Select the appropriate lettered meaning for each numbered line.

_____ 1. arthroscope

_____ 2. carpal tunnel syndrome

_____ 3. clawfoot

_____ 4. gout

_____ 5. hammertoe

_____ 6. kyphosis

_____ 7. metacarpal

_____ 8. rickets

_____ 9. tennis elbow

_____ 10. ulnar

a. A deficiency condition in children primarily caused by a lack of vitamin D

b. An acquired flexion deformity of the interphalangeal joint

c. A hereditary metabolic disease that is a form of acute arthritis

d. A chronic condition characterized by pain that is caused by excessive pronation and supination activities of the forearm

e. A deformity of the foot characterized by an abnormally high arch

f. Pertaining to the elbow

g. Pertaining to the bones of the hand

h. Humpback

i. An instrument used to examine the interior of a joint

j. A condition caused by compression of the median nerve by the carpal ligament

k. Pertaining to the knee

Abbreviations

Place the correct word, phrase, or abbreviation in the space provided.

_____ 1. congenital dislocation of hip

_____ 2. degenerative joint disease

_____ 3. LLC

_____   4. OA

_____   5. pulsing electromagnetic fields

_____   6. RA

_____   7. single-photon emission computed tomography

_____   8. T-1

_____   9. TMJ

_____   10. traction

Diagnostic and Laboratory Test

Select the best answer to each multiple choice question. Circle the letter of your choice.

1. _____ is a diagnostic examination of a joint in which air and, then, a radiopaque contrast medium is injected into the joint space, x-rays are taken, and internal injuries of the meniscus, cartilage, and ligaments may be seen, if present.

    a. Arthroscopy

    b. Goniometry

    c. Arthrography

    d. Thermography

2. The process of recording heat patterns of the body's surface is:

    a. arthrography

    b. arthroscopy

    c. goniometry

    d. thermography

3. _____ is increased in gout, arthritis, multiple myeloma, and rheumatism.

    a. Calcium

    b. Phosphorus

    c. Uric acid

    d. Alkaline phosphatase

4. _____ level of the blood may be increased in osteoporosis and fracture healing.

    a. Antinuclear antibodies

    b. Phosphorus

    c. Uric acid

    d. Alkaline phosphatase

5. _____ is/are present in a variety of immunologic diseases.

    a. Alkaline phosphatase

    b. Antinuclear antibodies

    c. C-Reactive protein

    d. Uric acid

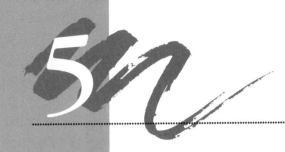

The Muscular System

The muscular system is composed of all the muscles in the human body. There are 700 skeletal muscles in the body and they make up approximately 42% of a person's body weight. Muscles are composed of long, slender cells known as fibers. Muscle fibers are of different lengths and shapes and vary in color from white to deep red.

MUSCLE vs BODY FAT

Percent Body-Fat Norms

	Male	Female
Lean	<8%	<15%
Healthy	8-15%	15-22%
Plump	16-19%	23-27%
Fat	20-24%	28-33%
Obese	>24%	>33%

Average College Male
  = 12-15%
Average College Female
  = 22-25%

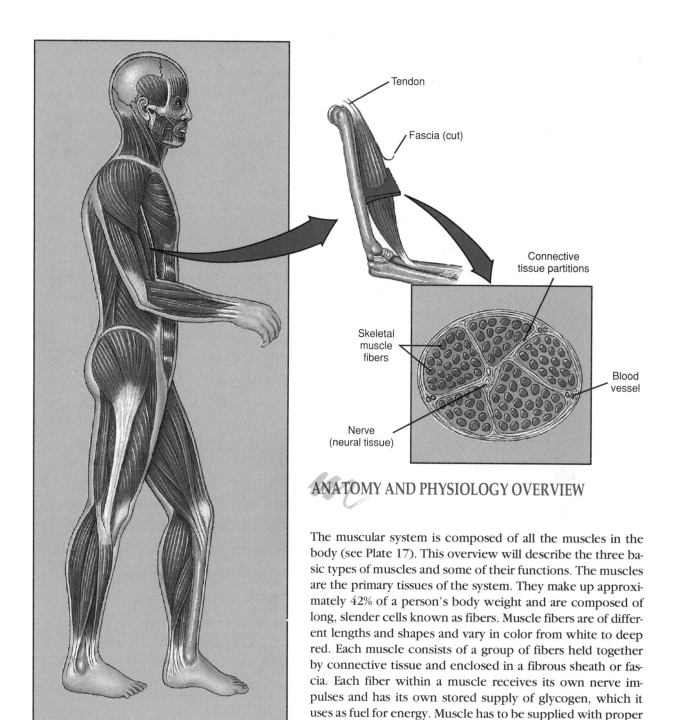

Tendon

Fascia (cut)

Connective
tissue partitions

Skeletal
muscle
fibers

Blood
vessel

Nerve
(neural tissue)

ANATOMY AND PHYSIOLOGY OVERVIEW

The muscular system is composed of all the muscles in the body (see Plate 17). This overview will describe the three basic types of muscles and some of their functions. The muscles are the primary tissues of the system. They make up approximately 42% of a person's body weight and are composed of long, slender cells known as fibers. Muscle fibers are of different lengths and shapes and vary in color from white to deep red. Each muscle consists of a group of fibers held together by connective tissue and enclosed in a fibrous sheath or fascia. Each fiber within a muscle receives its own nerve impulses and has its own stored supply of glycogen, which it uses as fuel for energy. Muscle has to be supplied with proper nutrition and oxygen to perform properly; therefore, blood and lymphatic vessels permeate its tissues.

THE MUSCULAR SYSTEM	
Organ	**Primary Functions**
Skeletal Muscles (700)	Provide skeletal movement, control entrances and exits of digestive tract, heat production, support skeletal position, protect soft tissues
Tendons, Aponeuroses	Harness forces of contraction to perform specific tasks

Types of Muscle Tissue

Skeletal muscle, smooth muscle, and cardiac muscle are the three basic types of muscle tissue classed according to their functions and appearance (Fig. 5-1).

SKELETAL MUSCLE

Also known as voluntary or striated muscles, skeletal muscles are controlled by the conscious part of the brain and attach to the bones. There are 700 skeletal muscles that, through contractility, extensibility, and elasticity, are responsible for the movement of the body. These muscles have a cross-striped appearance and thus are known as striated muscles. They vary in size, shape, arrangement of fibers, and means of attachment to bones. Selected skeletal muscles are listed with their functions in Tables 5-1 and 5-2, and shown in Figures 5-2 and 5-3.

Skeletal muscles have two or more attachments. The more fixed attachment is known as the origin, and the point of attachment of a muscle to the part that it moves is the insertion. The means of attachment is called a tendon, which can vary in length from less than 1 inch to more than 1 foot. A wide, thin, sheet-like tendon is known as an aponeurosis.

FIGURE 5–1

Types of muscle tissue. *(Adapted from Evans WF. Anatomy and Physiology, 3rd ed. Englewood Cliffs, NJ: Prentice-Hall, 1983, with permission.)*

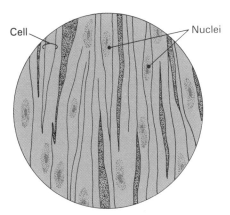

Visceral smooth muscle tissue

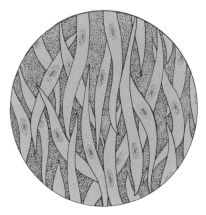

Multi-unit smooth muscle tissue

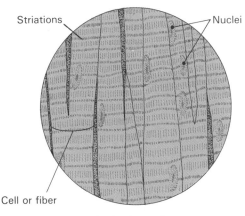

Skeletal muscle

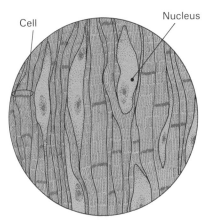

Cardiac muscle

TABLE 5–1. SELECTED SKELETAL MUSCLES (ANTERIOR VIEW)

Muscle	Action
Sternocleidomastoid	Rotates and laterally flexes neck
Trapezius	Draws head back and to the side, rotates scapula
Deltoid	Raises and rotates arm
Rectus femoris	Extends leg and assists flexion of thigh
Sartorius	Flexes and rotates the thigh and leg
Tibialis anterior	Dorsiflexes foot and increases the arch in the beginning process of walking
Pectoralis major	Flexes, adducts and rotates arm
Biceps brachii	Flexes arm and forearm and supinates forearm
Rectus abdominis	Compresses or flattens abdomen
Gastrocnemius	Plantar flexes foot and flexes knee
Soleus	Plantar flexes foot

A muscle has three distinguishable parts: the body or main portion, an origin, and an insertion. The skeletal muscles move body parts by pulling from one bone across its joint to another bone with movement occurring at the diarthrotic joint. The types of body movement occurring at the diarthrotic joints are described in the chapter entitled The Skeletal System.

Muscles and nerves function together as a unit. For skeletal muscles to contract, it is necessary to have stimulation by impulses from motor nerves. Muscles perform in groups and are classified as follows:

Antagonist. A muscle that counteracts the action of another muscle

Prime mover. A muscle that is primary in a given movement. Its contraction produces the movement

Synergist. A muscle that acts with another muscle to produce movement

SMOOTH MUSCLE

Also called involuntary, visceral, or unstriated, smooth muscles are not controlled by the conscious part of the brain. They are under the control of the autonomic nervous system and, in most cases, produce relatively slow contraction with greater degree of extensibility. These muscles lack the cross-striped appearance of skeletal muscle and are smooth. Included in this type are the muscles of internal organs of the digestive, respiratory, and urinary tract, plus certain muscles of the eye and skin.

CARDIAC MUSCLE

The muscle of the heart is involuntary but striated in appearance. It is controlled by the autonomic nervous system and specialized neuromuscular tissue located within the right atrium. Refer to the chapter entitled The Cardiovascular System for additional information.

TABLE 5–2. SELECTED SKELETAL MUSCLES (POSTERIOR VIEW)

Muscle	Action
Trapezius	Draws head back and to the side, rotates scapula
Deltoid	Raises and rotates arm
Triceps	Extends forearm
Latissimus dorsi	Adducts, extends and rotates arm. Used during "swimming"
Gluteus maximus	Extends and rotates thigh
Biceps femoris	Flexes knee and rotates it outward
Gastrocnemius	Plantar flexes foot and flexes knee
Semitendinosus	Flexes and rotates leg, extends thigh

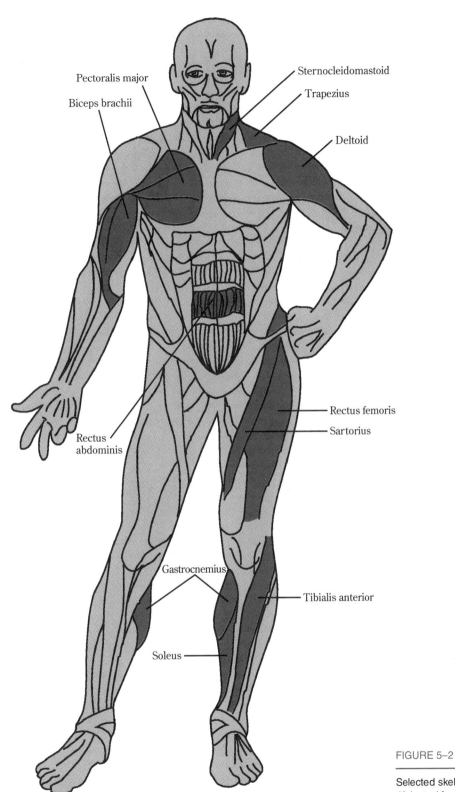

Pectoralis major

Biceps brachii

Sternocleidomastoid

Trapezius

Deltoid

Rectus
abdominis

Rectus femoris

Sartorius

Gastrocnemius

Tibialis anterior

Soleus

FIGURE 5–2

Selected skeletal muscles (anterior view).
(Adapted from MediClip Art, *Alpha Media,*
1992, with permission from Charles McColgan.)

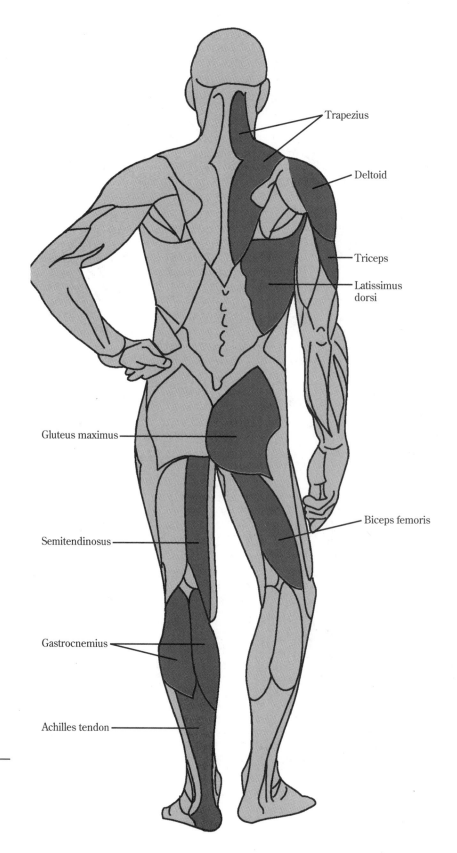

FIGURE 5–3

Selected skeletal muscles and the
Achilles tendon (posterior view).
(Adapted from MediClip Art, *Alpha
Media, 1992, with permission from
Charles McColgan.)*

Functions of Muscles

The following is a list of the primary functions of the muscular system:

1. Muscles are responsible for movement. The types of movement are locomotion, propulsion of substances through tubes as in circulation and digestion, and changes in the size of openings as in the contraction and relaxation of the iris of the eye.
2. Muscles help to maintain posture through a continual partial contraction of skeletal muscles. This process is known as tonicity.
3. Muscles help to produce heat through the chemical changes involved in muscular action.

Insights

EXERCISE—Benefits and Injuries

Each year, more and more evidence indicates that regular physical activity can help the human body maintain, repair, and improve itself. Regular aerobic and weight-bearing exercises, such as aerobic dance, brisk walking, weight-lifting, and bicycling, improve heart and lung function, and muscle tone. To maintain aerobic fitness, one needs to exercise three times a week for 20 to 30 minutes at his or her target heart rate.

Other benefits of exercise are:

- It reduces the risk for heart disease.
- It may slow down the progression of osteoporosis.
- It reduces the levels of triglycerides, and raises the "good" cholesterol (high density lipoproteins)
- It can lower systolic and diastolic blood pressure.
- It may improve blood glucose levels in the diabetic patient.
- Combined with a low-fat, low-calorie diet, it is effective in preventing obesity, and helping individuals maintain a proper body weight.
- It strengthens muscles and keeps joints, tendons, and ligaments more flexible.
- It can elevate one's mood and reduce anxiety and tension.

Although there are many benefits of exercise, it carries a number of risks due to the stresses placed on joints, muscles, tendons, and connective tissue. Injuries caused by sports and/or exercise are very common. Some of the most common types of injuries are bone bruise, bursitis, tendonitis, muscle cramps, sprains, stress fractures, strains, bone spurs, and pulled muscles.

In basketball, tennis, track, running, and brisk walking, the Achilles' tendon is most commonly injured. This tendon can become inflamed and/or torn. In baseball and swimming, the tendons of the shoulder are commonly injured. In tennis, players are susceptible to tennis elbow, as are politicians who shake the hands of many people. Knee injuries account for many sports injuries, as well as presenting problems for many patients who engage in strenuous physical activity.

The best way to prevent injuries due to exercise and/or sports is to build muscle strength gradually. Muscles respond to increased use by becoming larger and stronger. Warm-up exercises are very important in conditioning the body and preparing it for exercise. Stretching exercises stimulate muscle circulation, and help keep joints and tendons flexible.

The Aerobics and Fitness Association of America recommends the following guidelines for stretching your workout:

(Insights continues on next page)

1. A warm-up should include a balanced combination of static stretching and rhythmic limbering.
2. End a workout with static stretching.
3. Follow aerobic workouts with a sufficient cool-down period including hamstring and calf stretches.
4. After completing exercises for a specific muscle group, always stretch those muscles.

When there is a minor musculoskeletal injury, the First Aid treatment is RICE (rest, ice, compression, and elevation). If the injury is severe, then medical and/or surgical treatment should begin as soon as possible.

Exercise has numerous benefits, but injuries do occur. It is wise to know one's body and to recognize any warning signs that could indicate injury. It is best to always seek advice from your physician before beginning any exercise program.

Terminology with Surgical Procedures & Pathology

Term	Word Parts			Definition
abductor (ăb-dŭk′ tōr)	ab	P	away from	A muscle that, on contraction, draws away from the middle
	duct	R	to lead	
	or	S	a doer	
adductor (ă-dŭk′ tōr)	ad	P	toward	A muscle that draws a part toward the middle
	duct	R	to lead	
	or	S	a doer	
antagonist (ăn-tăg′ ō-nĭst)	ant	P	against	A muscle that counteracts the action of another muscle
	agon	R	agony, a contest	
	ist	S	agent	
aponeurorrhaphy (ăp″ ō-nū-ror′ ă-fē)	apo	P	separation	Suture of an aponeurosis
	neuro	CF	nerve	
	rrhaphy	S	suture	
aponeurosis (ăp″ ō-nū-rō′ sĭs)	apo	P	separation	A fibrous sheet of connective tissue that serves to attach muscle to bone or to other tissues
	neur	R	nerve	
	osis	S	condition of	
ataxia (ă-tăks′ ĭ-ă)	a	P	lack of	A lack of muscular coordination
	taxia	S	order	
atonic (ă-tŏn′ ĭk)	a	P	lack of	Pertaining to a lack of normal tone or tension
	ton	R	tone, tension	
	ic	S	pertaining to	
atrophy (ăt′ rō-fē)	a	P	lack of	A lack of nourishment; a wasting of muscular tissue caused by lack of use
	trophy	S	nourishment, development	
biceps (bī′ sĕps)	bi	P	two	A muscle with two heads or points of origin
	ceps	S	head	
brachialgia (brā″ kĭ-ăl′ jĭ-ă)	brachi	CF	arm	Pain in the arm
	algia	S	pain	
bradykinesia (brăd″ ĭ-kĭ-nē′ sĭ-ă)	brady	P	slow	Slowness of motion or movement
	kinesia	S	motion	
clonic (klŏn′ ĭk)	clon	R	turmoil	Pertaining to alternate contraction and relaxation of muscles
	ic	S	pertaining to	
contraction (kŏn-trăk′ shŭn)	con	P	with, together	The process of drawing up and thickening of a muscle fiber
	tract	R	to draw	
	ion	S	process	

(Terminology—continued)

Term	Word Parts			Definition
dactylospasm (dăk′ tĭ-lō-spăzm)	dactylo spasm	CF S	finger or toe tension, spasm	Cramp of a finger or toe
diaphragm (dī′ ă-frăm)	dia phragm	P S	through a fence, partition	The partition, of muscles and membranes, that separates the chest cavity and the abdominal cavity
dystonia (dĭs′ tō′ nĭ-ă)	dys ton ia	P R S	difficult tone, tension condition	A condition of impaired muscle tone
dystrophy (dĭs′ trō-fē)	dys trophy	P S	difficult nourishment, development	Faulty muscular development caused by lack of nourishment
fascia (făsh′ ĭ-ă)	fasc ia	R S	a band condition	A thin layer of connective tissue covering, supporting, or connecting the muscles or inner organs of the body
fasciectomy (făsh″ ĭ-ĕk′ tō-mē)	fasci ectomy	CF S	a band excision	Surgical excision of fascia
fasciodesis (făsh ĭ-ŏd′ ĕ-sĭs)	fascio desis	CF S	a band binding	Surgical binding of a fascia to a tendon or another fascia
fascioplasty (făsh ′ ĭ-ō-plăs ″ tē)	fascio plasty	CF S	a band surgical repair	Surgical repair of a fascia
fascitis (fă-sī′ tĭs)	fasc itis	R S	a band inflammation	Inflammation of a fascia
fibromyitis (fī″ brō-mī-ī′ tĭs)	fibro my itis	CF R S	fiber muscle inflammation	Inflammation of muscle and fibrous tissue
insertion (ĭn″ sûr′ shŭn)	in sert ion	P R S	into to gain process	The point of attachment of a muscle to the part that it moves
intramuscular (ĭn″ tră-mŭs′kū-lər)	intra muscul ar	P R S	within muscle pertaining to	Pertaining to within a muscle
isometric (ī″ sō-mĕt′ rĭk)	iso metr ic	CF R S	equal to measure pertaining to	Pertaining to having equal measure
isotonic (ī″ sō-tŏn′ ĭk)	iso ton ic	CF R S	equal tone, tension pertaining to	Pertaining to having the same tone or tension

(Terminology—continued)

Term	Word Parts			Definition
levator (lē-vā′ tər)	levat or	R S	lifter a doer	A muscle that raises or elevates a part
lordosis (lòr-dō′ sĭs)	lord osis	R S	bending condition of	Abnormal anterior curve of the spine
myalgia (mī-ăl′ jĭ-ă)	my algia	R S	muscle pain	Pain in the muscle
myasthenia (mī-ăs-thē′ nĭ-ă)	my asthenia	R S	muscle weakness	Muscle weakness
myitis (mī-ī′ tĭs)	my itis	R S	muscle inflammation	Inflammation of a muscle
myoblast (mī′ ō blăst)	myo blast	CF S	muscle immature cell, germ cell	An embryonic cell that develops into a cell of muscle fiber
myofibroma (mī″ ō fĭ-brō′ mă)	myo fibr oma	CF R S	muscle fiber tumor	A tumor that contains muscle and fiber
myogenesis (mī″ ō-jĕn′ ĕ-sĭs)	myo genesis	CF F	muscle formation, produce	Formation of muscle tissue
myograph (mī′ ō-grăf)	myo graph	CF S	muscle to write, record	An instrument used to record muscular contractions
myoid (mī′ oid)	my oid	R S	muscle resemble	Resembling muscle
myokinesis (mī″ ō-kĭn-ē′ sĭs)	myo kinesis	CF S	muscle motion	Muscular motion or activity
myology (mĭ-ŏl ō-jē)	myo logy	CF S	muscle study of	The study of muscles
myolysis (mī-ŏl′ ĭ-sĭs)	myo lysis	CF S	muscle destruction	Destruction of muscle tissue
myoma (mī-ō′ mă)	my oma	R S	muscle tumor	A tumor containing muscle tissue
myomalacia (mī″ ō-mă-lā′ sĭ-ă)	myo malacia	CF S	muscle softening	Softening of muscle tissue
myomelanosis (mī″ ō-mĕl-ă-nō′ sĭs)	myo melan osis	CF R S	muscle black condition of	A condition of abnormal darkening of muscle tissue

(Terminology—continued)

Term	Word Parts			Definition
myoparesis (mī″ō-păr′ĕ-sĭs)	myo paresis	CF S	muscle weakness	Weakness or slight paralysis of a muscle
myopathy (mī-ŏp′ă-thē)	myo pathy	CF S	muscle disease	Muscle disease
myoplasty (mī′-ŏ-plăs″tē)	myo plasty	CF S	muscle surgical repair	Surgical repair of a muscle
myorrhaphy (mī-ŏr′ă-fē)	myo rrhaphy	CF S	muscle suture	Suture of a muscle wound
myorrhexis (mī-ŏr-ĕk′sĭs)	myo rrhexis	CF S	muscle rupture	Rupture of a muscle
myosarcoma (mī″ō-sar-kō′mă)	myo sarc oma	CF R S	muscle flesh tumor	A malignant tumor derived from muscle tissue
myosclerosis (mī″ō-sklĕr-ō′sĭs)	myo scler osis	CF R S	muscle hardening condition of	A condition of hardening of muscle
myospasm (mī″ō-spăzm)	myo spasm	CF S	muscle tension, spasm	Spasmodic contraction of a muscle
myotenositis (mī″ō-tĕn″ō-sī′tĭs)	myo tenos itis	CF R S	muscle tendon inflammation	Inflammation of a muscle and its tendon
myotome (mī′ō-tōm)	myo tome	CF S	muscle instrument to cut	An instrument used to cut muscle
myotomy (mī″ŏt′ō-mē)	myo tomy	CF S	muscle incision	Incision into a muscle
myotrophy (mī″ŏt′rō-fē)	myo trophy	CF S	muscle nourishment, development	Nourishment of muscle tissue
neuromuscular (nū″rō-mŭs′kū-lăr)	neuro muscul ar	CF R S	nerve muscle pertaining to	Pertaining to both nerves and muscles
neuromyopathic (nū″rō-mī″ō-păth′ĭk)	neuro myo path ic	CF CF R S	nerve muscle disease pertaining to	Pertaining to disease of both nerves and muscles
neuromyositis (nū″rō-mī″ō-sī′tĭs)	neuro myos itis	CF R S	nerve muscle inflammation	Inflammation of nerves and muscles

(Terminology—continued)

Term	Word Parts			Definition
polymyoclonus (pŏl″ ē-mī ŏk′ lō-nŭs)	poly myo clon us	P CF R S	many muscle turmoil pertaining to	Pertaining to a shock-like muscular contraction occurring in various muscles at the same time
polyplegia (pŏl″ ē-plē′ jĭ-ă)	poly plegia	P S	many stroke, paralysis	Paralysis affecting many muscles
quadriceps (kwŏd′ rĭ-sĕps)	quadri ceps	CF S	four head	A muscle that has four heads or points of origin
relaxation (rē-lăk-sā′ shŭn)	relaxat ion	R S	to loosen process	The process in which a muscle loosens and returns to a resting stage
rhabdomyoma (răb″ dō-mī-ō′ mă)	rhabdo my oma	CF R S	rod muscle tumor	A tumor of striated muscle tissue
rotation (rō-tā′ shŭn)	rotat ion	R S	to turn process	The process of moving a body part around a central axis
sarcitis (sar-sī′ tĭs)	sarc itis	R S	flesh inflammation	Inflammation of muscle tissue
sarcolemma (sar″ kō-lĕm′ ă)	sarco lemma	CF R	flesh a rind	A plasma membrane surrounding each striated muscle fiber
spasticity (spăs-tĭs′ ĭ-tē)	spastic ity	R S	convulsive condition	A condition of increased muscular tone causing stiff and awkward movements
sternocleidoma-stoid (stur″ nō-klī″ dō-măs′ toyd)	sterno cleido mast oid	CF CF R S	sternum clavicle breast resemble	Muscle arising from the sternum and clavicle with its insertion in the mastoid process
synergetic (sin″ ĕr-jĕt′ ĭk)	syn erget ic	P R S	with, together work pertaining to	Pertaining to certain muscles that work together
tenodesis (tĕn-ōd′ ĕ-sĭs)	teno desis	CF S	tendon binding	Surgical binding of a tendon
tenodynia (tĕn″ ō-dĭn-ĭ-ă)	teno dynia	CF S	tendon pain	Pain in a tendon
tenorrhaphy (tĕn-ōr′ ă-fē)	teno rrhaphy	CF S	tendon suture	Suture of a tendon

(Terminology—continued)

Term	Word Parts			Definition
tenotomy (tĕn-ŏt′ ō-mē)	teno tomy	CF S	tendon incision	Surgical incision of a tendon
tonic (tŏn′ ĭk)	ton ic	R S	tone, tension pertaining to	Pertaining to tone, especially muscular tension
torticollis (tŏr″ tĭ-kŏl′ ĭs)	torti collis	CF R	twisted neck	Stiff neck caused by spasmodic contraction of the muscles of the neck; wry neck
triceps (trī′ sĕps)	tri ceps	P S	three head	A muscle having three heads with a single insertion
voluntary (vŏl′ ŭn-tĕr″ ē)	volunt ary	R S	will pertaining to	Pertaining to under the control of one's will

Vocabulary Words

Vocabulary words are terms that have not been divided into component parts. They are common words or specialized terms associated with the subject of this chapter. These words are provided to enhance your medical vocabulary.

Word	Definition
acetylcholine (ă″ sĕt-ĭl-kō′ lēn)	An ester of choline that is stored in vesicles of the nerve terminal; acts on the membrane of the muscle fiber causing generation of impulse
amputation (ăm″ pū-tā′ shŭn)	Surgical excision of a limb, part, or other appendage
contracture (kŏn-trăk′ chūr)	A condition in which a muscle shortens and renders the muscle resistant to the normal stretching process
degeneration (dē-gĕn″ ĕ-rā′ shŭn)	The process of deteriorating; to change from a higher to a lower form
dermatomyositis (dĕr″ mă-tō-mī″ ō-sī′ tĭs)	Inflammation of the muscles and the skin; a connective tissue disease characterized by edema, dermatitis, and inflammation of the muscles
diathermy (dī′ ă-thĕr″ mē)	Treatment using high-frequency current to produce heat within a part of the body; used to increase blood flow and should not be used in acute stage of recovery from trauma. Types: **Microwave.** Electromagnetic radiation is directed to specified tissues **Short-wave.** High-frequency electric current (wavelength of 3–30 m) is directed to specified tissues **Ultrasound.** High-frequency sound waves (20,000–10 billion cycles/sec) are directed to specified tissues

(Vocabulary—continued)

Word	Definition
Dupuytren's contracture (dū-pwē-trăn′ kŏn-trăk′ chūr)	A slow, progressive contracture of the palmar fascia causing the ring and little fingers to bend into the palm so that they cannot be extended
dystrophin (dĭs-trŏf′ ĭn)	A protein found in muscle cells; when the gene that is responsible for this protein is defective and sufficient dystrophin is not produced, muscle wasting occurs
exercise (ĕk′ sĕr-sīz)	Performed activity of the muscles for improvement of health or correction of deformity. Types: **Active.** The patient contracts and relaxes his or her muscles **Assistive.** The patient contracts and relaxes his or her muscles with the assistance of a therapist **Isometric.** Active muscular contraction performed against stable resistance, thereby not shortening the muscle length **Passive.** Exercise is performed by another individual without the assistance of the patient **Range of Motion.** Movement of each joint through its full range of motion. Used to prevent loss of motility or to regain usage after an injury or fracture **Relief of Tension.** Technique used to promote relaxation of the muscles and provide relief from tension
extrinsic (ĕks-trĭn′ sĭk)	Pertaining to external origin; a muscle or muscles partly attached to the trunk and partly to a limb
fatigue (fă-tēg′)	A state of tiredness or weariness occurring in a muscle as a result of repeated contractions
fibromyalgia (fī″ brō-mī-ăl′ jē-ă)	A condition with widespread muscular pain and debilitating fatigue; believed to have an organic or biochemical cause. Diagnosis may be made by testing for unusual tenderness at specific body points
First Aid Treatment—RICE Rest Ice Compression Elevation	Cryotherapy (use of cold) is the treatment of choice for soft tissue injuries and muscle injuries. It causes vasoconstriction of blood vessels and is effective in diminishing bleeding and edema. Ice should not be placed directly onto the skin **Compression** by an elastic bandage is generally determined by the type of injury and the preference of the physician. Some experts disagree on the use of elastic bandages. When used, the bandage should be 3 to 4 inches wide and applied firmly, and toes or fingers should be periodically checked for blue or white discoloration, indicating that the bandage is too tight **Elevation** is used to reduce swelling. The injured part should be elevated on two or three pillows
flaccid (flăs′ sĭd)	Lacking muscle tone; weak, soft, and flabby
heat (hēt)	**Thermotherapy.** The treatment using scientific application of heat may be used 48 to 72 hours after the injury. Types: heating pad, hot water bottle, hot packs, infrared light, and immersion of body part in warm water. Extreme care should be followed when using or applying heat

(Vocabulary—continued)

Word	Definition
hydrotherapy (hī-drō-thĕr′ ă-pē)	Treatment using scientific application of water; types: hot tub, cold bath, whirlpool, and vapor bath
intrinsic (ĭn-trĭn′ sĭk)	Pertaining to internal origin; a muscle or muscles that have their origin and insertion within a structure
involuntary (ĭn-vŏl′ ŭn-tăr″ ē)	Pertaining to action independent of the will
manipulation (măh-nĭp″ ŭ-lā′ shŭn)	The process of using the hands to handle or manipulate as in massage of the body
massage (măh-săhzh)	To knead, apply pressure and friction to external body tissues
muscular dystrophy (mŭs′ kū-lăr dĭs′ trō-fē)	A chronic, progressive wasting and weakening of muscles. It is a familial disease and onset is usually at an early age
myositis (mī-ō-sī′ tĭs)	Inflammation of muscle tissue
origin (ȯr′ ĭ-jĭn)	The beginning of anything; the more fixed attachment of a skeletal muscle
position (pō-zĭsh′ ŭn)	Bodily posture or attitude; the manner in which a patient's body may be arranged for examination Types of positions and their descriptions: **Anatomic.** Body is erect, head facing forward, arms by the sides with palms to the front; used as the position of reference in designating the site or direction of a body structure **Dorsal Recumbent.** Patient is on back with lower extremities flexed and rotated outward; used in application of obstetric forceps, vaginal and rectal examination, and bimanual palpation **Fowler's.** The head of the bed or examining table is raised about 18 inches or 46 cm, and the patient sits up with knees also elevated **Knee-Chest.** Patient on knees, thighs upright, head and upper part of chest resting on bed or examining table, arms crossed and above head; used in sigmoidoscopy, displacement of prolapsed uterus, rectal exams, and flushing of intestinal canal **Lithotomy.** Patient is on back with lower extremities flexed and feet placed in stirrups; used in vaginal examination, Pap smear, vaginal operations, and diagnosis and treatment of diseases of the urethra and bladder **Orthopneic.** Patient sits upright or erect; used for patients with dyspnea **Prone.** Patient lying face downward; used in examination of the back, injections, and massage **Sims'.** Patient is lying on left side, right knee and thigh flexed well up above left leg that is slightly flexed, left arm behind the body, and right arm forward, flexed at elbow; used in examination of rectum, sigmoidoscopy, enema, and intrauterine irrigation after labor

(Vocabulary—continued)

Word	Definition
	Supine. Patient lying flat on back with face upward and arms at the sides; used in examining the head, neck, chest, abdomen, and extremities and in assessing vital signs
	Trendelenburg. Patient's body is supine on a bed or examining table that is tilted at about 45° angle with the head lower than the feet; used to displace abdominal organs during surgery and in treating cardiovascular shock; also called the "shock position"
prosthesis (prŏs′ thē-sĭs)	An artificial device, organ, or part such as a hand, arm, leg, or tooth
rheumatism (roo′ mă-tĭzm)	A general term used to describe conditions characterized by inflammation, soreness and stiffness of muscles, and pain in joints
rigor mortis (rĭg′ ur mȯr tĭs)	Stiffness of skeletal muscles seen in death
rotator cuff (rō-tā′ tor kŭf)	A term used to describe the muscles immediately surrounding the shoulder joint. They stabilize the shoulder joint while the entire arm is moved
strain (strān)	Excessive, forcible stretching of a muscle or the musculotendinous unit
synovectomy (sĭn″ ō-vĕk′ tō-mē)	Surgical excision of a synovial membrane
tendon (tĕn′ dŭn)	A band of fibrous connective tissue serving for the attachment of muscles to bones
torsion (tȯr′ shŭn)	The process of being twisted

ABBREVIATIONS

ADP	adenosine diphosphate	**FROM**	full range of motion
AE	above elbow	**Ht**	height
AK	above knee	**IM**	intramuscular
ALD	aldolase	**LDH**	lactic dehydrogenase
AST	aspartate transaminase	**LOM**	limitation or loss of motion
ATP	adenosine triphosphate	**MS**	musculoskeletal
BE	below elbow	**NSAID**	nonsteroidal anti-inflammatory drug
BK	below knee		
Ca	calcium	**PM**	physical medicine
CPK	creatine phosphokinase	**PMR**	physical medicine and rehabilitation
CPM	continuous passive motion		
DTR's	deep tendon reflexes	**ROM**	range of motion
EMG	electromyography		

SGOT	serum glutamic oxaloacetic transaminase	**sh**	shoulder
		TBW	total body weight
SGPT	serum glutamic pyruvic transaminase	**TJ**	triceps jerk
		Wt	weight

Drug Highlights

Drugs that are generally used for muscular system diseases and disorders include skeletal muscle relaxants and stimulants, neuromuscular blocking agents, anti-inflammatory agents, and analgesics. See Chapter 4, The Skeletal System, Drug Highlights for a description of anti-inflammatory agents and analgesics.

Skeletal Muscle Relaxants

Used to treat painful muscle spasms that may result from strains, sprains, and musculoskeletal trauma or disease. Centrally acting muscle relaxants act by depressing the central nervous system (CNS) and can be administered either orally or by injection. The patient must be informed of the sedative effect produced by these drugs. Drowsiness, dizziness, and blurred vision may diminish the patient's ability to drive a vehicle, operate equipment, or climb stairs.

Examples: Paraflex (chlorzoxazone), Flexeril (cyclobenzaprine HCl), and Robaxin (methocarbamol).

Skeletal Muscle Stimulants

Used in the treatment of myasthenia gravis. This disease is characterized by progressive weakness of skeletal muscles and their rapid fatiguing. Skeletal muscle stimulants act by inhibiting the action of acetylcholinesterase, the enzyme that halts the action of acetylcholine at the neuromuscular junction. By slowing the destruction of acetylcholine, these drugs foster accumulation of higher concentrations of this neurotransmitter and increase the number of interactions between acetylcholine and the available receptors on muscle fibers.

Examples: Mytelase (ambenonium chloride), Tensilon (edrophonium chloride), and Prostigmin Bromide (neostigmine bromide).

Neuromuscular Blocking Agents

Used to provide muscle relaxation. These agents are used in patients undergoing surgery and/or electroconvulsive therapy, endotracheal intubation, and to relieve laryngospasm.

Examples: Tracrium (atracurium besylate), Flaxedil (gallamine triethiodide), and Norcuron (vecuronium).

Communication Enrichment

This segment is provided for those who wish to enhance their ability to communicate in either English or Spanish.

RELATED TERMS

English	Spanish
muscle	músculo (*mūs*-kū-lō)
muscle spasm	espasmo muscular (ĕs-*păs*-mō *mŭs*-kū-lăr)
raise your:	levante su: (lĕ-*văn*-tĕ sū:)
arm	brazo (*bră*-zō)
leg	pierna (pĭ-*ĕr*-nă)
muscle biopsy	biopsia muscular (bĭ-*ōp*-sĭ-ă *mŭs*-kū-lăr)
weight	peso (*pĕ*-sō)
height	altura (ăl-*tū*-ră)
malaise	malestar (*mă*-lĕs-tăr)
painful	doloroso (dō-lō-*rō*-sō)
shoulder	hombro (*ōm*-brō)
stiffness	tiesura (tĭ-ĕ-*sū*-ră)
contraction	contracción (cōn-trăk-sĭ-*ōn*)
twitch	crispamiento (*krĭs*-pă-mĭ-ĕn-tō)
tighten	estrechar (ĕs-trĕ-*chăr*)
walk	caminar (*kă*-mĭ-năr)
limitation of movement	limitación de movimiento (lĭ-mĭ-tă-sĭ-*ōn* dĕ *mō*-vĭ-mĭ-ĕn-tō)
tendon	tendón (*tĕn*-dōn)
neck	cuello (*kwā*-yō)
finger, toe	dedo (*dĕ*-dō)

English	Spanish
fiber	fibra (*fĭ*-bră)
bend	vuelta (*vū*-ĕl-tă)
motion	moción (*mō*-sĭ-ōn)
weakness	debilidad (dĕ-bĭ-lĭ-*dăd*)
fatigue	fatiga (*fă*-tĭ-gă)
tone	tono (*tō*-nō)
flaccid	flacido (*flă*-sĭ-dō)
position	posición (pō-sĭ-sĭ-*ōn*)
development	desarrollo (dĕ-să-*rō*-jō)
exercise	ejercicio (ĕ-hĕr-*sĭ*-sĭ-ō)
amputate	amputar (ăm-pū-*tăr*)
sport	deporte (dĕ-*pōr*-tĕ)
heat	calor (kă-*lōr*)
massage	masaje (mă-*să*-hĕ)
harden	endurecer (ĕn-*dū*-rĕ-sĕr)
tense	tenso (*tĕn*-sō)
nourishment	nutrimento (nū-trĭ-mĭ-*ĕn*-tō)
two	dos (dōs)
slow	lento (*lĕn*-tō)

DIAGNOSTIC AND LABORATORY TESTS

Test	Description
aldolase (ALD) blood test (ăl′ dō-lāz blod test)	A test performed on serum that measures ALD enzyme present in skeletal and heart muscle. It is helpful in the diagnosis of Duchenne's muscular dystrophy before symptoms appear.
calcium blood test (kăl′ sē-ŭm blod test)	A test performed on serum to determine levels of calcium. Calcium is essential for muscular contraction, nerve transmission, and blood clotting.
creatine phosphokinase (CPK) (krē′ ă-tĭn fŏs″ fō-kĭn′ āz)	A blood test to determine the level of CPK. It is increased in necrosis or atrophy of skeletal muscle, traumatic muscle injury, strenuous exercise, and progressive muscular dystrophy.
electromyography (EMG) (ē-lĕk″ trō-mī-ŏg′ ră-fē)	A test to measure electrical activity across muscle membranes by means of electrodes that are attached to a needle that is inserted into the muscle. Electrical activity can be heard over a loudspeaker, viewed on an oscilloscope, or printed on a graph (electromyogram). Abnormal results may indicate myasthenia gravis, amyotrophic lateral sclerosis, muscular dystrophy, peripheral neuropathy, and anterior poliomyelitis.
lactic dehydrogenase (LDH) (lăk′ tĭk dē-hī-drŏj′ ĕ-nāz)	A blood test to determine the level of LDH enzyme. It is increased in muscular dystrophy, damage to skeletal muscles, after a pulmonary embolism, and during skeletal muscle malignancy.
muscle biopsy (mŭs′ ĕl bī′ ŏp-sē)	An operative procedure in which a small piece of muscle tissue is excised and then stained for microscopic examination. Lower motor neuron disease, degeneration, inflammatory reactions, or involvement of specific muscle fibers may indicate myopathic disease.
serum glutamic-oxaloacetic transaminase (SGOT) (sē′ rŭm gloo-tăm′ ĭk ŏks″ ăl-ō-ă-sē′ tĭk trăns ăm′ ĭn-āz)	A blood test to determine the level of SGOT enzyme. It is increased in skeletal muscle damage and muscular dystrophy. This test is also called aspartate transaminase (AST).
serum glutamic pyruvic transaminase (SGPT) (sē′ rŭm gloo-tăm′ ĭk pī-roo′ vĭk trăns-ăm′ ĭn-āz)	A blood test to determine the level of SGPT enzyme. It is increased in skeletal muscle damage. This test is also called alanine aminotransferase (ALT).

Learning Exercises

Anatomy and Physiology

Write your answers to the following questions. Do not refer back to the text.

1. The muscular system is made up the three types of muscle tissue. Name the three types.

   a. _____   b. _____

   c. _____

2. Muscles make up approximately _____ percent of a person's body weight.

3. Name the two essential ingredients that are needed for a muscle to perform properly.

   a. _____   b. _____

4. Name the two points of attachment for a skeletal muscle.

   a. _____   b. _____

5. Skeletal muscle is also known as _____ or _____ .

6. A wide, thin, sheet-like tendon is known as an _____.

7. Name the three distinguishable parts of a muscle.

   a. _____   b. _____

   c. _____

8. Define the following:

   a. Antagonist _____

   b. Prime Mover _____

   c. Synergist _____

9. Smooth muscle is also called _____, _____, or _____ .

10. Smooth muscles are found in the internal organs. Name five examples of these locations.

    a. _____   b. _____

    c. _____   d. _____

    e. _____

11. _____ is the muscle of the heart.

12. Name the three primary functions of the muscular system.

    a. _____   b. _____

    c. _____

Word Parts

1. In the spaces provided, write the definition of these prefixes, roots, combining forms, and suffixes. Do not refer to the listings of terminology words. Leave blank those terms you cannot define.

2. After completing as many as you can, refer back to the terminology word listings to check your work. For each word missed or left blank, write the term and its definition several times on the margins of these pages or on a separate sheet of paper.
3. To maximize the learning process, it is to your advantage to do the following exercises as directed. To refer to the terminology listings before completing these exercises invalidates the learning process.

PREFIXES

Give the definitions of the following prefixes:

1. a- _____   2. ab- _____

3. ad- _____   4. ant- _____

5. apo- _____   6. bi- _____

7. brady- _____ 8. con- _____

9. dia- _____   10. dys- _____

11. in- _____   12. intra- _____

13. poly- _____ 14. syn- _____

15. tri- _____

ROOTS AND COMBINING FORMS

Give the definitions of the following roots and combining forms:

1. agon _____   2. brachi _____

3. cleido _____   4. clon _____

5. collis _____   6. dactylo _____

7. duct _____   8. erget _____

9. fasc _____   10. fasci _____

11. fascio _____ 12. fibr _____

13. fibro _____   14. iso _____

15. lemma _____   16. levat _____

17. lord _____   18. mast _____

19. melan _____   20. metr _____

21. muscul _____ 22. my _____

23. myo _____   24. myos _____

25. neur _____   26. neuro _____

27. path _____   28. quadri _____

29. relaxat _____ 30. rhabdo _____

31. rotat _____   32. sarc _____

33. sarco _____   34. scler _____

35. sert _____   36. spastic _____

37. sterno _____ 38. teno _____

39. tenos _____	40. ton _____
41. torti _____	42. tract _____
43. volunt _____	

SUFFIXES

Give the definitions of the following suffixes:

1. -algia _____	2. -ar _____
3. -ary _____	4. -asthenia _____
5. -blast _____	6. -ceps _____
7. -desis _____	8. -dynia _____
9. -ectomy _____	10. -genesis _____
11. -graph _____	12. -ia _____
13. -ic _____	14. -ion _____
15. -ist _____	16. -itis _____
17. -ity _____	18. -kinesia _____
19. -kinesis _____	20. -logy _____
21. -lysis _____	22. -malacia _____
23. -oid _____	24. -oma _____
25. -or _____	26. -osis _____
27. -paresis _____	28. -pathy _____
29. -phragm _____	30. -plasty _____
31. -plegia _____	32. -rrhaphy _____
33. -rrhexis _____	34. -spasm _____
35. -taxia _____	36. -tome _____
37. -tomy _____	38. -trophy _____
39. -us _____	

Identifying Medical Terms

In the spaces provided, write the medical terms for the following meanings:

1. _____ Suture of an aponeurosis
2. _____ Pertaining to a lack of normal tone or tension
3. _____ Slowness of motion or movement
4. _____ Cramp of a finger or toe
5. _____ Faulty muscular development caused by lack of nourishment
6. _____ Surgical repair of a fascia
7. _____ Pertaining to within a muscle

8. _____ A muscle that raises or elevates a part

9. _____ Muscle weakness

10. _____ Formation of muscle tissue

11. _____ Study of muscles

12. _____ Weakness or slight paralysis of a muscle

13. _____ Surgical repair of a muscle

14. _____ A malignant tumor derived from muscle tissue

15. _____ Inflammation of a muscle and its tendon

16. _____ Incision into a muscle

17. _____ Inflammation of nerves and muscles

18. _____ Paralysis affecting many muscles

19. _____ Surgical binding of a tendon

20. _____ Pertaining to certain muscles that work together

21. _____ A muscle having three heads with a single insertion

Spelling

In the spaces provided, write the correct spelling of these misspelled terms:

1. facia _____   2. mykinesis _____

3. polymyclonus _____   4. rhadomyoma _____

5. sarclemma _____   6. sterncleidomastoid _____

7. tentomy _____   8. torticolis _____

Review Questions

Matching

Select the appropriate lettered meaning for each numbered line.

_____ 1. dermatomyositis

_____ 2. fibromyalgia

_____ 3. muscular dystrophy

_____ 4. myositis

_____ 5. prosthesis

_____ 6. rotator cuff

_____ 7. strain

_____ 8. tenodynia

_____ 9. torsion

_____ 10. voluntary

a. A term used to describe the muscles immediately surrounding the shoulder joint

b. The process of being twisted

c. Pain in a tendon

d. Inflammation of the muscles and the skin

e. Inflammation of muscle tissue

f. Pertaining to under the control of one's will

g. A chronic, progressive wasting and weakening of muscles

h. Excessive, forcible stretching of a muscle or the musculotendinous unit

i. A condition with widespread muscular pain and debilitating fatigue

j. An artificial device, organ, or part

k. Pain in a joint

Abbreviations

Place the correct word, phrase, or abbreviation in the space provided.

_____ 1. AE

_____ 2. AST

_____ 3. calcium

_____ 4. electromyography

_____ 5. FROM

_____ 6. MS

_____ 7. range of motion

_____ 8. shoulder

_____ 9. TBW

_____ 10. TJ

Diagnostic and Laboratory Tests

Select the best answer to each multiple choice question. Circle the letter of your choice.

1. A diagnostic test to help diagnose Duchenne's muscular dystrophy before symptoms appear.

    a. creatine phosphokinase

    b. aldolase blood test

    c. calcium blood test

    d. muscle biopsy

2. A test to measure electrical activity across muscle membranes by means of electrodes that are attached to a needle that is inserted into the muscle.

    a. muscle biopsy

    b. lactic dehydrogenase

    c. creatine phosphokinase

    d. electromyography

3. This test is also called aspartate transaminase.

    a. lactic dehydrogenase

    b. serum glutamic oxaloacetic transaminase

    c. serum glutamic pyruvic transaminase

    d. creatine phosphokinase

4. This test is also called alanine aminotransferase.

    a. lactic dehydrogenase

    b. serum glutamic oxaloacetic transaminase

    c. serum glutamic pyruvic transaminase

    d. creatine phosphokinase

5. A/An _____ is where a small piece of muscle tissue is excised and then stained for microscopic examination.

    a. muscle biopsy

    b. electromyography

    c. bone biopsy

    d. electrocardiography

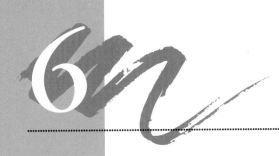

The Digestive System

The digestive system is composed of the mouth, pharynx, esophagus, stomach, and the large and small intestines. Its accessory organs are the salivary glands, the liver, gallbladder, and the pancreas.

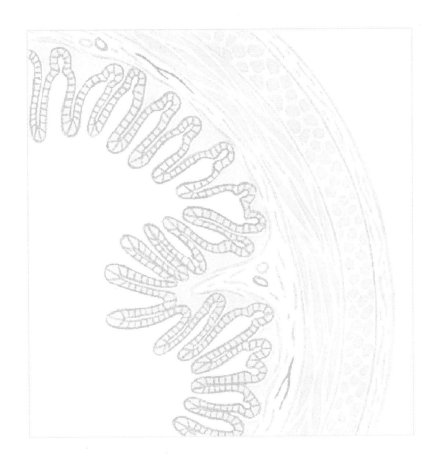

133

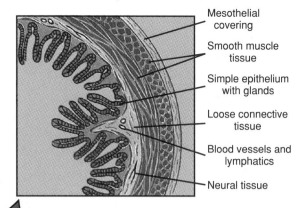

- Mesothelial covering
- Smooth muscle tissue
- Simple epithelium with glands
- Loose connective tissue
- Blood vessels and lymphatics
- Neural tissue

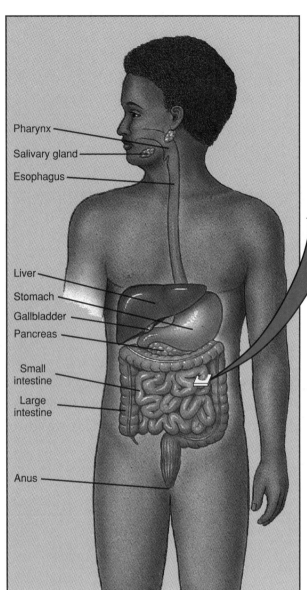

- Pharynx
- Salivary gland
- Esophagus
- Liver
- Stomach
- Gallbladder
- Pancreas
- Small intestine
- Large intestine
- Anus

ANATOMY AND PHYSIOLOGY OVERVIEW

A general description of the digestive system is that of a continuous tube beginning with the mouth and ending at the anus. This tube is known as the alimentary canal and/or gastrointestinal tract. It measures about 30 feet in adults and contains both primary and accessory organs for the conversion of food and fluids into a semiliquid that can be absorbed for use by the body. The three main functions of the digestive system are digestion, absorption, and elimination. Each of the various organs commonly associated with digestion is described in this chapter. The organs of digestion are shown in Figure 6–1 and Plates 9 and 18, as well as in the figure and table on this page.

THE DIGESTIVE SYSTEM

Organ	Functions
Mouth	Breaks food apart by the action of the teeth, moistens and lubricates food with saliva, food formed into a bolus
Pharynx	Common passageway for both respiration and digestion, muscular constrictions move the bolus into the esophagus
Esophagus	Peristalsis moves the food down the esophagus into the stomach
Stomach	Reduces food to a digestible state, converts the food to a semiliquid form
Small Intestine	Digestion and absorption takes place. Nutrients are absorbed into tiny capillaries and lymph vessels in the walls of the small intestine and transmitted to body cells by the circulatory system
Large Intestine	Removes water from the fecal material, stores, and then eliminates waste from the body via the rectum and anus
Salivary Glands	Secretes saliva to moisten and lubricate food
Liver	Changes glucose to glycogen and stores it until needed, changes glycogen back to glucose, desaturates fats, assists in protein catabolism, manufactures bile, fibrinogen, prothrombin, heparin, and blood proteins, stores vitamins, produces heat, and detoxifies substances
Gallbladder	Stores and concentrates bile
Pancreas	Secretes pancreatic juice into the small intestine, contains cells that produce digestive enzymes, secretes insulin and glucagon

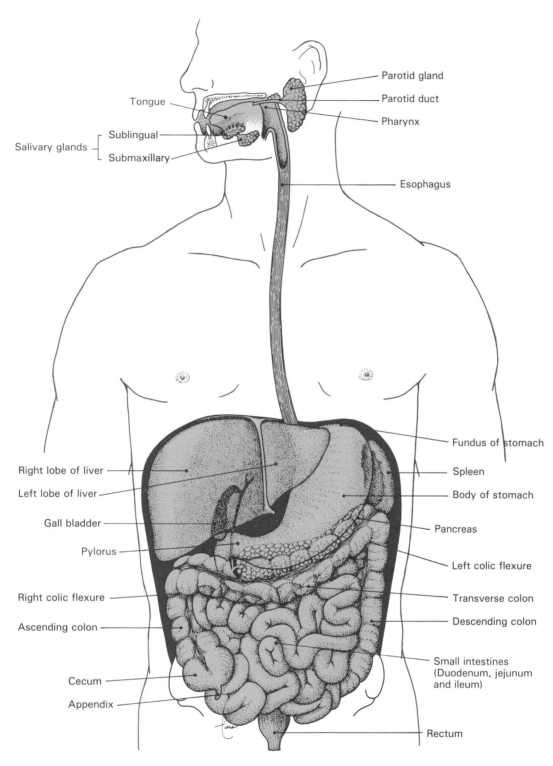

FIGURE 6–1

The digestive system. *(Adapted from Evans WF. Anatomy and Physiology, 3rd ed. Englewood Cliffs, NJ: Prentice-Hall, 1983, with permission.)*

The Mouth

The mouth is the cavity formed by the palate or roof, the lips and cheeks on the sides, and the tongue at its floor. Contained within are the teeth and salivary glands. The cheeks form the lateral walls and are continuous with the lips. The vestibule includes the space between the cheeks and the teeth. The gingivae (gums) surrounds the necks of the teeth. The hard and soft palates provide a roof for the oral cavity, with the tongue at its floor. The free portion of the tongue is connected to the underlying epithelium by a thin fold of mucous membrane, the lingual frenulum. The tongue is made of skeletal muscle and is covered with mucous membrane. The tongue can be divided into a blunt rear portion called the root, a pointed tip, and a central body. Located on the surface of the tongue are papillae (elevations) and taste buds (sweet, salt, sour, and bitter). Three pairs of salivary glands secrete fluids into the oral cavity. These glands are the parotid, sublingual, and the submandibular. The posterior margin of the soft palate supports the dangling uvula and two pairs of muscular pharyngeal arches. On either side, a palatine tonsil lies between an anterior palatoglossal arch and a posterior palatopharyngeal arch. A curving line that connects the palatoglossal arches and uvula forms the boundaries of the fauces, the passageway between the oral cavity and the pharynx (Figure 6–2). Digestion begins as food is broken apart by the action of the teeth, moistened and lubricated by saliva, and formed into a bolus. A bolus is a small mass of masticated food ready to be swallowed.

The Pharynx

Just beyond the mouth, at the beginning of the tube leading to the stomach, is the pharynx. Simply put, the pharynx is a common passageway for both respiration and digestion. Both

FIGURE 6–2

The oral cavity. **A.** The oral cavity as seen in sagittal section. **B.** An anterior view of the oral cavity, as seen through the open mouth. (*From Martini F.* Fundamentals of Anatomy and Physiology, *2nd ed. Englewood Cliffs, NJ: Prentice-Hall, 1992, with permission*.)

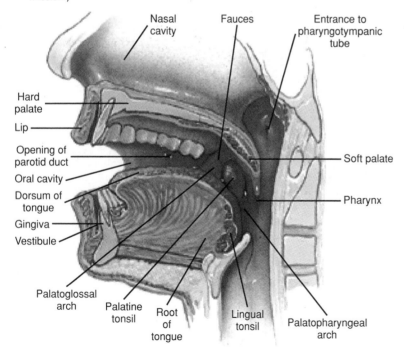

A

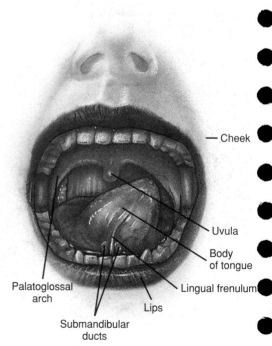

B

the larynx or voicebox and the esophagus begin in the pharynx. Food that is swallowed passes through the pharynx into the esophagus reflexively. Muscular constrictions move the ball of food into the esophagus while, at the same time, blocking the opening to the larynx and preventing the food from entering the airway leading to the trachea or wind-pipe.

The Esophagus

The esophagus is a collapsible tube about 10 inches long that leads from the pharynx to the stomach. Food passes down the esophagus and into the stomach. Food is carried along the esophagus by a series of wave-like muscular contractions call peristalsis.

The Stomach

The stomach is a large sac-like organ into which food passes from the esophagus for storage while undergoing the early processes of digestion. In the stomach, food is further reduced to a digestible state. Hydrochloric acid and gastric juices convert the food to a semiliquid state, which is passed, at intervals, into the small intestine.

The Small Intestine

The small intestine is about 21 feet long and 1 inch in diameter. It extends from the pyloric orifice at the base of the stomach to the entrance of the large intestine. The small intestine is considered to have three parts: the duodenum, the jejunum, and the ileum. The duodenum is the first 12 inches just beyond the stomach. The jejunum is the next 8 feet or so, and the ileum is the remaining 12 feet of the tube. Semiliquid food (called chyme) is received from the stomach through the pylorus and mixed with bile from the liver and gallbladder along with pancreatic juice from the pancreas. Digestion and absorption take place chiefly in the small intestine. Nutrients are absorbed into tiny capillaries and lymph vessels in the walls of the small intestine and transmitted to body cells by the circulatory system.

The Large Intestine

The large intestine is about 5 feet long and 2.5 inches in diameter. It extends from the ileocecal orifice at the small intestine to the anus. The large intestine may be divided into the cecum, the colon, the rectum, and the anal canal. The cecum is a pouch-like structure forming the beginning of the large intestine. It is about 3 inches long and has the appendix attached to it. The colon makes up the bulk of the large intestine and is divided into several parts—the ascending colon, the transverse colon, the descending colon, and, at its end, the sigmoid colon. Digestion and absorption continue in the large intestine on a reduced scale. The waste products of digestion are eliminated from the body via the rectum and the anus.

Accessory Organs

The salivary glands, the liver, the gallbladder, and the pancreas are not actually part of the digestive tube; however, they are closely related to it in their functions. These organs and their functions related to digestion are described below.

THE SALIVARY GLANDS

Located in or near the mouth, the salivary glands secrete saliva in response to the sight, smell, taste, or mental image of food. The various salivary glands are the parotid, located on

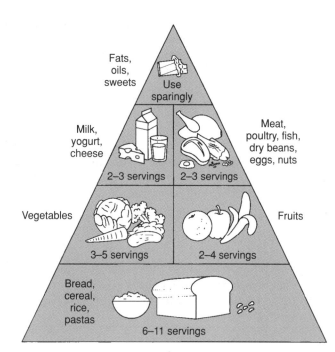

FIGURE 6–3

The Food Guide Pyramid. (*From Martini F.* Fundamentals of Anatomy and Physiology, *2nd ed. Englewood Cliffs, NJ: Prentice-Hall, 1992, with permission.*)

either side of the face slightly below the ear; the submandibular, located in the floor of the mouth; and the sublingual, located below the tongue. All salivary glands secrete through openings into the mouth to moisten and lubricate food.

THE LIVER

The largest glandular organ in the body, the liver weighs about 3 lb and is located in the upper right part of the abdomen. The liver plays an essential role in the normal metabolism of carbohydrates, fats, and proteins. In carbohydrate metabolism, it changes glucose to glycogen and stores it until needed by body cells. It also changes glycogen back to glucose. In fat metabolism, the liver serves as a storage place and acts to desaturate fats before releasing them into the bloodstream. In protein metabolism, the liver acts as a storage place and assists in protein catabolism.

The liver manufactures the following important substances:

1. Bile—a digestive juice
2. Fibrinogen and Prothrombin—coagulants essential for blood clotting
3. Heparin—an anticoagulant that helps to prevent the clotting of blood
4. Blood Proteins—albumin, gamma globulin

Additionally, the liver stores iron and vitamins B_{12}, A, D, E, and K. It also produces body heat and detoxifies many harmful substances such as drugs and alcohol.

THE GALLBLADDER

The gallbladder is a membranous sac attached to the liver in which excess bile is stored and concentrated. Bile leaving the gallbladder is six to ten times as concentrated as that which comes to it from the liver. Concentration is accomplished by absorption of water from the bile into the mucosa of the gallbladder.

THE PANCREAS

The pancreas is a large, elongated gland situated behind the stomach and secreting pancreatic juice into the small intestine. The pancreas is 6 to 9 inches long and contains cells that produce digestive enzymes. Other cells in the pancreas secrete the hormones insulin and glucagon directly into the bloodstream.

Insights

PROPER NUTRITION—A Plan To Improve Health

You have heard the saying, "you are what you eat." The correlation between dietary habits and health has become a much researched topic. Much has been learned about fat intake and heart disease; calcium intake and osteoporosis; sodium and hypertension; and fiber-containing grain products, fruits, and vegetables and cancer. According to the National Institutes of Health, over one third of cancer deaths in 1992 may be related to diet. This Institute has launched a program called "5 A Day for Better Health." It recommends eating at least five servings of fruits and vegetables daily, as a way of reducing the risk of cancer.

Some dietary substances showing anticarcinogenic activity in animal studies include vitamins A, C, E, and beta-carotene, the minerals calcium and selenium, and some forms of fiber.

Some foods are better than others, and the following are foods that you should include in your diet, at least once a week.

1. Broccoli contains a nutrient that is believed to help protect against cancer. If you do not like broccoli try cauliflower, cabbage, and/or turnips.
2. Dry beans provide protein, without fat or cholesterol.
3. Nonfat yogurt is a good source of calcium.
4. Fish (most) provides protein without excess fat. Some fish, such as tuna, salmon, mackerel, herring, and sardines, contain small amounts of omega-3 oils, that help fight heart disease.
5. Whole wheat bread, pasta, and cereals are high in fiber that aids in digestion and helps prevent constipation, and possible colorectal cancer.
6. Oatmeal is high in soluble fiber, and it is believed to help lower cholesterol. Other sources of soluble fiber are apples, peas, dried beans, prunes, and lentils.

In 1992, the United States Department of Agriculture unveiled the new "Food Guide Pyramid," made up of six food groups. This pyramid, provides a guide to choosing the proper foods, one should eat on a daily basis. See Figure 6–3.
The six food groups are:
- Bread, Cereal, Rice, and Pasta (6–11 servings/day)
- Fruit (2–4 servings/day)
- Vegetable (3–5 servings/day)
- Milk, Yogurt, and Cheese (2–3 servings/day)
- Meat, Poultry, Fish, Dry Beans, Eggs, and Nuts (2–3 servings/day)
- Fats, Oils, and Sweets (use sparingly).

The positive benefits of proper nutrition are many. It is believed that if one eats a variety of foods, maintains desirable weight, avoids too much fat, sugar, and sodium, eats high-fiber foods, and drinks alcoholic beverages in moderation, the quality of life will be improved, and certain diseases may be prevented.

Terminology with Surgical Procedures & Pathology

Term	Word Parts			Definition
amylase (ăm′ ĭ-lās)	amyl ase	R S	starch enzyme	An enzyme that breaks down starch
anabolism (ă-năb′ ō-lĭzm)	ana bol ism	P R S	up to cast, throw condition of	Literally "a throwing upward"; the building up of the body substance
anorexia (ăn″ ō-rĕks′ ĭ-ă)	an orexia	P S	lack of appetite	Lack of appetite
anoscope (ā′ nō-skōp)	ano scope	CF S	anus instrument	An instrument used to examine the anus
appendectomy (ăp″ ĕn-dĕk′ tō-mē)	append ectomy	R S	appendix excision	Surgical excision of the appendix
appendicitis (ă-pĕn″ dĭ-sī′ tĭs)	appendic itis	R S	appendix inflammation	Inflammation of the appendix
biliary (bĭl′ ĭ-ār″ ē)	bili ary	CF S	gall, bile pertaining to	Pertaining to or conveying bile
buccal (bək′ əl)	bucc al	R S	cheek pertaining to	Pertaining to the cheek
catabolism (kă-tăb′ ō-lĭzm)	cata bol ism	P R S	down to cast, throw condition of	Literally "a throwing down"; a breaking of complex substances into more basic elements
celiac (sē′ lĭ-ăk)	celi ac	R S	abdomen, belly pertaining to	Pertaining to the abdomen
cheilosis (kī-lō′ sĭs)	cheil osis	R S	lip condition of	An abnormal condition of the lip as seen in riboflavin and other B-complex deficiencies
cholecystectomy (kō″ lē-sĭs-tĕk′ tō-mē)	chole cyst ectomy	CF R S	gall, bile bladder excision	Surgical excision of the gallbladder
cholecystitis (kō″ lē-sĭs-tī′ tĭs)	chole cyst itis	CF R S	gall, bile bladder inflammation	Inflammation of the gallbladder
choledochotomy (kō-lĕd″ ō-kŏt′ ō-mē)	choledocho tomy	CF S	common bile duct incision	Surgical incision of the common bile duct

(Terminology—continued)

Term	Word Parts			Definition
colectomy (kō-lĕk′ tō-mē)	col ectomy	R S	colon excision	Surgical excision of part of the colon
colonic (kō-lŏn′ ĭk)	colon ic	R S	colon pertaining to	Pertaining to the colon
colonoscopy (kō-lŏn-ŏs′ kō-pē)	colono scopy	CF S	colon to view, examine	Examination of the upper portion of the colon
colorrhaphy (kŏ-lōr′ ăh-fē)	colo rrhaphy	CF S	colon suture	Suture of the colon
colostomy (kō-lŏs′ tō-mē)	colo stomy	CF S	colon new opening	The creation of a new opening into the colon
dentalgia (dĕn-tăl′ jĭ-ā)	dent algia	R S	tooth pain	Pain in a tooth; toothache
dentibuccal (dĕn″ tĭ-bŭk′ l)	denti bucc al	CF R S	tooth cheek pertaining to	Pertaining to the teeth and the cheek
dentist (dĕn′ təst)	dent ist	R S	tooth one who specializes	One who specializes in dentistry
diverticulitis (dī″ vĕr-tĭk″ ū-lī′ tĭs)	diverticul itis	R S	diverticula inflammation	Inflammation of the diverticula in the colon
duodenal (dū″ ō-dē′ năl)	duoden al	R S	duodenum pertaining to	Pertaining to the duodenum; the first part of the small intestine
dyspepsia (dĭs-pĕp′ sĭ-ā)	dys pepsia	P S	difficult to digest	Difficulty in digestion; indigestion
dysphagia (dĭs-fā′ jĭ-ā)	dys phagia	P S	difficult to eat	Difficulty in swallowing
enteric (ĕn-tĕr′ ĭk)	enter ic	R S	intestine pertaining to	Pertaining to the intestine
enteritis (ĕn″ tĕr-ī′ tĭs)	enter itis	R S	intestine inflammation	Inflammation of the intestine
enteroclysis (ĕn″ tĕr-ŏk′ lĭ-sĭs)	entero clysis	CF S	intestine injection	Injection of a solution into the intestine
enterostomy (ĕn″ tĕr-ŏs′ tō-mē)	entero stomy	CF S	intestine new opening	The creation of a permanent opening into the intestine

(Terminology—continued)

Term	Word Parts			Definition
epigastric (ĕp′ ĭ-găs′ trĭc)	epi gastr ic	P R S	above stomach pertaining to	Pertaining to the region above the stomach
esophageal (ē-sŏf″ ă-jē′ ăl)	esophage al	CF S	esophagus pertaining to	Pertaining to the esophagus
esophagoscope (ĕ-sŏf′ ă-gō-skōp″)	esophago scope	CF S	esophagus instrument	An instrument used to examine the esophagus
gastralgia (găs-trăl′ jĭ-ă)	gastr algia	R S	stomach pain	Pain in the stomach
gastrectomy (găs-trĕk′ tō-mē)	gastr ectomy	R S	stomach excision	Surgical excision of a part or the whole stomach
gastric (găs′ trĭk)	gastr ic	R S	stomach pertaining to	Pertaining to the stomach
gastrodynia (găs″ trō-dĭn′ ĭ-ă)	gastro dynia	CF S	stomach pain	Pain in the stomach
gastroenterology (găs″ trō-ĕn″ tĕr-ŏl ′ ō-jē)	gastro entero logy	CF CF S	stomach intestine study of	Study of the stomach and the intestines
gastropexy (găs′ trō-pĕk″ sē)	gastro pexy	CF S	stomach fixation	Surgical fixation of the stomach to the abdominal wall
gastroscope (găs′ trō-skōp)	gastro scope	CF S	stomach instrument	An instrument used to view the interior of the stomach
gastrotomy (găs-trŏt′ ō-mē)	gastro tomy	CF S	stomach incision	Surgical incision into the stomach
gingivitis (jĭn″ jĭ-vī′ tĭs)	gingiv itis	R S	gums inflammation	Inflammation of the gums
glossotomy (glŏ-sŏt′ ō-mē)	glosso tomy	CF S	tongue incision	Surgical incision into the tongue
glycogenesis (glī″ kŏ-jĕn′ ĕ-sĭs)	glyco genesis	CF S	sweet, sugar formation, produce	The formation of glycogen from glucose
hematemesis (hĕm″ ăt-ēm′ ĕ-sĭs)	hemat emesis	R S	blood vomiting	Vomiting of blood
hepatitis (hĕp″ ă-tī′ tĭs)	hepat itis	R S	liver inflammation	Inflammation of the liver

(Terminology—continued)

Term	Word Parts			Definition
hepatoma (hĕp″ ă-tŏ′ mă)	hepat oma	R S	liver tumor	A tumor of the liver
hepatomegaly (hĕp″ ă-tō-mĕg′ ă-lē)	hepato megaly	CF S	liver enlargement, large	Enlargement of the liver
hepatotoxin (hĕp″ ă-tō-tŏk′sĭn)	hepato tox in	CF R S	liver poison pertaining to	Pertaining to a substance that is poisonous to the liver
herniotomy (hĕr″ nĭ-ŏt′ ō-mē)	hernio tomy	CF S	hernia incision	Surgical incision for the repair of a hernia
hyperemesis (hī″ pĕr-ĕm′ ĕ-sĭs)	hyper emesis	P S	excessive, above vomiting	Excessive vomiting
hypogastric (hī″ pō-găs′ trĭk)	hypo gastr ic	P R S	deficient, below stomach pertaining to	Pertaining to below the stomach
ileitis (īl″ ē-ī′ tis)	ile itis	R S	ileum inflammation	Inflammation of the ileum
ileostomy (īl″ ē-ŏs′ tō-mē)	ileo stomy	CF S	ileum new opening	The creation of a new opening through the abdominal wall into the ileum
labial (lā′ bĭ-ăl)	labi al	R S	lip pertaining to	Pertaining to the lip
laparotomy (lăp″ ăr-ŏt′ ō-mē)	laparo tomy	CF S	flank, abdomen incision	Surgical incision into the abdomen
laxative (lăk′ să-tĭv)	laxat ive	R S	to loosen nature of, quality of	A substance that acts to loosen the bowels
lingual (lĭng′ gwal)	lingu al	R S	tongue pertaining to	Pertaining to the tongue
lipolysis (lĭp-ŏl′ ĭ-sĭs)	lipo lysis	CF S	fat destruction, to separate	The destruction of fat
malabsorption (măl″ ăb-sōrp′ shŭn)	mal absorpt ion	P R S	bad to suck in process	The process of bad or inadequate absorption of nutrients from the intestinal tract

(Terminology—continued)

Term	Word Parts			Definition
megacolon (mĕg′ ă-kō′ lŏn)	mega colon	P R	large, great colon	A condition in which the colon is extremely enlarged
mesentery (mĕs′ ĕn-tĕr″ ē)	mes enter y	R R S	middle intestine pertaining to	Pertaining to the peritoneal fold encircling the small intestines and connecting the intestines to the abdominal wall
pancreatectomy (păn″ krē-ăt-ĕk′ tō-mē)	pancreat ectomy	R S	pancreas excision	Surgical excision of the pancreas
pancreatitis (păn″ krē-ă-tī′ tĭs)	pancreat itis	R S	pancreas inflammation	Inflammation of the pancreas
peptic (pĕp′ tĭk)	pept ic	R S	to digest pertaining to	Pertaining to gastric digestion
peristalsis (pĕr″ ĭ-stăl′ sĭs)	peri stalsis	P S	around contraction	A wave-like contraction that occurs involuntarily in hollow tubes of the body, especially the alimentary canal
pharyngeal (făr-ĭn′ jē-ăl)	pharynge al	CF S	pharynx pertaining to	Pertaining to the pharynx
postprandial (pōst-prăn′ dĭ-ăl)	post prandi al	P CF S	after meal pertaining to	Pertaining to after a meal
proctalgia (prŏk-tăl′ jĭ-ă)	proct algia	R S	rectum, anus pain	Pain in the rectum and anus
proctologist (prŏk-tŏl′ ō-jĭst)	procto log ist	CF R S	rectum, anus study of one who specializes	One who specializes in the study of the anus and the rectum
proctoscope (prŏk′ tō-scōp)	procto scope	CF S	rectum, anus instrument	An instrument used to view the anus and rectum
pyloric (pī-lōr′ ĭk)	pylor ic	R S	pylorus, gatekeeper pertaining to	Pertaining to the gatekeeper, the opening between the stomach and the duodenum
pyloroplasty (pī-lōr′ ō-plăs″ tē)	pyloro plasty	CF S	pylorus, gatekeeper surgical repair	Surgical repair of the pylorus
rectocele (rĕk′ tō-sēl)	recto cele	CF S	rectum hernia	A hernia of part of the rectum into the vagina

(Terminology—continued)

Term	Word Parts			Definition
retrolingual	retro	P	backward	Pertaining to behind the
(rĕt″ rō-lĭng′gwăl)	lingu	R	tongue	tongue
	al	S	pertaining to	
sialadenitis	sial	R	saliva	Inflammation of the salivary
(sī″ ăl-ăd″ ĕ-nī′tĭs)	aden	R	gland	gland
	itis	S	inflammation	
sigmoidoscope	sigmoido	CF	sigmoid	An instrument used to view
(sĭg-moy′ dō-skōp)	scope	S	instrument	the sigmoid
splenomegaly	spleno	CF	spleen	Enlargement of the spleen
(splē″ nō-mĕg′ă-lē)	megaly	S	enlargement, large	
splenopathy	spleno	CF	spleen	Any disease of the spleen
(splē-nŏp′ ă-thē)	pathy	S	disease	
stomatitis	stomat	R	mouth	Inflammation of the mouth
(stō″ mă-tī′ tĭs)	itis	S	inflammation	
sublingual	sub	P	below	Pertaining to below the tongue
(sŭb-lĭng′ gwăl)	lingu	R	tongue	
	al	S	pertaining to	
vagotomy	vago	CF	vagus	Incision into the vagus nerve
(vā-gŏt′ ō-mē)	tomy	S	incision	
vermiform	vermi	CF	worm	Shaped like a worm
(vĕr′ mĭ-form)	form	S	shape	

Vocabulary Words

Vocabulary words are terms that have not been divided into component parts. They are common words or specialized terms associated with the subject of this chapter. These words are provided to enhance your medical vocabulary.

Word	Definition
absorption (ăb-sōrp′ shŭn)	The process whereby nutrient material is taken into the bloodstream or lymph
ascites (ă-sī′ tēz)	An accumulation of serous fluid in the peritoneal cavity
bilirubin (bĭl″ ĭ-roo′ bĭn)	The orange-colored bile pigment produced by the separation of hemoglobin into parts that are excreted by the liver cells

(Vocabulary—continued)

Word	Definition
bowel (bou′ əl)	The intestine, gut, entrail
chyle (kīl)	The milky fluid of intestinal digestion, composed of lymph and emulsified fats
cirrhosis (sĭ–rō′ sĭs)	A chronic degenerative liver disease characterized by changes in the lobes; parenchymal cells and the lobules are infiltrated with fat
constipation (kon″ stĭ-pā′ shŭn)	Infrequent passage of unduly hard and dry feces; difficult defecation
defecation (dĕf-ĕ-kā′ shŭn)	The evacuation of the bowel
deglutition (dē″ glo͞o-tĭsh′ ŭn)	The act or process of swallowing
diarrhea (dī′ ă-rē′ ă)	Frequent passage of unformed watery stools
digestion (dī-jĕst′ chŭn)	The process by which food is changed in the mouth, stomach, and intestines by mechanical and physical action so that it can be absorbed by the body
dysentery (dĭs′ ĕn-tĕr″ ē)	An intestinal disease characterized by inflammation of the mucous membrane
emesis (ĕm′ ĕ-sĭs)	Vomiting
enzyme (ĕn′ zīm)	A protein substance capable of causing chemical changes in other substances without being changed itself
eructation (ē-rŭk-tā′ shŭn)	Belching
esophageal reflux (ē-sŏf″ ă-jē-ăl rē′ flŭks)	A return or backward flow of gastric contents into the esophagus
feces (fē′ sēz)	Body waste expelled from the bowels; stools, excreta
fiberscope (fī′ bĕr-skōp)	A flexible scope that is equipped with fiberoptic lens; useful in endoscopic examination of the colon (fibercolonoscope) and the stomach (fibergastroscope)
flatus (flā′ tŭs)	Gas in the stomach or intestines
gavage (gă-văzh′)	To feed liquid or semiliquid food via a tube (stomach or nasogastric)

(Vocabulary—continued)

Word	Definition
halitosis (hăl″ ĭ-tō′ sĭs)	Bad breath
hemorrhoid (hĕm′ ō-royd)	A mass of dilated, tortuous veins in the anorectum; may be internal or external
hernia (hĕr′ nē-ă)	The abnormal protrusion of an organ or a part of an organ through the wall of the body cavity that normally contains it
hyperalimentation (hī″ pĕr-ăl″ mĕn-tā′ shŭn)	An intravenous infusion of a hypertonic solution to sustain life; used in patients whose gastrointestinal tracts are not functioning properly
lavage (lă-văzh′)	To wash out a cavity
liver transplant (lĭv′ ĕr trăns′ plănt)	The surgical process of transferring the liver from a donor to a patient
mastication (măs″ tĭ-kā′ shŭn)	Chewing
melena (mĕl′ ĕ-nă)	Black feces caused by the action of intestinal juices on blood
nausea (naw′ sē-ă)	The feeling of the inclination to vomit
pancreas transplant (păn′ krē-ăs trăns plănt)	The surgical process of transferring the pancreas from a donor to a patient
paralytic ileus (păr″ ă-lĭt′ ĭk ĭl′ ē-ŭs)	A paralysis of the intestines that causes distention and symptoms of acute obstruction and prostration
pilonidal cyst (pī″ lō-nī′ dăl sĭst)	A closed sac in the crease of the sacrococcygeal region caused by a developmental defect that permits epithelial tissue and hair to be trapped below the skin
volvulus (vŏl′ vū-lŭs)	A twisting of the bowel on itself that causes an obstruction
vomit (vŏm′ ĭt)	To eject stomach contents through the mouth

ABBREVIATIONS

a.c.	before meals (ante cibum)	**HAV**	hepatitis A virus
A/G	albumin/globulin (ratio)	**HBIG**	hepatitis B immune globulin
ALP	alkaline phosphatase		
ATP	adenosine triphosphate	**HBV**	hepatitis B virus
Ba	barium	**HCl**	hydrochloric acid
BaE	barium enema	**IBS**	irritable bowel syndrome
BAO	basal acid output	**ICG**	indocyanine green
BM	bowel movement	**IVC**	intravenous cholangiography
BRP	bathroom privileges		
BS	bowel sounds	**LDH**	lactic dehydrogenase
BSP	bromsulphalein	**NANBH**	non-A, non-B hepatitis virus
CCK-PZ	cholecystokinin-pancreozymin		
		NG	nasogastric (tube)
CDCA	chenodeoxycholic acid	**NH$_4$**	ammonia
CHO	carbohydrate	**NPO**	nothing by mouth
chol	cholesterol	**OCG**	oral cholecystography
cib	food (cibus)	**O&P**	ova and parasites
CUC	chronic ulcerative colitis	**p.c.**	after meals (post cibum)
E. coli	*Escherichia coli*	**PEG**	percutaneous endoscopic gastrostomy
ERCP	endoscopic retrograde cholangiopancreatography		
		PO	per os (by mouth)
GB	gallbladder	**PP**	postprandial (after meals)
GGT	gamma-glutamyl transferase	**PTC**	percutaneous transhepatic cholangiography
GI	gastrointestinal	**RDA**	recommended dietary or daily allowance
GIP	gastric inhibitory peptide		
GTT	glucose tolerance test	**TPN**	total parenteral nutrition
HAA	hepatitis-associated antigen	**UDCA**	ursodeoxycholic acid

Drug Highlights

Drugs that are generally used for digestive system diseases and disorders include antacids, antacid mixtures, histamine H$_2$-receptor antagonist, other ulcer medicines, laxatives, antidiarrheal agents, and antiemetics.

Antacids — Neutralize hydrochloric acid in the stomach. Antacids are classified as nonsystemic and systemic.

Nonsystemic — *Examples: Amphojel (aluminum hydroxide), Tums (calcium carbonate), Riopan (magaldrate), and Milk of Magnesia (magnesium hydroxide).*

Systemic — *Example: sodium bicarbonate.*

Antacid Mixtures

Products that combine aluminum (may cause constipation) and/or calcium compounds with magnesium (may cause diarrhea) salts. By combining the antacid properties of two single-entity agents, these products provide the antacid action of both, yet tend to counter the adverse effects of each other.

Examples: Gaviscon, Gelusil, Maalox Plus, and Mylanta.

Histamine H₂-Receptor Antagonist

Inhibit both daytime and nocturnal basal gastric acid secretion and inhibit gastric acid stimulated by food, histamines, caffeine, insulin, and pentagastrin. These drugs are used in the treatment of active duodenal ulcer.

Examples: Tagamet (cimetidine), Pepcid (famotidine), Axid (nizatidine), and Zantac (ranitidine).

Other Ulcer Medications

Include *Carafate (sucralfate)* that is a cytoprotective agent that is used to prevent further damage by ulcers, and to promote the healing process by coating the surface of the damaged mucosa. *Cytotec (misoprostol)* is an antiulcer agent that is used to prevent nonsteroidal anti-inflammatory drug (NSAID)-induced gastric ulcers.

In February 1994, it was announced that a bacterium called *Helicobacter pylori* plays a role in peptic ulcer disease. It is recommended that patients with peptic ulcer disease who test positive for *H. pylori* be treated with *bismuth* and a combination of antibiotic drugs, such as *tetracycline, metronidazole or amoxicillin* for a period of 2 weeks.

Laxatives

Used to relieve constipation and to facilitate the passage of feces through the lower gastrointestinal tract.

Examples: Dulcolax (bisacodyl), Milk of Magnesia (magnesium hydroxide), Metamucil (psyllium hydrophilic muciloid), and Ex-Lax (phenolphthalein).

Antidiarrheal Agents

Used to treat diarrhea.

Examples: Pepto-Bismol (bismuth subsalicylate), Kaopectate (kaolin mixture with pectin), and Imodium (loperamide HCl).

Antiemetics

Prevent or arrest vomiting. These drugs are also used in the treatment of vertigo, motion sickness, and nausea.

Examples: Dramamine (dimenhydrinate), Phenergan (promethazine HCl), Tigan (trimethobenzamide), and Transderm-Scop (scopolamine).

Communication Enrichment

This segment is provided for those who wish to enhance their ability to communicate in either English or Spanish.

RELATED TERMS

English	Spanish	English	Spanish
swallowing	tragar (tră-*găr*)	beans	frijoles (frĭ-*hō*-lĕs)
nausea	nausea (*nă*-ū-sĕ-ă)	beer	cerveza (sĕr-*vĕ*-ză)
vomit	vomitos (*vō*-mĭ-tōs)	bread	pan (păn)
belch	eructos (ĕ-*rūk*-tōs)	butter	mantequilla (măn-tĕ-*kĭ*-jă)
constipation	estreñimiento (ĕs-trĕ-ñĭ-mĭ-*ĕn*-tō)	cheese	queso (*kĕ*-sō)
diarrhea	diarrea (dĭ-ă-*rĕ*-ă)	coffee	café (că-*fĕ*)
gallbladder	vesicula biliar (vĕ-*sĭ*-kū-lă bĭ-lĭ-*ăr*)	cream	crema (*crĕ*-mă)
gallstones	cálculos biliares (*kăl*-kū-lōs bĭ-lĭ-ă-rĕs)	cup	taza (*tă*-să)
gingiva; gum	encias (*ĕn*-sĭ-ăs)	eggs	huevos (*wĕ*-vōs)
intestine	intestino (ĭn-tĕs-*tĭ*-nō)	diet	dieta (dĭ-*ē*-tă)
lips	labios (*lă*-bĭ-ōs)	fatty foods	comida grasosa (kō-*mĭ*-dă gră-*sō*-să)
liver	higado (*ĭ*-gă-dō)	fish	pescado (pĕs-*kă*-dō)
mouth	boca (*bō*-kă)	food	comida (kō-*mĭ*-dă)
rectum	recto (*rĕk*-tō)	fried	frito (*frĭ*-tō)
stomach	estomago (ĕs-*tō*-mă-gō)	fruit	fruta (*frū*-tă)
teeth	dientes (dĭ-*ĕn*-tĕs)	meat	carne (*kăr*-nĕ)
tongue	lengua (*lĕn*-gwă)	milk	leche (*lĕ*-chĕ)
chewing	masticar (*măs*-ti-kăr)	hunger	hambre (*ăm*-brĕ)

English	Spanish	English	Spanish
jaundice	ictericia (ĭk-tĕ-rĭ-*sĭ*-ă)	vegetable	vegetal (*vĕ*-hĕ-tăl)
laxative	purgante (pūr-*gán*-tĕ)	vitamins	vitaminas (*vĭ*-tă-mĭ-năs)
appetite	apetito (ă-pĕ-*tĭ*-tō)	bitter taste	sabor amargo (*să*-bōr ă-*măr*-gō)

DIAGNOSTIC AND LABORATORY TESTS

Test	Description
alcohol toxicology (ethanol and ethyl) (ăl ′ kō-hōl tŏks ″ ĭ-kŏl ′ ō-jē)	A test performed on blood serum or plasma to determine levels of alcohol. Legally, 0.05% or 50 mg/dL is considered not under the influence. Increased values indicate alcohol consumption that may lead to cirrhosis of the liver, gastritis, malnutrition, vitamin deficiencies, and other gastrointestinal disorders
ammonia (NH_4) (ă-mō ′ nē-ă)	A test performed on blood plasma to determine the level of ammonia (end product of protein breakdown). Increased values may indicate hepatic failure, hepatic encephalopathy, portacaval anastomosis, high protein diet in hepatic failure, and Reye's syndrome
barium enema (bă ′ rē-ūm ĕn ′ ĕ-mă)	A test performed by administering barium via the rectum to determine the condition of the colon. X-rays are taken to ascertain the structure and to check the filling of the colon. Abnormal results may indicate cancer of the colon, polyps, fistulas, ulcerative colitis, diverticulitis, hernias, and intussusception
bilirubin blood test (total) (bĭl-ĭ-roo ′ bĭn blod test)	A test done on blood serum to determine if bilirubin is conjugated and excreted in the bile. Abnormal results may indicate obstructive jaundice, hepatitis, and cirrhosis
carcinoembryonic antigen (CEA) (kăr ″ sĭn-ō-ĕm ″ brē-ōn ′ ĭk ăn ′ tĭ-jĕn)	A test performed on whole blood or plasma to determine the presence of CEA (antigens originally isolated from colon tumors). Increased values may indicate stomach, intestinal, rectal, and various other cancers and conditions. This test is nonspecific and must be combined with other tests for a final diagnosis. It is being used to monitor the course of cancer therapy
cholangiography (kō-lăn ″ jē-ŏg ′ ră-fē)	X-ray examination of the common bile duct, cystic duct, and hepatic ducts. A radiopaque dye is injected, and then films are taken. Abnormal results may indicate obstruction, stones, and tumors
cholecystography (kō ″ lē-sĭs-tŏg ′ ră-fē)	X-ray examination of the gallbladder. A radiopaque dye is injected, and then films are taken. Abnormal results may indicate cholecystitis, cholelithiasis, and tumors

Test	Description
colonofiberoscopy (kŏ′lō-nŏ-fī″bĕr-ŏs′kō-pē)	Fiberoptic colonoscopy. The direct visual examination of the colon via a flexible colonoscope; used as a diagnostic aid, for removal of foreign bodies, polyps, and tissue
endoscopic retrograde cholangiopancreatography (ERCP) (ĕn′dō-skŏp-ĭk rĕt′rō-grād kō-lăn″jē-ō-păn″krē-ă-tŏg′ră-fē)	X-ray examination of the biliary and pancreatic ducts. A contrast medium is injected, and then films are taken. Abnormal results may indicate fibrosis, biliary or pancreatic cysts, strictures, stones, and chronic pancreatitis
esophagogastroduodenoscopy (ĕ-sŏf″ă-gō′găs″trō-dū″ō-dĕ-nŏs′kō-pē)	An endoscopic examination of the esophagus, stomach, and small intestine. During the procedure, photographs, biopsy, or brushings may be done
gamma-glutamyl tranferase (GGT) (găm′ă gloo-tăm′ĭl trăns′fĕr-ās)	A test performed on blood serum to determine the level of GGT (enzyme found in the liver, kidney, prostate, heart, and spleen). Increased values may indicate cirrhosis, liver necrosis, hepatitis, alcoholism, neoplasms, acute pancreatitis, acute myocardial infarction, nephrosis, and acute cholecystitis
gastric analysis (găs′trĭk ă-năl′ĭ sĭs)	A test performed to determine quality of secretion, amount of free and combined HCl, and absence or presence of blood, bacteria, bile, and fatty acids. Increased level of HCl may indicate peptic ulcer disease, Zollinger-Ellison syndrome, and hypergastremia. Decreased level of HCl may indicate stomach cancer, pernicious anemia, and atrophic gastritis
gastrointestinal (GI) series (găs″trō-ĭn-tes′tĭn″ăl sēr′ēz)	Fluoroscopic examination of the esophagus, stomach, and small intestine. Barium is given orally, and it is observed as it flows through the GI system. Abnormal results may indicate esophageal varices, ulcers, gastric polyps, malabsorption syndrome, hiatal hernias, diverticuli, pyloric stenosis, and foreign bodies
Hemo Quant test (hē″mō kwant test)	A quantitative assay test that detects heme (iron-containing portion of hemoglobin) in the stool
hepatic antigen (HAA) (hĕ-păt′ĭk ăn′tĭ-jĕn)	A test performed to determine the presence of the hepatitis B virus
liver biopsy (lĭv′ĕr bī-ŏp-sē)	Microscopic examination of liver tissue. Abnormal results may indicate cirrhosis, hepatitis, and tumors
occult blood (ŭ-kŭlt blod)	A test performed on feces to determine gastrointestinal bleeding that is invisible (hidden). Positive results may indicate gastritis, stomach cancer, peptic ulcer, ulcerative colitis, bowel cancer, bleeding esophageal varices, portal hypertension, pancreatitis, and diverticulitis
ova and parasites (O&P) (o′vă păr′ă-sīts)	A test performed on stool to identify ova and parasites. Positive results indicate protozoa infestation
stool culture (stool kŭl′tūr)	A test performed on stool to identify the presence of organisms

Test	Description
ultrasonography, gallbladder (ŭl-tră-sŏn-ŏg ′ ră-fē găl ″ blăd′ dĕr)	A test to visualize the gallbladder by using high-frequency sound waves. The echoes are recorded on an oscilloscope and film. Abnormal results may indicate biliary obstruction, cholelithiasis, and acute cholecystitis
ultrasonography, liver (ŭl-tră-sŏn-ŏg ′ ră-fē lĭv ′ ĕr)	A test to visualize the liver by using high-frequency sound waves. The echoes are recorded on an oscilloscope and film. Abnormal results may indicate hepatic tumors, cysts, abscess, and cirrhosis
upper gastrointestinal fiberoscopy (ŭp ′ ir găs ′ trō-ĭn-tĕs ′ tĭn ″ ăl fī ′ bĕr-ŏs ′ kō-pē)	The direct visual examination of the gastric mucosa via a flexible fiberscope. Colored photographs or motion pictures can be taken during the procedure; used when gastric neoplasm is suspected

Learning Exercises

Anatomy and Physiology

Write your answers to the following questions. Do not refer back to the text.

1. Name the primary organs commonly associated with digestion.

    a. _____ b. _____

    c. _____ d. _____

    e. _____ f. _____

2. Name four accessory organs of digestion.

    a. _____ b. _____

    c. _____ d. _____

3. State the three main functions of the digestive system.

    a. _____

    b. _____

    c. _____

4. Define bolus. _____
    _____

5. Define peristalsis. _____
    _____

6. _____ _____ and _____ _____

    convert the food into a semiliquid state.

7. The _____ is the first portion of the small intestine.

8. Semiliquid food is called _____.

9. The _____ _____ transports nutrients to body cells.

10. The large intestine can be divided into four distinct sections called the _____

    _____ , the _____ ,

    the _____ , and the _____ .

11. The _____ is the largest glandular organ in the body.

12. State the function of the gallbladder. _____

13. Name an important function of the pancreas. _____

14. State three functions of the liver.

    a. _____ b. _____

    c. _____

15. Where does digestion and absorption chiefly take place? _____
    _____

16. The salivary glands located in and about the mouth are called the _____

    _____ , the _____ , and the _____ .

17. Name the two hormones secreted into the bloodstream by the pancreas.

a. _____   b. _____

Word Parts

1. In the spaces provided, write the definition of these prefixes, roots, combining forms, and suffixes. Do not refer to the listings of terminology words. Leave blank those terms you cannot define.
2. After completing as many as you can, refer back to the terminology word listings to check your work. For each word missed or left blank, write the term and its definition several times on the margins of these pages or on a separate sheet of paper.
3. To maximize the learning process, it is to your advantage to do the following exercises as directed. To refer to the terminology listings before completing these exercises invalidates the learning process.

PREFIXES

Give the definitions of the following prefixes:

1. an- _____   2. ana- _____

3. cata- _____   4. dys- _____

5. epi- _____   6. hyper- _____

7. hypo- _____   8. mal- _____

9. mega- _____   10. peri- _____

11. post- _____   12. retro- _____

13. sub- _____

ROOTS AND COMBINING FORMS

Give the definitions of the following roots and combining forms:

1. absorpt _____   2. aden _____

3. amyl _____   4. ano _____

5. append _____   6. appendic _____

7. bili _____   8. bol _____

9. bucc _____   10. celi _____

11. cheil _____   12. chole _____

13. choledocho _____   14. col _____

15. colo _____   16. colon _____

17. colono _____   18. cyst _____

19. dent _____   20. denti _____

21. diverticul _____   22. duoden _____

23. enter _____   24. entero _____

25. esophage _____   26. esophago _____

27. gastr _____   28. gastro _____

29. gingiv _____   30. glosso _____

31. glyco _____   32. hemat _____

33. hepat _____   34. hepato _____

35. hernio _____   36. ile _____

37. ileo _____   38. labi _____

39. laparo _____   40. laxat _____

41. lingu _____   42. lipo _____

43. log _____   44. mes _____

45. pancreat _____   46. pept _____

47. pharynge _____   48. prandi _____

49. proct _____   50. procto _____

51. pylor _____   52. recto _____

53. sial _____   54. sigmoido _____

55. spleno _____   56. stomat _____

57. tox _____   58. vago _____

59. vermi _____

SUFFIXES

Give the definitions of the following suffixes:

1. -ac _____   2. -al _____

3. -algia _____   4. -ary _____

5. -ase _____   6. -cele _____

7. -clysis _____   8. -dynia _____

9. -ectomy _____   10. -emesis _____

11. -form _____   12. -genesis _____

13. -ic _____   14. -in _____

15. -ion _____   16. -ism _____

17. -ist _____   18. -itis _____

19. -ive _____   20. -logy _____

21. -lysis _____   22. -megaly _____

23. -oma _____   24. -orexia _____

25. -osis _____   26. -pathy _____

27. -pepsia _____   28. -pexy _____

29. -phagia _____   30. -plasty _____

31. -rrhaphy _____   32. -scope _____

33. -scopy _____   34. -stalsis _____

35. -stomy _____   36. -tomy _____

37. -y _____

Identifying Medical Terms

In the spaces provided, write the medical terms for the following meanings:

1. _____ An enzyme that breaks down starch
2. _____ The building up of the body substances
3. _____ Lack of appetite
4. _____ Surgical excision of the appendix
5. _____ Inflammation of the appendix
6. _____ Pertaining to or conveying bile
7. _____ Pertaining to the abdomen
8. _____ Suture of the colon
9. _____ Difficulty in swallowing
10. _____ Inflammation of the liver
11. _____ Surgical incision for the repair of a hernia
12. _____ Pertaining to after meals
13. _____ Pain in the rectum and anus
14. _____ Enlargement of the spleen
15. _____ Instrument used to view the sigmoid

Spelling

In the spaces provided, write the correct spelling of these misspelled terms:

1. bilery _____   2. colonscopy _____

3. enteroclsis _____   4. gastorentreology _____

5. heptotoxin _____   6. laxtive _____

7. persitalsis _____   8. salademitis _____

9. vaogtomy _____   10. verimform _____

Review Questions

Matching

Select the appropriate lettered meaning for each numbered line.

_____ 1. cirrhosis

2. constipation

_____ 3. diarrhea

_____ 4. gavage

_____ 5. hemorrhoid

_____ 6. hernia

_____ 7. hyperalimentation

_____ 8. lavage

_____ 9. pilonidal cyst

_____ 10. volvulus

a. To wash out a cavity

b. To feed liquid or semiliquid food via a tube

c. A twisting of the bowel on itself

d. Frequent passage of unformed watery stools

e. A chronic degenerative liver disease

f. Infrequent passage of unduly hard and dry feces

g. A closed sac in the crease of the sacrococcygeal region

h. The abnormal protrusion of an organ or a part of an organ through the wall of the body cavity that normally contains it

i. A mass of dilated, tortuous veins in the anorectum

j. An intravenous infusion of a hypertonic solution to sustain life

k. The evacuation of the bowel

Abbreviations

Place the correct word, phrase, or abbreviation in the space provided.

_____ 1. before meals

_____ 2. BM

_____ 3. BS

_____ 4. food

_____ 5. gallbladder

_____ 6. hepatitis A virus

_____ 7. NG

_____ 8. NPO

_____ 9. after meals

_____ 10. total parenteral nutrition

Diagnostic and Laboratory Tests

Select the best answer to each multiple choice question. Circle the letter of your choice.

1. X-ray examination of the common bile duct, cystic duct, and hepatic ducts.

    a. cholangiography

    b. cholecystography

    c. cholangiopancreatography

    d. ultrasonography

2. The direct visual examination of the colon via a flexible colonoscope.

    a. cholangiography

    b. ultrasonography

    c. colonofiberoscopy

    d. cholecystography

3. Fluoroscopic examination of the esophagus, stomach, and small intestine.

    a. barium enema

    b. ultrasonography

    c. cholangiography

    d. gastrointestinal series

4. An endoscopic examination of the esophagus, stomach, and small intestine.

    a. cholangiography

    b. gastroduodenoesophagoscopy

    c. esophagogastroduodenoscopy

    d. gastric analysis

5. A quantitative assay test that detects heme in the stool.

    a. occult blood test

    b. stool culture

    c. Hemo Quant test

    d. ova and parasites test

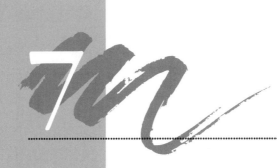

The Cardiovascular System

The heart, arteries, veins, and capillaries make up the cardiovascular system. Through this system blood is circulated to all parts of the body by the action of the heart. The heart is a four-chambered, hollow, muscular pump that circulates blood throughout the cardiovascular system. In an average, healthy adult the heart beats approximately 100,000 times a day.

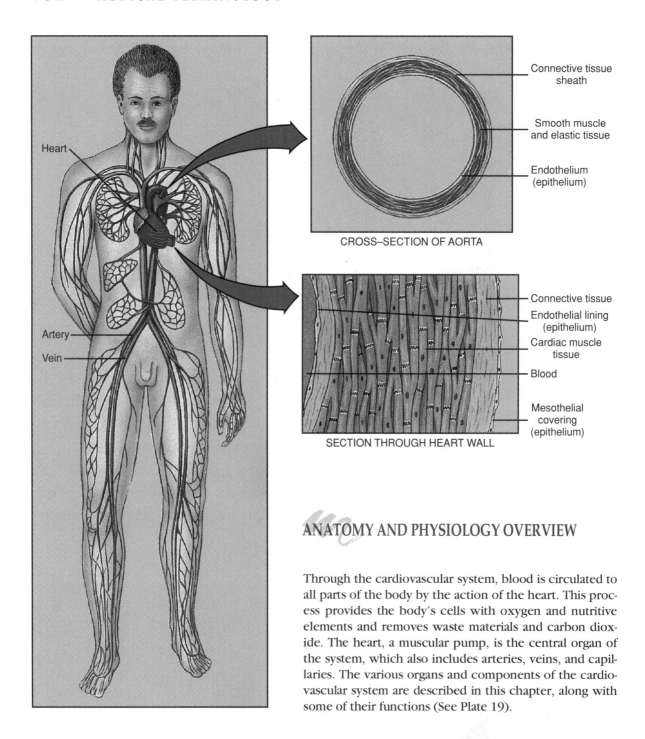

Heart

Artery

Vein

Connective tissue
sheath

Smooth muscle
and elastic tissue

Endothelium
(epithelium)

CROSS–SECTION OF AORTA

Connective tissue
Endothelial lining
(epithelium)
Cardiac muscle
tissue
Blood

Mesothelial
covering
(epithelium)

SECTION THROUGH HEART WALL

ANATOMY AND PHYSIOLOGY OVERVIEW

Through the cardiovascular system, blood is circulated to all parts of the body by the action of the heart. This process provides the body's cells with oxygen and nutritive elements and removes waste materials and carbon dioxide. The heart, a muscular pump, is the central organ of the system, which also includes arteries, veins, and capillaries. The various organs and components of the cardiovascular system are described in this chapter, along with some of their functions (See Plate 19).

THE CARDIOVASCULAR SYSTEM

Organ	Primary Functions
Heart	Propels blood, maintains blood pressure
Blood Vessels	Distribute blood around the body
Arteries	Carry blood from heart to capillaries
Capillaries	Site of diffusion between blood and interstitial fluids
Veins	Return blood from capillaries to the heart
Blood	Transports oxygen and carbon dioxide, delivers nutrients, removes waste products, assists in defense against disease
Bone Marrow	Primary site of blood cell production

The Heart

The heart is a four-chambered, hollow muscular pump that circulates blood throughout the cardiovascular system. The heart is the center of the cardiovascular system from which the various blood vessels originate and later return. It is slightly larger than a man's fist and weighs approximately 300 g in the average adult male. It lies slightly to the left of the midline of the body and is shaped like an inverted cone with its apex downward. The heart has three layers or linings:

1. **Endocardium.** The inner lining of the heart
2. **Myocardium.** The muscular, middle layer of the heart
3. **Pericardium.** The outer, membranous sac surrounding the heart

CHAMBERS OF THE HEART

The human heart acts as a double pump and is divided into the right and left heart by a partition called the septum. Each side contains an upper and lower chamber. The atria or upper chambers are separated by the interatrial septum. The ventricles or lower chambers are separated by the interventricular septum. The atria receive blood from the various parts of the body, whereas the ventricles pump blood to body parts. A description of the heart's four chambers and some of their functions is given below.

The Right Atrium

The right upper portion of the heart is called the right atrium. It is a thin-walled space that receives blood from all body parts except the lungs. Two large veins bring the blood into the right atrium and are known as the superior and inferior vena cavae.

The Right Ventricle

The right lower portion of the heart is called the right ventricle. It receives blood from the right atrium through the atrioventricular valve and pumps it through a semilunar valve to the lungs.

The Left Atrium

The left upper portion of the heart is called the left atrium. It receives blood rich in oxygen as it returns from the lungs via the left and right pulmonary veins.

The Left Ventricle

The left lower portion of the heart is called the left ventricle. It receives blood from the left atrium through an atrioventricular valve and pumps it through a semilunar valve to a large artery known as the aorta and from there to all parts of the body except the lungs.

HEART VALVES

The valves of the heart are located at the entrance and exit of each ventricle. The functions of each of the four heart valves are described below.

The Tricuspid Valve

The right atrioventricular or tricuspid valve guards the opening between the atrium and the right ventricle. The tricuspid valve allows the flow of blood into the ventricle and prevents its return to the right atrium.

The Pulmonary Semilunar Valve

The exit point for blood leaving the right ventricle is called the pulmonary semilunar valve. Located between the right ventricle and the pulmonary artery, it allows blood to flow from the right ventricle through the pulmonary artery to the lungs.

The Bicuspid or Mitral Valve

The left atrioventricular valve between the left atrium and ventricle is called the bicuspid or mitral valve. It allows blood to flow to the left ventricle and closes to prevent its return to the left atrium.

The Aortic Semilunar Valve

Blood exits from the left ventricle through the aortic semilunar valve. Located between the left ventricle and the aorta, it allows blood to flow into the aorta and prevents its return to the ventricle.

VASCULAR SYSTEM OF THE HEART

Due to the membranous lining of the heart (endocardium) and the thickness of the myocardium, it is essential that the heart have its own vascular system. The coronary arteries supply the heart with blood, and the cardiac veins, draining into the coronary sinus, collect the blood and return it to the right atrium (Fig. 7–1).

The Flow of Blood

Blood flows through the heart, to the lungs, back to the heart, and on to the various body parts as indicated in Figure 7–2 and Plate 2. Blood from the superior and inferior vena cavae enters the right atrium and subsequently passes through the tricuspid valve and into the right ventricle, which pumps it through the pulmonary semilunar valve into the left and right pulmonary arteries, which carry it to the lungs. In the lungs, the blood gives up wastes and takes on oxygen as it passes through capillaries into veins. Blood leaves the lungs through the left and right pulmonary veins, which carry it to the heart's left atrium. The oxygenated blood then passes through the bicuspid or mitral valve into the left ventricle, which pumps it out through the aortic valve and into the aorta. This large artery supplies a branching system of smaller arteries that connect to tiny capillaries throughout the body.

FIGURE 7–1

Coronary circulation. **(A)** A cast of the coronary vessels, showing the complexity and extent of the coronary circulation. **(B)** Coronary vessels supplying the anterior surface of the heart. (*From Martini F.* Fundamentals of Anatomy and Physiology, *2nd ed. Englewood Cliffs, NJ: Prentice-Hall, 1992, with permission.*)

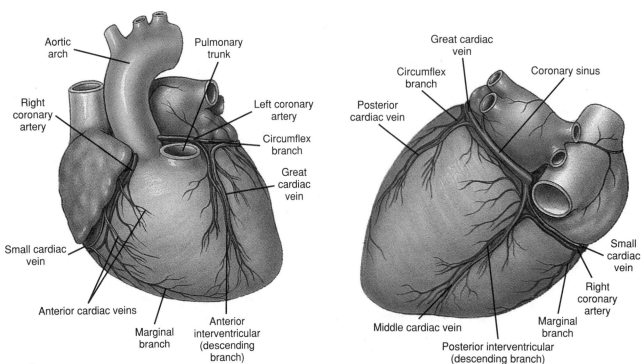

A

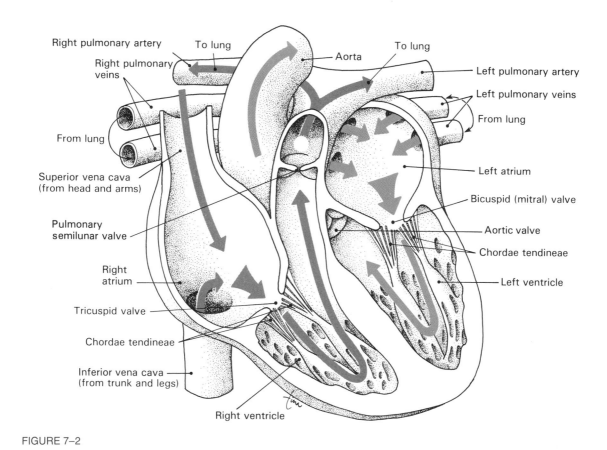

FIGURE 7–2

Structure of the heart showing blood flow. *(Adapted from Evans WF. Anatomy and Physiology, 3rd ed. Englewood Cliffs, NJ: Prentice-Hall, 1983, with permission.)*

Capillaries are microscopic blood vessels with thin walls that allow the passage of oxygen and nutrients to the body and let the blood pick up waste and carbon dioxide. Veins lead away from the capillaries as tiny vessels and increase in size until they join the superior and inferior vena cavae as they return to the heart.

THE HEARTBEAT

The heartbeat is controlled by the autonomic nervous system. It is normally generated by specialized neuromuscular tissue of the heart that is capable of causing cardiac muscle to contract rhythmically. The neuromuscular tissue of the heart comprises the sinoatrial node, the atrioventricular node, and the atrioventricular bundle (Fig. 7-3).

Sinoatrial Node (SA Node)
Often called the pacemaker of the heart, the SA node is located in the upper wall of the right atrium, just below the opening of the superior vena cava. It consists of a dense network of Purkinje fibers (atypical muscle fibers) considered to be the source of impulses initiating the heartbeat. Electrical impulses discharged by the SA node are distributed to the right and left atria and cause them to contract.

Atrioventricular Node (AV Node)
Located beneath the endocardium of the right atrium, the AV node transmits electrical impulses to the bundle of His (atrioventricular bundle).

Atrioventricular Bundle (Bundle of His)
The bundle of His forms a part of the conducting system of the heart. It extends from the AV node into the intraventricular septum where it divides into two branches within the two

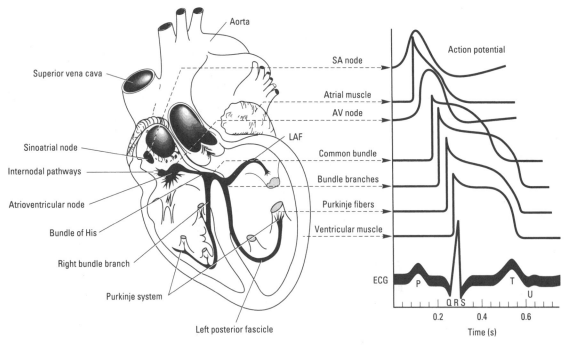

FIGURE 7–3

Conducting system of the heart. Typical transmembrane action potentials for the SA and AV nodes, other parts of the conduction system, and the atrial and ventricular muscles are shown along with the correlation to the extracellularly recorded electrical activity, ie, the electrocardiogram (ECG). The action potentials and ECG are plotted on the same time axis but with different zero points on the vertical scale. LAF, left anterior fascicle. (*From Ganong WF.* Review of Medical Physiology, *16th ed. Norwalk, CT: Appleton & Lange, 1993.*)

ventricles. The Purkinje system includes the bundle of His and the peripheral fibers. These fibers end in the ventricular muscles where the excitation of muscle is initiated causing contraction. The average heartbeat (pulse) is between 60 and 100 beats per minute for the average adult. The rate of heartbeat may be affected by emotions, smoking, disease, body size, age, stress, the environment, and many other factors.

ELECTROCARDIOGRAM

An electrocardiogram (ECG, EKG) records the electrical activity of the heart. A standard electrocardiogram consists of 12 different leads. With electrodes placed on the patient's arms, legs, and six positions on the chest, a 12-lead ECG can be recorded. The leads that are recorded on an electrocardiograph are I, II, III, aVR, aVL, aVF, and six chest leads V_1, V_2, V_3, V_4, V_5, and V_6. The standard limb leads, leads I, II, and III, each record the differences in potential between two limbs. Augmented limb leads, aVR, aVL, and aVF record between one limb and the other two limbs. There are six unipolar chest leads that record electrical activity of different parts of the heart. An ECG provides valuable information in the diagnosing of cardiac abnormalities, such as myocardial damage and arrhythmias (Fig. 7-4).

Arteries

The arteries constitute a branching system of vessels that transports blood from the right and left ventricles of the heart to all body parts (Table 7-1, Fig. 7-5, and Plate 20). In a normal state, arteries are elastic tubes that recoil and carry blood in pulsating waves. All arteries have a pulse reflecting the rhythmical beating of the heart; however, certain points

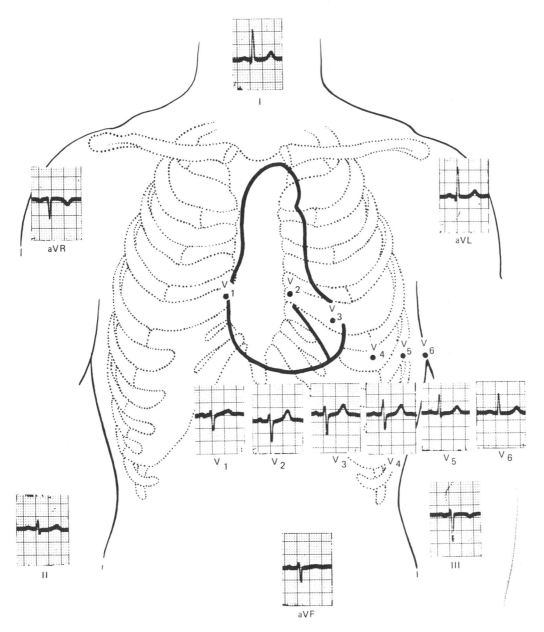

FIGURE 7–4

Normal ECG. (*From Goldman MJ*. Principles of Clinical Electrocardiography, *12th ed. Lange, 1986, with permission.*)

are commonly used to check the rate, rhythm, and condition of the arterial wall. These checkpoints are listed below and shown in Figure 7-6.

Radial. Located on the radial (thumb side) of the wrist. This is the most common site for taking a pulse

Brachial. Located in the antecubital space of the elbow. This is the most common site used to check blood pressure

Carotid. Located in the neck. In an emergency (cardiac arrest), this site is the most readily accessible

Temporal. Located at the temple

Femoral. Located in the groin

TABLE 7–1. SELECTED ARTERIES

Artery	Tissue Supplied
Right common carotid	Right side of the head and neck
Left common carotid	Left side of the head and neck
Left subclavian	Left upper extremity
Brachiocephalic	Head and arm
Aortic arch	Branches to head, neck, and upper extremities
Celiac	Stomach, spleen, and liver
Renal	Kidneys
Superior mesenteric	Lower half of large intestine
Inferior mesenteric	Small intestines and first half of the large intestine
Axillary	Axilla (armpit)
Brachial	Arm
Radial	Lateral side of the hand
Ulnar	Medial side of the hand
Internal iliac	Pelvic viscera and rectum
External iliac	Genitalia and lower trunk muscles
Deep femoral	Deep thigh muscles
Femoral	Thigh
Popliteal	Leg and foot
Anterior tibial	Leg
Dorsalis pedis	Foot

Popliteal. Located behind the knee

Dorsalis Pedis. Located on the upper surface of the foot

Blood Pressure

Blood pressure, generally speaking, is the pressure exerted by the blood on the walls of the vessels. The term most commonly refers to the pressure exerted in large arteries at the peak of the pulse wave. This pressure is measured with a sphygmomanometer used in concert with a stethoscope. Pressure is reported in millimeters of mercury as observed on a graduated column. With the use of a pressure cuff, circulation is interrupted in the brachial artery just above the elbow. Pressure from the cuff is shown on the graduated column of the sphygmomanometer, and as the pressure is released, blood again flows past the cuff. At this point, using a stethoscope, one hears a heartbeat and records the systolic pressure. Continued release of pressure results in a change in the heartbeat sound from loud to soft, at which point one records the diastolic pressure. This method results in a ratio of systolic over diastolic readings expressed in millimeters of mercury (mm Hg). In the average adult, the systolic pressure usually ranges from 100 to 140 mm Hg and the diastolic from 60 to 90 mm Hg. A typical blood pressure showing systolic over diastolic readings might be expressed as 120/80. Two types of sphygmomanometers are shown in Figure 7–7.

PULSE PRESSURE

The pulse pressure is the difference between the systolic and diastolic readings. This reading is an indication of the tone of the arterial walls. The normal pulse pressure is found when the systolic pressure is about 40 points higher than the diastolic reading. For example, if the blood pressure is 120/80, the pulse pressure would be 40.

Veins

The vessels that transport blood from peripheral tissues to the heart are the veins (See Table 7-2, Fig. 7-8, and Plate 21). In a normal state, veins have thin walls and valves that prevent

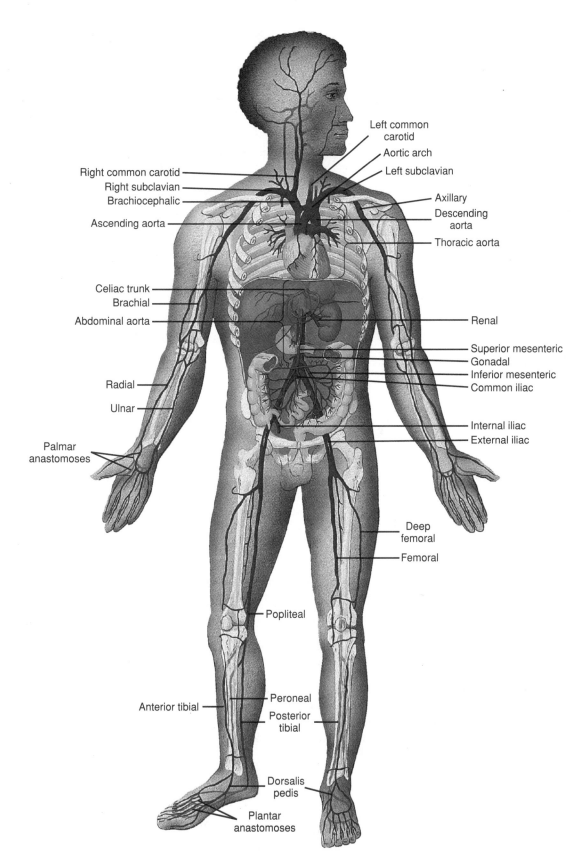

FIGURE 7–5

An overview of the arterial system. *(From Martini F. Fundamentals of Anatomy and Physiology, 2nd ed. Englewood Cliffs, NJ: Prentice-Hall, 1992, with permission.)*

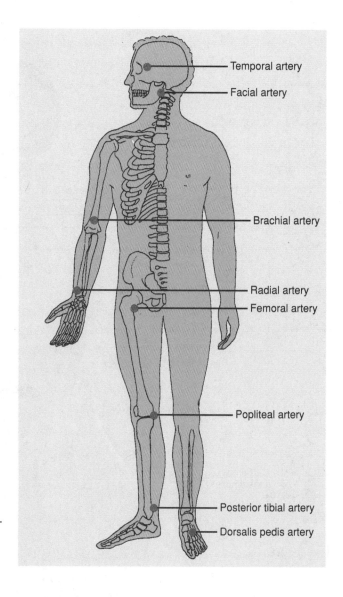

FIGURE 7–6

Pulse points. (*From Martini F. Fundamentals of Anatomy and Physiology, 2nd ed. Englewood Cliffs, NJ: Prentice-Hall, 1992, with permission.*)

the backflow of blood. Veins are the vessels used when blood is removed for analysis. The process of removing blood from a vein is called venipuncture.

Capillaries

The capillaries are microscopic blood vessels with single-celled walls that connect arterioles (small arteries) with venules (small veins). Blood, passing through capillaries, gives up the oxygen and nutrients carried to this point by the arteries and picks up waste and carbon dioxide as it enters veins. The extremely thin walls of capillaries facilitate passage of life-sustaining fluids containing oxygen and nutrients to cell bodies and the removal of accumulated waste and carbon dioxide.

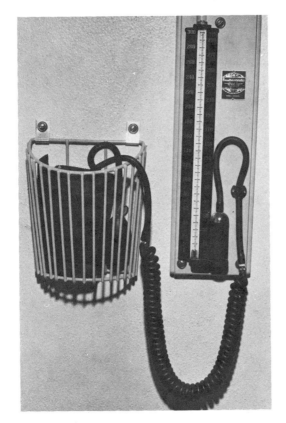

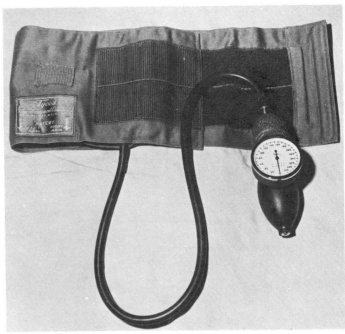

A

B

FIGURE 7–7

Sphygmomanometers used for indirect measurement of systemic blood pressure. **(A)** Mercury type. **(B)** Aneroid type. (*From Burns K, Johnson P. Health Assessment in Clinical Practice, Englewood Cliffs, NJ: Prentice-Hall, 1980, with permission.*)

TABLE 7–2. SELECTED VEINS

Vein	Tissue Drained
External jugular	Superficial tissues of the head and neck
Internal jugular	Sinuses of the brain
Subclavian	Upper extremities
Superior vena cava	Head, neck, and upper extremities
Inferior vena cava	Lower body
Hepatic	Liver
Hepatic portal	Liver and gallbladder
Superior mesenteric	Small intestine and most of the colon
Inferior mesenteric	Descending colon and rectum
Cephalic	Lateral arm
Axillary	Axilla and arm
Basilic	Medial arm
External iliac	Lower limb
Internal iliac	Pelvic viscera
Femoral	Thigh
Great saphenous	Leg
Popliteal	Lower leg
Peroneal	Foot
Anterior tibial	Deep anterior leg and dorsal foot

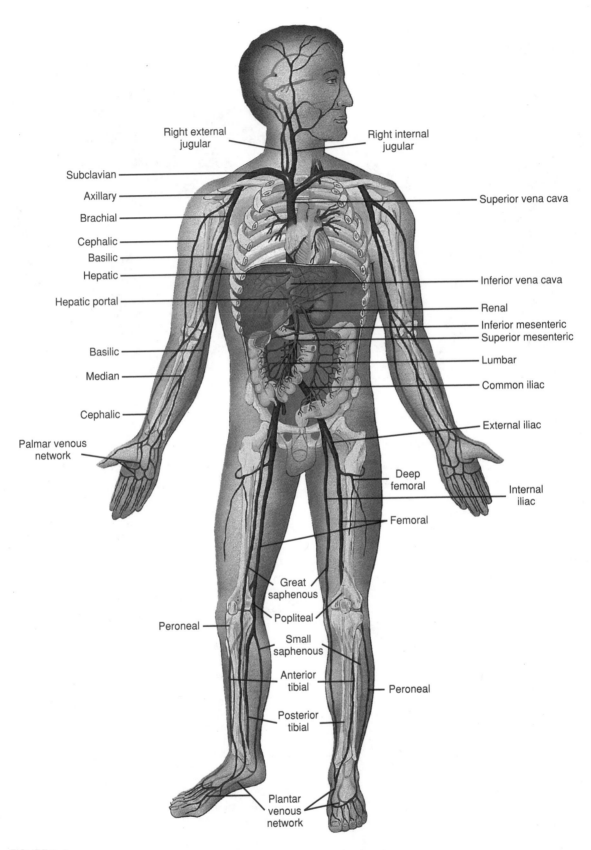

FIGURE 7–8

An overview of the venous system. (*From Martini F.* Fundamentals of Anatomy and Physiology, *2nd ed. Englewood Cliffs, NJ: Prentice-Hall, 1992, with permission.*)

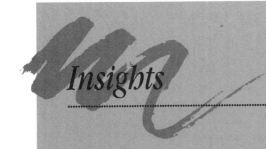

Insights

TRANSESOPHAGEAL ECHOCARDIOGRAPHY (TEE)

Transesophageal echocardiography (TEE) is an invasive test that produces high-quality computerized images of the heart by means of a probe that is threaded through the mouth and into the esophagus. Because the esophagus sits right behind the left atrium and the other cardiac chambers, the TEE can provide high-quality images of the heart and great vessels that cannot be provided by surface or transthoracic echocardiography. It is valuable in assessing cardiac mass lesions, congenital defects, and prosthetic heart valves, clots within the cardiac chambers, shunts, disease of the aorta, and infections affecting the heart valves. It is also of particular benefit in patients who have chronic pulmonary disease, thoracic cage deformities, or who are obese.

PATIENT PREPARATION

- The patient is asked to read and sign a consent form.
- The patient should not eat or drink anything for 6 to 8 hours before the procedure; however, prescribed medication may be taken with sips of water.
- If the patient has dentures and/or wears eyeglasses, these should be removed before the exam. If the patient wears a hearing aid, it should not be removed for the exam.
- The bladder should be emptied right before the test.
- If the patient has a nasoenteral tube in place, it is usually removed to prevent entanglement with the endoscopic probe.
- An intravenous line is usually started and the patient is sedated, but kept awake for the procedure.
- Electro pads are placed on the patient's chest and connected to a monitor. A blood pressure cuff is applied to the patient's arm, and a probe that monitors blood oxygen level is placed on one of the patient's fingers.
- The heart rhythm, blood pressure, and blood oxygen level are carefully assessed during the procedure.

The TEE has proven to be very useful to heart surgeons during valve repair surgery. When performed before valve surgery, it shows exactly what is wrong with the valve and then, when performed directly after the surgery (before the chest is closed), it can show if the valve is correctly and completely repaired.

This procedure may also be performed at the bedside of a critically ill patient or in the Intensive or Coronary Care Unit for the patient who suddenly begins to experience heart failure. It can show a physician that a patient is suddenly deteriorating because there is a hole in the heart, an acute rupture in the mitral valve, or an aortic dissection. By pinpointing the cause of the deterioration, the heart surgeon can perform surgery immediately and possibly save the life of the pa-

(Insights continues on next page)

tient. Prior to the availability of the TEE procedure, there was no other test that could quickly pinpoint the cause of sudden heart failure.

TEE is contraindicated in patients who have esophageal problems such as dysphagia, strictures, or varices. It is also contraindicated in patients with a history of mediastinal radiation.

THE PROCEDURE: A topical anesthetic is sprayed into the back of the throat to diminish the gag reflex. Next, the patient gargles a viscous xylocaine solution for several seconds and swallows it, to further numb the throat and esophagus, and to suppress the gag reflex. A guard may be inserted between the patient's teeth to prevent biting down on the endoscope or the examiner's fingers. The patient is placed on his or her left side, with a pillow under the head and a wedged cushion behind the neck. The patient is instructed to take slow, deep breaths and to put his or her chin to his or her chest and to open his or her mouth. The probe is lubricated with xylocaine jelly, and inserted through the patient's mouth. The patient is asked to swallow to assist insertion. The procedure takes approximately 15 to 30 minutes and several views of the heart will be transmitted during the procedure.

AFTER CARE: The patient should be carefully assessed for 15 to 30 minutes to assure that blood pressure and respirations are stable. The patient should rest for about 2 hours and not eat or drink anything since his throat will still be numb and swallowing may be impaired.

Terminology with Surgical Procedures & Pathology

Term	Word Parts			Definition
anginal (ăn′ jĭ-năl)	angin	R	to choke, quinsy	Pertaining to attacks of choking or suffocation
	al	S	pertaining to	
angioblast (ăn′ jĭ-ō-blăst)	angio	CF	vessel	The germ cell from which blood vessels develop
	blast	S	immature cell, germ cell	
angiocardio-graphy (ăn″ jĭ-ō-kăr″ dĭ-ŏg′ ră-fē)	angio	CF	vessel	The process of recording the heart and vessels after an intravenous injection of a radiopaque solution
	cardio	CF	heart	
	graphy	S	recording	
angiocarditis (ăn″ jĭ-ō-kăr-dī′ tĭs)	angio	CF	vessel	Inflammation of the heart and its great vessels
	card	R	heart	
	itis	S	inflammation	
angioma (ăn″ jĭ-ō′ mă)	angi	CF	vessel	A tumor of a blood vessel
	oma	S	tumor	
angionecrosis (ăn″ jĭ-ō-nēc-rō′ sĭs)	angio	CF	vessel	A condition of the death of blood vessels
	necr	R	death	
	osis	S	condition of	
angiopathy (ăn″ jĭ-ŏp′ ă-thē)	angio	CF	vessel	Disease of blood vessels
	pathy	S	disease	
angioplasty (ăn′ jĭ-ō-plăs″ tē)	angio	CF	vessel	Surgical repair of a blood vessel or vessels
	plasty	S	surgical repair	
angiorrhaphy (ăn″ jĭ-or′ ă-fē)	angio	CF	vessel	Suture of a blood vessel or vessels
	rrhaphy	S	suture	
angiospasm (ăn′ jĭ-ō-spăzm)	angio	CF	vessel	Contraction or spasm of a blood vessel
	spasm	S	contraction, spasm	
angiostenosis (ăn″ jĭ-ō-stĕ-nō′ sĭs)	angio	CF	vessel	A condition of narrowing of a blood vessel
	sten	R	narrowing	
	osis	S	condition of	
aortitis (ā″ ōr-tī′ tĭs)	aort	R	aorta	Inflammation of the aorta
	itis	S	inflammation	
aortomalacia (ā-ōr″ tō-mă-lā′ shĭ-ă)	aorto	CF	aorta	Softening of the walls of the aorta
	malacia	S	softening	

(Terminology—continued)

Term	Word Parts			Definition
arrhythmia (ă-rĭth′ mĭ-ă)	a	P	lack of	A condition in which there is a lack of rhythm of the heart beat
	rrhythm	R	rhythm	
	ia	S	condition	
arterectomy (ăr″ tĕ-rĕk′ tō-mē)	arter	R	artery	Surgical excision of an artery
	ectomy	S	excision	
arterial (ăr-tē′ rĭ-ăl)	arteri	CF	artery	Pertaining to an artery
	al	S	pertaining to	
arteriolith (ăr-tē′ rĭ-ō-lĭth)	arterio	CF	artery	An arterial stone
	lith	S	stone	
arteriosclerosis (ăr-tē″ rĭ-ō-sklĕ-rō′ sĭs)	arterio	CF	artery	A condition of hardening of an artery
	scler	R	hardening	
	osis	S	condition of	
arteriotome (ăr-tē′ rĭ-ō-tōm)	arterio	CF	artery	An instrument used to cut an artery
	tome	S	instrument to cut	
arteriotomy (ăr″ tē-rĭ-ŏt′ ō-mē)	arterio	CF	artery	Incision into an artery
	tomy	S	incision	
arteritis (ăr″ tĕ-rī′ tĭs)	arter	R	artery	Inflammation of an artery
	itis	S	inflammation	
atheroma (ăth″ ĕr-ō′ mă)	ather	R	fatty substance, porridge	Tumor of an artery containing a fatty substance
	oma	S	tumor	
atherosclerosis (ăth″ ĕr-ō-sklĕ-rō′ sĭs)	athero	CF	fatty substance, porridge	A condition of the arteries characterized by the buildup of fatty substances and hardening of the walls
	scler	R	hardening	
	osis	S	condition of	
atrioventricular (ăt″ rĭ-ō-vĕn-trĭk′ ū-lăr)	atrio	CF	atrium	Pertaining to the atrium and the ventricle
	ventricul	R	ventricle	
	ar	S	pertaining to	
bicuspid (bī-kŭs′ pĭd)	bi	P	two	Having two points or cusps; pertaining to the mitral valve
	cuspid	S	point	
bradycardia (brăd″ ĭ-kăr′ dĭ-ă)	brady	P	slow	A condition of slow heartbeat
	card	R	heart	
	ia	S	condition	
cardiac (kăr′ dĭ-ăk)	cardi	CF	heart	Pertaining to the heart
	ac	S	pertaining to	

(Terminology—continued)

Term	Word Parts			Definition
cardiocentesis (kăr″ dĭ-ō-sĕn-tē′ sĭs)	cardio centesis	CF S	heart surgical puncture	Surgical puncture of the heart
cardiodynia (kăr″ dĭ-ō-dĭn′ ĭ-ă)	cardio dynia	CF S	heart pain	Pain in the heart
cardiokinetic (kăr″ dĭ-ō-kĭ-nĕt′ ĭk)	cardio kinet ic	CF R S	heart motion pertaining to	Pertaining to heart motion
cardiologist (kăr-dē-ŏl′ ō-jĭst)	cardio log ist	CF R S	heart study of one who specializes	One who specializes in the study of the heart
cardiology (kăr″ dĭ-ŏl′ ō-jē)	cardio logy	CF S	heart study of	The study of the heart
cardiomegaly (kăr″ dĭ-ō-mĕg′ ă-lē)	cardio megaly	CF S	heart enlargement, large	Enlargement of the heart
cardiometer (kăr″ dĭ-ōm′ ĕ-tĕr)	cardio meter	CF S	heart instrument to measure	An instrument used to measure the action of the heart
cardiopathy (kăr″ dĭ-ŏp′ ă-thē)	cardio pathy	CF S	heart disease	Heart disease
cardioplegia (kăr″ dĭ-ō-plē′ jĭ-ă)	cardio plegia	CF S	heart stroke, paralysis	Paralysis of the heart
cardioptosis (kăr″ dĭ-ō-tō′ sĭs)	cardio ptosis	CF S	heart prolapse, drooping	Prolapse of the heart; a downward displacement
cardiopulmonary (kăr″ dĭ-ō-pŭl′ mō-nĕr-ē)	cardio pulmonar y	CF R S	heart lung pertaining to	Pertaining to the heart and lungs
cardioscope (kăr′ dĭ-ō-skōp″)	cardio scope	CF S	heart instrument	An instrument used to examine the interior of the heart
cardiotonic (kăr″ dĭ-ō-tŏn′ ĭk)	cardio ton ic	CF R S	heart tone pertaining to	Pertaining to increasing the tone of the heart; a type of medication

(Terminology—continued)

Term	Word Parts			Definition
cardiovascular (kăr″ dĭ-ō-văs′ kū-lar)	cardio vascul ar	CF R S	heart small vessel pertaining to	Pertaining to the heart and small blood vessels
carditis (kăr-dī′ tĭs)	card itis	R S	heart inflammation	Inflammation of the heart
constriction (kən-strĭk′ shən)	con strict ion	P R S	together, with to draw, to bind process	The process of drawing together as in the narrowing of a vessel
cyanosis (sī-ăn-ō′ sĭs	cyan osis	R S	dark blue condition of	A dark blue condition of the skin and mucus membranes caused by oxygen deficiency
dextrocardia (dĕks″ trō-kăr′ dĭ-ă)	dextro card ia	CF R S	to the right heart condition	The condition of the heart being on the right side of the body
electrocardio-graph (ē-lĕk″ trō-kăr′ dĭ-ō-grăf)	electro cardio graph	CF CF S	electricity heart to write, record	A device used for recording the electrical impulses of the heart muscle
electrocardio-phonograph (ē-lĕk″ trō-kăr″ dĭ-ō-fō′ nō-grăf)	electro cardio phono graph	CF CF CF S	electricity heart sound to write, record	A device used to record heart sounds
embolism (ĕm′ bō-lĭzm)	embol ism	R S	a throwing in condition of	A condition in which a blood clot obstructs a blood vessel; a moving blood clot
endarterectomy (ĕn″ dăr-tĕr-ĕk′ tō-mē)	end arter ectomy	P R S	within artery excision	Surgical excision of the inner portion of an artery
endocarditis (ĕn″ dō-kăr-dī′ tĭs)	endo card itis	P R S	within heart inflammation	Inflammation of the endocardium
endocardium (ĕn″ dō-kăr′ dē-ŭm)	endo cardi um	P CF S	within heart tissue	The inner lining of the heart
extrasystole (ĕks″ tră-sĭs′ tō-lē)	extra systole	P S	outside contraction	A cardiac contraction caused by an impulse arising outside the sinoatrial node

(Terminology—continued)

Term	Word Parts			Definition
hemangiectasis (hē″ măn-jĭ-ĕk′ tă-sĭs)	hem	R	blood	Dilatation of a blood vessel
	angi	CF	vessel	
	ectasis	S	dilatation	
hemangioma (hē-măn″ jĭ-ō′ mă)	hem	R	blood	A benign tumor of a blood vessel
	angi	CF	vessel	
	oma	S	tumor	
hypertension (hī″ pĕr-tĕn′ shŭn)	hyper	P	excessive, above	High blood pressure; a disease of the arteries caused by such pressure
	tens	R	pressure	
	ion	S	process	
hypotension (hī″ pō-tĕn′ shŭn)	hypo	P	deficient, below	Low blood pressure
	tens	R	pressure	
	ion	S	process	
ischemia (ĭs-kē′ mĭ-ă)	isch	R	to hold back	A condition in which there is a lack of blood supply to a part caused by constriction or obstruction of a blood vessel
	emia	S	blood condition	
mitral stenosis (mī′ trăl stĕ-nō′ sĭs)	mitr	R	mitral valve	A condition of narrowing of the mitral valve
	al	S	pertaining to	
	sten	R	narrowing	
	osis	S	condition of	
myocardial (mī″ ō-kăr′ dĭ-ăl)	myo	CF	muscle	Pertaining to the heart muscle
	cardi	CF	heart	
	al	S	pertaining to	
myocarditis (mī″ ō-kăr-dī′ tĭs)	myo	CF	muscle	Inflammation of the heart muscle
	card	R	heart	
	itis	S	inflammation	
oxygen (ŏk′ sĭ-jĕn)	oxy	R	sour, sharp, acid	A colorless, odorless, tasteless gas essential in the respiration of plants and animals
	gen	S	formation, produce	
pericardial (pĕr″ ĭ-kăr′ dĭ-ăl)	peri	P	around	Pertaining to the pericardium; the sac surrounding the heart
	cardi	CF	heart	
	al	S	pertaining to	
pericardio-rrhaphy (pĕr″ ĭ-kăr″ dĭ-ōr′ ă-fē)	peri	P	around	Suture of the pericardium
	cardio	CF	heart	
	rrhaphy	S	to suture	

(Terminology—continued)

Term	Word Parts			Definition
pericarditis (pĕr″ ĭ-kăr-dī′ tĭs)	peri	P	around	Inflammation of the pericardium
	card	R	heart	
	itis	S	inflammation	
phlebitis (flĕ-bī′ tĭs)	phleb	R	vein	Inflammation of a vein
	itis	S	inflammation	
phlebolith (flĕb′ ō-lĭth)	phlebo	CF	vein	A stone within a vein
	lith	S	stone	
phlebotomy (flĕ-bŏt′ ō-mē)	phlebo	CF	vein	Incision into a vein
	tomy	S	incision	
presystolic (prē″ sĭs-tōl′ ĭk)	pre	P	before	Pertaining to before the systole (regular contraction) of the heart
	systol	R	contraction	
	ic	S	pertaining to	
semilunar (sĕm″ ĭ-lū′ năr)	semi	P	half	Valves of the aorta and pulmonary artery
	lun	R	moon	
	ar	S	pertaining to	
sinoatrial (sīn″ ō-ā′ trĭ-ăl)	sino	CF	a curve	Pertaining to the sinus venosus and the atrium
	atri	R	atrium	
	al	S	pertaining to	
sphygmomano-meter (sfĭg″ mō-măn-ōm ĕt-ĕr)	sphygmo	CF	pulse	An instrument used to measure the arterial blood pressure
	mano	CF	thin	
	meter	S	instrument to measure	
stethoscope (stĕth′ ō-skōp)	stetho	CF	chest	An instrument used to listen to the sounds of the heart, lungs, and other internal organs
	scope	S	instrument	
tachycardia (tăk″ ĭ-kăr′ dĭ-ă)	tachy	P	fast	A fast heartbeat
	card	R	heart	
	ia	S	condition	
thrombosis (thrŏm-bō′ sĭs)	thromb	R	clot of blood	A condition in which there is a blood clot within the vascular system; a stationary blood clot
	osis	S	condition of	
tricuspid (trī-kŭs′ pĭd)	tri	P	three	Having three points; pertaining to the tricuspid valve
	cuspid	S	a point	

(Terminology—continued)

Term	Word Parts			Definition
triglyceride	tri	P	three	Pertaining to a compound
(trī-glĭs′ ĕr-īd)	glyc	R	sweet, sugar	consisting of three molecules
	er	S	relating to	of fatty acids
	ide	S	having a particular quality	
vasoconstrictive	vaso	CF	vessel	The drawing together, as in
(văs″ ō-kŏn-strĭk′	con	P	together	the narrowing of a blood
tĭv)	strict	R	to draw, to bind	vessel
	ive	S	nature of, quality of	
vasodilator	vaso	CF	vessel	A widening of a blood vessel
(văs″ ō-dī-lā′ tor)	dilat	R	to widen	
	or	S	one who, a doer	
vasospasm	vaso	CF	vessel	Contraction of a blood vessel
(văs′ ō-spăzm)	spasm	S	contraction, spasm	
vasotonic	vaso	CF	vessel	Pertaining to the tone of vessel
(văs″ ō-tŏn′ ĭk)	ton	R	tone	
	ic	S	pertaining to	
vasotripsy	vaso	CF	vessel	The crushing of a blood vessel
(văs′ ō-trĭp″ sē)	tripsy	S	crushing	to arrest hemorrhaging
vectorcardiogram	vector	R	a carrier	A record of the direction and
(vĕk″ tor-kăr′	cardio	CF	heart	magnitude of the
dĭ-ō-grăm)	gram	S	a mark, record	electromotive forces of the heart during one complete cycle
venipuncture	veni	CF	vein	To pierce a vein
(vĕn′ ĭ-pŭnk″ chūr)	puncture	S	to pierce	
venoclysis	veno	CF	vein	The injection of medicine or
(vē-nŏk′ lĭ-sĭs)	clysis	S	injection	nutritional fluid via a vein
venotomy	veno	CF	vein	Incision into a vein
(vē-nŏt′ ō-mē)	tomy	S	incision	
ventricular	ventricul	R	ventricle	Pertaining to a ventricle
(vĕn-trĭk′ ū-lăr)	ar	S	pertaining to	

Vocabulary Words

Vocabulary words are terms that have not been divided into component parts. They are common words or specialized terms associated with the subject of this chapter. These words are provided to enhance your medical vocabulary.

Word	Definition
anastomosis (ă-năs″ tō-mō′ sĭs)	A surgical connection between blood vessels or the joining of one hollow or tubular organ to another
aneurysm (ăn′ ū-rĭzm)	A sac formed by a local widening of the wall of an artery or a vein; usually caused by injury or disease
artificial pacemaker (ăr″ tĭ-fĭsh′ ăl pās′ māk-ĕr)	An electronic device that stimulates impulse initiation within the heart
auscultation (ŏs″ kool-tā′ shŭn)	A method of physical assessment using a stethoscope to listen to sounds within the chest, abdomen, and other parts of the body
bruit (broōt)	Noise, a sound of venous or arterial origin heard on auscultation
cardiocybernetics (kăr″ dē-ō-sī″ bĕr-nĕt′ ĭks)	An exercise program that combines a daily workout with relaxation therapy and guided imagery
cardiomyopathy (kăr″ dē-ō-mī-ŏp′ ă-thē)	Disease of the heart muscle that may be caused by a viral infection, a parasitic infection, or overconsumption of alcohol
catheterization (kăth″ ĕ-tĕr-ĭ-zā′ shŭn)	The process of inserting a catheter into the heart or the urinary bladder
cholesterol (kō-lĕs′ tĕr-ŏl)	A waxy, fat-like substance in the bloodstream of all animals. It is believed to be dangerous when it builds up on arterial walls and contributes to the risk of coronary heart disease
circulation (sər″-kyə lā′ shən)	The process of moving the blood in the veins and arteries throughout the body
claudication (klaw-dĭ-kā′ shŭn)	The process of lameness, limping; may result from inadequate blood supply to the muscles in the leg
coronary bypass (kŏr′ ō-nă-rē bī′ păs)	A surgical procedure performed to increase blood flow to the myocardium by using a section of a saphenous vein or internal mammary artery to bypass the obstructed or occluded coronary artery
diastole (dī-ăs′ tō-lē)	The relaxation phase of the heart cycle during which the heart muscle relaxes and the heart chambers fill with blood

(Vocabulary—continued)

Word	Definition
dysrhythmia (dĭs-rĭth′ mē-ă)	An abnormal, difficult, or bad rhythm
echocardio-graphy (ĕk″ ō-kăr″ dē-ŏg′ rah-fē)	A noninvasive ultrasound method for evaluating the heart for valvular or structural defects and coronary artery disease
extracorporeal circulation (ĕks-tră-kȯr-pōr′ ē-ăl sər″-kyə lā′ shən)	Pertaining to the circulation of the blood outside the body via a heart-lung machine or hemodialyzer
fibrillation (fĭ″ brĭl-ā′ shŭn)	Quivering of muscle fiber; may be atrial or ventricular
flutter (flŭt′ ər)	A condition of the heartbeat in which the contractions become extremely rapid
harvest (hăr′ vĭst)	To gather an organ and make it ready for transplantation
heart-lung transplant (hart-lŭng trăns′ plănt)	The surgical process of transferring the heart and lungs from a donor to a patient
heart transplant (hart trăns′ plănt)	The surgical process of transferring the heart from a donor to a patient
hemodynamic (hē″ mō-dī-năm′ ĭk)	Pertaining to the study of the heart's ability to function as a pump; the movement of the blood and its pressure
infarction (ĭn-fărk′ shŭn)	Process of development of an infarct, which is necrosis of tissue resulting from obstruction of blood flow
Korotkoff sounds (kor′ ŏt-kŏf sowndz)	Tapping sounds heard during auscultation of blood pressure
laser angioplasty (lā′ zĕr ăn′ jĭ-ō-plăs″ tē)	The use of light beams to clear a path through a blocked artery. Once the blockage is located, a laser probe is inserted into the blood vessel and advanced to the clogged area. The laser is activated by a qualified physician and, in an instant, the blockage is vaporized and blood flow is restored in the artery
lipoproteins (lĭp-ō-prō′ tēns)	Fat (lipid) and protein molecules that are bound together. They are classified as: VLDL—very low density lipoproteins; LDL—low density lipoproteins; and HDL—high density lipoproteins. High levels of VLDL and LDL are associated with cholesterol and triglyceride deposits in arteries, which could lead to coronary artery disease, hypertension, and atherosclerosis

(Vocabulary—continued)

Word	Definition
lubb-dupp (lŭb-dŭp)	The two separate heart sounds that can be heard with the use of a stethoscope
murmur (mər′ mər)	A soft blowing or rasping sound heard by auscultation of various parts of the body, especially in the region of the heart
occlusion (ŏ-kloo′ zhŭn)	The process or state of being closed
palpitation (păl-pĭ-tā′ shŭn)	Rapid throbbing or fluttering of the heart
percutaneous transluminal coronary angioplasty (pĕr″ kū-tā′ nē-ŭs trăns-lū′ mĭ-năl kŏr′ ŏ-nă-rē ăn′ jĭ-ō-plăs″ tē)	The use of a balloon-tipped catheter to compress fatty plaques against an artery wall. When successful, the plaques remain compressed, and this permits more blood to flow through the artery, thereby relieving the symptoms of heart disease
rheumatic heart disease (roo-măt′ ĭk hart dĭ-zēz′)	Endocarditis or valvular heart disease as a result of complications of acute rheumatic fever
septum (sĕp′ tŭm)	A wall or partition that divides or separates a body space or cavity
shock (shŏk)	A state of disruption of oxygen supply to the tissues and a return of blood to the heart
stroke (strōk)	A sudden severe attack such as a blockage or rupture of a blood vessel within the brain
systole (sĭs′ tō-lē)	The contractive phase of the heart cycle during which blood is forced into the aorta and the pulmonary artery
tissue plasminogen activator (tĭsh′ ū plăz-mĭn′ ō-jĕn ăk′ tĭ-vā″ tor)	A drug that is used within the first 6 hours of a myocardial infarction to dissolve fibrin clots. It reduces the chance of dying after a myocardial infarction by 50%. Examples are Kabikinase (streptokinase) and Activase (alteplase recombinant)

ABBREVIATIONS

ACG	angiocardiography	**IHSS**	idiopathic hypertrophic subaortic stenosis
AI	aortic insufficiency		
AMI	acute myocardial infarction	**LA**	left atrium
AS	aortic stenosis	**LBBB**	left bundle branch block
ASD	atrial septal defect	**LD**	lactic dehydrogenase
ASH	asymmetrical septal hypertrophy	**LDL**	low density lipoproteins
		LV	left ventricle
ASHD	arteriosclerotic heart disease	**MI**	myocardial infarction
AST	aspartate aminotransferase	**MS**	mitral stenosis
A-V, AV	atrioventricular	**MVP**	mitral valve prolapse
BBB	bundle branch block	**OHS**	open heart surgery
BP	blood pressure	**PAT**	paroxysmal atrial tachycardia
CAD	coronary artery disease		
CC	cardiac catheterization	**PMI**	point of maximum impulse
CCU	coronary care unit		
CHF	congestive heart failure	**PTCA**	percutaneous transluminal coronary angioplasty
CK	creatine kinase		
CO	cardiac output		
CPR	cardiopulmonary resuscitation	**PVCs**	premature ventricular contractions
CVP	central venous pressure	**RA**	right atrium
DVTs	deep vein thromboses	**RV**	right ventricle
ECC	extracorporeal circulation	**S-A, SA**	sinoatrial
ECG	electrocardiogram	**SCD**	sudden cardiac death
EKG	electrocardiogram	**TEE**	transesophageal echocardiography
FHS	fetal heart sound		
HDL	high density lipoproteins	**tPA**	tissue plasminogen activator
H&L	heart and lungs	**VLDL**	very low density lipoproteins
		VSD	ventricular septal defect

Drug Highlights

Drugs that are generally used for cardiovascular diseases and disorders include digitalis preparations, antiarrhythmic agents, vasopressors, vasodilators, antihypertensive agents, and antilipemic agents.

Digitalis Drugs   Strengthen the heart muscle, increase the force and velocity of myocardial systolic contraction, slow the heart rate, and decrease conduction velocity through the atrioventricular (AV) node. These drugs are used in the treatment of congestive heart failure, atrial fibrillation, atrial flutter, and paroxysmal atrial tachycardia. With the administration of digitalis, toxicity may occur. The most common early symptoms of digitalis toxicity are anorexia, nausea, vomiting, and arrhythmias.

Examples: digitalis leaf, Crystodigin (digitoxin), Lanoxin (digoxin), and Cedilanid-D (deslanoside).

Antiarrhythmic Agents

Used in the treatment of cardiac arrhythmias.

Examples: Tambocor (flecainide acetate), Tonocard (tocainide HCl), Inderal (propranolol HCl), and Quinidex (quinidine sulfate).

Vasopressors

Cause contraction of the muscles associated with capillaries and arteries, thereby narrowing the space through which the blood circulates. This narrowing results in an elevation of blood pressure. Vasopressors are useful in the treatment of patients suffering from shock.

Examples: Dopastat (dopamine HCl), Aramine (metaraminol bitartrate), and Levophed Bitartrate (norepinephrine).

Vasodilators

Cause relaxation of blood vessels and lower blood pressure. Coronary vasodilators are used for the treatment of angina pectoris.

Examples: Sorbitrate (isosorbide dinitrate), nitroglycerin, amyl nitrate, and Cardilate (erythrityl tetranitrate).

Antihypertensive Agents

Used in the treatment of hypertension.

Examples: Catapres (clonidine HCl), Aldomet (methyldopa), Lopressor (metoprolol tartrate), and Capoten (captopril).

Antilipemic Agents

Used to lower abnormally high blood levels of fatty substances (lipids) when other treatment regimens fail.

Examples: niacin (Nicolar, Nicobid), Mevacor (lovastatin), Lopid (gemfibrozil), Atromid-S (clofibrate), and Questran (cholestyramine).

Communication Enrichment

This segment is provided for those who wish to enhance their ability to communicate in either English or Spanish.

RELATED TERMS

English	Spanish
blood pressure	presión sanguinea (*prĕ*-sĭ-ōn săn-gĭ-nĕ-ă)
cholesterol	colesterol (*kō*-lĕs-tĕ-rōl)
clot	coagulo (kō-ă-gŭ-lō)
heart	corazón (*kō*-ră-zōn)
heart disease	enfermedad del corazón (ĕn-fĕr-*mĕ*-dăd dĕl *kō*-ră-zōn)

English	Spanish
high blood pressure	presion alta (*prĕ*-sĭ-ōn ăl-tă)
murmur	murmullo (*mūr*-mū-jō)
palpitations	palpitaciónes (*păl*-pĭ-tă-sĭ-ō-nĕs)
pulse	pulso (*pŭl*-sō)
system	sistema (sĭs-*tĕ*-mă)
varicose veins	venas varicosas (*vĕ*-năs vă-rĭ-*kō*-săs)
veins	venas (*vĕ*-năs)
heartbeat	latidos del corazón (*lă*-tĭ-dōs dĕl kō-*ră*-zōn)
artery	arteria (ăr-*tĕ*-rĭ-ă)
capillary	capilar (*că*-pĭ-lăr)
vessel	vaso (*vă*-sō)
choke, suffocate	sofocar (sō-*fō*-kăr)
injection	inyeccion (*ĭn*-jĕc-sĭ-ōn)
record	registro (*rĕ*-hĭs-trō)
motion	moción (*mō*-sĭ-ōn)
inflammation	inflamación (ĭn-*flă*-mă-sĭ-ōn)
spasm	espasmo (ĕs-*păs*-mō)
oxygen	oxigeno (ōx-sĭ-*hĕ*-nō)
narrowing	estrecho (ĕs-*trĕ*-chō)
puncture	pinchazo (pĭn-*chă*-sō)
soften	ablandar (*ă*-blăn-dăr)
rhythm	ritmo (*rĭt*-mō)

DIAGNOSTIC AND LABORATORY TESTS

Test	Description
angiogram (ăn′ jē-ō-grăm)	A test used to determine the size and shape of arteries and veins of organs and tissues. A radiopaque substance is injected into the blood vessel, and x-rays are taken
angiography (ăn″ jē-ŏg′ ră-fē)	The x-ray recording of a blood vessel after the injection of a radiopaque substance. Used to determine the condition of the blood vessels, organ, or tissue being studied. Types: aortic, cardiac, cerebral, coronary, digital subtraction (use of a computer technique), peripheral, pulmonary, selective, and vertebral
cardiac catheterization (kăr′ dĭ-ăk kăth″ ĕ-tĕr-ĭ-zA′ shŭn)	A test used in diagnosis of heart disorders. A tiny catheter is inserted into an artery in the groin area of the patient and is fed through this artery to the heart. Dye is then pumped through the catheter, enabling the physician to locate by x-ray any blockages in the arteries supplying the heart
cardiac enzymes (kăr′ dĭ-ăk ĕn′ zīmz)	Blood tests performed to determine cardiac damage in an acute myocardial infarction
alanine aminotransferase (ALT)	Levels begin to rise 6–10 hours after a MI and peak at 24–48 hours
aspartate aminotransferase (AST)	Levels begin to rise 6–10 hours after a MI and peak at 24–48 hours
creatine phosphokinase (CPK)	Used to detect area of damage
creatine kinase (CK)	Level may be 5–8 times normal
creatine kinase isoenzymes	Used to indicate area of damage; CK-MB heart muscle, CK-MM skeletal muscle, and CK-BB brain
cholesterol (kōl-lĕs′ tĕr-ŏl)	A blood test to determine the level of cholesterol in the serum. Elevated levels may indicate an increased risk of coronary heart disease. Any level greater than 200 mg/dL is considered too high for good heart health
electrophysiology (ē-lĕk″ trō-fĭz″ ĭ-ŏl′ ō-jē)	A cardiac procedure that maps the electrical activity of the heart from within the heart itself
Holter monitor (hōlt′ ər mŏn′ ĭ-tər)	A method of recording a patient's ECG for 24 hours. The device is portable and small enough to be worn by the patient during normal activity
lactic dehydrogenase (LDH) (lăk′ tĭk dē-hī-drŏj′ ĕ-nās)	Increased 6–12 hours after cardiac injury
stress test (strĕs test)	A method of evaluating cardiovascular fitness. The ECG is monitored while the patient is subjected to increasing levels of work. A treadmill or ergometer is used for this test
triglycerides (trī-glĭs′ ĕr-īds)	A blood test to determine the level of triglycerides in the serum. Elevated levels (greater than 200 mg/dL) may indicate an increased risk of coronary heart disease and diabetes mellitus
ultrasonography (ŭl-tră-sŏn-ŏg′ ră-fē)	A test used to visualize an organ or tissue by using high-frequency sound waves. It may be used as a screening test or as a diagnostic tool to determine abnormalities of the aorta, arteries and veins, and the heart

Learning Exercises

Anatomy and Physiology

Write your answers to the following questions. Do not refer back to the text.

1. The cardiovascular system includes:

   a. _____   b. _____

   c. _____   d. _____

2. Name the three layers of the heart.

   a. _____   b. _____

   c. _____

3. The heart weighs approximately _____ grams.

4. The _____ or upper chambers of the heart are separated by the _____ septum.

5. The _____ or lower chambers of the heart are separated by the _____ septum.

6. By listing each cardiovascular part in the proper order, trace the flow of blood through the heart, to the lungs, back to the heart, and on to the various body parts.

   a. _____   b. _____

   c. _____   d. _____

   e. _____   f. _____

   g. _____   h. _____

   i. _____   j. _____

   k. _____   l. _____

   m. _____   n. _____

7. The _____ _____ _____ controls the heartbeat.

8. The _____ _____ is called the pacemaker of the heart.

9. The _____ _____ includes the bundle of His and the peripheral fibers.

10. Name the three primary pulse points and state their locations on the body.

    a. _____   located _____

    b. _____   located _____

    c. _____   located _____

11. Define the following terms:

    a. Blood pressure _____

    b. Pulse pressure _____

12. The average adult heart is about the size of a _____ and normally beats at a pulse rate of _____ to _____ beats per minute.

13. The average adult usually has a systolic pressure between _____ and _____ mm Hg and a diastolic pressure between _____ and _____ mm Hg.

14. Give the purpose and function of arteries. _____
_____

15. Give the purpose and function of veins. _____
_____

Word Parts

1. In the spaces provided, write the definition of these prefixes, roots, combining forms, and suffixes. Do not refer to the listing of terminology words. Leave blank those terms you cannot define.
2. After completing as many as you can, refer back to the terminology word listings to check your work. For each word missed or left blank, write the term and its definition several times on the margins of these pages or on a separate sheet of paper.
3. To maximize the learning process, it is to your advantage to do the following exercises as directed. To refer to the terminology listings before completing these exercises invalidates the learning process.

PREFIXES

Give the definitions of the following prefixes:

1. a- _____
2. bi- _____
3. brady- _____
4. con- _____
5. end- _____
6. endo- _____
7. extra- _____
8. hyper- _____
9. hypo- _____
10. peri- _____
11. pre- _____
12. semi- _____
13. tachy- _____
14. tri- _____

ROOTS AND COMBINING FORMS

Give the definitions of the following roots and combining forms:

1. angi _____
2. angin _____
3. angio _____
4. aort _____
5. aorto _____
6. arter _____
7. arteri _____
8. arterio _____
9. ather _____
10. athero _____
11. atri _____
12. atrio _____
13. card _____
14. cardi _____
15. cardio _____
16. cyan _____
17. dextro _____
18. dilat _____

19. electro _____
20. embol _____
21. glyc _____
22. hem _____
23. isch _____
24. kinet _____
25. log _____
26. lun _____
27. mano _____
28. mitr _____
29. myo _____
30. necr _____
31. oxy _____
32. phleb _____
33. phlebo _____
34. phono _____
35. pulmonar _____
36. rrhythm _____
37. scler _____
38. sino _____
39. sphygmo _____
40. sten _____
41. stetho _____
42. strict _____
43. systol _____
44. tens _____
45. thromb _____
46. ton _____
47. vascul _____
48. vaso _____
49. vector _____
50. veni _____
51. veno _____
52. ventricul _____

SUFFIXES

Give the definitions of the following suffixes:

1. -ac _____
2. -al _____
3. -ar _____
4. -blast _____
5. -centesis _____
6. -clysis _____
7. -cuspid _____
8. -dynia _____
9. -ectasis _____
10. -ectomy _____
11. -emia _____
12. -er _____
13. -gen _____
14. -gram _____
15. -graph _____
16. -graphy _____
17. -ia _____
18. -ic _____
19. -ide _____
20. -ion _____
21. -ism _____
22. -ist _____
23. -itis _____
24. -ive _____
25. -lith _____
26. -logy _____
27. -malacia _____
28. -megaly _____
29. -meter _____
30. -oma _____
31. -or _____
32. -osis _____
33. -pathy _____
34. -plasty _____

35. -plegia _____   36. -ptosis _____

37. -puncture _____   38. -rrhaphy _____

39. -scope _____   40. -spasm _____

41. -systole _____   42. -tome _____

43. -tomy _____   44. -tripsy _____

45. -um _____   46. -y _____

Identifying Medical Terms

In the spaces provided, write the medical terms for the following meanings:

1. _____ A tumor of a blood vessel

2. _____ The germ cell from which blood vessels develop

3. _____ Surgical repair of a blood vessel or vessels

4. _____ A condition of narrowing of a blood vessel

5. _____ Surgical excision of an artery

6. _____ An arterial stone

7. _____ Incision into an artery

8. _____ Inflammation of an artery

9. _____ Having two points or cusps; pertaining to the mitral valve

10. _____ Pain in the heart

11. _____ One who specializes in the study of the heart

12. _____ Enlargement of the heart

13. _____ Pertaining to the heart and lungs

14. _____ The process of drawing together as in the narrowing of a vessel

15. _____ A condition in which a blood clot obstructs a blood vessel

16. _____ Inflammation of a vein

17. _____ A stone within a vein

18. _____ A fast heartbeat

19. _____ A widening of a blood vessel

Spelling

In the spaces provided, write the correct spelling of these misspelled terms:

1. artrectomy _____   2. athrosclerosis _____

3. atriventrcular _____   4. endcarditis _____

5. extrsystole   _____   6. iscemia   _____

7. mycardial   _____   8. oxygen   _____

9. phelebitis   _____   10. persystolic   _____

Review Questions

Matching

Select the appropriate lettered meaning for each numbered line.

_____ 1. cholesterol

_____ 2. claudication

_____ 3. dysrhythmia

_____ 4. harvest

_____ 5. laser angioplasty

_____ 6. lipoproteins

_____ 7. lubb-dupp

_____ 8. palpitation

_____ 9. percutaneous transluminal coronary angioplasty

_____ 10. tissue plasmino-gen activator

a. The two separate heart sounds that can be heard with the use of a stethocope

b. The use of light beams to clear a path through a blocked artery

c. Fat and protein molecules that are bound together

d. A waxy, fat-like substance in the bloodstream of all animals

e. The process of lameness, limping

f. An abnormal, difficult, or bad rhythm

g. To gather an organ and make it ready for transplantation

h. A drug that is used within the first 6 hours of a myocardial infarction to dissolve fibrin clots

i. Rapid throbbing or fluttering of the heart

j. The use of a balloon-tipped catheter to compress fatty plaques against an artery wall

k. The process of being closed

Abbreviations

Place the correct word, phrase, or abbreviation in the space provided.

_____ 1. acute myocardial infarction

_____ 2. atrioventricular

_____ 3. BP

_____ 4. CAD

_____ 5. cardiac catheterization

_____ 6. ECG, EKG

_____ 7. HDL

_____ 8. heart and lungs

_____   9. MI

_____   10. tPA

Diagnostic and Laboratory Test

Select the best answer to each multiple choice question. Circle the letter of your choice.

1. _____ is a cardiac procedure that maps the electrical activity of the heart from within the heart itself.

    a. electrocardiogram

    b. electrocardiomyogram

    c. electrophysiology

    d. cardiac catheterization

2. Blood tests performed to determine cardiac damage in an acute myocardial infarction.

    a. cardiac enzymes

    b. cholesterol

    c. triglycerides

    d. angiogram

3. A method of recording a patient's ECG for 24 hours.

    a. stress test

    b. Holter monitor

    c. ultrasonography

    d. angiography

4. A test used to determine the size and shape of arteries and veins of organs and tissues.

    a. electrophysiology

    b. stress test

    c. angiogram

    d. cholesterol

5. The x-ray recording of a blood vessel after the injection of a radiopaque substance.

    a. angiogram

    b. angiography

    c. stress test

    d. cardiac catheterization

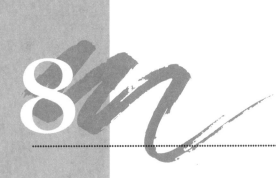

Blood and the Lymphatic System

Blood and lymph are two of the body's main fluids. Blood is circulated by the action of the heart, but lymph does not actually circulate. It is propelled in one direction, away from its source, through increasingly larger lymph vessels. Numerous valves within the lymph vessels permit one-directional flow.

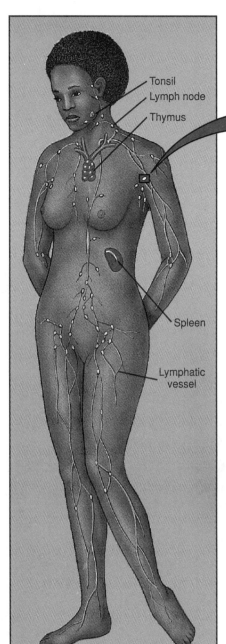

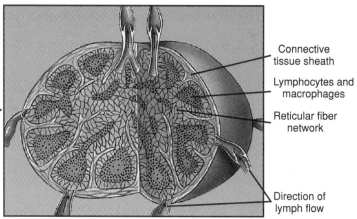

LYMPH NODE STRUCTURE

ANATOMY AND PHYSIOLOGY OVERVIEW

Blood and lymph are two of the body's main fluids and are circulated through two separate but interconnected vessel systems. Blood is circulated, by the action of the heart, through the circulatory system consisting largely of arteries, veins, and capillaries. Lymph does not actually circulate. It is propelled in one direction, away from its source, through increasingly larger lymph vessels, to drain into large veins of the circulatory system located in the neck region. Numerous valves within the lymph vessels permit one-directional flow, opening and closing as a consequence of pressure caused by the massaging action of muscles on the vessels and the fluid they contain. The various organs and components of blood and the lymphatic system are described in this chapter (See Plate 22).

THE LYMPHATIC SYSTEM	
Organ	**Primary Functions**
Lymphatic Vessels	Carry lymph from peripheral tissues to the veins of the cardiovascular system
Lymph Nodes	Monitor the composition of lymph, engulf pathogens, stimulate immune response
Spleen	Monitors circulating blood, engulfs pathogens, stimulates immune response
Thymus	Controls development and maintenance of lymphocytes

Blood

Blood is a fluid consisting of formed elements and plasma, both of which are continuously produced by the body for the purpose of transporting respiratory gases (oxygen and carbon dioxide), chemical substances (foods, salts, hormones), and cells that act to protect the body from foreign substances. The blood volume within an individual depends on body weight. An individual weighing 154 lb (70 kg) has a blood volume of about 5 qt or 5 L.

FORMED ELEMENTS

The formed elements in blood are the red blood cells or erythrocytes, platelets or thrombocytes, and white blood cells or leukocytes. Formed elements compromise about 45% of the total volume of blood and are sometimes referred to as whole blood (Table 8–1).

Erythrocytes

Erythrocytes are doughnut-shaped cells without nuclei. They transport oxygen (most of which is bound to hemoglobin contained in the cell) and carbon dioxide. There are approximately 5 million erythrocytes per cubic millimeter, and they have a life span of 80 to 120 days. Erythrocytes are formed in the red bone marrow and are commonly called red blood cells (Fig. 8–1).

Thrombocytes

Thrombocytes are disk-shaped cells about half the size of erythrocytes. They play an important role in the clotting process by releasing thrombokinase, which, in the presence of calcium, reacts with prothrombin to form thrombin. There are approximately 200,000 to 500,000 thrombocytes per cubic millimeter. Thrombocytes are fragments of certain giant cells called megakaryocytes, which are formed in the red bone marrow. Thrombocytes are commonly called platelets (Fig. 8–1).

Leukocytes

Leukocytes are sphere-shaped cells containing nuclei of varying shapes and sizes. Leukocytes are the body's main defense against the invasion of pathogens. At the time pathogens enter the tissue, the leukocytes leave the blood vessels through their walls and move in an ameba-like motion to the area of infection where they perform phagocytosis. There are approximately 8000 leukocytes per cubic millimeter. There are five types of leukocytes: neutrophils, eosinophils, basophils, lymphocytes, and monocytes.

Except for the lymphocytes, leukocytes are formed in the red bone marrow. Lymphocytes are formed in lymph nodes and other lymphoid tissue. Leukocytes are commonly called white blood cells (Fig. 8–1).

TABLE 8–1. TYPES OF BLOOD CELLS AND FUNCTIONS

Blood Cell	Function
Erythrocyte (red blood cell)	Transport oxygen and carbon dioxide
Thrombocyte (platelet)	Blood clotting
Leukocyte (white blood cell)	Body's main defense against invasion of pathogens
Types of leukocytes	
Neutrophil	Protection against infection, phagocytosis
Eosinophil	Destroy parasitic organisms, plays a key role in allergic reactions
Basophil	Key role in releasing histamine and other chemicals that act on blood vessels, essential to nonspecific immune response to inflammation
Monocyte	One of the first lines of defense in the inflammatory process, phagocytosis
Lymphocyte	Provides the body with immune capacity
B-lymphocyte	Identify foreign antigens and differentiate into antibody-producing plasma cells (source for immunoglobulins-antibodies)
T-lymphocyte	Essential for the specific immune response of the body

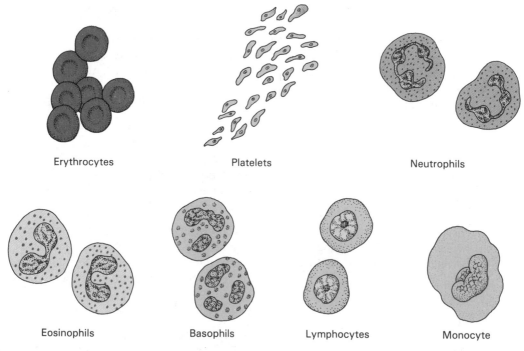

Erythrocytes   Platelets   Neutrophils

Eosinophils   Basophils   Lymphocytes   Monocyte

FIGURE 8–1

The formed elements in blood. *(Adapted from Evans WF. Anatomy and Physiology, 3rd ed. Englewood Cliffs, NJ: Prentice-Hall, 1983, with permission.)*

BLOOD GROUPING

There are four recognized blood types, and each is named for the antigens contained in the red cells. The four blood types identified are types A, B, AB, and O.

Rh FACTOR

The presence of a substance called an agglutinogen in the red blood cells is responsible for what is known as the Rh factor. It was first discovered in the blood of the rhesus monkey from which the factor gets its name. About 85% of the population have the Rh factor and are called Rh positive. The other 15% lack the Rh factor and are designated Rh negative.

PLASMA

The fluid part of the blood is called plasma. It comprises about 55% of the total volume of blood, is clear and somewhat straw-colored, and is composed of water (91%) and chemical compounds (9%). Plasma is the medium for circulation of blood cells, it provides nutritive substances to various body structures, and it removes waste products of metabolism from body structures. There are four major plasma proteins: albumin, globulin, fibrinogen, and prothrombin.

The Lymphatic System

The lymphatic system is a vessel system apart from, but connected to, the circulatory system. The lymphatic system returns fluids from tissue spaces to the bloodstream. The lymphatic system is composed of lymph capillaries, lymphatic vessels, lymphatic ducts, and lymph nodes. The system conveys lymph from the tissues to the blood. Lymph is a clear, colorless, alkaline fluid that is about 95% water. The principal component of lymph is fluid from plasma that has seeped out of capillary walls into spaces among the body tissues. Lymph contains white blood cells, particularly lymphocytes. Figure 8–2 shows the major lymphatics of the body. The three main functions of the lymphatic system are as follows:

1. It transports proteins and fluids, lost by capillary seepage, back to the bloodstream.
2. It protects the body against pathogens by phagocytosis and immune response.
3. It serves as the pathway for the absorption of fats from the small intestines into the bloodstream.

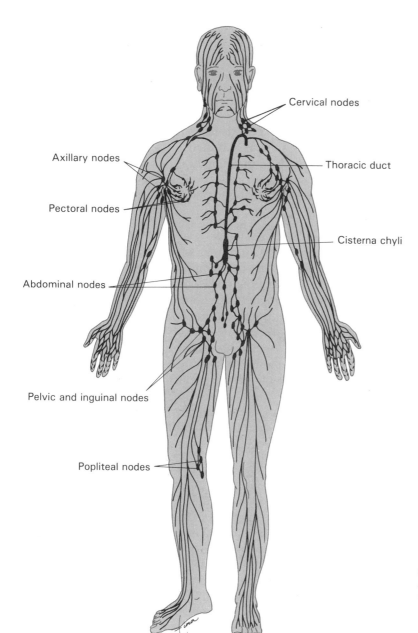

FIGURE 8–2

Major lymphatics of the body. (*Adapted from Evans WF.* Anatomy and Physiology, *3rd ed. Englewood Cliffs, NJ: Prentice-Hall, 1983, with permission.*)

Accessory Organs

The spleen, the tonsils, and the thymus are not actually part of the lymphatic system; however, they are closely related to it in their functions. These organs and their functions as they relate to the lymphatic system are described below.

THE SPLEEN

The spleen is a soft, dark red oval body lying in the upper left quadrant of the abdomen. The spleen is the major site of erythrocyte destruction. It serves as a reservoir for blood. The spleen plays an essential role in the immune response and acts as a filter, removing microorganisms from the blood.

THE TONSILS

The tonsils are lymphoid masses located in depressions of the mucous membranes of the face and pharynx. They consist of the palatine tonsils, nasopharyngeal tonsil (adenoids), and the lingual tonsil. The tonsils filter bacteria and aid in the formation of white blood cells.

THE THYMUS

The thymus is considered as one of the endocrine glands, but because of its function and appearance, it is a part of the lymphoid system. It is located in the mediastinal cavity. The thymus plays an essential role in the formation of antibodies and the development of the immune response in the newborn. It manufactures infection-fighting T cells and helps distinguish normal T cells from those that attack the body's own tissue. T cells are important in the body's cellular immune response.

The Immune System/Response

All of us live in a virtual "sea" of microorganisms, organisms so tiny that they cannot be seen with the naked eye. Many of these organisms are not harmful to humans, while others are pathogenic, capable of causing disease. Each day our bodies are faced with microorganisms, potential harmful toxins in the environment, and even some of our own cells that may change into cancer. Fortunately, the average, healthy human body is equipped with natural defenses that assist the body in fighting off disease and cancer. These natural defenses are intact skin, the cleansing action of the body's secretions (such as tears, mucus), white blood cells, body chemicals (such as hormones, enzymes), and antibodies. As long as the immune system is intact and functioning properly, it can defend the body against invading foreign substances and cancer.

The immune system consists of the tissues, organs and physiological processes used by the body to identify abnormal cells, foreign substances, and foreign tissue cells that may have been transplanted into the body. Many of these tissues and organs are part of the lymphatic system.

The Immune Response

The immune response is the reaction of the body to foreign substances and the means by which it protects the body. The following is an overview of this response.

The immune response may be described as humoral immunity or antibody-mediated immunity, and cellular immunity or cell-mediated immunity.

Humoral (pertaining to body fluids or substances contained in them) immunity or antibody-mediated immunity, involves the production of plasma lymphocytes (B cells) in response to antigen exposure with subsequent formation of antibodies. Antibodies are protein substances that are developed in response to a specific antigen. An antigen is a substance such as bacteria, toxins, or certain allergens that induces the formation of antibodies. Humoral immunity is a major defense against bacterial infections.

Cellular immunity or cell-mediated immunity, involves the production of lymphocytes (T cells) that responds to any form of injury and NK (natural killer) cells that attack foreign cells, normal cells infected with viruses, and cancer cells. Cellular immunity constitutes a major defense against infections caused by viruses, fungi and a few bacteria, such as the tubercle bacillus that causes tuberculosis. It also helps defend against the formation of tumors, especially cancer.

There are four general phases associated with the body's immune response to a foreign substance and these are:

1. The recognition of the foreign substance or the invader (enemy).
2. Activation of the body's defenses by producing more white blood cells that are designed to seek and destroy the invader(s), especially the macrophages that eat and engulf the foreign substances and lymphocytes, B cells and T cells (See Table 8-2).

    T cells of the helper type identify the enemy and rush to the spleen and lymph nodes, where they stimulate the production of other cells to aid in the fight of the foreign substance.

    T cells of the natural killer (NK) type are large granular lymphocytes that also specialize in killing cells of the body that have been invaded by foreign substances and fighting cells that have turned cancerous.

    The B cells reside in the spleen or lymph nodes and produce antibodies for specific antigens.
3. The attack phase is where the above defenders of the body produce antibodies and/or seek out to kill and/or remove the foreign invader. This is done by phagocytosis, where the macrophages squeeze out between the cells in the capillaries and crawl into the tissue to the site of the infection. Here they surround and eat the foreign substances that caused the infection. Other white blood cells respond to infection by producing antibodies. Antibodies are released into the bloodstream and carried to the site of the infection, where they surround and immobilize the invaders. Later, both antibody and invader may be eaten by the phagocytes.
4. The slowdown phase is where the number of defenders returns to normal, following victory over the foreign invader.

TABLE 8–2. SUMMARY OF FUNCTIONS OF LYMPHOCYTES

Type of cell	Functions
T cells (thymus-dependent)	Cellular immunity
B cells (bone marrow-derived)	Humoral immunity
NK cells (natural killers)	Attack foreign cells, normal cells infected with viruses, and cancer cells

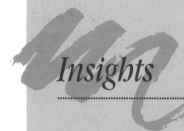

Insights

IMMUNIZATION

Immunity is the state of being protected from or resistant to a particular disease due to the development of antibodies. The mechanisms of immunity involve an antigen–antibody response. When an antigen enters the body, complex activities are set into motion. These activities involve chemical and mechanical forces that defend and protect the body's cells and tissues. Antibodies are formed and released from plasma cells, after which they enter the body fluids where they react with the invading antigen.

Immunization is a term denoting the process of inducing or providing immunity artificially by administering an immunobiologic (immunizing agent). Immunization can be active or passive.

Vaccine	Schedule
Diphtheria, Tetanus, and Pertussis (DTP)	Primary: 2, 4, 6, and 18 months. Boosters: 4 to 6 years, then every 10 years.
Haemophilus influenza type b (Hib)	Primary: 2 and 4 months, and 6 months (depending on type). Boosters: 15 months.
DTP and Hib combination (Tetramune)	Primary: 2, 4, 6, and 15 to 18 months.
Polio	Primary: 2, 4, 6, and 18 months. Boosters: 4 to 6 years.
Mumps	Primary: 15 months. Booster: 4 to 6 years or 11 to 12 years.
Rubeola	Primary: 15 months. Booster: 4 to 6 years or 11 to 12 years.
Rubella	Primary: 15 months. Booster: 4 to 6 years or 11 to 12 years.
Hepatitis B	Regimen consists of 3 doses: initial, 1 month, and 6 months from initial dose. Recommended: persons of all ages at risk of contracting the virus.
Pneumococcus	Single dose given to high-risk children over 2 years, all high-risk adults, and adults at age 50 and again at age 65.
Influenza Type A and Type B	Given during the fall of the year, usually in early October.
Bacille Calmette-Guerin (BCG)	Given in high incidence of tuberculosis.
Menomune (meningococcus serogroup C)	Given during outbreaks and for specific populations at high risk of infection.

(Insights continues on next page)

- Active immunization denotes the production of antibody or antitoxin in response to the administration of a vaccine or toxoid.
- Passive immunization denotes the provision of temporary immunity by the administration of preformed antitoxins or antibodies.

Three types of immunobiologics are used for passive immunization and these are pooled human immune globulin, specific immune globulin preparations, and antitoxin.

Recommendations for immunization of infants, children, and adults are based on facts about immunobiologics and scientific knowledge about the principles of active and passive immunization, and on judgments by public health officials and specialists in clinical and preventive medicine. Benefits and risks are associated with the use of all products, as no vaccine is completely safe or completely effective. The benefits range from partial to complete protection from the consequences of disease, and the risks range from inconvenient side effects to rare, severe, and life-threatening conditions.

Hypersensitivity to vaccine components may occur in susceptible individuals, so careful screening of persons should be done before the administration of any vaccine.

President Clinton's National Immunization Program is set to begin in October 1994. The federal immunization program will cover children on Medicaid, uninsured children, children whose insurance doesn't cover immunizations, and Native American children. Those covered by private health insurance are ineligible.

The Centers for Disease Control recommends children be vaccinated against diphtheria, polio, whooping cough, mumps, rubella, hepatitis B, measles and tetanus. The CDC offers a 24-hour hotline (404–332–4559) on disease control and prevention.

The chickenpox vaccine may become a standard vaccine for children. The CDC's Advisory Committee on Immunization Practices recommends that all children should be immunized between 12 and 18 months of age. Also, adult health care workers and family members of immunocompromised people, such as those who have AIDS, should be vaccinated.

Terminology with Surgical Procedures & Pathology

Term	Word Parts			Definition
agglutination (ă-gloo″ tĭ-nā′ shŭn)	agglutinat ion	R S	clumping process	The process of clumping together, as of blood cells that are incompatible
allergy (ăl′ ĕr-jē)	all ergy	R S	other work	Individual hypersensitivity to a substance that is usually harmless
anemia (ăn-nē′ mĭ-ă)	an emia	P S	lack of blood condition	A condition of a lack of red blood cells
angiology (ăn″ jĭ-ŏl′ ō-jē)	angio logy	CF S	vessel study of	The study of the blood vessels and the lymphatics
anisocytosis (ăn-ī″ sō-sī-tō′ sĭs)	aniso cyt osis	CF R S	unequal cell condition of	A condition in which the erythrocytes are unequal in size and shape
antibody (ăn′ tĭ-bŏd″ ē)	anti body	P S	against body	A protein substance produced in the body in response to an invading foreign substance (antigen)
anticoagulant (ăn″ tĭ-kō-ăg′ ū-lănt)	anti coagul ant	P R S	against clots forming	An agent that works against the formation of blood clots
antigen (ăn′ tĭ-jĕn)	anti gen	P S	against formation, produce	An invading foreign substance that induces the formation of antibodies
antihemophilic (ăn″ tĭ-hē″ mō-fĭl′ ĭk)	anti hemo phil ic	P CF S S	against blood attraction pertaining to	Pertaining to an agent that is effective against the bleeding tendency in hemophilia
antihemorrhagic (ăn″ tĭ-hĕm″ ō-răj′ ĭk)	anti hemo rrhag ic	P CF S S	against blood bursting forth pertaining to	Pertaining to an agent that prevents or arrests hemorhage, the bursting forth of blood
autohemotherapy (ăw″ tō-hĕ″ mō-thĕr′ ăh-pē)	auto hemo therapy	P CF S	self blood treatment	Treatment of a patient by using the patient's own blood
basocyte (bā′ sō-sīt)	baso cyte	CF S	base cell	A base cell leukocyte

(Terminology—continued)

Term	Word Parts			Definition
basophil (bā′ sō-fĭl)	baso phil	CF S	base attraction	A cell that has an attraction for a base dye
coagulable (kō-ăg′ ū-lăb-l)	coagul able	R S	to clot capable	Capable of forming a clot
creatinemia (krē″ ă-tĭn-ē′ mĭ-ă)	creatin emia	R S	flesh, creatine blood condition	A condition of excess creatine in the blood
dysemia (dĭs-ē′ mĕ-ăh)	dys emia	P S	bad blood condition	A bad blood condition A blood disease
dysglycemia (dĭs″ glī-sē′ mĕ-ăh)	dys glyc emia	P R S	bad sweet, sugar blood condition	A condition of abnormal blood sugar metabolism
eosinophil (ē″ ŏ-sĭn′ ō-fĭl)	eosino phil	CF S	rose-colored attraction	A cell that stains readily with the acid stain; attraction for the rose-colored stain
erythroblast (ĕ-rĭth′ rō-blăst)	erythro blast	CF S	red immature cell, germ cell	An immature red blood cell
erythroclastic (ĕ-rĭth″ rō-klăs′ tĭk)	erythro clast ic	CF R S	red destruction pertaining to	Pertaining to the destruction of red blood cells
erythrocyte (ĕ-rĭth′ rō-sīt)	erythro cyte	CF S	red cell	A red blood cell
erythrocytosis (ĕ-rĭth″ rō-sī-tō′ sĭs)	erythro cyt osis	CF R s	red cell condition of	An abnormal condition in which there is an increase in red blood cells
erythropathy (ĕ-rĭth″ rōp′ ă-thē)	erythro pathy	CF S	red disease	Disease of the red blood cells
erythropenia (ĕ-rĭth″ rō-pē′ nĭ-ă)	erythro penia	CF S	red lack of	Lack of red blood cells
erythropoiesis (ĕ-rĭth″ rō-poy-ē′ sĭs)	erythro poiesis	CF S	red formation	Formation of red blood cells
granulocyte (grăn′ ū-lō-sīt″)	granulo cyte	CF S	little grain, granular cell	A granular leukocyte

(Terminology—continued)

Term	Word Parts			Definition
hematocele (hē″ mă-tō-sēl′)	hemato cele	CF S	blood hernia	A blood cyst, hernia
hematocrit (hē-măt′ ō-krĭt)	hemato crit	CF S	blood to separate	A blood test that separates solids from plasma in the blood by centrifuging the blood sample
hematologist (hē″ mă-tŏl′ ō-jĭst)	hemato log ist	CF R S	blood study of one who specializes	One who specializes in the study of the blood
hematology (hē″ mă-tŏl′ ō-jē)	hemato logy	CF S	blood study of	The study of the blood
hematoma (hē″ mă-tō′ mă)	hemat oma	R S	blood tumor	A blood tumor
hemoglobin (hē″ mō-glō′ bĭn)	hemo globin	CF S	blood globe, protein	Blood protein; the iron-containing pigment of red blood cells
hemolysis (hē-mŏl′ ĭ-sĭs)	hemo lysis	CF S	blood destruction	Destruction of red blood cells
hemophilia (hē″ mō-fĭl′ ĭ-ă)	hemo philia	CF S	blood attraction	A hereditary blood disease characterized by prolonged coagulation and tendency to bleed
hemophobia (hē″ mō-fō′ bē-ă)	hemo phobia	CF S	blood fear	Fear of blood
hemopoiesis (hē″ mō-poy-ē′ sĭs)	hemo poiesis	CF S	blood formation	Formation of blood cells
hemorrhage (hĕm′ ĕ-rĭj)	hemo rrhage	CF S	blood bursting forth	Excessive bleeding; bursting forth of blood
hemostasis (hē-mŏs′ tā-sĭs)	hemo stasis	CF S	blood control, stopping	The control or stopping of bleeding
hypercalcemia (hī″ pĕr-kăl-sē′ mĭ-ă)	hyper calc emia	P R S	excessive lime, calcium blood condition	A condition of excessive amounts of calcium in the blood
hypercapnia (hī″ pĕr-kăp′ nē-ăh)	hyper capn ia	P R S	excessive smoke condition	A condition of excessive amounts of carbon dioxide in the blood

(Terminology—continued)

Term	Word Parts			Definition
hyperglycemia (hī″ pĕr-glī-sē′ mĭ-ă)	hyper glyc emia	P R S	excessive sweet, sugar blood condition	A condition of excessive amounts of sugar in the blood
hyperlipemia (hī″ pĕr-lĭp-ē′ mĭ-ă)	hyper lip emia	P R S	excessive fat blood condition	A condition of excessive amounts of fat in the blood
hypoglycemia (hī″ pō-glī-sē′ mĭ-ă)	hypo glyc emia	P R S	deficient sweet, sugar blood condition	A condition of deficient amounts of sugar in the blood
leukapheresis (loo″ kă-fē-rē′ sĭs)	leuka pheresis	CF S	white removal	Removal of white blood cells from the circulation
leukemia (loo-kē′ mē-ă)	leuk emia	R S	white blood condition	A disease of the blood characterized by overproduction of leukocytes. The disease may be malignant, acute, or chronic
leukocyte (loo′ kō-sīt)	leuko cyte	CF S	white cell	A white blood cell
leukocytopenia (loo″ kō-sī″ tō-pē′ nĭ-ă)	leuko cyto penia	CF CF S	white cell lack of	A lack of white blood cells
lymphadenitis (lĭm-făd″ ĕn-ī′ tĭs)	lymph aden itis	R R S	lymph gland inflammation	Inflammation of the lymph glands
lymphadenotomy (lĭm-făd″ ĕ-nō tō-mē)	lymph adeno tomy	R CF S	lymph gland incision	Incision into a lymph gland
lymphangiology (lĭm-făn″ jē-ŏl′ ō-jē)	lymph angio logy	R CF S	lymph vessel study of	The study of the lymphatic vessels
lymphostasis (lĭm-fō′ stā-sĭs)	lympho stasis	CF S	lymph control, stopping	The control or stopping of the flow of lymph
macrocyte (măk′ rō-sīt)	macro cyte	CF S	large cell	An abnormally large erythrocyte
monocyte (mŏn′ ō-sīt)	mono cyte	P S	one cell	The largest leukocyte, which has one nucleus

(Terminology—continued)

Term	Word Parts			Definition
mononucleosis (mŏn″ ō-nū″ klē-ō′ sĭs)	mono	P	one	A condition of excessive amounts of mononuclear leukocytes in the blood
	nucle	R	kernel, nucleus	
	osis	S	condition	
neutrophil (nū′ trō-fĭl)	neutro	CF	neither	A leukocyte that stains with neutral dyes
	phil	S	attraction	
pancytopenia (păn″ sī-tō-pē′ nĭ-ă)	pan	P	all	A lack of the cellular elements of the blood
	cyto	CF	cell	
	penia	S	lack of	
phagocytosis (făg″ ō-sī-tō′ sĭs)	phago	CF	eat, engulf	A condition of the engulfing and eating of bacteria by the phagocytes
	cyt	R	cell	
	osis	S	condition of	
plasmapheresis (plăz″ mă-fĕr-ē′ sĭs)	plasma	R	a thing formed, plasma	Removal of blood from the body and centrifuging it to separate the plasma from the blood
	pheresis	S	removal	
polycythemia (pŏl″ ē-sī-thē′ mĭ-ă)	poly	P	many	A condition of too many red blood cells
	cyth	R	cell	
	emia	S	blood condition	
prothrombin (prō-thrŏm′ bĭn)	pro	P	before	A chemical substance that interacts with calcium salts to produce thrombin
	thromb	R	clot	
	in	S	chemical	
reticulocyte (rĕ-tĭk′ ū-lō-sīt)	reticulo	CF	net	A red blood cell containing a network of granules
	cyte	S	cell	
septicemia (sĕp″ tĭ-sē′ mĭ-ă)	septic	R	putrefying	A condition in which pathogenic bacteria are present in the blood
	emia	S	blood condition	
seroculture (sē′ rō-kŭl″ chūr)	sero	CF	whey, serum	A bacterial culture of blood serum
	culture	S	cultivation	
serodiagnosis (sē″ rō-dī″ ăg-nō′ sĭs)	sero	CF	whey, serum	Diagnosis of disease by observing the reactions of blood serum
	dia	P	through	
	gnosis	S	knowledge	
serologist (sē-rŏl′ ō-jĭst)	sero	CF	whey, serum	One who specializes in the study of serum
	log	R	study of	
	ist	S	one who specializes	
serology (sē-rŏl′ ō-jē)	sero	CF	whey, serum	The study of serum
	logy	S	study of	

(Terminology—continued)

Term	Word Parts			Definition
sideropenia (sĭd″ ĕr-ō-pē′ nĭ-ă)	sidero penia	CF S	iron lack of	Lack of iron in the blood
splenemia (splē-nē′ mĭ-ă)	splen emia	R S	spleen blood condition	A condition in which the spleen is congested with blood
splenomegaly (splē″ nō-mĕg′ ă-lē)	spleno megaly	CF S	spleen enlargement	Enlargement of the spleen
splenopexy (splē′ nō-pĕk″ sē)	spleno pexy	CF S	spleen fixation	Surgical fixation of a movable spleen
thalassemia (thăl-ă-sē′ mĭ-ă)	thalass emia	R S	sea blood condition	Hereditary anemias occurring in populations bordering the Mediterranian Sea and in Southeast Asia
thrombectomy (thrŏm-bĕk′ tō-mē)	thromb ectomy	R S	clot excision	Surgical excision of a blood clot
thrombocyte (thrŏm′ bō-sīt)	thrombo cyte	CF S	clot cell	A clotting cell; a blood platelet
thrombogenic (thrŏm″ bō-jĕn′ ĭk)	thrombo genic	CF S	clot formation, produce	Formation of a blood clot
thrombolysis (thrŏm-bŏl′ ĭ-sĭs)	thrombo lysis	CF S	clot destruction	Destruction of a blood clot
thrombosis (thrŏm-bō′ sĭs)	thromb osis	R S	clot condition of	Condition of a blood clot
thymitis (thī-mī′ tĭs)	thym itis	R S	thymus inflammation	Inflammation of the thymus gland
thymocyte (thī′ mō-sīt)	thymo cyte	CF S	thymus cell	A lymphocyte derived from the thymus
thymoma (thī-mō′ mă)	thym oma	R S	thymus tumor	A tumor of the thymus
tonsillectomy (tŏn″ sĭl-ĕk′ tō-mē)	tonsill ectomy	R S	tonsil excision	Surgical excision of the tonsil

Vocabulary Words

Vocabulary words are terms that have not been divided into component parts. They are common words or specialized terms associated with the subject of this chapter. These words are provided to enhance your medical vocabulary.

Word	Definition
acquired immunodeficiency syndrome (AIDS) (ă-kwĭrd ĭm″ ū-nō-dĕ-fĭsh′ ĕn-sē sĭn-drōm)	AIDS is a disease caused by the human immunodeficiency virus (HIV). This virus is transmitted through sexual contact, through exposure to infected blood or blood components, and perinatally from mother to infant. The HIV virus invades the T4 lymphocytes, and as the disease progresses the body's immune system becomes paralyzed. The patient becomes severely weakened, and potentially fatal infections can occur. *Pneumocystis carinii* pneumonia and Kaposi's sarcoma account for many of the deaths of AIDS patients
albumin (ăl-bū′ mĭn)	One of a group of simple proteins found in blood plasma and serum
autoimmune disease (aw″ tō-ĭm-mūn dĭ-zēz)	A condition in which the body's immune system becomes defective and produces antibodies against itself. Hemolytic anemia, rheumatoid arthritis, myasthenia gravis, and scleroderma are considered as autoimmune diseases
autotransfusion (aw″ tō-trăns-fū′ zhŭn)	The process of reinfusing a patient's own blood. Methods used are: "harvesting" the blood 1–3 weeks before elective surgery; "salvaging" intraoperative blood; and collecting blood from trauma or selected surgical patients for reinfusion within 4 hours
blood (blud)	The fluid that circulates through the heart, arteries, veins, and capillaries
corpuscle (kŏr′ pŭs-ĕl)	A blood cell
embolus (ĕm′ bō-lŭs)	A blood clot carried in the bloodstream
erythropoietin (ĕ-rĭth″ rō-poy′ ĕ-tĭn)	A hormone that stimulates the production of red blood cells
extravasation (ĕks-tră″ vă-sā′ shŭn)	The process whereby fluids and/or medications (IVs) escape into surrounding tissue
fibrin (fī′ brĭn)	An insoluble protein formed from fibrinogen by the action of thrombin in the blood-clotting process
fibrinogen (fī-brĭn′ ō-gĕn)	A blood protein converted to fibrin by the action of thrombin in the blood-clotting process

(Vocabulary—continued)

Word	Definition
globulin (glŏb′ ū-lĭn)	An albuminous protein found in body fluids and cells
hemochromatosis (hē″ mō-krō″ mă-tō′ sĭs)	A disease condition in which iron is not metabolized properly and it accumulates in body tissues. The skin has a bronze hue, and liver becomes enlarged, and diabetes and cardiac failure may occur
heparin (hĕp′ ă-rĭn)	A substance found in the liver, lungs, and other body tissues that inhibits blood clotting
immunoglobulin **(Ig)** (ĭm″ ū-nō-glŏb′ ū-lĭn)	A blood protein capable of acting as an antibody. The five major types are; IgA, IgD, IgE, IgG, and IgM
lymph (lĭmf)	A clear, colorless, alkaline fluid found in the lymphatic vessels
opportunistic **infection** (ŏp″ ŏr-too-nĭs′ tĭk ĭn-fĕk′ shŭn)	A protozoal, fungal, viral, or bacterial infection that occurs when one's immune system is compromised. AIDS patients are very vulnerable and develop one or more opportunistic infections
plasma (plăz′ mă)	The fluid part of the blood
Pneumocystis *carinii* (nū″ mō-sĭs′ tĭs kăr′ ī-nī)	A protozoan that causes pneumocystis pneumonia (PCP)
pneumocystis **pneumonia** (nū″ mō-sĭs′ tĭs nū-mō′ nē-ă)	An opportunistic infection that is prevalent in AIDS patients. If not treated, the mortality rate is high
radioimmuno- **assay** (rā″ dē-ō-ĭm″ ū-nō-ăs′ ā)	A method of determining the concentration of protein-bound hormones in the blood plasma
serum (sē′ rŭm)	The clear, yellowish fluid that separates from the clot when blood clots
stem cell (stĕm sĕl)	A cell in the bone marrow that gives rise to various types of blood cells
thrombin (thrŏm′ bĭn)	A blood enzyme that causes clotting by forming fibrin

(Vocabulary—continued)

Word	Definition
thromboplastin (thrŏm″ bō-plăs′ tĭn)	An essential factor in the production of thrombin and blood clotting
transfusion (trăns-fū′ zhŭn)	The process whereby blood is transferred from one individual to the vein of another

ABBREVIATIONS

ABO	blood group	**HIV**	human immunodeficiency virus
AHF	antihemophilic factor	**lymphs**	lymphocytes
AIDS	acquired immuno-deficiency syndrome	**MCH**	mean corpuscular hemoglobin
ALL	acute lymphocytic leukemia	**MCHC**	mean corpuscular hemoglobin concentration
ARC	AIDS-related complex	MCV	mean corpuscular volume
BAC	blood alcohol concentration	metamyl	metamyelocyte
baso	basophils	mon, mono	monocyte
BSI	body systems isolation	myelocyt	myelocyte
CBC	complete blood count	**PCP**	pneumocystis pneumonia
CLL	chronic lymphocytic leukemia	PCV	packed cell volume
CML	chronic myelogenous leukemia	**PMN**	polymorphonuclear neutrophil
diff	differential count	**poly**	polymorphonuclear
EBV	Epstein-Barr virus	PT	prothrombin time
ELISA	enzyme-linked immuno-sorbent assay	**PTT**	partial thromboplastin time
eosins	eosinophils	**RBC**	red blood cell (count)
ESR	erythrocyte sedimentation rate	**Rh**	Rhesus (factor)
Hb, Hgb	hemoglobin	**RIA**	radioimmunoassay
Hct	hematocrit	**segs**	segmented (mature RBCs)
		WBC	white blood cell (count)

Drug Highlights

Drugs that are generally used in blood and lymphatic diseases and disorders include anticoagulants, antiplatelet drug (aspirin), thrombolytic agents, hemostatic agents, hematinic agents, epoetin alfa, and drugs used in treating megaloblastic anemias.

Anticoagulants

Used in inhibiting or preventing a blood clot formation. Hemorrhage can occur at almost any site in patients on anticoagulant therapy.

Examples: heparin sodium, dicumarol, Coumadin (warfarin sodium), and Athrombin-K (warfarin potassium).

Antiplatelet Drug
(aspirin)

May be recommended by physicians to reduce the risk of a second heart attack and/or to reduce the risk of having a heart attack and/or stroke. It is generally recommended that an individual take aspirin 80, 160, or 326 mg per day to prevent thromboembolic disorders.

Thrombolytic Agents

Act to dissolve existing thrombus when administered soon after its occurrence. These agents dissolve the clot, reopen the artery, restore blood flow to the heart, and prevent further damage to the myocardium. Unless contraindicated, thrombolytic therapy is the treatment of choice for an acute myocardial infarction patient who reaches the hospital within 6 hours of the onset of chest pain.

Examples: streptokinase (Kabikinase, Streptase), anistreplase (APSAC; Eminase), and alteplase (Activase).

Hemostatic Agents

Used to control bleeding and may be administered systemically or topically.

Examples: Humafac, Proplex, Amicar, vitamin K, and Surgicel.

Hematinic Agents
(irons)

Used to treat iron deficiency anemia. Oral iron preparations interfere with the absorption of oral tetracycline antibiotics. These products should not be taken within 2 hours of each other.

Examples: ferrous fumarate (Eldofe, Fecot, Feostat), ferrous gluconate (Fergon, Ferralet, Simiron), and ferrous sulfate (Feosol, Mol-Iron, Slow-Fe).

Epoetin Alfa
(Epogen, Amgen)

A genetically engineered hemopoietin that stimulates the production of red blood cells. It is a recombinant version of erythropoietin and is indicated for treating anemia in patients with chronic renal failure and AIDS patients taking zidovudine (AZT).

Agents

Used in treating megaloblastic anemias; include *folic acid (Folvite) and vitamin B_{12}.*

Communication Enrichment

This segment is provided for those who wish to enhance their ability to communicate in either English or Spanish.

RELATED TERMS

English	Spanish
AIDS	SIDA (sĭ-dǎ)
allergies	alergias (ă-lĕr-hĭ-ăs)
anemia	anemia (ă-nĕ-mĭ-ă)
bleeding tendency	tendencia a sangrar (tĕn-dĕn-sĭ-ă ă săn-grăr)
blood	sangre (săn-grăr)
blood test	prueba de sangre (prū-ĕ-bă de săn-grăr)
blood transfusion	transfusión de sangre (trăns-fū-sĭ-ōn dĕ săn-grĕ)
blood type	tipo de sangre (tĭ-pō dĕ săn-grĕ)
hematologic system	sistema hematologico (sĭs-tĕ-mă ĕ-mă-tō-lō-hĭ-kō)
hemorrhage	hemorragia (ĕ-mō-ră-hĭ-ă)
immunization	inmunización (ĭn-mū-nĭ-ză-sĭ-ōn)
lymph	linfo (lĭn-fō)
lymphadenitis	linfadenitis (lĭn-fă-dĕ-nĭ-tĭs)
lymphangitis	linfangitis (lĭn-făn-hĭ-tĭs)
lymphatic	linfático (lĭn-fă-tĭ-kō)
lymph gland	ganglio linfático (găn-glĭ-ō lĭn-fă-tĭ-kō)
lymph node	nódulo linfático (nō-dū-lō lĭn-fă-ti-kō)
lymphocyte	linfocito (lĭn-fō-sĭ-tō)
spleen	baso (bă-sō)

English	Spanish
tonsil	tonsila; amigdala (tōn-*sĭ*-lă; *ă*-mĭg-dă-lă)
tonsillectomy	tonsilectómia (tōn-sĭ-*lĕc*-tō-mĭ-ă)
vaccination	vacunación (vă-*kū*-nă-sĭ-ōn)
vaccine	vacuna (vă-*kū*-nă)

Have you had vaccinations for:	Le han puesto vacunación de: (¿ Le *ăn* pū-ĕs-tō vă-*kū*-nă-sĭ-ōn dĕ)
1. diphtheria?	1. difteria? (dĭf-*tĕ*-rĭ-ă)
2. whooping cough?	2. tosferina? (tōs-*fĕ*-rĭ-nă)
3. polio?	3. polio? (*pō*-lĭ-ō)
4. tetanus?	4. tétanos? (tĕ-*tă*-nōs)
5. smallpox?	5. viruela? (vĭ-rū-*ĕ*-lă)
6. typhoid fever?	6. fiebre tifoidea? (fĭ-ĕ-brĕ tĭ-fō-ĭ-dĕ-ă)
7. cholera?	7. cólera? (*kō*-lĕ-ră)
8. BCG?	8. BCG? (bĕ- sĕ- hĕ)
9. yellow fever?	9. fiebre amarilla? (fĭ-ĕ-brĕ ă-mă-rĭ-jă)
10. measles?	10. sarampion? (să-*răm*-pĭ-ōn)
11. hepatitis?	11. hepatitis? (ĕ-*pă*-tĭ-tĭs)
12. mumps?	12. paperas? (*pă*-pĕ-răs)

DIAGNOSTIC AND LABORATORY TESTS

Test	Description
antinuclear antibodies (ANA) (ăn″ tĭ-nū′ klē-ăr ăn′ tĭ-bŏd″ ēs)	A blood test to identify antigen–antibody reactions. ANA antibodies are present in a number of autoimmune diseases
bleeding time (blēd′ ĭng tīm)	A puncture of the ear lobe or forearm to determine the time required for blood to stop flowing. Duke method (ear lobe) 1–3 min is the normal time, and with the Ivy (forearm), 1–9 min is the normal time for the flow of blood to cease. Times greater than these may indicate

Test	Description
	thrombocytopenia, aplastic anemia, leukemia, decreased platelet count, hemophilia, and potential hemorrhage. Anticoagulant drugs delay the bleeding time
blood typing (ABO group and Rh factor) (blod tīp′ ĭng)	A blood test to determine an individual's blood type and Rh factor. Blood types are A, B, AB, and O. Rh factor may be negative or positive
bone marrow aspiration (bōn măr′ ō ăs-pĭ-rā′ shŭn)	Removal of bone marrow for examination; may be performed to determine aplastic anemia, leukemia, certain cancers, and polycythemia
complete blood count (CBC) (kom-plēt′ blod kount)	This blood test includes a hematocrit, hemoglobin, red and white blood cell count, and differential. This test is usually a part of a complete physical examination and a good indicator of hematologic system functioning
hematocrit (Hct) (hē-măt′ ō-krĭt)	A blood test performed on whole blood to determine the percentage of red blood cells in the total blood volume
hemoglobin (Hb, Hgb) (hē″ mō-glō′ bĭn)	A blood test to determine the amount of iron-containing pigment of the red blood cells
immunoglobulins (Ig) (ĭm″ ū-nō-glŏb′ ū-lĭns)	A serum blood test to determine the presence of IgA, IgD, IgE, IgG, and/or IgM. Lymphocytes and plasma cells produce immunoglobulins in response to antigen exposure. Increased and/or decreased values may indicate certain disease conditions
partial thromboplastin time (PTT) (păr′ shāl thrŏm″ bō-plăs′ tĭn tĭm)	A test performed on blood plasma to determine how long it takes for fibrin clots to form; used to regulate heparin dosage and to detect clotting disorders
platelet count (plāt′ lĕt kount)	A test performed on whole blood to determine the number of thrombocytes present. Increased and/or decreased amounts may indicate certain disease conditions
prothrombin time (PT) (prō-thrŏm′ bĭn tĭm)	A test performed on blood plasma to determine the time needed for oxalated plasma to clot; used to regulate anticoagulant drug therapy and to detect clotting disorders
red blood count (RBC) (red blod kount)	A test performed on whole blood to determine the number of erythrocytes present. Increased and/or decreased amounts may indicate certain disease conditions
sedimentation rate (ESR) (sĕd″ ĭ-mĕn-tā′ shŭn rāt)	A blood test to determine the rate at which red blood cells settle in a long, narrow tube. The distance the RBCs settle in 1 hour is the rate. Increased and/or decreased level may indicate certain disease conditions
white blood count (WBC) (hwīt blod kount)	A blood test to determine the number of leukocytes present. Increased level indicates infection and/or inflammation and decreased level indicates aplastic anemia, pernicious anemia, and malaria

Learning Exercises

Anatomy and Physiology

Write your answers to the following questions. Do not refer back to the text.

1. Name the three formed elements of blood.

    a. _____   b. _____

    c. _____

2. State the function of erythrocytes. _____

    _____

3. There are approximately _____ million erythrocytes per cubic millimeter of blood.

4. The life span of an erythrocyte is _____.

5. State the function of leukocytes. _____

    _____

6. There are approximately _____ thousand leukocytes per cubic millimeter of blood.

7. Name the five types of leukocytes.

    a. _____   b. _____

    c. _____   d. _____

    e. _____

8. State the function of thrombocytes. _____

    _____

9. There are approximately _____ _____ thrombocytes per cubic millimeter of blood.

10. Name the four blood types.

    a. _____   b. _____

    c. _____   d. _____

11. State the three main functions of the lymphatic system.

    a. _____

    b. _____

    c. _____

12. Name the three accessory organs of the lymphatic system.

    a. _____

    b. _____

    c. _____

Word Parts

1. In the spaces provided, write the definition of these prefixes, roots, combining forms, and suffixes. Do not refer to the listings of terminology words. Leave blank those terms you cannot define.
2. After completing as many as you can, refer back to the terminology word listings to check your work. For each word missed or left blank, write the term and its definition several times on the margins of these pages or on a separate sheet of paper.
3. To maximize the learning process, it is to your advantage to do the following exercises as directed. To refer to the terminology listings before completing these exercises invalidates the learning process.

PREFIXES

Give the definitions of the following prefixes:

1. an- _____   2. anti- _____
3. auto- _____   4. dia- _____
5. dys- _____   6. hyper- _____
7. hypo- _____   8. mono- _____
9. pan- _____   10. poly- _____
11. pro- _____

ROOTS AND COMBINING FORMS

Give the definitions of the following roots and combining forms:

1. aden _____   2. adeno _____
3. agglutinat _____   4. all _____
5. angio _____   6. aniso _____
7. baso _____   8. calc _____
9. capn _____   10. clast _____
11. coagul _____   12. creatin _____
13. cyt _____   14. cyth _____
15. cyto _____   16. eosino _____
17. erythro _____   18. glyc _____
19. granulo _____   20. hemat _____
21. hemato _____   22. hemo _____
23. leuk _____   24. leuko _____
25. lip _____   26. log _____
27. lymph _____   28. lympho _____
29. macro _____   30. neutro _____
31. nucle _____   32. phago _____
33. plasma _____   34. reticulo _____

35. septic   _____   36. sero   _____

37. sidero   _____   38. splen   _____

39. spleno   _____   40. thalass   _____

41. thromb   _____   42. thrombo   _____

43. thym   _____   44. thymo   _____

45. tonsill   _____

SUFFIXES

Give the definitions of the following suffixes:

1. -able   _____   2. -ant   _____

3. -blast   _____   4. -body   _____

5. -cele   _____   6. -crit   _____

7. -culture   _____   8. -cyte   _____

9. -ectomy   _____   10. -emia   _____

11. -ergy   _____   12. -gen   _____

13. -genic   _____   14. -globin   _____

15. -gnosis   _____   16. -ia   _____

17. -ic   _____   18. -in   _____

19. -ion   _____   20. -ist   _____

21. -itis   _____   22. -logy   _____

23. -lysis   _____   24. -megaly   _____

25. -oma   _____   26. -osis   _____

27. -pathy   _____   28. -penia   _____

29. -pexy   _____   30. -pheresis   _____

31. -phil   _____   32. -philia   _____

33. -phobia   _____   34. -poiesis   _____

35. -rrhag   _____   36. -rrhage   _____

37. -stasis   _____   38. -therapy   _____

39. -tomy   _____

Identifying Medical Terms

In the spaces provided, write the medical terms for the following meanings:

1. _____ Process of clumping together, as of blood cells that are incompatible

2. _____ Individual hypersensitivity to a substance that is usually harmless

3. _____ A protein substance produced in the body in response to an invading foreign substance

4. _____ An agent that works against the formation of blood clots

5. _____ An invading foreign substance that induces the formation of antibodies

6. _____ Pertaining to an agent that prevents or arrests hemorrhage

7. _____ A base cell, leukocyte

8. _____ Capable of forming a clot

9. _____ Excess of creatine in the blood

10. _____ A cell that readily stains with the acid stain

11. _____ Pertaining to the destruction of red blood cells

12. _____ A granular leukocyte

13. _____ One who specializes in the study of the blood

14. _____ Blood protein

15. _____ Excessive amounts of sugar in the blood

16. _____ Excessive amounts of fat in the blood

17. _____ A white blood cell

18. _____ The control or stopping of the flow of lymph

19. _____ Condition of excessive amounts of mononuclear leukocytes in the blood

20. _____ A chemical substance that interacts with calcium salts to produce thrombin

21. _____ Surgical fixation of a movable spleen

22. _____ A clotting cell; a blood platelet

23. _____ Formation of a blood clot

24. _____ Inflammation of the thymus

Spelling

In the spaces provided, write the correct spelling of these misspelled terms:

1. allregy _____   2. cretinemia _____

3. dyglycema _____   4. erythcytosis _____

5. hemacele _____   6. hemacrit _____

7. hemorhage _____   8. lukemia _____

9. lymphadnotomy _____   10. serlogy _____

Review Questions

Matching

Select the appropriate lettered meaning for each numbered line.

_____ 1. autotransfusion

_____ 2. erythrocyte

_____ 3. erythropoietin

_____ 4. extravasation

_____ 5. hemorrhage

_____ 6. immunoglobulin

_____ 7. hemochromatosis

_____ 8. radioimmunoassay

_____ 9. reticulocyte

_____ 10. thrombectomy

a. A method of determining the concentration of protein-bound hormones in the blood plasma

b. A disease condition in which iron is not metabolized properly and accumulates in body tissues

c. A blood protein capable of acting as an antibody

d. A red blood cell

e. A hormone that stimulates the production of red blood cells

f. Excessive bleeding

g. The process whereby fluids and/or medications escape into surrounding tissue

h. The process of reinfusing a patient's own blood

i. Surgical excision of a blood clot

j. A red blood cell containing a network of granules

k. A white blood cell

Abbreviations

Place the correct word, phrase, or abbreviation in the space provided.

_____ 1. acquired immunodeficiency syndrome

_____ 2. body systems isolation

_____ 3. CML

_____ 4. hemoglobin

_____ 5. Hct

_____ 6. human immunodeficiency virus

_____ 7. PCP

_____ 8. PT

_____ 9. RBC

_____ 10. radioimmunoassay

Diagnostic and Laboratory Tests

Select the best answer to each multiple choice question. Circle the letter of your choice.

1. A blood test to identify antigen–antibody reactions.

    a. sedimentation rate

    b. hematocrit

    c. immunoglobulins

    d. antinuclear antibodies

2. This blood test includes a hematocrit, hemoglobin, red and white blood cell count, and differential.

    a. blood typing

    b. sedimentation rate

    c. CBC

    d. Hb, Hgb

3. A blood test performed on whole blood to determine the percentage of red blood cells in the total blood volume.

    a. RBC

    b. WBC

    c. Hct

    d. PTT

4. A blood test to determine the number of leukocytes present.

    a. RBC

    b. WBC

    c. Hct

    d. PTT

5. A puncture of the ear lobe or forearm to determine the time required for blood to stop flowing.

    a. bleeding time

    b. platelet count

    c. prothrombin time

    d. PTT

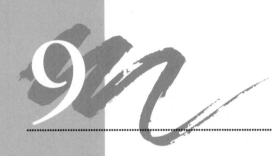

The Respiratory System

The respiratory system consists of the nose, pharynx, larynx, trachea, bronchi, and lungs. The primary function of the respiratory system is to furnish oxygen for use by individual tissue cells and to take away their gaseous waste product, carbon dioxide, This process is accomplished through the act of respiration.

TB ON THE RISE

Tuberculosis killed 4 million people in the US during the first half of the century. The disease was effectively erradicated in the 40s and 50s due to antibiotics. It is again on the rise. In 1993, the Centers for Disease Control spent more than $104 million to control TB. The disease is transmitted from person to person and its initial site of infection is the lung. Symptoms include:

- *Fever*
- *Fatigue*
- *Night Sweats*
- *Weight Loss*

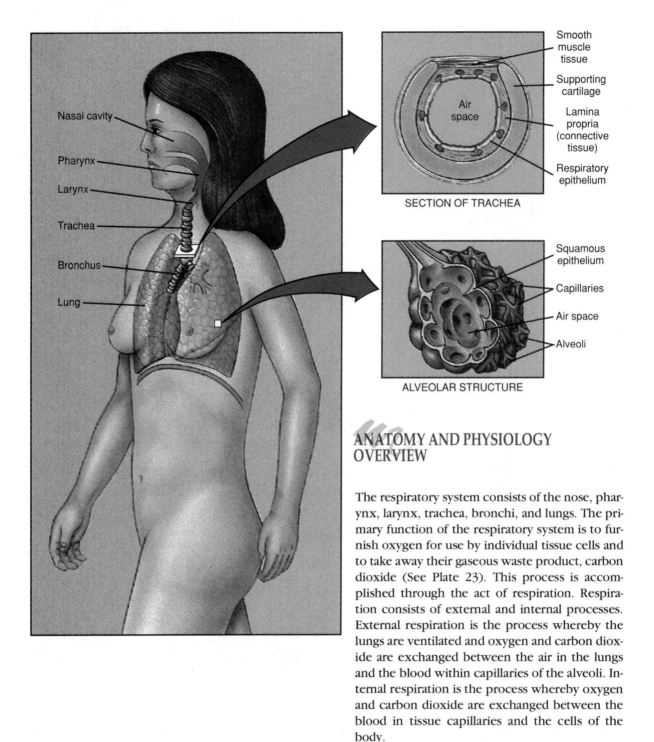

SECTION OF TRACHEA

- Smooth muscle tissue
- Supporting cartilage
- Lamina propria (connective tissue)
- Respiratory epithelium
- Air space

ALVEOLAR STRUCTURE

- Squamous epithelium
- Capillaries
- Air space
- Alveoli

Labels on body diagram: Nasal cavity, Pharynx, Larynx, Trachea, Bronchus, Lung

ANATOMY AND PHYSIOLOGY OVERVIEW

The respiratory system consists of the nose, pharynx, larynx, trachea, bronchi, and lungs. The primary function of the respiratory system is to furnish oxygen for use by individual tissue cells and to take away their gaseous waste product, carbon dioxide (See Plate 23). This process is accomplished through the act of respiration. Respiration consists of external and internal processes. External respiration is the process whereby the lungs are ventilated and oxygen and carbon dioxide are exchanged between the air in the lungs and the blood within capillaries of the alveoli. Internal respiration is the process whereby oxygen and carbon dioxide are exchanged between the blood in tissue capillaries and the cells of the body.

THE RESPIRATORY SYSTEM	
Organ	Primary Functions
Nasal Cavities	Filter, warm, humidify air, detect smells
Pharynx	Chamber shared with digestive tract, conducts air to larynx
Larynx	Protects opening to trachea and contains vocal cords
Trachea	Filters air, traps particles in mucus, cartilages keep airway open
Bronchi	Same as trachea
Alveoli	Sites of gas exchange between air and blood

The Nose

The nose is the projection in the center of the face and consists of an external and internal portion. The external portion is a triangle of cartilage and bone that is covered with skin and lined with mucous membrane. The external entrance of the nose is known as the nostrils or anterior nares. The internal portion of the nose is divided into two chambers by a partition, the septum, separating it into a right and a left cavity. These cavities are divided into three air passages: the superior, middle, and inferior conchae. These passages lead to the pharynx, are connected by openings with the paranasal sinuses, with the ears by the eustachian tube, and with the region of the eyes by the nasolacrimal ducts.

The palatine bones separate the nasal cavities from the mouth cavity. When the palatine bones fail to unite during fetal development, a congenital defect known as cleft palate occurs. This defect may be corrected by surgery. The nose, as well as the rest of the respiratory system, is lined with mucous membrane, which is covered with cilia. The nasal mucosa produces about 946 mL or 1 qt of mucus per day. Four pairs of paranasal sinuses drain into the nose. These are the frontal, maxillary, ethmoidal, and sphenoidal sinuses (Fig. 9-1).

FUNCTIONS OF THE NOSE

Five functions have been attributed to the nose. These functions are as follows:

1. It serves as an air passageway.
2. It warms and moistens inhaled air.
3. Its cilia and mucous membrane trap dust, pollen, bacteria, and other foreign matter.
4. It contains olfactory receptors, which sort out odors.
5. It aids in phonation and the quality of voice.

The Pharynx

The pharynx or throat is a musculomembranous tube about 5 inches long that extends from the base of the skull, lies anterior to the cervical vertebrae, and becomes continuous with the esophagus. It is divided into three portions: the nasopharynx located behind the nose, the oropharynx located behind the mouth, and the laryngopharynx located behind the larynx. Seven openings are found in the pharynx: two openings from the eustachian tubes, two openings from the posterior nares into the nasopharynx, the fauces or opening from the mouth into the oropharynx, and the openings from the larynx and the esophagus into the laryngopharynx. Associated with the pharynx are three pairs of lymphoid tissues, which are the tonsils. The nasopharynx contains the adenoids or pharyngeal tonsils. The oropharynx contains the faucial or palatine tonsils and the lingual tonsils. The tonsils are accessory organs of the lymphatic system and aid in filtering bacteria and other foreign substances from the circulating lymph (Fig. 9-2).

FUNCTIONS OF THE PHARYNX

The following three functions are associated with the pharynx:

1. It serves as a passageway for air.
2. It serves as a passageway for food.
3. It aids in phonation by changing its shape.

The Larynx

The larynx or voicebox is a muscular, cartilaginous structure lined with mucous membrane. It is the enlarged upper end of the trachea below the root of the tongue and hyoid bone (Fig. 9-2 and Plate 8).

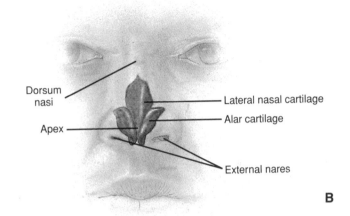

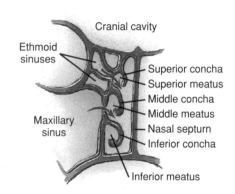

A

B

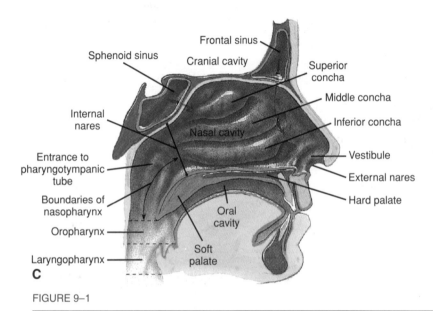

C

FIGURE 9–1

The nose, nasal cavity, and pharynx. **A.** The nasal cartilages and external landmarks on the nose. **B.** The meatuses and the positions of the entrances to the maxillary and ethmoidal sinuses. **C.** The nasal cavity and pharynx as seen in sagittal section, with the nasal septum removed. The openings draining the frontal and sphenoidal sinuses are shown. (*From Martini F.* Fundamentals of Anatomy and Physiology, *2nd ed. Englewood Cliffs, NJ: Prentice-Hall, 1992, with permission.*)

CARTILAGE OF THE LARYNX

The larynx is composed of nine cartilages bound together by muscles and ligaments. The three unpaired cartilages, each of which is described below, are the thyroid, cricoid, and epiglottic, and the three paired cartilages are the arytenoid, cuneiform, and corniculate.

The Thyroid Cartilage

The thyroid cartilage is the largest cartilage in the larynx and forms the structure commonly called the "Adam's apple." This structure is usually larger and more prominent in men than in women and contributes to the deeper male voice.

The Epiglottic Cartilage

The epiglottic cartilage is a small cartilage attached to the superior border of the thyroid cartilage. Known as the epiglottis, it covers the entrance of the larynx, and during swallowing, it acts as a lid to prevent aspiration of food into the trachea. When the epiglottis fails to cover the entrance to the larynx, food or liquid intended for the esophagus may enter, causing irritation, coughing, or in extreme cases, choking.

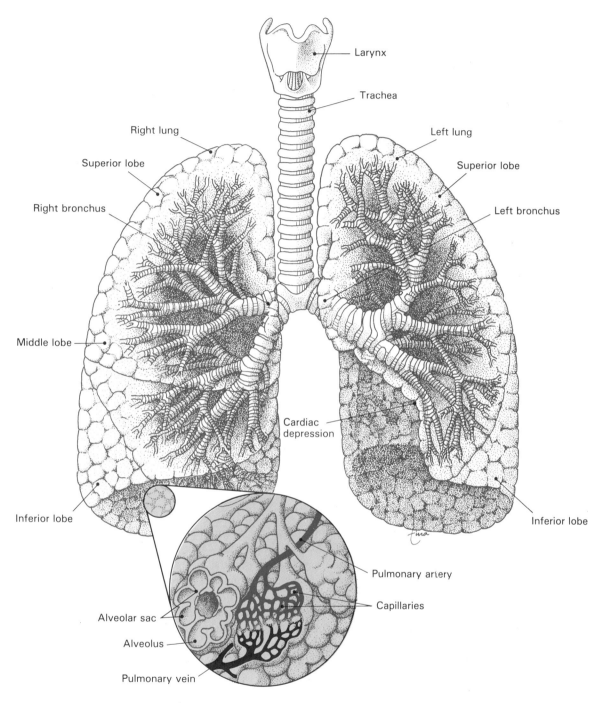

FIGURE 9–2

The larynx, trachea, bronchi, and lungs with an exploded view of clusters of alveoli showing the pulmonary blood vessels. (*From Evans WF. Anatomy and Physiology, 3rd ed. Englewood Cliffs, NJ: Prentice-Hall, 1983, with permission.*)

The Cricoid Cartilage

The cricoid cartilage is the lowermost cartilage of the larynx. It is shaped like a signet ring with the broad portion being posterior and the anterior portion forming the arch and resembling the ring's band.

The cavity of the larynx contains a pair of ventricular folds (false vocal cords) and a pair of vocal folds or true vocal cords. The cavity is divided into three regions: the vestibule, the ventricle, and the entrance to the glottis. The glottis is a narrow slit at the opening between the true vocal folds.

FUNCTION OF THE LARYNX

The function of the larynx is the production of vocal sounds. High notes are formed by short, tense vocal cords. Low notes are produced by long, relaxed vocal cords. The nose, mouth, pharynx, and bony sinuses aid in phonation.

The Trachea

The trachea or windpipe is a cylindrical cartilaginous tube that is the air passageway extending from the pharynx and larynx to the main bronchi. It is about 1 inch wide and 4 inches long. It is composed of smooth muscle that is reinforced at the front and sides by C-shaped rings of cartilage. Mucous membrane lining the trachea contains cilia, which sweep foreign matter out of the passageway. The function of the trachea is to provide an open passageway for air to the lungs (see Fig. 9–2 and Plate 8).

The Bronchi

The bronchi are the two main branches of the trachea, which provide the passageway for air to the lungs. The trachea divides into the right bronchus and the left bronchus. The right bronchus is larger and extends down in a more vertical direction than the left bronchus. When a foreign body is inhaled or aspirated, it frequently lodges in the right bronchus or enters the right lung. Each bronchus enters the lung at a depression, the hilum. They then subdivide into the bronchial tree composed of smaller bronchi, bronchioles, and alveolar ducts. The bronchial tree terminates in the alveoli, which are tiny air sacs supporting a network of capillaries from pulmonary blood vessels. The function of the bronchi is to provide a passageway for air to and from the lungs (see Fig. 9–2 and Plate 8).

The Lungs

The lungs are cone-shaped, spongy organs of respiration lying on either side of the heart within the pleural cavity of the thorax. They occupy a large portion of the thoracic cavity and are enclosed in the pleura, a serous membrane composed of several layers. The six layers of the pleura are the costal, parietal, pericardiaca, phrenica, pulmonalis, and visceral. The parietal pleura extends from the roots of the lungs and lines the walls of the thorax and the superior surface of the diaphragm. The visceral pleura covers the surface of the lungs and enters into and lines the interlobar fissures. The pleural cavity is a space between the parietal and visceral pleura and contains a serous fluid that lubricates and prevents friction caused by the rubbing together of the two layers. The thoracic cavity is separated from the abdominal cavity by a musculomembranous wall, the diaphragm. The central portion of the thoracic cavity, between the lungs, is a space called the mediastinum, containing the heart and other structures.

The lungs consist of elastic tissue filled with interlacing networks of tubes and sacs that carry air and with blood vessels carrying blood. The broad inferior surface of the lung is the base, which rests on the diaphragm, while the apex, or pointed upper margin, rises from 2.5 to 5 cm above the sternal end of the first rib. The lungs are divided into lobes with the right lung having three lobes and the left lung having only two lobes. The left lung has an indentation, the cardiac depression, for the normal placement of the heart. In an average adult male, the right lung weighs approximately 625 g and the left about 570 g. In an average adult male, the total lung capacity is 3.6 to 9.4 L, whereas in an average adult female it is 2.5 to 6.9 L. The lungs contain around 300 million alveoli, which are the air cells where the exchange of oxygen and carbon dioxide takes place. The main function of the lungs is to bring air into intimate contact with blood so that oxygen and carbon dioxide can be exchanged in the alveoli (see Fig. 9–2 and Plate 8).

Respiration

VOLUME

The following terms are used by physiologists and respiratory specialists to describe the volume of air exchanged in breathing:

Tidal Volume. The amount of air in a single inspiration or expiration. In the average adult male, about 500 cc of air enters the respiratory tract during normal quiet breathing

Supplemental Air. The amount of air that may be forcibly expired after a normal quiet respiration. This is also the expiratory reserve volume and measures approximately 1600 cc

Complemental Air. The amount of air that may be forcibly inspired over and above a normal inspiration. This is known as the inspiratory reserve volume

Residual Volume. The amount of air remaining in the lungs after maximal expiration—about 1500 cc

Minimal Air. The small amount of air that remains in the alveoli. After death, if the thorax is opened and the lungs collapse, the minimal air pressure will allow the lungs to float

Vital Capacity. The volume of air that can be exhaled after a maximal inspiration. This amount equals the sum of the tidal air, complemental air, and the supplemental air

Functional Residual Capacity. The volume of air that remains in the lungs at the end of a normal expiration

Total Lung Capacity. The maximal volume of air in the lungs after a maximal inspiration

THE VITAL FUNCTION OF RESPIRATION

Temperature, pulse, respiration, and blood pressure are the vital signs that are essential elements for determining an individual's state of health. A deviation from normal of one or all of the vital signs denotes a state of illness. Evaluation of an individual's response to changes occurring within the body can be measured by taking his or her vital signs. Through careful analysis of these changes in the vital signs, a physician may determine a diagnosis, a prognosis, and a plan of treatment for the patient. The variations of certain vital signs signify a typical disease process and its stages of development. For example, in a patient who has pneumonia the temperature is elevated to 101° to 106°F, and pulse and respiration increase to almost twice their normal rates. When the patient's temperature falls, he or she will perspire profusely and his or her pulse and respiration will begin to return to normal rates.

The process of respiration is interrelated with other systems of the body. The medulla oblongata and the pons of the central nervous system regulate and control respiration. The rate, rhythm, and depth of respiration are controlled by nerve impulses from the medulla oblongata and the pons via the spinal cord and nerves to the muscles of the diaphragm, abdomen, and rib cage.

RESPIRATORY RATES

Individuals of different ages breathe at different respiratory rates. Respiratory rate is regulated by the respiratory center located in the medulla oblongata. The following are respiratory rates for some different age groups:

Newborn	30–80 per minute
1st year	20–40 per minute
5th year	20–25 per minute
15th year	15–20 per minute
Adult	15–20 per minute

230   MEDICAL TERMINOLOGY

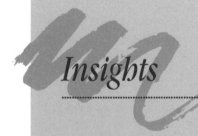

TUBERCULOSIS

Tuberculosis (TB) is a contagious disease caused by the bacillus *Mycobacterium tuberculosis.* This bacillus is carried in airborne particles, known as droplet nuclei, that can be generated when persons with pulmonary or laryngeal tuberculosis sneeze, cough, speak, or sing and can settle on food, clothing, walls, and floors.

Tuberculosis, once called "consumption," is not a new disease. At one time, it was the number one killer in the United States and it is still a major cause of death worldwide. One of public health's oldest enemies is back, and with a vengeance. An estimated 10 million Americans are infected with the TB bacterium. Compounding the problem is drug-resistant strains of TB that can shrug off as many as seven of the antibiotics traditionally used to treat this disease.

At the present time, TB is occurring primarily among AIDS patients, the homeless, drug abusers, prison inmates, and immigrants. Health officials are concerned about the rapid spread of this disease and the risks for the general public. Virtually anyone who comes in contact with an infected person is at risk of contracting TB. Studies show that exposure to an infected person in confined quarters such as in homes and classrooms increases an individual's risk.

CDC Guidelines

The Centers for Disease Control has published a booklet on Guidelines for Preventing the Transmission of Tuberculosis in Health-Care Settings. In the booklet, it gives the following specific actions to reduce the risk of tuberculosis transmission:

- Screening patients for active TB and TB infection.
- Providing rapid diagnostic services.
- Prescribing appropriate curative and preventive therapy.
- Maintaining physical measures to reduce microbial contamination of the air.
- Providing isolation rooms for persons with, or suspected of having, infectious TB.
- Screening health-care-facility personnel for TB infection.
- Promptly investigating and controlling outbreaks.

Symptoms:

Symptoms include a chronic cough, fatigue, low grade fever, night sweats, weakness, chills, anorexia, weight loss, hemoptysis, and in the early stages scanty, whitish, or grayish-yellow, frothy sputum. During the early stages of TB the sputum is expectorated in small quantities, but later when consolidation takes place it becomes more copious, tenacious, and yellowish-gray. In the late stages of TB, the sputum becomes mucopurulent, musty and fetid, containing fibers and tubercle bacilli, and blood-tinged or mixed with blood.

(Insights continues on next page)

Diagnosis:

To determine a diagnosis of tuberculosis, a careful history is taken and a complete physical examination is performed. After evaluation of the patient, the physician may order a tuberculin test (if the patient has not had a previous positive reaction), chest x-ray, a bronchoscopy or a sputum analysis for a positive diagnosis.

Treatment:

Treatment of TB requires long-term drug therapy (9 to 12 months), often using a regimen that includes a combination of antituberculosis agents. The use of multiple drugs is indicated in all but a few active cases, because any large population of *Mycobacterium tuberculosis* will have naturally occurring mutants that are resistant to each of the drugs administered. The primary drug regimen for active tuberculosis combines the drugs isoniazid, rifampin, and ethambutol. Diet and rest are also important aspects of treatment for this disease.

Terminology with Surgical Procedures & Pathology

Term	Word Parts			Definition
aerophore (air′ ō-for)	aero phore	CF S	air bearing	An apparatus for inflating the lungs of stillborn infants
aeropleura (air′ ō-ploo″ră)	aero pleura	CF R	air pleura	Air in the pleural cavity
alveolus (ăl-vē′ ō-lŭs)	alveol us	R S	small, hollow air sac pertaining to	Pertaining to a small air sac in the lungs
anosmia (ăn-ŏz′ mĭ-ă)	an osm ia	P R S	lack of smell condition	A condition in which there is a lack of the sense of smell
anoxia (ăn-ŏks′ ĭ-ă)	an ox ia	p R S	lack of oxygen condition	A condition in which there is a lack of oxygen
anthracosis (ăn″ thră-kō′ sĭs)	anthrac osis	R S	coal condition of	Black lung; a lung condition caused by inhalation of coal dust and silica
aphonia (ă-fō′ nĭ-ă)	a phon ia	P R S	lack of voice condition	A condition of inability to produce vocal sounds
aphrasia (ă-frā-′ zĭ-ă)	a phras ia	P R S	lack of speech condition	A condition of inability to speak
apnea (ăp′ -nē ă)	a pnea	P S	lack of breathing	Temporary cessation of breathing
atelectasis (ăt″ ĕ-lĕk′ tă-sĭs)	atel ectasis	R S	imperfect dilation	A condition of imperfect dilation of the lungs
bronchiectasis (brŏng″ kĭ-ĕk′ tă-sĭs)	bronchi ectasis	CF S	bronchi dilation	Dilation of the bronchi
bronchiolitis (brŏng″ kĭ-ō-lī′ tĭs)	bronchiol itis	R S	bronchiole inflammation	Inflammation of the bronchioles
bronchitis (brŏng-kī′ tĭs)	bronch itis	R S	bronchi inflammation	Inflammation of the bronchi
bronchomycosis (brŏng″ kō-mī-kō′ sĭs)	broncho myc osis	CF R S	bronchi fungus condition of	A fungus condition of the bronchi

(Terminology—continued)

Term	Word Parts			Definition
bronchoplasty (brŏng′ kō-plăs″ tē)	broncho	CF	bronchi	Surgical repair of the bronchi
	plasty	S	surgical repair	
bronchoscope (brŏng′ kō-skōp)	broncho	CF	bronchi	An instrument used to examine the bronchi
	scope	S	instrument	
cyanosis (sī″ ăn-ō′ -sĭs)	cyan	R	dark blue	A dark blue condition of the skin and mucous membrane caused by oxygen deficiency
	osis	S	condition of	
diaphragmalgia (dī″ ă-frăg-măl′ jĭ-ă)	dia	P	through	Pain in the diaphragm
	phragm	R	partition	
	algia	S	pain	
diaphragmatocele (dī″ ă-frăg-măt′ ō-sēl)	dia	P	through	A hernia of the diaphragm
	phragmato	CF	partition	
	cele	S	hernia	
dysphonia (dĭs-fō′ nĭ-ă)	dys	P	difficult	A condition of difficulty in speaking
	phon	R	voice	
	ia	S	condition	
dyspnea (dĭsp-nē′ ă)	dys	P	difficult	Difficulty in breathing
	pnea	S	breathing	
endotracheal (ĕn″ dō-trā′ kē-ăl)	endo	P	within	Pertaining to within the trachea
	trache	CF	trachea	
	al	S	pertaining to	
eupnea (ūp-nē′ ă)	eu	P	good, normal	Good or normal breathing
	pnea	S	breathing	
exhalation (ĕks″ hə-lā′ shən)	ex	P	out	The process of breathing out
	halat	R	breathe	
	ion	S	process	
expectoration (ĕk-spĕk″ tə′ rā′ shən)	ex	P	out	The process by which saliva, mucus, or phlegm is expelled from the air passages
	pectorat	R	breast	
	ion	S	process	
hemoptysis (hē-mŏp′ tĭ-sĭs)	hemo	CF	blood	The spitting up of blood
	ptysis	S	to spit	
hemothorax (hē″ mō-thō-răks)	hemo	CF	blood	Blood in the chest cavity
	thorax	R	chest	
hyperpnea (hī″ pĕrp-nē′ ă)	hyper	P	excessive	Excessive or rapid breathing
	pnea	S	breathing	

(Terminology—continued)

Term	Word Parts			Definition
hypoxia (hī-pŏks′ ĭ-ă)	hyp	P	below, deficient	A condition of deficient amounts of oxygen in the inspired air
	ox	R	oxygen	
	ia	S	condition	
inhalation (ĭn″ hă-lă′ shŭn)	in	P	in	The process of breathing in
	halat	R	breathe	
	ion	S	process	
laryngeal (lăr-ĭn′ jĭ-ăl)	larynge	CF	larynx	Pertaining to the larynx
	al	S	pertaining to	
laryngectomy (lăr″ ĭn-jĕk′ tō-mē)	laryng	R	larynx	Surgical excision of the larynx
	ectomy	S	excision	
laryngitis (lăr″ ĭn-jī′ tĭs)	laryng	R	larynx	Inflammation of the larynx
	itis	S	inflammation	
laryngoplasty (lăr-ĭn′ gō-plăs″ tē)	laryngo	CF	larynx	Surgical repair of the larynx
	plasty	S	surgical repair	
laryngoscope (lăr-ĭn′ gō-skōp)	laryngo	CF	larynx	An instrument used to examine the larynx
	scope	S	instrument	
laryngostenosis (lăr-ĭng″ gō-stĕ-nō′ sĭs)	laryngo	CF	larynx	A condition of narrowing of the larynx
	sten	R	narrowing	
	osis	S	condition of	
laryngostomy (lăr″ ĭn-gŏs′ tō-mē)	laryngo	CF	larynx	Establishing a new opening in the larynx
	stomy	S	new opening	
lobectomy (lō-bĕk′ tō-mē)	lob	R	lobe	Surgical excision of a lobe of any organ or gland, such as the lung
	ectomy	S	excision	
nasomental (nā″ zō-mĕn′ tăl)	naso	CF	nose	Pertaining to the nose and chin
	ment	R	chin	
	al	S	pertaining to	
nasopharyngitis (nā″ zō-făr′ ĭn-jī′ tĭs)	naso	CF	nose	Inflammation of the nose and pharynx
	pharyng	R	pharynx	
	itis	S	inflammation	
orthopnea (or″ thŏp-nē′ ă)	ortho	CF	straight	Inability to breathe unless in an upright or straight position
	pnea	S	breathing	
palatoplegia (păl″ ă-tō-plē′ jĭ-ă)	palato	CF	palate	Paralysis of the muscles of the soft palate
	plegia	S	stroke, paralysis	
pharyngalgia (făr″ ĭn-găl′ jĭ-ă)	pharyng	R	pharynx	Pain in the pharynx
	algia	S	pain	

(Terminology—continued)

Term	Word Parts			Definition
pharyngitis (făr″ ĭn-jī′ tĭs)	pharyng itis	R S	pharynx inflammation	Inflammation of the pharynx
pleuritis (ploo-rī′ tĭs)	pleur itis	R S	pleura inflammation	Inflammation of the pleura
pleurodynia (ploo″ rō-dĭn′ ĭ-ă)	pleuro dynia	CF S	pleura pain	Pain in the pleura
pneumoconiosis (nū″ mō-kō″ nĭ-ō′ sĭs)	pneumo coni osis	CF R S	lung dust condition of	A condition of the lung caused by the inhalation of dust
pneumonitis (nū″ mō-nī′ tĭs)	pneumon itis	R S	lung inflammation	Inflammation of the lung
pneumothorax (nū″ mō-thō′ răks)	pneumo thorax	CF R	air chest	A collection of air in the chest cavity
pulmometer (pŭl-mŏm′ ĕ-tĕr)	pulmo meter	CF S	lung instrument to measure	An instrument used to measure lung capacity
pulmonectomy (pŭl″ mō-nĕk′ tō-mē)	pulmon ectomy	R S	lung excision	Surgical excision of the lung or a part of a lung
pyothorax (pī″ ō-thō′ răks)	pyo thorax	CF R	pus chest	Pus in the chest cavity
rhinoplasty (rī′ nō-plăs″ tē)	rhino plasty	CF S	nose surgical repair	Surgical repair of the nose
rhinorrhagia (rī″ nō-ră′ jĭ-ă)	rhino rrhagia	CF S	nose bursting forth	The bursting forth of blood from the nose
rhinorrhea (rī″ nō-rē′ ă)	rhino rrhea	CF S	nose flow, discharge	Discharge from the nose
rhinostenosis (rī″ nō-stĕn-ō′ sĭs)	rhino sten osis	CF R S	nose narrowing condition of	A condition of narrowing of the nasal passages
rhinotomy (rī-nŏt′ ō-mē)	rhino tomy	CF S	nose incision	Incision of the nose
sinusitis (sī″ nŭs-ī′ tĭs)	sinus itis	R S	a curve, hollow inflammation	Inflammation of a sinus

(Terminology—continued)

Term	Word Parts			Definition
spirogram (spī′ rō-grăm)	spiro	CF	breath	A record made by a spirograph showing respiratory movements
	gram	S	a mark, record	
spirometer (spī-rŏm′ ĕt-ĕr)	spiro	CF	breath	An instrument used to measure the volume of respired air
	meter	S	instrument to measure	
tachypnea (tăk″ ĭp-nē′ ă)	tachy	P	fast	Fast breathing
	pnea	S	breathing	
thoracocentesis (thō″ răk-ō-sĕn-tē′ sĭs)	thoraco	CF	chest	Surgical puncture of the chest for removal of fluid
	centesis	S	surgical puncture	
thoracopathy (thō″ răk-ŏp′ ă-thē)	thoraco	CF	chest	Any disease of the chest
	pathy	S	disease	
thoracoplasty (thō′ ră-kō-plăs″ tē)	thoraco	CF	chest	Surgical repair of the chest
	plasty	S	surgical repair	
thoracotomy (thō″ răk-ŏt′ ō-mē)	thoraco	CF	chest	Incision of the chest
	tomy	S	incision	
tonsillectomy (tŏn″ sĭl-ĕk′ tō-mē)	tonsill	R	almond, tonsil	Surgical excision of the tonsils
	ectomy	S	excision	
tonsillitis (tŏn″ sĭl-ī′ tĭs)	tonsill	R	almond, tonsil	Inflammation of the tonsils
	itis	S	inflammation	
tracheal (trā′ kē-ăl)	trache	R	trachea	Pertaining to the trachea
	al	S	pertaining to	
trachealgia (trā″ kē-ăl′ jĭ-ă)	trache	R	trachea	Pain in the trachea
	algia	S	pain	
tracheitis (trā″ kē-ī′ tĭs)	trache	R	trachea	Inflammation of the trachea
	itis	S	inflammation	
tracheolaryngo-tomy (trā″ kē-ō-lăr″ ĭn-gŏt′ ō-mē)	tracheo	CF	trachea	Incision into the larynx and trachea
	laryngo	CF	larynx	
	tomy	S	incision	
tracheostomy (trā″ kē-ŏs′ tō-mē)	tracheo	CF	trachea	New opening into the trachea
	stomy	S	new opening	

Vocabulary Words

Vocabulary words are terms that have not been divided into component parts. They are common words or specialized terms associated with the subject of this chapter. These words are provided to enhance your medical vocabulary.

Word	Definition
artificial respiration (ăr″ tĭ-fĭsh′ ăl rĕs″ pĭr-ā′ shŭn)	The process of using artificial means to cause air to flow into and out of an individual's lungs when breathing is inadequate or ceases
asphyxia (ăs-fĭk′ sĭ-ă)	A condition in which there is a depletion of oxygen in the blood with an increase of carbon dioxide in the blood and tissues. First-aid treatment is by artificial respiration
aspiration (ăs″ pĭ-rā′ shŭn)	The process of taking substances in or out by means of suction
asthma (ăz′ mă)	A disease of the bronchi characterized by wheezing, dyspnea, and a feeling of constriction in the chest
atelectasis (ăt″ ĕ-lĕk′ tă-sĭs)	A condition in which the lung is collapsed or airless
carbon dioxide (kăr bən dī-ŏk′ sīd)	A colorless, odorless gas used with oxygen to stimulate respiration
Cheyne-Stokes respiration (chān′ stōks′ rĕs″ pĭr-ā′ shŭn)	A rhythmic cycle of breathing with a gradual increase in respiration followed by apnea (which may last from 10–60 sec), then a repeat of the same cycle
coryza (kŏr-rī′ ză)	The common cold characterized by sneezing, nasal discharge, coughing, and malaise
cough (kawf)	Sudden, forceful expulsion of air from the lungs. It is an essential protective response that clears irritants, secretions, or foreign objects from the trachea, bronchi, and/or lungs
croup (croop)	A respiratory disease characterized by a "barking" cough, dyspnea, hoarseness, and laryngeal spasm
cystic fibrosis (sĭs′ tĭk fĭ-brō′ sĭs)	An inherited disease that affects the pancreas, respiratory system, and sweat glands. The etiology is unknown, and the prognosis is generally poor
emphysema (ĕm″ fĭ-sē′ mă)	A chronic pulmonary disease in which the bronchioles become obstructed with mucus
empyema (ĕm″ pī-ē′ mă)	Pus in a body cavity, especially the pleural cavity
epistaxis (ĕp″ ĭ-stăk′ sĭs)	Nosebleed

(Vocabulary—continued)

Word	Definition
Heimlich maneuver (hīm′ lĭk)	A technique for removing a foreign body (usually a bolus of food) that is blocking the trachea
hyperbaric oxygenation (hī″ pĕr-băr′ ĭk ŏk″ sĭ-jĕn-ā′ shŭn)	The process of administering oxygen in a closed chamber at a pressure greater than one and one-half to three times absolute atmospheric pressure
hyperventilation (hī″ pĕr-vĕn″ tĭ-lā′ shŭn)	The process of excessive ventilating, thereby increasing the air in the lungs beyond the normal limit
influenza (ĭn″ flū-ĕn′ ză)	An acute, contagious respiratory infection caused by a virus. Onset is usually sudden, and symptoms are fever, chills, headache, myalgia, cough, and sore throat
Kussmaul's breathing (koos′ mowlz brēth′ ĭng)	A distressing, deep gasping type of breathing associated with metabolic acidosis and coma; also called air hunger
legionnaire's disease (lē jə naerz′ dĭ-zēz′)	A severe pulmonary pneumonia caused by *Legionella pneumophilia*
mesothelioma (mĕs″ ō-thē″ lĭ-ō′ mă)	A malignant tumor of mesothelium (serous membrane of the pleura) caused by the inhalation of asbestos
nares (nā′ rĕs)	The nostrils
olfaction (ŏl-făk′ shŭn)	The process of smelling
oropharynx (or″ ō-făr′ ĭnks)	The central portion of the throat that lies between the soft palate and upper portion of the epiglottis
palatopharyngo-plasty (păl″ ăt-ō-făr″ ĭn′ gō-plăs″ tē)	A type of surgery that cures snoring and sleep apnea by removing the uvula and the tonsils and reshaping the lining at the back of the throat to enlarge the air passageway
pertussis (pĕr-tŭs′ ĭs)	An acute, infectious disease characterized by coryza, an explosive paroxysmal cough ending in a "crowing" or "whooping" sound; also called whooping cough
pleurisy (ploo′ rĭs-ē)	Inflammation of the pleura caused by injury, infection, or a tumor

(Vocabulary—continued)

Word	Definition
pneumonia (nū-mō′ nĭ-ā)	Inflammation of the lung caused by bacteria, viruses, or chemical irritants
pollinosis (pŏl-ĭn-ō′ sĭs)	Hay fever; nasal congestion of mucous membranes caused by an allergic reaction to a pollen or pollens
polyp (pŏl′ ĭp)	A tumor with a stem; may occur where there are mucous membranes, such as the nose, ears, mouth, uterus, and intestines
rale (rahl)	An abnormal sound heard on auscultation of the chest; a crackling, rattling, or bubbling sound
respirator (rĕs′ pĭ-rā″ tor)	A type of machine used for prolonged artificial respiration
respiratory distress syndrome (hyaline membrane disease) (rĕs′ pĭ-ră-tō″ rē dĭs-trĕs′ sĭn′ drōm)	A condition that may occur in a premature infant in which the lungs are not matured to the point of manufacturing lecithin, a pulmonary surfactant. This results in collapse of the alveoli, which leads to cyanosis and hypoxia
rhinovirus (rī″ nō-vī′ rŭs)	One of a subgroup of viruses that causes the common cold in humans
rhonchus (rŏng′ kŭs)	A rale or rattling sound in the throat or bronchial tubes caused by a partial obstruction
sputum (spū′ tŭm)	Substance coughed up from the lungs; may be watery, thick, purulent, clear, or bloody and may contain microorganisms
stridor (strī′ dōr)	A high-pitched sound caused by obstruction of the air passageway
tuberculosis (tū-bĕr″ kū-lō′ sĭs)	An infectious disease caused by the tubercle bacillus, *Mycobacterium tuberculosis*
wheeze (hwēz)	A whistling sound caused by obstruction of the air passageway

ABBREVIATIONS

ABGs	arterial blood gases	**IRV**	inspiratory reserve volume
AFB	acid-fast bacilli	**MBC**	maximal breathing capacity
ARD	acute respiratory disease	**MV**	minute volume
ARDS	adult respiratory distress syndrome	**MVV**	maximal voluntary ventilation
CF	cystic fibrosis	**O₂**	oxygen
CO₂	carbon dioxide	**PEEP**	positive end expiratory pressure
COLD	chronic obstructive lung disease	**PND**	postnasal drip
COPD	chronic obstructive pulmonary disease	**PPD**	purified protein derivative
		R	respiration
CXR	chest x-ray	**RD**	respiratory disease
ENT	ear, nose, and throat	**RDS**	respiratory distress syndrome
ERV	expiratory reserve volume	**SIDS**	sudden infant death syndrome
ET	endotracheal	**SOB**	shortness of breath
FEF	forced expiratory flow	**T & A**	tonsillectomy and adenoidectomy
FEV	forced expiratory volume	**TB**	tuberculosis
HBOT	hyperbaric oxygen therapy	**TLC**	total lung capacity
HMD	hyaline membrane disease	**TV**	tidal volume
IPPB	intermittent positive-pressure breathing	**URI**	upper respiratory infection
IRDS	infant respiratory distress syndrome	**VC**	vital capacity

Drug Highlights

Drugs that are generally used in respiratory system diseases and disorders include antihistamines, decongestants, antitussives, expectorants, mucolytics, bronchodilators, inhalational corticosteroids, and antituberculosis agents.

Antihistamines   Act to counter the effects of histamine by blocking histamine 1 (H_1) receptors. They are used in the treatment of allergy symptoms, for preventing or controlling motion sickness, and in combination with cold remedies to decrease mucus secretion and produce bedtime sedation.

Examples: Benadryl (diphenhydramine), Seldane (terfenadine), Hismanal (astemizole), and Dimetane (brompheniramine maleate).

Decongestants   Act to constrict dilated arterioles in the nasal mucosa. These agents are used for the temporary relief of nasal congestion associated with the common cold, hay fever, other upper respiratory allergies, and sinusitis.

Examples: Sudafed (pseudoephedrine HCl), Coricidin (phenylephrine HCl), Sinutab Long-Lasting Sinus Spray (xylometazoline HCl), and Afrin (oxymetazoline HCl).

Antitussives
Non-narcotic agents

May be classified as non-narcotic and narcotic.
Anesthetize the stretch receptors located in the respiratory passages, lungs, and pleura by dampening their activity and thereby reducing the cough reflex at its source.

Examples: Tessalon (benzonatate), Benylin (diphenhydramine HCl), and dextromethorphan hydrobromide.

Narcotic agents

Depress the cough center that is located in the medulla, thereby raising its threshold for incoming cough impulse.

Examples: codeine and Codone (hydrocodone bitartrate).

Expectorants

Promote and facilitate the removal of mucus from the lower respiratory tract.

Examples: Robitussin (guaifenesin) and terpin hydrate.

Mucolytics

Break chemical bonds in mucus, thereby lowering its thickness.

Example: Mucomyst (acetylcysteine).

Bronchodilators

Are used to improve pulmonary airflow.

Examples: Adrenalin (epinephrine), Proventil (albuterol), ephedrine sulfate, aminophylline, and Tedral SA (theophylline).

Inhalational Corticosteroids

Used in the treatment of bronchial asthma, and in seasonal or perennial allergic conditions when other forms of treatment are not effective.

Examples: Decadron (dexamethasone phosphate), Beclovent (beclomethasone dipropionate), and Azmacort (triamcinolone acetonide).

Antituberculosis Agents

Used in the long-term treatment of tuberculosis (9 months to 1 year). They are often used in *combination of two or more drugs and the primary drug regimen for active tuberculosis combines the drugs ethambutol HCl (Myambutol), isoniazid (INH; Nydrazid), and rifampin (Rifadin; Rimactane).*

Communication Enrichment

This segment is provided for those who wish to enhance their ability to communicate in either English or Spanish.

RELATED TERMS

English	Spanish
asthma	asma (ăs-mă)
breath	aliento; respiro (ă-lĭ-ĕn-tō; rĕs-pĭ-rō)
bronchitis	bronquitis (brōn-kĭ-tĭs)
chest	pecho (pĕ-chō)
cough	tos (tōs)
deep breath	rispire profundo (rĕs-pĭ-rĕ prō-fūn-dō)
diaphragm	diafragma (dĭ-ă-frăg-mă)
difficulty in breathing	dificultad en respirar (dĭ-fĭ-cŭl-tăd ĕn rĕs-pĭ-răr)
dust	polvo (pōl-vō)
hoarseness	ronquedad; ronquera (rōn-kĕ-dăd; rōn-kay-ră)
lungs	pulmónes (pŭl-mō-nĕs)
nose	nariz (nă-riz)
nosebleed	hemorragia nasal (ĕ-mōr-ră-hĭ-ă nă-săl)
phlegm	flema (flĕ-mă)
pneumonia	neumonía; pulmonía (nĕ-ū-mō-nĭ-ă; pŭl-mō-nĭ-ă)
pollen	polen (pō-lĕn)
throat	garganta (găr-găn-tă)
sore throat	dolor de garganta (dō-lōr dĕ găr-găn-tă)

English	Spanish
tuberculosis	tuberculosis (tŭ-*bĕr*-kū-lōs-ĭs)
voice	voz (vōz)
whooping cough	tosferina (tōs-*fĕ*-rĭ-nă)
respiration	respiración (rĕs-pĭ-*ră*-sĭ-ōn)
thorax	tórax (*tō*-răx)
hoarse	ronco (*rōn*-kō)
snore	ronquido (rōn-*kĭ*-dō)
influenza	gripe (*ġrĭ*-pĕ)
pleurisy	pleuritis (plĕ-ū-rĭ-tĭs)
exhale	exhalar (ex-*hă*lăr)
inhale	inhalar (*ĭn*-hă-lăr)
larynx	laringe (*lă*-rĭn-hĕ)
tonsil	tonsila; amigdala (tōn-*sĭ*-lă; ă-mĭg-*dă*lă)
tonsillitis	tonsilitis; amigdalitis (tōn-*sĭ*-lĭ-tĭs; ă-mĭg-*dă*lĭ-tĭs)
croup	crup (crūp)
aspiration	aspiración (*ăs*-pĭ-ră-sĭ-ōn)
asphyxia	asfixia (ăs-*fix*-ĭ-ă)
common cold	resfriado común (rĕs-*frĭ*-ă-dō cō-mūn)

DIAGNOSTIC AND LABORATORY TESTS

Test	Description
acid-fast bacilli (AFB) (ăs ĭd-făst″ bă-sĭl′ ī)	A test performed on sputum to detect the presence of *Mycobacterium tuberculosis,* an acid-fast bacilli. Positive results indicate tuberculosis
antistreptolysin O (ASO) (ăn″ tĭ-strĕp-tŏl′ ĭ-sĭn)	A test performed on blood serum to detect the presence of streptolysin enzyme O, which is secreted by beta-hemolytic streptococcus. Positive results indicate streptococcal infection
arterial blood gases (ABGs) (ăr-tē′ rē-ăl blod găs′ ĕs)	A series of tests performed on arterial blood to establish acid-base balance. Important in determining respiratory acidosis and/or alkalosis, metabolic acidosis and/or alkalosis
bronchoscopy (brŏng-kŏs′ kō-pē)	Visual examination of the larynx, trachea, and bronchi via a flexible bronchoscope. With the use of biopsy forceps, tissues and secretions can be removed for further analysis
culture, sputum (kŭl′ tūr, spū′ tŭm)	Examination of the sputum to determine the presence of microorganisms. Abnormal results may indicate tuberculosis, bronchitis, pneumonia, bronchiectasis, and other infectious respiratory diseases
culture, throat (kŭl′ tūr, thrōt)	A test done to identify the presence of microorganisms in the throat, especially beta-hemolytic streptococci
laryngoscopy (lăr″ ĭn-gŏs′ kō-pē)	Visual examination of the larynx via a laryngoscope
nasopharyngography (nā″ zō-făr-ĭn-ŏg′ ră-fē)	X-ray examination of the nasopharynx
pulmonary function test (pŭl′ mō-nĕ-rē fũng′ shŭn test)	A series of tests performed to determine the diffusion of oxygen and carbon dioxide across the cell membrane in the lungs. Tests included are: tidal volume (TV), vital capacity (VC), expiratory reserve volume (ERV), inspiratory capacity (IC), residual volume (RV), forced inspiratory volume (FIV), functional residual capacity (FRC), maximal voluntary ventilation (MVV), total lung capacity (TLC), and flow volume loop (F-V loop). Abnormal results may indicate various respiratory diseases and conditions
rhinoscopy (rī-nŏs′ kō-pē)	Visual examination of the nasal passages

Learning Exercises

Anatomy and Physiology

Write your answers to the following questions. Do not refer back to the text.

1. List the organs of the respiratory system.

   a. _____   b. _____

   c. _____   d. _____

   e. _____   f. _____

2. State the primary function of the respiratory system. _____
   _____

3. Define external respiration. _____

4. Define internal respiration. _____

5. List the five functions of the nose.

   a. _____

   b. _____

   c. _____

   d. _____

   e. _____

6. Name the three divisions of the pharynx.

   a. _____   b. _____

   c. _____

7. List the three functions of the pharynx.

   a. _____

   b. _____

   c. _____

8. State the function of the epiglottis. _____

9. Define glottis. _____

10. State the function of the larynx. _____

11. State the function of the trachea. _____

12. The trachea divides into the _____ _____ and
    the _____ _____ .

13. State the function of the bronchi. _____

14. Give a brief description of the lungs. _____
    _____

15. Define pleura. _____

16. The thoracic cavity is separated from the abdominal cavity by a musculomembranous
    wall commonly known as the _____ .

17. The central portion of the thoracic cavity, between the lungs, is a space called the _____.

18. The right lung has _____ lobes and the left lung has _____ lobes.

19. The air cells of the lungs are the _____.

20. State the main function of the lungs. _____
_____

21. The vital signs, which are essential elements for determining an individual's state of health, are _____, _____, _____, and _____.

22. Define the following terms:

   a. Tidal Volume _____

   b. Residual Volume _____

   c. Vital Capacity _____

23. The _____ _____ and the _____ of the central nervous system regulate and control respiration.

24. The respiratory rate for a newborn is _____ to _____ breaths per minute.

25. The respiratory rate for an adult is _____ to _____ breaths per minute.

Word Parts

1. In the spaces provided, write the definition of these prefixes, roots, combining forms, and suffixes. Do not refer to the listings of terminology words. Leave blank those terms you cannot define.
2. After completing as many as you can, refer back to the terminology word listings to check your work. For each word missed or left blank, write the term and its definition several times on the margins of these pages or on a separate sheet of paper.
3. To maximize the learning process, it is to your advantage to do the following exercises as directed. To refer to the terminology listings before completing these exercises invalidates the learning process.

PREFIXES

Give the definitions of the following prefixes:

1. a- _____ 2. an- _____
3. dia- _____ 4. dys- _____
5. endo- _____ 6. eu- _____
7. ex- _____ 8. hyp- _____
9. hyper- _____ 10. in- _____
11. tachy- _____

ROOTS AND COMBINING FORMS

Give the definitions of the following roots and combining forms:

1. aero _____
2. alveol _____
3. anthrac _____
4. atel _____
5. bronch _____
6. bronchi _____
7. bronchiol _____
8. broncho _____
9. coni _____
10. cyan _____
11. halat _____
12. hemo _____
13. laryng _____
14. larynge _____
15. laryngo _____
16. lob _____
17. ment _____
18. myc _____
19. naso _____
20. ortho _____
21. osm _____
22. ox _____
23. palato _____
24. pectorat _____
25. pharyng _____
26. phon _____
27. phragm _____
28. phragmato _____
29. phras _____
30. pleur _____
31. pleura _____
32. pleuro _____
33. pneumo _____
34. pneumon _____
35. pulmo _____
36. pulmon _____
37. pyo _____
38. rhino _____
39. sinus _____
40. spiro _____
41. sten _____
42. thoraco _____
43. thorax _____
44. tonsill _____
45. trache _____
46. tracheo _____

SUFFIXES

Give the definitions of the following suffixes:

1. -al _____
2. -algia _____
3. -cele _____
4. -centesis _____
5. -dynia _____
6. -ectasis _____
7. -ectomy _____
8. -gram _____
9. -ia _____
10. -ion _____
11. -itis _____
12. -meter _____
13. -osis _____
14. -pathy _____
15. -phore _____
16. -plasty _____
17. -plegia _____
18. -pnea _____

19. -ptysis   _____   20. -rrhagia   _____

21. -rrhea   _____   22. -scope   _____

23. -stomy   _____   24. -tomy   _____

25. -us   _____

Identifying Medical Terms

In the spaces provided, write the medical terms for the following meanings:

1. _____ Air in the pleural cavity

2. _____ Pertaining to a small air sac in the lungs

3. _____ Inability to produce vocal sounds

4. _____ Dilation of the bronchi

5. _____ Inflammation of the bronchi

6. _____ Surgical repair of the bronchi

7. _____ Difficulty in speaking

8. _____ Good or normal breathing

9. _____ The spitting up of blood

10. _____ The process of breathing in

11. _____ Inflammation of the larynx

12. _____ A condition of narrowing of the larynx

13. _____ Pertaining to the nose and chin

14. _____ Pain in the pharynx

15. _____ A collection of air in the chest cavity

16. _____ Surgical repair of the nose

17. _____ Discharge from the nose

18. _____ Inflammation of a sinus

19. _____ Any disease of the chest

Spelling

In the spaces provided, write the correct spelling of these misspelled terms:

1. bronchscope   _____   2. diaphramatcele   _____

3. expectorion   _____   4. laryngal   _____

5. orthpnea   _____   6. peluritis   _____

7. pulmnectomy   _____   8. rhintomy   _____

9. trachypnea   _____   10. trachal   _____

Review Questions

Matching

Select the appropriate lettered meaning for each numbered line.

_____ 1. cough   a. Substance coughed up from the lungs

_____ 2. cystic fibrosis   b. Hay fever

_____ 3. influenza   c. The process of smelling

_____ 4. nares   d. One of a subgroup of viruses that causes the
                                             common cold in humans
_____ 5. olfaction
                                         e. Fast breathing
_____ 6. pollinosis
                                         f. The nostrils
_____ 7. rhinovirus
                                         g. Surgical puncture of the chest for removal of fluid
_____ 8. sputum
                                         h. Sudden, forceful expulsion of air from the lungs
_____ 9. tachypnea
                                         i. An inherited disease that affects the pancreas,
_____ 10. thoracocentesis   respiratory system, and sweat glands

                                         j. Slow breathing

                                         k. An acute, contagious respiratory infection caused
                                             by a virus

Abbreviations

Place the correct word, phrase, or abbreviation in the space provided.

_____ 1. acid-fast bacilli

_____ 2. CF

_____ 3. Chest x-ray

_____ 4. chronic obstructive lung disease

_____ 5. ET

_____ 6. PND

_____ 7. respiration

_____ 8. SIDS

_____ 9. shortness of breath

_____ 10. TB

Diagnostic and Laboratory Tests

Select the best answer to each multiple choice question. Circle the letter of your choice.

1. A test performed on sputum to detect the presence of *Mycobacterium tuberculosis.*

   a. antistreptolysin O

   b. acid-fast bacilli

   c. pulmonary function test

   d. bronchoscopy

2. The visual examination of the nasal passages.

   a. bronchoscopy

   b. laryngoscopy

   c. rhinoscopy

   d. nasopharyngography

3. _____ are important in determining respiratory acidosis and/or alkalosis, metabolic acidosis and/or alkalosis.

   a. Acid-fast bacilli

   b. Antistreptolysin O

   c. Arterial blood gases

   d. Pulmonary function test

4. A series of tests to determine the diffusion of oxygen and carbon dioxide across the cell membrane in the lungs.

   a. acid-fast bacilli

   b. antistreptolysin O

   c. arterial blood gases

   d. pulmonary function test

5. The visual examination of the larynx, trachea, and bronchi via a flexible scope.

   a. bronchoscopy

   b. laryngoscopy

   c. nasopharyngography

   d. rhinoscopy

10 The Urinary System

The urinary system consists of two kidneys, two ureters, one bladder, and one urethra. It is referred to as the excretory system, genitourinary system, or urogenital system. The vital function of the urinary system is extraction of certain wastes from the bloodstream, conversion of these materials to urine, transport of the urine from the kidneys via the ureters to the bladder, and elimination of it at appropriate intervals via the urethra.

URINARY TRACT INFECTIONS

Left untreated, bladder and other urinary tract infections can travel into the kidneys and cause serious complications. Each year, approximately 10 million patients seek treatment for urinary tract infections, with cystitis being most common. Prevalence of urinary tract infections according to age and sex:

Age Group	Prevalence	Sex Ratio Male: Female
Preschool	2–3%	1:10
School age	1–2%	1:30
Reproductive age	2.5%	1:50
Elderly (65–70)	20%	1:10

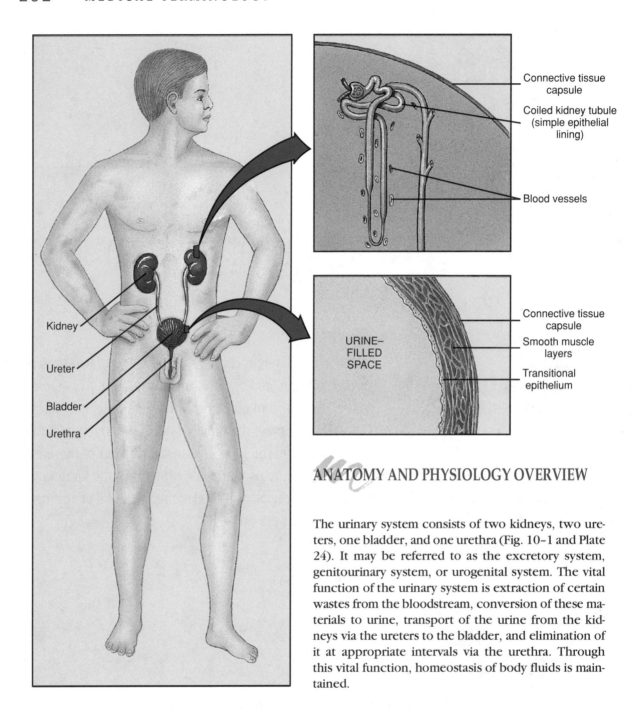

Connective tissue capsule

Coiled kidney tubule (simple epithelial lining)

Blood vessels

Connective tissue capsule

Smooth muscle layers

Transitional epithelium

URINE–FILLED SPACE

Kidney

Ureter

Bladder

Urethra

ANATOMY AND PHYSIOLOGY OVERVIEW

The urinary system consists of two kidneys, two ureters, one bladder, and one urethra (Fig. 10–1 and Plate 24). It may be referred to as the excretory system, genitourinary system, or urogenital system. The vital function of the urinary system is extraction of certain wastes from the bloodstream, conversion of these materials to urine, transport of the urine from the kidneys via the ureters to the bladder, and elimination of it at appropriate intervals via the urethra. Through this vital function, homeostasis of body fluids is maintained.

THE URINARY SYSTEM

Organ	Primary Function
Kidneys	Form and concentrate urine, regulate blood pH and ion concentrations
Ureters	Conduct urine from kidneys to urinary bladder
Urinary Bladder	Stores urine for eventual elimination
Urethra	Carries urine to exterior

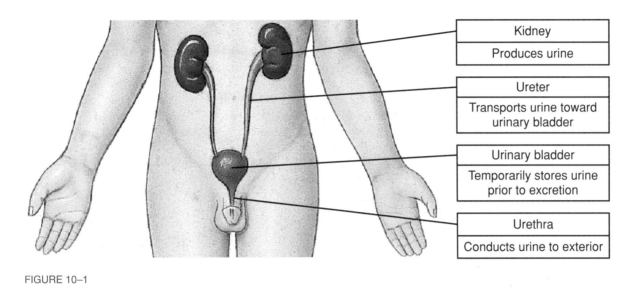

Kidney
Produces urine

Ureter
Transports urine toward urinary bladder

Urinary bladder
Temporarily stores urine prior to excretion

Urethra
Conducts urine to exterior

FIGURE 10–1

Components of the urinary system. (*From Martini F.* Fundamentals of Anatomy and Physiology, *2nd ed. Englewood Cliffs, NJ: Prentice-Hall, 1992, with permission.*)

The Kidneys

The kidneys are purplish-brown, bean-shaped organs located at the back of the abdominal cavity (retroperitoneal area). They lie, one on each side of the spinal column, just above the waistline, against the muscles of the back. Each kidney is surrounded by three capsules; the true capsule, the perirenal fat, and the renal fascia. The true capsule is a smooth, fibrous connective membrane that is loosely adherent to the surface of the kidney. The perirenal fat is the adipose capsule that embeds each kidney in fatty tissue. The renal fascia is a sheath of fibrous tissue that helps to anchor the kidney to the surrounding structures and helps to maintain its normal position.

EXTERNAL STRUCTURE

Each kidney has a concave border and a convex border. The center of the concave border opens into a notch called the hilum. The renal artery and vein, nerves, and lymphatic vessels enter and leave through the hilum. The ureter enters the kidney through the hilum into a sac-like collecting portion called the renal pelvis.

INTERNAL STRUCTURE

When a cross section is made through the kidney, two distinct areas are seen comprising its anterior: the cortex, which is the outer layer, and the medulla or inner portion. The cortex contains the arteries, veins, convoluted tubules, and glomerular capsules. The medulla contains the renal pyramids, cone-like masses with papillae projecting into calyces of the pelvis.

MICROSCOPIC ANATOMY

Microscopic examination of the kidney reveals about 1 million nephrons, which are the structural and functional units of the organ. Each nephron consists of a renal corpuscle and tubule. The renal corpuscle or malpighian corpuscle consists of a glomerulus and Bowman's capsule. Extending from each Bowman's capsule is a tubule consisting of the proximal convoluted portion, the loop of Henle, and a distal convoluted portion that opens into a collecting tubule.

THE NEPHRON

The vital function of the nephron is to remove the waste products of metabolism from the blood plasma. These waste products are urea, uric acid, and creatinine, plus any excess sodium, chloride, and potassium ions and ketone bodies. The nephron plays a vital role in the maintenance of normal fluid balance in the body by allowing for reabsorption of water and some electrolytes back into the blood. Approximately 1000 to 1200 mL of blood passes through the kidney per minute. At a rate of 1000 mL of blood per minute about 1.5 million mL pass through the kidney in each 24-hour day (Fig. 10–2 and Plate 3).

The Ureters

There are two ureters, one for each kidney. They are narrow, muscular tubes that transport urine from the kidneys to the bladder. They are from 28 to 34 cm long and vary in diameter from 1 mm to 1 cm. The walls of the ureters consist of three layers: an inner coat of mucous membrane, a middle coat of smooth muscle, and an outer coat of fibrous tissue.

The Urinary Bladder

The urinary bladder is the muscular, membranous sac that serves as a reservoir for urine. It is located in the anterior portion of the pelvic cavity and consists of a lower portion, the neck, which is continuous with the urethra, and an upper portion, the apex, which is connected with the umbilicus by the median umbilical ligament. The trigone is a small triangular area near the base of the bladder. The wall of the bladder consists of four layers: an inner layer of epithelium, a muscular coat of smooth muscle, an outer layer comprised of longitudinal muscle (detrusor urinae), and a fibrous layer. An empty bladder feels firm as the muscular wall becomes thick. As the bladder fills with urine, the muscular wall becomes thinner and it distends according to the amount of urine present.

The Urethra

The urethra is the musculomembranous tube extending from the bladder to the outside of the body. The external urinary opening is the urinary meatus. The male urethra is approximately 8 inches long and is divided into three sections: prostatic, membranous, and penile. It conveys both urine and semen. The female urethra is approximately 1.5 inches long. The urinary meatus is situated between the clitoris and the opening of the vagina. The female urethra conveys only urine.

Urine

THE FORMATION OF URINE

Urine is formed by the process of filtration and reabsorption in the nephron. Blood enters the nephron via the afferent arteriole. As it passes through the glomerulus, water and dissolved substances are filtered through the glomerular membrane and collect in the Bowman's capsule. The glomerular filtrate passes through the proximal tubule, into the loop of Henle, into the distal tubule, and then into the collecting tubule. Water and some selected substances are reabsorbed into the capillaries surrounding the tubules. Substances such as uric acid and hydrogen ions, through the process of secretion, may be added to the fluid now known as urine. Urine consists of 95% water and 5% solid substances. It is secreted by the kidneys and transported by the ureters to the bladder, where it is stored before being discharged from the body via the urethra. An average normal adult feels the need to void when the bladder contains around 300 to 350 mL of urine. An average of 1000 to 1500 mL

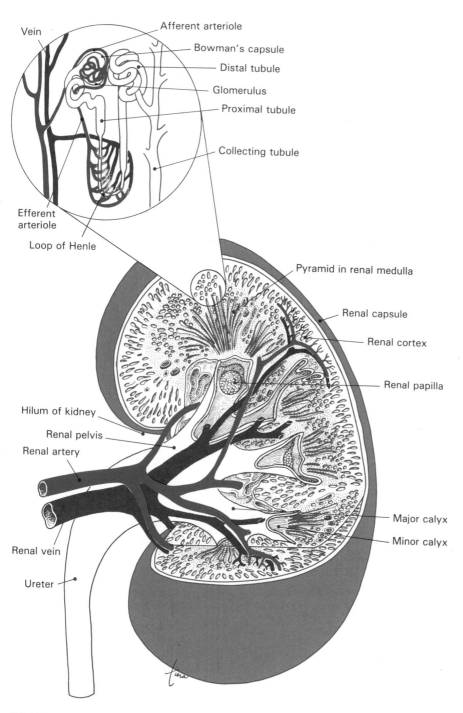

FIGURE 10–2

The kidney with an exploded view of a nephron. *Adapted from Evans WF.* Anatomy and Physiology, *3rd ed. Englewood Cliffs, NJ: Prentice-Hall, 1983, with permission.)*

of urine is voided daily. Normal urine is clear, yellow to amber in color, has a faintly aromatic odor, a specific gravity of 1.015 to 1.025, and a slightly acid pH.

URINALYSIS

Urinalysis is a laboratory procedure that may involve the physical, chemical, and microscopic examination of urine. A freshly voided urine specimen will provide for more accurate test results as certain changes may occur in urine that is left standing. If the urinalysis cannot be performed on the specimen within 1 hour of the time voided, it should be refrigerated, with the time of collection written on the label of the container. Urine should be collected in a clean, dry container. A disposable container is preferred. When a bacteriologic culture is to be done on urine, the specimen is collected by catheterization.

Urinalysis is a valuable diagnostic tool, as abnormal conditions or diseases may be quickly and easily detected because of the fact that the physical and chemical constituents of normal urine are constant.

NORMAL CONSTITUENTS

The following are the normal constituents of urine as detected by various examinations of the specimen:

Under Physical Examination

1. Color—should be yellow to amber in color because of the presence of urochrome
2. Appearance—normal urine is described as being clear
3. Reaction—acid, between 5.0 and 7.0 pH with an average pH of 6.0
4. Specific gravity—between 1.015 and 1.025
5. Odor—faintly aromatic
6. Quantity—around 1000 to 1500 mL per day

Under Chemical Examination

1. pH—5.0 to 7.0
2. Protein—negative
3. Glucose—negative
4. Ketones—negative
5. Bilirubin—negative
6. Blood—negative
7. Nitrites—negative
8. Urobilinogen—0.1 to 1.0

Under Microscopic Examination

1. Red blood cells—not normally found in urine although they may be present as a result of menstrual contamination or trauma of catheterization
2. White blood cells—usually present, especially in females; normal to find zero to five white blood cells
3. Epithelial cells—normally found in urine. There are three kinds of epithelial cells: renal from the renal cells of the kidney; transitional from the pelvis of the kidney, ureters, and bladder; and the third type, squamous from the urethra and vagina
4. Yeast—not normally found in urine
5. Urinary casts—not normally found in urine. When present, they are highly diagnostic as they are molded in the shape of the kidney tubules in which they are formed and are seen in urine with a pH of 6.0 or less
6. Trichomonas—not normally found in urine
7. Crystals—not normally found in urine
8. Other features—cotton fibers, powder, oil, spermatozoa, and hair may be seen in normal urine

ABNORMAL CONSTITUENTS

The following are the indications of abnormal constituents that may be found in urine during urinalysis:

Under Physical Examination

1. Color—red or reddish tint may be caused by the presence of hemoglobin, dyes, or phenophthalein. Orange may be due to pyridum or santonin. Greenish-yellow to greenish-brown or black may be caused by bile pigments or thymol indigo. The color of urine darkens on standing
2. Appearance—a milky appearance may be caused by fat globules, pus, or bacteria. A smoky appearance may be caused by blood cells. Haze or turbidity may be caused by refrigeration
3. Reaction: High acidity—diabetic acidosis, fever, pulmonary emphysema, diarrhea, and dehydration
Alkalinity—chronic cystitis, urinary tract infection, renal failure, pyloric obstruction, and salicylate intoxication; also may indicate an old urine specimen
4. Specific Gravity: Low—dilute urine 1.001 to 1.010, diabetes insipidus
High—concentrated urine 1.025 to 1.030, diabetes mellitus, hepatic disease, congestive heart failure
5. Odor: Fruity sweet—acetone, associated with diabetes mellitus
Unpleasant—decomposition of certain chemicals, drugs, foods, alcohol, or beer
6. Quantity: High—diabetes mellitus, diabetes insipidus, nervousness, diuretics, excessive intake of fluids
Low—acute nephritis, heart disease, fever, diarrhea, vomiting
None—uremia, acute nephritis, renal failure

Under Chemical Examination

1. Protein—an important sign of renal disease, acute glomerulonephritis, pyelonephritis
2. Glucose—diabetes mellitus, pain, excitement, acromegaly, liver damage
3. Ketones—uncontrolled diabetes mellitus, an increase in metabolic needs as during a high-protein–low-carbohydrate diet, during vomiting, diarrhea, and starvation
4. Bilirubin—liver disease, biliary obstruction, congestive heart failure
5. Blood—renal disease or disorders, trauma
6. Nitrites—bacteriuria
7. Urobilinogen: Absent—biliary obstruction
Reduced—antibiotic therapy
Increased—early warning of hepatic or hemolytic diseases

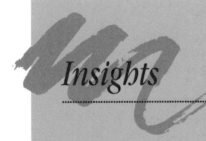

Insights

URINARY TRACT INFECTION (UTI): Cystitis

Cystitis is an inflammation of the urinary bladder. The urinary bladder is a muscular, membranous sac that serves as a reservoir for urine. It is located in the anterior portion of the pelvic cavity and consists of a lower portion, the neck, which is continuous with the urethra, and an upper portion, the apex, which is connected with the umbilicus by the median umbilical ligament. The urethra is the musculomembranous tube extending from the bladder to the outside of the body. The external urinary opening is the urinary meatus. The male urethra is approximately 8 inches long and the female urethra is approximately 1.5 inches long.

Guidelines to Help Avoid Cystitis (Female)

- Drink plenty of fluids (8 glasses or more) a day.
- Females should wipe themselves from front to back after a bowel movement to avoid contaminating the urinary meatus.
- Females who have repeated infections (cystitis) should drink a glass of water before engaging in sexual intercourse, and then urinate right after intercourse. This helps flush out any bacteria that could have entered the urethra.
- Have your sexual partner wear a condom.
- Do not use vaginal deodorants, bubble baths, colored toilet paper, and other substances that could cause irritation to the urinary meatus.
- Wear cotton underclothes and keep the genital area dry.

Each year, in the United States, approximately 10 million patients seek treatment for urinary tract infections, with cystitis being the most common. Cystitis is most often caused by an ascending infection from the urethra and it is more common in the female, because of the short length of the urethra that promotes the transmission of bacteria from the skin and genitals to the internal bladder. The most common type of bacteria that causes cystitis in the female is *Escherichia coli (E. coli)*, the colon bacillus. This bacillus is constantly present in the alimentary canal and is normally nonpathogenic, but when it enters the urinary tract and is transmitted to the bladder, it can cause infection. Cystitis in men is usually secondary to some other type of infection such as epididymitis, prostatitis, gonorrhea, syphilis, and/or kidney stones.

Diagnosis
History of symptoms
Microscopic urinalysis
Urine culture
Dipstick
Gram stain

Symptoms
Frequency
Hematuria
Pain or spasm in the region of the bladder
    and pelvic area
Urgency
Pyuria
Chills and fever
Burning sensation and pain during urination

(Insights continues on next page)

Treatment

Treatment of cystitis usually consists of taking an antibiotic or antibacterial agent for a specified number of times and days, depending on the type of infection and its severity. The sulfonamides and antibiotics such as penicillins, cephalosporins, tetracyclines, and aminoglycosides are generally the drugs of first choice. Always ask the patient if he or she is allergic to any medication before the initiation of drug therapy. Note: if there is any question about a person's hypersensitivity to an antibiotic and/or sulfa drugs, an appropriate skin test should be performed before the initiation of drug therapy.

The patient should be informed about possible adverse reactions to the prescribed medication and be instructed to report any signs to his or her physician. Advise the patient to take the medication as prescribed until all of the drug has been taken.

Interstitial Cystitis

Interstitial cystitis (IC) is a painful inflammation of the bladder wall. Approximately 450,000 people suffer from this condition and 90% are women. Research showed that the median age of onset was 40, with many women experiencing symptoms as early as their twenties and thirties.

Symptoms can vary from mild to severe and are similar to a urinary tract infection (cystitis). There is usually pelvic pain and pressure, frequent urination, sometimes as often as 50 times a day. Diagnosis is difficult because the standard blood tests, urine tests, and x-rays come up negative. The cause is unknown and IC does not respond to antibiotic therapy. Women with IC often live in chronic pain. They are always tired, because they are going to the bathroom often and their sexual, social, and work life are affected.

FYI: In 1993, the United States Congress earmarked $4 million for research into this condition, and the National Institutes of Health has started a data base that will collect information on IC patients. For a referral to a data base center, send a self- addressed, stamped, business-size envelope to the Interstitial Cystitis Association, P.O. Box 1553, Madison Square Station, New York, NY 10159.

Terminology with Surgical Procedures & Pathology

Term	Word Parts			Definition
albuminuria (ăl-bū″ mĭn-oo′rĭ-ă)	albumin uria	R S	protein urine	Presence of serum protein in the urine
antidiuretic (ăn″ tĭ-dī″ ū-rĕt′ĭk)	anti di(a) uret ic	P P R S	against through urine pertaining to	Pertaining to a medication that decreases urine secretion
anuria (ăn-ū′ rĭ-ă)	an uria	P S	without urine	Without the formation of urine
bacteriuria (băk-tē″ rĭ-ū′ rĭ-ă)	bacteri uria	R S	bacteria urine	Presence of bacteria in the urine
calciuria (kăl″ sĭ-ū′ rĭ-ă)	calci uria	R S	calcium urine	Presence of calcium in the urine
cystectasy (sĭs-tĕk′ tă-sē)	cyst ectasy	R S	bladder dilation	Dilation of the bladder
cystectomy (sĭs-tĕk′ tō-mē)	cyst ectomy	R S	bladder excision	Surgical excision of the bladder or part of the bladder
cystistaxia (sĭs″ tĭ-stăk′ sĭ-ă)	cysti staxia	CF S	bladder dripping, trickling	The oozing of blood from the mucous membrane of the bladder
cystitis (sĭs-tī′ tĭs)	cyst itis	R S	bladder inflammation	Inflammation of the bladder
cystocele (sĭs′ tō-sēl)	cysto cele	CF S	bladder hernia	Hernia of the bladder that protrudes into the vagina
cystodynia (sĭs″ tō-dĭn′ ĭ-ă)	cysto dynia	CF S	bladder pain	Pain in the bladder
cystogram (sĭs′ tō-grăm)	cysto gram	CF S	bladder a mark, record	An x-ray record of the bladder
cystolithectomy (sĭs″ tō-lĭ-thĕk′ tō-mē)	cysto lith ectomy	CF S S	bladder stone excision	Surgical excision of a stone from the bladder
cystopexy (sĭs′ tō-pĕk″ sē)	cysto pexy	CF S	bladder fixation	Surgical fixation of the bladder to the abdominal wall
cystoplasty (sĭs′ tō-plăs″ tē)	cysto plasty	CF S	bladder surgical repair	Surgical repair of the bladder

(Terminology—continued)

Term	Word Parts			Definition
cystoplegia (sĭs″ tō-plē′ jĭ-ă)	cysto	CF	bladder	Paralysis of the bladder
	plegia	S	paralysis	
cystopyelitis (sĭs″ tō-pī″ ĕ-lī′ tĭs)	cysto	CF	bladder	Inflammation of the bladder and renal pelvis
	pyel	R	renal pelvis	
	itis	S	inflammation	
cystorrhagia (sĭs″ tō-rā′ jĭ-ă)	cysto	CF	bladder	Bursting forth of blood from the bladder
	rrhagia	S	bursting forth	
cystorrhaphy (sĭst-ōr′ ā-fē)	cysto	CF	bladder	Surgical suture of the bladder
	rrhaphy	S	suture	
cystoscope (sĭst′ ō-skōp)	cysto	CF	bladder	An instrument used for examination of the bladder
	scope	S	instrument	
dialysis (dī-ăl′ ĭ-sĭs)	dia	P	through	A procedure to separate waste material from the blood and to maintain fluid, electrolyte, and acid-base balance in impaired kidney function or in the absence of the kidney
	lysis	S	destruction, to separate	
diuresis (dī″ ū-rē′ sĭs)	di(a)	P	through	A condition of increased or excessive flow of urine
	ure	R	urinate	
	sis	S	condition	
dysuria (dĭs-ū′ rĭ-ă)	dys	P	difficult, painful	Difficult or painful urination
	uria	S	urine	
enuresis (ĕn″ ū-rē′ sĭs)	en	P	within	A condition of involuntary emission of urine; bedwetting
	ure	R	urinate	
	sis	S	condition of	
glomerular (glō-mĕr′ ū-lăr)	glomerul	R	glomerulus, little ball	Pertaining to the glomerulus
	ar	S	pertaining to	
glomerulitis (glō-mĕr″ ū-lī′ tĭs)	glomerul	R	glomerulus, little ball	Inflammation of the renal glomeruli
	itis	S	inflammation	
glomerulone-phritis (glō-mĕr″ ū-lō-nĕ-frī′ tĭs)	glomerulo	CF	glomerulus, little ball	Inflammation of the kidney involving primarily the glomeruli
	nephr	R	kidney	
	itis	S	inflammation	
glycosuria (glī″ kō-soo′ rĭ-ă)	glycos	R	sweet, sugar	Presence of glucose in the urine
	uria	S	urine	

(Terminology—continued)

Term	Word Parts			Definition
hematuria (hē″ mă-tū′ rĭ-ă)	hemat uria	R S	blood urine	Presence of blood in the urine
hydronephrosis (hī″ drō-nĕf-rō′ sĭs)	hydro nephr osis	P R S	water kidney condition of	A condition in which urine collects in the renal pelvis because of an obstructed outflow
hypercalciuria (hī″ pĕr-kăl″ sĭ-ū′ rĭ-ă)	hyper calci uria	P R S	excessive calcium urine	An excessive amount of calcium in the urine
incontinence (ĭn-kən′ tĭn-əns)	in continence	P R	not to hold	The inability to hold urine
ketonuria (kē″ tō-nū′ rĭ-ă)	keton uria	R S	ketone urine	Presence of ketone in the urine
meatal (mē″ā′ tăl)	meat al	R S	passage pertaining to	Pertaining to a passage
meatoscopy (mē″ ă-tŏs′ kō-pē)	meato scopy	CF S	passage to veiw, examine	Instrumental examination of the meatus of the urethra
meatotomy (mē″ ă-tŏt′ ō-mē)	meato tomy	CF S	passage incision	Incision of the urinary meatus to enlarge the opening
micturition (mĭk′ tū-rĭ′ shŭn)	micturit ion	R S	to urinate process	The process of urination
nephradenoma (nĕf″ răd-ĕ-nō′ mă)	nephr aden oma	R R S	kidney gland tumor	Glandular tumor of the kidney
nephratony (nĕ-frăt′ ō-nē)	nephr a tony	R P S	kidney not, lack of tension	Lack of normal kidney tone
nephrectasia (nĕf″ rĕk-tā′ zĭ-ă)	nephr ectasia	R S	kidney distention	Distention of the kidney
nephrectomy (nĕ-frĕk′ tō-mē)	nephr ectomy	R S	kidney excision	Surgical excision of a kidney
nephremia (nĕf-rē′ mĭ-ă)	nephr emia	R S	kidney blood condition	A condition in which the kidney is congested with blood
nephritis (nĕf-rī′ tĭs)	nephr itis	R S	kidney inflammation	Inflammation of the kidney

(Terminology—continued)

Term	Word Parts			Definition
nephrocystitis (něf″ rō-sĭs′tĭ′ tĭs)	nephro cyst itis	CF R S	kidney bladder inflammation	Inflammation of the bladder and the kidney
nephrohyper-trophy (něf″ rō-hī-pěr′ trō-fē)	nephro hyper trophy	CF P S	kidney excessive nourishment, development	Excessive development of the kidney
nephrolith (něf′ rō-lĭth)	nephro lith	CF S	kidney stone	Kidney stone
nephrology (ně-frŏl′ ō-jē)	nephro logy	CF S	kidney study of	The study of the kidney
nephroma (ně-frō′ mă)	nephr oma	R S	kidney tumor	Kidney tumor
nephromalacia (něf″ rō-mă-lā′ sĭ-ă)	nephro malacia	CF S	kidney softening	Abnormal softening of the kidney
nephromegaly (něf″ rō-měg′ ă-lē)	nephro megaly	CF S	kidney enlargement	Enlargement of the kidney
nephropathy (ně-frŏp′ ă-thē)	nephro pathy	CF S	kidney disease	Disease of the kidney
nephropexy (něf′ rō-pěks″ ē)	nephro pexy	CF S	kidney fixation	Surgical fixation of a floating kidney
nephroptosis (něf″ rŏp-tō′ sĭs)	nephro ptosis	CF S	kidney prolapse, drooping	Prolapse of the kidney
nephropyosis (něf″ rō-pī-ō′ sĭs)	nephro py osis	CF R S	kidney pus condition of	A condition of pus in the kidney
nephrosclerosis (něf″ rō-sklē-rō′ sĭs)	nephro scler osis	CF R S	kidney hardening condition of	A condition of hardening of the kidney
nocturia (nŏk-tū′ rĭ-ă)	noct uria	R S	night urine	Excessive urination during the night
oliguria (ŏl-ĭg-ū′ rĭ-ă)	olig uria	P S	scanty urine	Scanty urination
paranephritis (păr″ ă-ně-frī′ tĭs)	para nephr itis	P R S	beside kidney inflammation	Inflammation of the suprarenal capsule

(Terminology—continued)

Term	Word Parts			Definition
periureteritis (pĕr″ ĭ-ū-rē″ tĕr- ĭ′ tĭs)	peri ureter itis	P R S	around ureter inflammation	Inflammation around the ureter
periurethral (pĕr″ ĭ-ū-rē′ thrăl)	peri urethr al	P R S	around urethra pertaining to	Pertaining to around the urethra
polyuria (pŏl″ ē-ū′ rĭ-ă)	poly uria	P S	excessive urine	Excessive urination
pyelocystitis (pī″ ĕ-lō-sĭs-tī′ tĭs)	pyelo cyst itis	CF R S	renal pelvis bladder inflammation	Inflammation of the bladder and renal pelvis
pyelocystosto-mosis (pī″ ĕ-lō-sĭs″ tō-stō-mō′ sĭs)	pyelo cysto stom osis	CF CF R S	renal pelvis bladder mouth condition of	Establishing a surgical opening between the renal pelvis and bladder
pyelolithotomy (pī″ ĕ-lō-lĭth-ŏt′ ō-mē)	pyelo litho tomy	CF CF S	renal pelvis stone incision	Surgical incision into the renal pelvis for removal of a stone
pyelonephritis (pī″ ĕ-lō-nĕ-frī′ tĭs)	pyelo nephr itis	CF R S	renal pelvis kidney inflammation	Inflammation of the kidney and renal pelvis
pyeloplication (pī″ ĕ-lō-plĭ-kā′ shŭn)	pyelo plicat ion	CF R S	renal pelvis to fold process	The process of shortening the wall of the renal pelvis by surgical folds
pyuria (pī-ū′ rĭ-ă)	py uria	R S	pus urine	Pus in the urine
renal (rē′ năl)	ren al	R S	kidney pertaining to	Pertaining to the kidney
trigonitis (trĭg″ ō-nī′ tĭs)	trigon itis	R S	trigone inflammation	Inflammation of the trigone of the bladder
ureagenetic (ū-rē″ ă-jĕn-ĕt′ ĭk)	urea genet ic	R R S	urea producing pertaining to	Pertaining to producing urea
uremia (ū-rē′ mĭ-ă)	ur emia	R S	urine blood condition	A condition of excess urea and other nitrogenous waste in the blood
ureterocolostomy (ū-rē″ tĕr-ō-kō- lŏs′ tō-mē)	uretero colo stomy	CF CF S	ureter colon new opening	Surgical implantation of the ureter into the colon

(Terminology—continued)

Term	Word Parts			Definition
ureteronephrec-tomy (ū-rē″ tĕr-ō-nĕf-rĕk′ tō-mē)	uretero nephr ectomy	CF R S	ureter kidney excision	Surgical excision of a kidney and its ureter
ureteropathy (ū-rē″ tĕr-ŏp′ ă-thē)	uretero pathy	CF S	ureter disease	Disease of the ureter
ureteroplasty (ū-rē′ tĕr-ō-plăs″ tē)	uretero plasty	CF S	ureter surgical repair	Surgical repair of the ureter
ureterorrhaphy (ū-rē″ tĕr-ōr′ ră-fē)	uretero rrhaphy	CF S	ureter suture	Suture of the ureter
ureterostenosis (ū-rē″ tĕr-ō-stĕn-ō′sĭs)	uretero sten osis	CF R S	ureter narrowing condition of	A condition of narrowing of the ureter
ureterovesical (ū-rē″ tĕr-ō-vĕs′ ĭ-kăl)	uretero vesic al	CF R S	ureter bladder pertaining to	Pertaining to a connection between the ureter and bladder
urethralgia (ū-rē-thrăl′ jĭ-ă)	urethr algia	R S	urethra pain	Pain in the urethra
urethropenile (ū-rē″ thrō-pē′ nīl)	urethro penile	CF R	urethra penis	Relating to the urethra and penis
urethroperineal (ū-rē″ thrō-pĕr″ ĭ nē′ ăl)	urethro perine al	CF R S	urethra perineum pertaining to	Pertaining to the urethra and perineum
urethropexy (ū-rēth′ rō-pĕks-ē)	urethro pexy	CF S	urethra fixation	Surgical fixation of the urethra
urethrophraxis (ū-rē″ thrō-frăks′ ĭs)	urethro phraxis	CF S	urethra to obstruct	Obstruction of the urethra
urethrospasm (ū-rē′ thrō-spăzm)	urethro spasm	CF S	urethra tension, spasm	Urethral spasm
urethrotome (ū-rē′ thrō-tōm)	urethro tome	CF S	urethra instrument to cut	An instrument used to cut an urethral stricture
urethrovaginal (ū-rē″ thrō-văg′ ĭ-năl)	urethro vagin al	CF R S	urethra vagina pertaining to	Pertaining to the urethra and vagina
urinal (ū′ rĭn-ăl)	urin al	R S	urine pertaining to	A container, toilet, or bathroom fixture into which one urinates

(Terminology—continued)

Term	Word Parts			Definition
urinalysis (ū′ rĭ-năl′ i-sĭs)	urin a lysis	R P S	urine apart destruction, to separate	Analysis of the urine; a separating of the urine for examination to determine the presence of abnormal elements
urination (ū″ rĭ-nā′ shŭn)	urinat ion	R S	urine process	The process of voiding urine
urinometer (ū″ rĭ-nŏm′ ĕ-tĕr)	urino meter	CF S	urine instrument to measure	An instrument used to measure the specific gravity of urine
urobilin (ū″ rō-bī′ lĭn)	uro bil in	CF R S	urine bile chemical	A brown pigment formed by the oxidation of urobilinogen; may be formed in the urine after exposure to air
urologist (ū-rŏl′ ō-jĭst)	uro log ist	CF R S	urine study of one who specializes	One who specializes in the study of the urinary system
urology (ū-rŏl′ ō-jē)	uro logy	CF S	urine study of	The study of the urinary system
uropoiesis (ū″ rō-poy-ē′ sĭs)	uro poiesis	CF S	urine formation	Formation of urine by the kidneys
uroporphyrin (ū″ rō-por′ fĭ-rĭn)	uro porphyr in	CF R S	urine purple chemical	A reddish-purple pigment present in urine in cases of porphyria or certain drugs

Vocabulary Words

Vocabulary words are terms that have not been divided into component parts. They are common words or specialized terms associated with the subject of this chapter. These words are provided to enhance your medical vocabulary.

Word	Definition
catheter (kăth′ ĕ-tĕr)	A tube of elastic, elastic web, rubber, glass, metal, or plastic that is inserted into a body cavity to remove fluid or to inject fluid
edema (ĕ-dē′ mă)	An abnormal condition in which the body tissues contain an accumulation of fluid
excretory (ĕks′ krə-tō-rē)	Pertaining to the elimination of waste products from the body
extracorporeal shock-wave lithotriptor (ĕks″ tră-kor-por′ ē-ăl lĭth′ ō-trip″ tor)	A device used to crush kidney stones (renal calculi). The patient is sedated and immersed in a water bath while shock waves pound the stones until they crumble into small pieces. These pieces are flushed out with urine
hemodialysis (hē″ mō-dī-ăl′ ĭ-sĭs)	The use of an artificial kidney to separate waste from the blood. The blood is circulated through tubes made of semipermeable membranes, and these tubes are continually bathed by solutions that remove waste
lithotripsy (lĭth′ ō trĭp″ sē)	The crushing of a kidney stone
meatus (mē-ā′ tŭs)	An opening or passage; the external opening of the urethra
nephron (nef′ rŏn)	The structural and functional unit of the kidney
percutaneous ultrasonic lithotripsy (pĕr″ kū-tā′ nē-ŭs)	The crushing of a kidney stone by using ultrasound. This is an invasive surgical procedure performed by using a nephroscope or fluoroscopy
peritoneal dialysis (pĕr″ i-tō-nē′ ăl dī-ăl′ ĭ-sĭs)	Separation of waste from the blood by using a peritoneal catheter and dialysis. Fluid is introduced into the peritoneal cavity, and wastes from the blood pass into this fluid. The fluid and waste are then removed from the body. Types of peritoneal dialysis are: IPD—intermittent and CAPD—continuous ambulatory
renal colic (rē′ năl kŏl′ ĭk)	An acute pain that occurs in the kidney area and is caused by blockage during the passage of a stone
renal failure (rē′ năl fāl′ yŭr)	Cessation of proper functioning of the kidney
renal transplant (rē′ năl trăns′ plănt)	To transfer a kidney from a donor to a patient

(Vocabulary—continued)

Word	Definition
renin (rĕn′ ĭn)	An enzyme produced by the kidney
residual urine (rē-zĭd′ ŭ-ăl ū′ rĭn)	Urine that is left in the bladder after urination
retention (rē-tĕn′ shŭn)	The holding back of a substance that should be excreted—urine, feces, or perspiration
sediment (sĕd′ ĭ-mĕnt)	The substance that settles at the bottom of a liquid; a precipitate
specific gravity (spĕ-sĭf′ ĭk grăv′ ĭ-tē)	The weight of a substance compared with an equal amount of water. Urine has a specific gravity of 1.015–1.025
specimen (spĕs′ ĭ-mĕn)	A sample of tissue, blood, or urine
sterile (stĕr′ ĭl)	A state of being free from living microorganisms; asepsis
stricture (strik′ chŭr)	An abnormal narrowing of a duct or passage such as the esophagus, ureter, or urethra
supernatant (sū″ pĕr-nā′ tănt)	The liquid floating on the surface after a precipitate settles
urea (ū-rē′ ă)	A compound found in urine, blood, and lymph
urethral stricture (ū-rē′ thrăl strĭk′ chŭr)	A narrowing or constriction of the urethra
urgency (ŭr-jĕn′ sē)	The sudden need to void, urinate
uric acid (ū′ rĭk ăs′ ĭd)	An end product of purine metabolism; a common component of urinary and renal stones
urine (ū′ rĭn)	The fluid and dissolved substances secreted by the kidneys, stored in the bladder, and excreted through the urethra
urochrome (ū′ rō-krōm)	The pigment that gives urine the normal yellow color
urolithiasis (ū″ rō-lĭ-thē″ ă-sĭs)	The formation of a urinary stone and its associated illness
void (voyd)	To empty the bladder

ABBREVIATIONS

ADH	antidiuretic hormone	**HCO₃**	bicarbonate
A/G	albumin/globulin ratio	**HD**	hemodialysis
AGN	acute glomerulonephritis	**H₂O**	water
ATN	acute tubular necrosis	**HPF**	high-power field
BUN	blood urea nitrogen	**I & O**	intake and output
CAPD	continuous ambulatory peritoneal dialysis	**IPD**	intermittent peritoneal dialysis
CC	clean catch	**IVP**	intravenous pyelogram
CGN	chronic glomerulonephritis	**K**	potassium
CRF	chronic renal failure	**KUB**	kidney, ureter, bladder
Cl	chloride	**LPF**	low-power field
CMG	cystometrogram	**Na**	sodium
C & S	culture and sensitivity	**PD**	peritoneal dialysis
cysto	cystoscopic examination	**pH**	potential of hydrogen
ECF	extracellular fluid	**PKU**	phenylketonuria
ESRD	end-stage renal disease	**PSP**	phenolsulfonphthalein
ESWL	extracorporeal shockwave lithotripsy	**PUL**	percutaneous ultrasonic lithotripsy
GBM	glomerular basement membrane	**RP**	retrograde pyelogram
		UA	urinalysis
GFR	glomerular filtration rate	**UTI**	urinary tract infection
GU	genitourinary	**VCUG**	voiding cystourethrogram

Drug Highlights

Drugs that are generally used for urinary system diseases and disorders include diuretics, urinary tract antibacterials and antiseptics, and other drugs.

Diuretics	Decrease reabsorption of sodium chloride by the kidneys, thereby increasing the amount of salt and water excreted in the urine. This action reduces the amount of fluid retained in the body and prevents edema. Diuretics are classified according to site and mechanism of action.
Thiazide	Appear to act by inhibiting sodium and chloride reabsorption in the early portion of the distal tubule.
	Examples: Naturetin (bendroflumethiazide), Diuril (chlorothiazide), HydroDIURIL (hydrochlorothiazide), and Renese (polythiazide).
Loop	Act by inhibiting the reabsorption of sodium and chloride in the ascending loop of Henle.
	Examples: Bumex (bumetanide) and Lasix (furosemide).

Potassium-sparing	Act by inhibiting the exchange of sodium for potassium in the distal tubule. They inhibit potassium excretion. *Examples: Aldactone (spironolactone) and Dyrenium (triamterene).*
Osmotic	Are capable of being filtered by the glomerulus, but have a limited capability of being reabsorbed into the bloodstream. *Example: Osmitrol (mannitol).*
Carbonic anhydrase inhibitor	Act to increase the excretion of bicarbonate ion, which carries out sodium, water, and potassium. *Example: Diamox (acetazolamide).*
Urinary Tract Antibacterials	Sulfonamides are generally the drugs of choice for treating acute, uncomplicated urinary tract infections, especially those caused by *Escherichia coli* and *Proteus mirabilis* bacterial strains. They exert a bacteriostatic effect against a wide range of gram-positive and gram-negative microorganisms. *Examples: Thiosulfil (sulfamethizole), Gantrisin (sulfisoxazole), Gantanol (sulfamethoxazole), Microsulfon (sulfadiazine), and Bactrim and Septra that are mixtures of trimethoprim and sulfamethoxazole.*
Urinary Tract Antiseptics	May inhibit the growth of microorganisms by bactericidal, bacteriostatic, anti-infective, and/or antibacterial action. *Examples: NegGram (nalidixic acid), Furadantin and Macrodantin (nitrofurantoin), Mandelamine and Hiprex (methenamine), and Cipro (ciprofloxacin).*
Other Drugs	Disorders of the lower urinary tract may be treated with drugs that either stimulate or inhibit smooth muscle activity, thereby improving urinary bladder functions. These functions are the storage of urine and its subsequent excretion from the body. *Examples: Cystospaz-M and Levsin (hyoscyamine sulfate), Urispas (flavoxate HCl), and Urecholine (bethanechol chloride).*
Rimso-50 (dimethyl sulfoxide)	Used in the treatment of interstitial cystitis.
Pyridium (phenazopyridine HCl)	Analgesic, anesthetic action on the urinary tract mucosa. This medication causes the urine to turn an orange color.

Communication Enrichment

This segment is provided for those who wish to enhance their ability to communicate in either English or Spanish.

RELATED TERMS

English	Spanish
bladder	vejiga (vĕ-*hĭ*-gă)
burning	ardiente (ăr-dĭ-*ĕn*-tĕ)
dialysis	diálisis (dĭ-*ă*-lĭs-ĭs)
dysuria	disuria (*dĭ*-sŭ-rĭ-ă)
kidney	riñón (rĭn-*yōn*)
kidney stone	cálculo renal (*căl*-cŭ-lō rĕ-*năl*)
urethral discharge	descargar uretral (dĕs-căr-*găr* ŭ-*rĕ*-trăl)
urinate	orinar (ō-rĭ-*năr*)
urine	orine (ō-*rĭ*-nĕ)
cloudy	nublado (nŭ-*blă*-dō)
pink	rosado (rō-*să*-dō)
loss of bladder control	perdida de control vejiga (per-*dĭ*-dă dĕ cōn-*trōl* vĕ-*hē*-gă)
fever	fiebre (fĭ-ĕ-brĕ)
urgent	urgente (ūr-*hĕn*-tĕ)
urethra	uretra (ū-*rĕ*-tra)
urethral	uretral (ū-*rĕ*-trăl)
urethritis	uretritis (ū-rĕ-*trĭ*-tĭs)
urethroscope	uretroscopio (ū-rĕ-trō-*scō*-pĭ-ō)
urethroscopy	uretroscopia (ū-rĕ-trō-*scō*-pĭ-ă)

English	Spanish
urinalysis	urinálisis (ū-rĭ-*nă*-lĭs-ĭs)
urinary	urinario (ū-rĭ-*nă*-rĭ-ō)
urinary calculus	cálculo urinario (*căl*-cŭ-lō ū-rĭ-*nă*-rĭ-ō)
urinary tract	vías urinarias (*vĭ*-ăs ū-rĭ-*nă*-rĭ-ăs)
urination	urinación (ū-rĭ-*nă*-sĭ-ōn)
urogenital	urogenital (ū-rō-*hĕ*-nĭ-tăl)
urolith	urolito (ū-rō-*lĭ*-tō)
urolithiasis	urolitiasis (ū-rō-lĭ-tĭ-*ăs*-ĭs)
urologic	urológico (ū-rō-*lō*-hĭ-kō)
urologist	urólogo (ū-rō-*lō*-hō)
urology	urología (ū-rō-lō-*hĭ*-ă)

DIAGNOSTIC AND LABORATORY TESTS

Test	Description
blood urea nitrogen (BUN) (blod ū-rē′ ă nĭ′ trō-jĕn)	A blood test to determine the amount of urea that is excreted by the kidneys. Abnormal results indicate urinary tract disease.
creatinine (krē′ ă-tĭn ēn)	A blood test to determine the amount of creatinine present. Abnormal results indicate kidney disease.
creatinine clearance (krē′ ă-tĭn ēn klir′ ăns)	A urine test to determine the glomerular filtration rate (GFR). Abnormal results indicate kidney disease.
culture, urine (kūl′ tūr, ū′ rĭn)	A urine test to determine the presence of microorganisms. Abnormal results indicate urinary tract infection.
cystoscopy (sĭs-tŏs′ kō-pē)	Visual examination of the bladder and urethra via a lighted cystoscope. Abnormal results may indicate the presence of renal calculi, a tumor, prostatic hyperplasia, and/or bleeding.
intravenous pyelography (pyelogram) (ĭn-tră-vē′ nŭs pĭ″ ĕ-lŏg′ ră-fē)	A test to visualize the kidneys, ureters, and bladder. A radiopaque substance is intravenously injected, and x-rays are taken. Abnormal results may indicate renal calculi, kidney or bladder tumors, and kidney disease.
kidney, ureter, bladder (KUB) (kĭd′ nē, ū′ rĕ-tĕr, blăd′ dĕr)	A flat-plate x-ray is taken of the abdomen to indicate the size and position of the kidneys, ureters, and bladder.

Test	Description
renal biopsy (rē′ năl bī′ ŏp-sē)	The removal of tissue from the kidney. Abnormal results may indicate kidney cancer, kidney transplant rejection, and glomerulonephritis.
retrograde pyelography (rĕt′ rō-grād pī″ ĕ-lŏg′ ră-fē)	The use of a contrast medium to visualize the kidneys, ureters, and bladder. Abnormal results may indicate renal calculi, kidney or bladder tumors, and kidney disease.
ultrasonography, kidneys (ŭ-tră-sŏn-ŏg′ ră-fē, kĭd′ nēs)	The use of high-frequency sound waves to visualize the kidneys. The sound waves (echoes) are recorded on an oscilloscope and film. Abnormal results may indicate kidney tumors, cysts, abscess, and kidney disease.

Learning Exercises

Anatomy and Physiology

Write your answers to the following questions. Do not refer back to the text.

1. List the organs of the urinary system.

   a. _____   b._____

   c. _____   d._____

2. State the vital function of the urinary system. _____
   _____

3. Name the three capsules that surround each kidney.

   a. _____   b._____

   c. _____

4. Define hilum. _____

5. Define renal pelvis. _____

6. The cortex of the kidney contains the _____, _____,
   _____, and _____ _____.

7. The medulla is the _____ portion of the kidney.

8. Define nephron. _____

9. Each nephron consists of a _____ _____ and
   _____.

10. The malpighian corpuscle consists of _____ and
    _____ _____.

11. State the vital function of the nephron. _____

12. Urine is formed by the process of _____ and
    _____ in the nephron.

13. Urine consists of _____ percent water and _____ percent solid
    substances.

14. An average of _____ to _____ mL of urine is voided daily.

15. Describe the ureters and state their function. _____
    _____

16. Describe the urinary bladder and state its function. _____
    _____

17. Define trigone. _____

18. State the function of the male urethra. _____

19. State the function of the female urethra. _____

20. The external urinary opening is the _____ _____.

21. Define urinalysis. _____
    _____

22. Give the normal constituents for the physical examination of urine.

    a. Color _____ b. Appearance _____

    c. Reaction _____ d. Specific gravity _____

    e. Odor _____ f. Quantity _____

23. Name the three types of epithelial cells that may be found in urine.

    a. _____ b._____

    c. _____

24. A urine that has a fruity sweet odor may indicate _____
_____.

25. Under chemical examination, the presence of protein in urine is an important sign of
_____
_____.

Word Parts

1. In the spaces provided, write the definition of these prefixes, roots, combining forms, and suffixes. Do not refer to the listings of terminology words. Leave blank those terms you cannot define.
2. After completing as many as you can, refer back to the terminology word listings to check your work. For each word missed or left blank, write the term and its definition several times on the margins of these pages or on a separate sheet of paper.
3. To maximize the learning process, it is to your advantage to do the following exercises as directed. To refer to the terminology listings before completing these exercises invalidates the learning process.

Prefixes

Give the definitions of the following prefixes:

1. a- _____ 2. an- _____
3. anti- _____ 4. di(a)- _____
5. dia- _____ 6. dys- _____
7. en- _____ 8. hydro- _____
9. hyper- _____ 10. in- _____
11. olig- _____ 12. para- _____
13. peri- _____ 14. poly- _____

Roots and Combining Forms

Give the definitions of the following roots and combining forms:

1. aden _____ 2. albumin _____
3. bacteri _____ 4. bil _____
5. calci _____ 6. colo _____
7. continence _____ 8. cyst _____
9. cysti _____ 10. cysto _____

11. genet _____   12. glomerul _____

13. glomerulo _____   14. glycos _____

15. hemat _____   16. keton _____

17. litho _____   18. log _____

19. meat _____   20. meato _____

21. micturit _____   22. nephr _____

23. nephro _____   24. noct _____

25. penile _____   26. perine _____

27. plicat _____   28. porphyr _____

29. py _____   30. pyel _____

31. pyelo _____   32. ren _____

33. scler _____   34. sten _____

35. stom _____   36. trigon _____

37. ur _____   38. ure _____

39. urea _____   40. uret _____

41. ureter _____   42. uretero _____

43. urethr _____   44. urethro _____

45. urin _____   46. urinat _____

47. urino _____   48. uro _____

49. vagin _____   50. vesic _____

SUFFIXES

Give the definitions of the following suffixes:

1. -al _____   2. -algia _____

3. -ar _____   4. -cele _____

5. -dynia _____   6. -ectasia _____

7. -ectasy _____   8. -ectomy _____

9. -emia _____   10. -gram _____

11. -ic _____   12. -in _____

13. -ion _____   14. -ist _____

15. -itis _____   16. -lith _____

17. -logy _____   18. -lysis _____

19. -malacia _____   20. -megaly _____

21. -meter _____   22. -oma _____

23. -osis _____   24. -pathy _____

25. -pexy _____   26. -phraxis _____

27. -plasty _____   28. -plegia _____

29. -poiesis _____   30. -ptosis _____

31. -rrhagia _____   32. -rrhaphy _____

33. -scope _____   34. -scopy _____

35. -sis _____   36. -spasm _____

37. -staxia _____   38. -stomy _____

39. -tome _____   40. -tomy _____

41. -tony _____   42. -trophy _____

43. -uria _____

Identifying Medical Terms

In the spaces provided, write the medical terms for the following meanings:

1. _____ Pertaining to a medication that decreases urine secretion

2. _____ Surgical excision of the bladder or part of the bladder

3. _____ Inflammation of the bladder

4. _____ Surgical fixation of the bladder to the abdominal wall

5. _____ Surgical suture of the bladder

6. _____ Difficult or painful urination

7. _____ Inflammation of the renal glomeruli

8. _____ An excessive amount of calcium in the urine

9. _____ Pertaining to a passage

10. _____ The process of urinating

11. _____ Lack of normal kidney tone

12. _____ Kidney stone

13. _____ Enlargement of the kidney

14. _____ Pertaining to around the urethra

15. _____ Pus in the urine

16. _____ Disease of the ureter

17. _____ Suture of the ureter

18. _____ Pain in the urethra

19. _____ Urethral system

20. _____ One who specializes in the study of the urinary system

Spelling

In the spaces provided, write the correct spelling of these misspelled terms:

1. cystplasty _____
2. cystorhagia _____
3. euresis _____
4. glycouria _____
5. hemauria _____
6. incontence _____
7. nephemia _____
8. nephrcysitis _____
9. nephrmalaca _____
10. nephrtosis _____
11. nocuria _____
12. ueteroplasty _____
13. urethropraxis _____
14. urinalsis _____
15. urbilin _____
16. uropoiesis _____

Review Questions

Matching

Select the appropriate lettered meaning for each numbered line.

_____ 1. lithotriptor

_____ 2. hemodialysis

_____ 3. lithotripsy

_____ 4. peritoneal dialysis

_____ 5. renal colic

_____ 6. urethral stricture

_____ 7. urgency

_____ 8. urination

_____ 9. urolithiasis

_____ 10. urinometer

a. An acute pain that occurs in the kidney area and is caused by blockage during the passage of a stone

b. The crushing of a kidney stone

c. The process of voiding urine

d. A device used to crush kidney stones

e. The use of an artificial kidney to separate waste from the blood

f. Separation of waste from the blood by using a peritoneal catheter and dialysis

g. A narrowing or constriction of the urethra

h. Formation of a urinary stone and its associated illness

i. An instrument used to measure the specific gravity of urine

j. The sudden need to void, urinate

k. Analysis of the urine

Abbreviations

Place the correct word, phrase, or abbreviation in the space provided.

_____ 1. antidiuretic hormone

_____ 2. BUN

_____ 3. chronic renal failure

_____ 4. cysto

_____ 5. GU

_____ 6. HD

_____ 7. intravenous pyelogram

_____ 8. PD

_____ 9. pH

_____ 10. urinalysis

Diagnostic and Laboratory Tests

Select the best answer to each multiple choice question. Circle the letter of your choice.

1. A urine test to determine the glomerular filtration rate.

   a. BUN

   b. creatinine

   c. creatinine clearance

   d. KUB

2. A urine test to determine the presence of microorganisms.

   a. BUN

   b. creatinine

   c. urine culture

   d. KUB

3. A test to visualize the kidneys, ureters, and bladder.

   a. cystoscopy

   b. intravenous pyelography

   c. KUB

   d. renal biopsy

4. The use of high-frequency sound waves to visualize the kidneys.

   a. retrograde pyelography

   b. intravenous pyelography

   c. ultrasonography

   d. cystoscopy

5. A flat-plate x-ray of the abdomen to indicate the size and position of the kidneys, ureters, and bladder.

   a. cystoscopy

   b. KUB

   c. BUN

   d. retrograde pyelography

11

The Endocrine System

The endocrine system consists of primary and secondary glands of internal secretion. The primary glands are the pituitary, pineal, thyroid, parathyroid, islets of Langerhans, adrenals, ovaries in the female, and testes in the male. The secondary glands are the thymus, the placenta during pregnancy, and the gastrointestinal mucosa. The vital function of the endocrine system involves the production and regulation of chemical substances called hormones.

DIABETES IQ

Did you know that the: Annual deaths among women due to breast cancer: 43,000 Annual deaths among women due to diabetes: 90,000 Percentage of women who think that more women die of breast cancer each year than diabetes: 82%

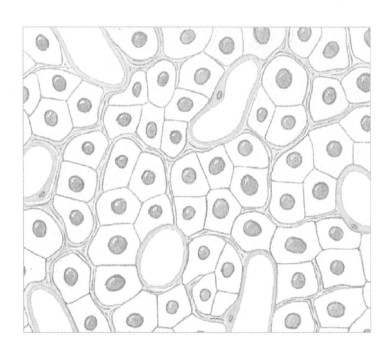

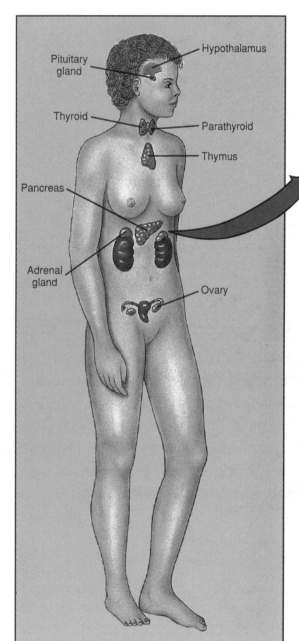

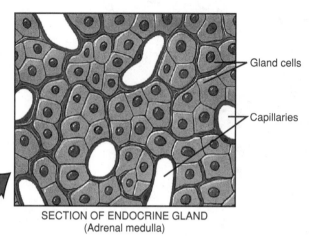

SECTION OF ENDOCRINE GLAND
(Adrenal medulla)

ANATOMY AND PHYSIOLOGY OVERVIEW

The endocrine system consists of primary and secondary glands of internal secretion. The primary glands are the pituitary (hypophysis), pineal, thyroid, parathyroid, pancreas, adrenals (suprarenals), ovaries, and testes. The secondary glands of the endocrine system are the thymus, the placenta during pregnancy, and the gastrointestinal mucosa. The endocrine glands are ductless and secrete their hormones directly into the bloodstream. The vital function of the endocrine system involves the production and regulation of chemical substances called hormones, which play an essential role in maintaining homeostasis (Fig. 11–1 and Plate 25).

THE ENDOCRINE SYSTEM	
Gland	**Primary Functions**
Pituitary (Hypophysis)	Master gland; regulatory effects on other endocrine glands
Anterior Lobe	Influences growth and sexual development, thyroid function, adrenocortical function, and regulates skin pigmentation
Posterior Lobe	Stimulates the reabsorption of water and elevates blood pressure, stimulates the release of milk and the uterus to contract during labor, delivery, and parturition
Pineal	Helps regulate the release of gonadotropin and controls body pigmentation
Thyroid	Vital role in metabolism and regulates the body's metabolic processes, influences bone and calcium metabolism, helps maintain plasma calcium homeostasis
Parathyroid	Maintenance of a normal serum calcium level, plays a role in the metabolism of phosphorus
Pancreas (Islets of Langerhans)	Regulates blood glucose levels and plays a vital role in metabolism of carbohydrates, proteins and fats
Adrenals (Suprarenals)	
Adrenal Cortex	Regulates carbohydrate metabolism, anti-inflammatory effect, helps body cope during stress, regulates electrolyte and water balance, promotes development of male characteristics
Adrenal Medulla	Synthesizes, secretes, and stores catecholamines (dopamine, epinephrine, norepinephrine)
Ovaries	Promotes growth, development, and maintenance of female sex organs
Testes	Promotes growth, development, and maintenance of male sex organs

The word **hormone** is derived from the Greek language and means "to excite" or "to urge on." A hormone is a chemical transmitter that is released in small amounts and transported via the bloodstream to a target organ or other cells. There are many hormones in the body, and their release is controlled by nerve stimulation. The release of hormones is either stimulated or retarded according to the feedback system regulating supply and demand. Hormones are either proteins, peptides, derivatives of amino acids, or steroids that are synthesized from cholesterol.

The endocrine system and the nervous system closely interact with each other. The hypothalamus, located in the brain, plays a vital role in regulating endocrine functions as it synthesizes and secretes releasing hormones such as thyrotropin-releasing hormone (TRH) and gonadotropin-releasing hormone (GnRH) and releasing factors such as corticotropin-releasing factor (CRF), growth hormone-releasing factor (GHRF), prolactin-releasing factor (PRF), and melanocyte-stimulating hormone-releasing factor (MRF). The hypothalamus also synthesizes and secretes release-inhibiting hormones such as growth hormone release-inhibiting hormone. It also produces release-inhibiting factors such as prolactin release-inhibiting factor (PIF) and melanocyte-stimulating hormone release-inhibiting factor (MIF). The hypothalamus also exerts direct nervous control over the anterior pituitary and the adrenal medulla and controls the secretion of the hormones epinephrine and norepinephrine.

The Pituitary Gland (Hypophysis)

The pituitary gland is a small gray gland located at the base of the brain. It lies or rests in a shallow depression of the sphenoid bone known as the sella turcica. It is attached by the infundibulum stalk to the hypothalamus. The pituitary is approximately 1 cm in diameter and weighs approximately 0.6 g. It is divided into the anterior lobe or adenohypophysis and the posterior lobe or neurohypophysis. The pituitary is called the master gland of the body because of its regulatory effects on the other endocrine glands (see Fig. 11–1 and Plate 4).

THE ANTERIOR LOBE

The adenohypophysis or anterior lobe secretes several hormones that are essential for the growth and development of bones, muscles, other organs, sex glands, the thyroid gland,

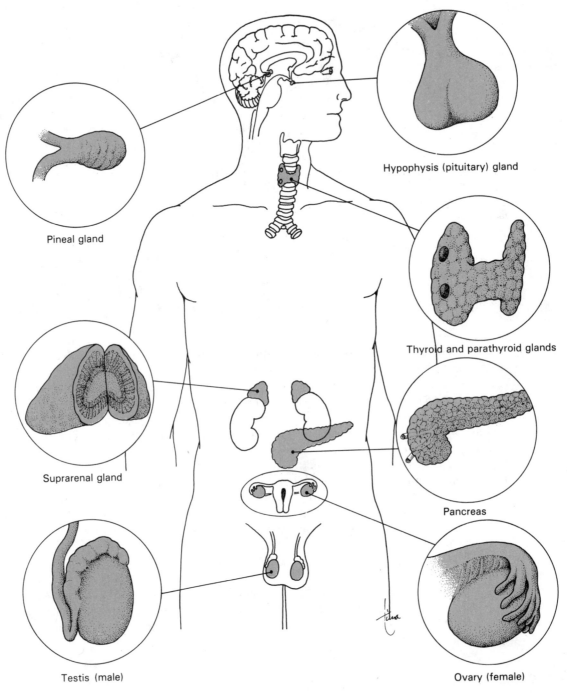

FIGURE 11–1

The endocrine glands and their locations in the body. *(Adapted from Evans WF.* Anatomy and Physiology, *3rd ed. Englewood Cliffs, NJ: Prentice-Hall, 1983, with permission.)*

and the adrenal cortex. The hormones secreted by the anterior lobe and their functions are described below and shown in Figure 11–2.

Growth Hormone (GH)

Growth hormone, also called somatotropin hormone (STH), is essential for the growth and development of bones, muscles, and other organs. It also enhances protein synthesis, decreases the use of glucose, and promotes fat destruction, lipolysis. Hyposecretion of this

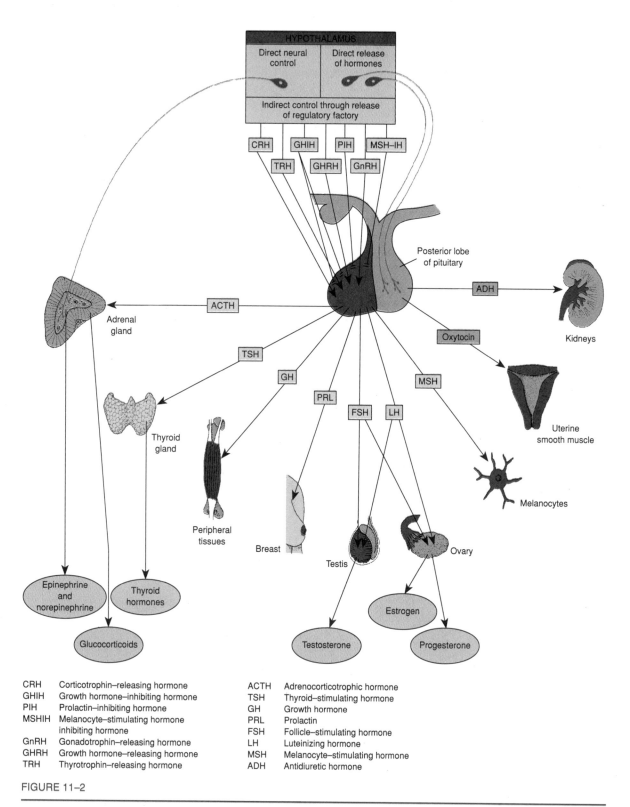

FIGURE 11–2

Pituitary hormones and their targets. (*From Martini F. Fundamentals of Anatomy and Physiology, 2nd ed. Englewood Cliffs, NJ: Prentice-Hall, 1992, with permission.*)

hormone may result in dwarfism and Simmond's disease. Hypersecretion of the hormone may result in gigantism during early life and acromegaly in adults.

Adrenocorticotropin (ACTH)

Adrenocorticotropin is essential for growth and development of the middle and inner zones of the adrenal cortex. The adrenal cortex secretes the glucocorticoids cortisol and corticosterone.

Thyroid-Stimulating Hormone (TSH)

Thyroid-stimulating hormone is essential for the growth and development of the thyroid gland. It stimulates the production of thyroxine and triiodothyronine. It also influences the body's metabolic processes and plays an important role in metabolism.

Follicle-Stimulating Hormone (FSH)

Follicle-stimulating hormone is a gonadotropic hormone that is essential in stimulating the growth of ovarian follicles in the female and the production of sperm in the male.

Luteinizing Hormone (LH)

Luteinizing hormone is a gonadotropic hormone that is essential in the maturation process of the ovarian follicles and stimulates the development of the corpus luteum in the female and the production of testosterone in the male.

Prolactin (PRL)

Prolactin is also known as lactogenic hormone (LTH). It is a gonadotropic hormone that stimulates the mammary glands to produce milk after childbirth.

Melanocyte-Stimulating Hormone (MSH)

Melanocyte-stimulating hormone regulates skin pigmentation and promotes the deposit of melanin in the skin after exposure to sunlight.

THE POSTERIOR LOBE

The neurohypophysis or posterior lobe secretes two known hormones: antidiuretic hormone and oxytocin (see Fig. 11-2). The following is a description of the functions of these hormones.

Antidiuretic Hormone (ADH)

Antidiuretic hormone is also known as vasopressin (VP). It stimulates the reabsorption of water by the renal tubules and has a pressor effect that elevates blood pressure. Hyposecretion of this hormone may result in diabetes insipidus.

Oxytocin

Oxytocin acts on the mammary glands to stimulate the release of milk and stimulates the uterus to contract during labor, delivery, and parturition.

The Pineal Gland (Body)

The pineal gland is a small, pine cone-shaped gland located near the posterior end of the corpus callosum. It is less than 1 cm in diameter and weighs approximately 0.1 g (see Fig. 11-1 and Plate 4). The pineal gland secretes melatonin and serotonin. Melatonin is a hormone that may be released at night to help regulate the release of gonadotropin. Serotonin is a hormone that is a neurotransmitter, vasoconstrictor, and smooth muscle stimulant and acts to inhibit gastric secretion.

The Thyroid Gland

The thyroid gland is a large, bilobed gland located in the neck. It is anterior to the trachea and just below the thyroid cartilage. The thyroid is approximately 5 cm long, 3 cm wide, and weighs approximately 30 g (see Fig. 11-1 and Plate 4). It plays a vital role in metabolism and regulates the body's metabolic processes. The hormones described below are stored and secreted by the thyroid gland.

Thyroxine (T$_4$)

Thyroxine is essential for the maintenance and regulation of the basal metabolic rate (BMR). It contains four iodine atoms, which are attached to its nucleus. Thyroxine influences growth and development, both physical and mental, and the metabolism of fats, proteins, carbohydrates, water, vitamins, and minerals. It can be synthetically produced or extracted from animal thyroid glands in crystalline form to be used in the treatment of thyroid dysfunction, especially cretinism, myxedema, and Hashimoto's disease.

Triiodothyronine (T$_3$)

Triiodothyronine is an effective thyroid hormone that contains three iodine atoms. It influences the basal metabolic rate and is more biologically active than thyroxine.

Calcitonin

Also known as thyrocalcitonin, calcitonin is a thyroid hormone that influences bone and calcium metabolism. It helps maintain plasma calcium homeostasis.

Hyposecretion of the thyroid hormones T$_3$ and T$_4$ results in cretinism during infancy, myxedema during adulthood, and Hashimoto's disease, which is a chronic thyroid disease. Hypersecretion of the thyroid hormones T$_3$ and T$_4$ results in hyperthyroidism, which is also called thyrotoxicosis, and Grave's disease, exophthalmic goiter, toxic goiter, or Basedow's disease. Simple or endemic goiter is an enlargement of the thyroid gland caused by a deficiency of iodine in the diet.

The Parathyroid Glands

The parathyroid glands are small, yellowish-brown bodies occurring as two pairs and located on the dorsal surface and lower aspect of the thyroid gland. Each parathyroid gland is approximately 6 mm in diameter and weighs approximately 0.033 g (Fig. 11-1 and Plate 4). The hormone secreted by the parathyroids is parathormone (PTH). This hormone is essential for the maintenance of a normal serum calcium level. It also plays a role in the metabolism of phosphorus. Hyposecretion of PTH may result in hypoparathyroidism, which may result in tetany. Hypersecretion of PTH may result in hyperparathyroidism, which may result in osteoporosis, kidney stones, and hypercalcemia.

The Pancreas (The Islets of Langerhans)

The islets of Langerhans are small clusters of cells located on the surface of the pancreas (see Fig. 11-1 and Plate 4). They are composed of three major types of cells: alpha, beta, and delta. The alpha cells secrete the hormone glucagon, which facilitates the breakdown of glycogen to glucose, thereby elevating blood sugar. The beta cells secrete the hormone insulin, which is essential for the maintenance of normal blood sugar (80–120 mg/100 mL of blood). Insulin is essential to life. It promotes the use of glucose in cells, thereby lowering the blood glucose level, and plays a vital role in carbohydrate, protein, and fat metabolism. Insulin can be synthetically produced in various types and was first discovered and used successfully by Sir F. G. Banting. Hyposecretion or inadequate use of insulin may result in diabetes mellitus. Hypersecretion of insulin may result in hyperinsulinism. The delta cells secrete a hormone, somatostatin, that suppresses the release of glucagon and insulin.

The Adrenal Glands (Suprarenals)

The adrenal glands are two small, triangular-shaped glands located on top of each kidney. Each gland weighs about 5 g and consists of an outer portion or cortex and an inner portion called the medulla (Fig. 11-1 and Plate 4).

THE ADRENAL CORTEX

The cortex is essential to life as it secretes a group of hormones, the glucocorticoids, the mineralocorticoids, and the androgens. These hormones and their effects on the body are described below.

The Glucocorticoids

The two glucocorticoid hormones are cortisol and corticosterone.

Cortisol. Cortisol (hydrocortisone) is the principal steroid hormone secreted by the cortex. The following are some of the known influences and functions of this hormone:

1. It regulates carbohydrate, protein, and fat metabolism.
2. It stimulates output of glucose from the liver (gluconeogenesis).
3. It increases the blood sugar level.
4. It regulates other physiological body processes.
5. It promotes the transport of amino acids into extracellular tissue, thereby making them available for energy.
6. It influences the effectiveness of catecholamines such as dopamine, epinephrine, and norepinephrine.
7. It has an anti-inflammatory effect.
8. It helps the body cope during times of stress.

Hyposecretion of this hormone may result in Addison's disease. Hypersecretion of cortisol may result in Cushing's disease.

Corticosterone. Corticosterone is a steroid hormone secreted by the adrenal cortex. It is essential for the normal use of carbohydrates, the absorption of glucose, and the process known as gluconeogenesis. It also influences potassium and sodium metabolism.

The Mineralocorticoids

Aldosterone is the principal mineralocorticoid secreted by the adrenal cortex. It is essential in regulating electrolyte and water balance by promoting sodium and chloride retention and potassium excretion. Hyposecretion of this hormone may result in a reduced plasma volume. Hypersecretion of this hormone may result in a condition known as primary aldosteronism.

The Androgens

Androgen refers to a substance or hormone that promotes the development of male characteristics. The two main androgen hormones are testosterone and androsterone. These hormones are essential for the development of the male secondary sex characteristics.

THE ADRENAL MEDULLA

The medulla synthesizes, secretes, and stores catecholamines, specifically, dopamine, epinephrine, and norepinephrine. A discussion of these substances and their effects on the body follows.

Dopamine

Dopamine acts to dilate systemic arteries, elevates systolic blood pressure, increases cardiac output, and increases urinary output. It is used in the treatment of shock and is a neurotransmitter in the nervous system.

Epinephrine

Epinephrine (Adrenalin, adrenaline) acts as a vasoconstrictor, vasopressor, cardiac stimulant, antispasmodic, and sympathomimetic. Its main function is to assist in the regulation of the sympathetic branch of the autonomic nervous system. It can be synthetically produced and may be administered parenterally (by an injection), topically (on a local area of the skin), or by inhalation (by nose or mouth). The following are some of the known influences and functions of this hormone:

1. It elevates the systolic blood pressure.
2. It increases the heart rate and cardiac output.
3. It increases glycogenolysis, thereby hastening the release of glucose from the liver. This action elevates the blood sugar level and provides the body with a spurt of energy.
4. It dilates the bronchial tubes.
5. It dilates the pupils.

Norepinephrine

Norepinephrine (noradrenalin) acts as a vasoconstrictor, vasopressor, and neurotransmitter. It elevates systolic and diastolic blood pressure, increases the heart rate and cardiac output, and increases glycogenolysis.

The Ovaries

The ovaries produce estrogens (estradiol, estrone, and estriol) and progesterone. Estrogen is the female sex hormone secreted by the Graafian follicles of the ovaries. Progesterone is a steroid hormone secreted by the corpus luteum. These hormones are essential for promoting the growth, development, and maintenance of secondary female sex organs and characteristics. They also prepare the uterus for pregnancy, promote development of the mammary glands, and play a vital role in a woman's emotional well-being and her sexual drive (see Fig. 11-1 and Plate 4).

The Testes

The testes produce the male sex hormone testosterone, which is essential for normal growth and development of the male accessory sex organs. Testosterone plays a vital role in the erection process of the penis and, thus, is necessary for the reproductive act, copulation (see Fig. 11-1 and Plate 4).

The Placenta

During pregnancy the placenta, a spongy structure joining mother and child, serves as an endocrine gland. It produces chorionic gonadotropin hormone, estrogen, and progesterone.

The Gastrointestinal Mucosa

The mucosa of the pyloric area of the stomach secretes the hormone gastrin, which stimulates gastric acid secretion. Gastrin also affects the gallbladder, pancreas, and small intestine secretory activities.

The mucosa of the duodenum and jejunum secretes the hormone secretin, which stimulates pancreatic juice, bile, and intestinal secretion. The mucosa of the duodenum also secretes pancreozymin-cholecystokinin, which stimulates the pancreas. Enterogastrone, a hormone that regulates gastric secretions, is also secreted by the duodenal mucosa.

The Thymus

The thymus is a bilobed body located in the mediastinal cavity in front of and above the heart (Fig. 11-3). It is composed of lymphoid tissue and is a part of the lymphoid system. It

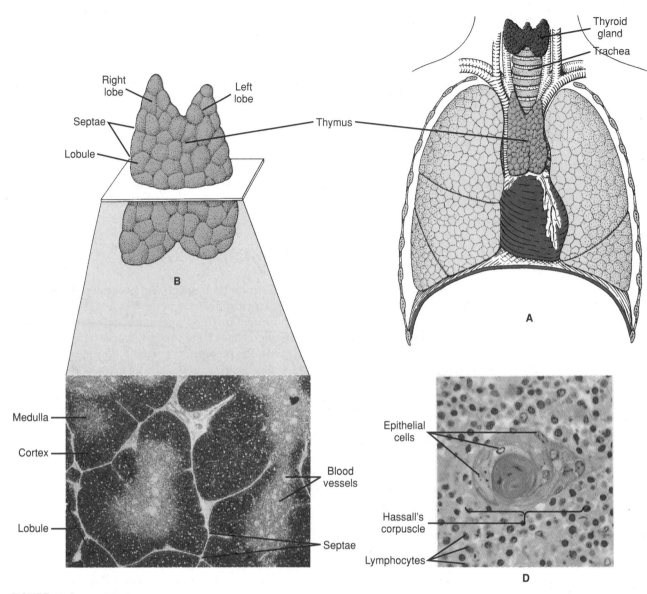

FIGURE 11–3

The thymus. **A.** Appearance and position of the thymus on gross dissection; note its relationship to other organs in the chest. **B.** Anatomical landmarks on the thymus. **C.** A low-power light micrograph of the thymus. Note the fibrous septae that divide the thymic tissue into lobes resembling interconnected lymphatic nodules. **D.** At higher magnification the unusual structure of Hassall's corpuscles can be examined. The small cells in view are lymphocytes in various stages of development (LM, x336). (*From Martini F. Fundamentals of Anatomy and Physiology, 2nd ed. Englewood Cliffs, NJ: Prentice-Hall, 1992, with permission.*)

is a ductless gland-like body and secretes the hormones thymosin and thymopoietin. Thymosin promotes the maturation process of T lymphocytes (thymus-dependent). Thymopoietin is a hormone that influences the production of lymphocyte precursors and aids in their process of becoming T lymphocytes.

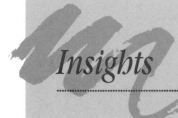

Insights

DIABETES MELLITUS

Diabetes mellitus is a complex disorder of metabolism. It affects 14 million Americans, with care and treatment costing $20 billion annually.

The National Diabetes Data Group of the National Institutes of Health has categorized the various forms of diabetes mellitus as: Type I—insulin-dependent diabetes mellitus (IDDM); Type II—noninsulin-dependent diabetes mellitus (NIDDM); Type III—women who have developed glucose intolerance in association with pregnancy; and Type IV—diabetes associated with pancreatic disease, hormonal changes, the adverse effects of drugs, and other anomalies.

One in ten people who have diabetes are Type I diabetics and must take insulin on a regular basis. Insulin was discovered in 1921 by Sir F. G. Banting. Insulin is essential for the proper metabolism of carbohydrates, fats, and proteins.

Warning Signs and Symptoms

Type I IDDM

- Frequent urination (polyuria)
- Excessive thirst (polydipsia)
- Extreme hunger (polyphagia)
- Unexplained weight loss
- Extreme fatigue
- Blurred vision

Type II NIDDM

- Any type I symptom
- Tingling or numbing in your feet
- Frequent vaginal or skin infection

The individual with Type I diabetes is faced with a lifetime commitment of trying to "juggle and balance" insulin, diet, exercise, other disease processes, stress, and all the other factors that are involved in one's life. Without proper treatment and control diabetes can lead to cardiovascular disease, nephropathy, neuropathy, retinopathy, and death.

The National Institute of Diabetes and Digestive and Kidney Diseases conducted a 10-year Diabetes Control and Complications Trial on how best to control the complications of insulin-dependent diabetes mellitus (IDDM) and found that those in the intensive-control group who tested their blood sugar four or more times a day and injected insulin three or more times a day, or who used an insulin pump, and followed a special diet showed reductions in complications.

The American Diabetes Association estimates that 7 million Americans have diabetes and do not know it. Are you at risk for diabetes? Do you have any, some, or many of the signs and symptoms of diabetes? If your answer is yes, you should see a physician and be carefully evaluated and tested for diabetes.

Promising Technology for the Detection and Treatment of Diabetes

SpectRx is a hand-held instrument that detects natural fluorescence in the eye associated with lens proteins, which are much higher in those with diabetes. It could be used as a screening tool for diabetes. This device needs Food and Drug Administration approval.

(Insights continues on next page)

In 1992, researchers at the University of Chicago discovered that a defect in a gene involved in glucose metabolism is responsible for one form of Type II diabetes. The gene is associated with an enzyme involved in regulating insulin secretion. It is anticipated that drugs can be developed through genetic engineering to compensate for this genetic defect.

Advances in miniaturization are bringing the "bionic" pancreas closer to reality. This device would be implanted in a patient's body and it would continuously monitor one's blood sugar levels, calculate the amount of insulin needed, and administer the exact amount.

Agents called surfactants can help transport insulin across mucous membranes and may be used to deliver insulin through the nose, eyes, or rectum. It is not known if this delivery method will be a feasible alternative to insulin injections.

The no-prick glucose meter uses a laser beam to test blood sugar. The light shines through the skin and blood vessels. A minicomputer calculates the blood sugar by measuring the amount of light absorbed. This device needs Food and Drug Administration approval.

Transplants of the pancreas and/or islet cells of the pancreas may someday be viable choices for a patient with diabetes. As with any type of transplant, the availability of a donor organ and/or cells, the immune system's response to such an organ and/or cells, plus all the other problems involved in transplants will have to be overcome for this to be a feasible choice for diabetics.

Terminology with Surgical Procedures & Pathology

Term	Word Parts			Definition
acidosis (ăs″ ĭ-dō′ sĭs)	acid	R	acid	A condition of excessive acidity of body fluids
	osis	S	condition of	
acromegaly (ăk″ rō-mĕg′ ă-lē)	acro	CF	extremity	Enlargement of the extremities caused by excessive growth hormone
	megaly	S	enlargement, large	
adenalgia (ăd″ ĕn-ăl′ jĭ-ă)	aden	R	gland	Pain in a gland
	algia	S	pain	
adenectomy (ăd″ ĕn-ĕk′ tō-mē)	aden	R	gland	Surgical excision of a gland
	ectomy	S	excision	
adenoma (ăd″ ĕ-nō′ mă)	aden	R	gland	A tumor of a gland
	oma	S	tumor	
adenomalacia (ăd″ ĕ-nō-mă-lā′ shĭ-ă)	adeno	CF	gland	A softening of a gland
	malacia	S	softening	
adenosclerosis (ăd″ ĕ-nō-sklĕ-rō′ sĭs)	adeno	CF	gland	A condition of hardening of a gland
	scler	R	hardening	
	osis	S	condition of	
adenosis (ăd″ ĕ-nō′ sĭs)	aden	R	gland	Any disease condition of a gland
	osis	S	condition of	
adrenal (ăd-rē′ năl)	ad	P	toward	Pertaining to toward the kidney
	ren	R	kidney	
	al	S	pertaining to	
adrenalectomy (ăd-rē″ năl-ĕk′ tō-mē)	ad	P	toward	Surgical excision of the adrenal gland
	ren	R	kidney	
	al	S	pertaining to	
	ectomy	S	excision	
adrenopathy (ăd″ rĕn-ŏp′ ă-thē)	ad	P	toward	Any disease of the adrenal gland
	reno	CF	kidney	
	pathy	S	disease	
adrenotropic (ăd-rē″ nō-trōp′ ĭk)	ad	P	toward	Pertaining to the nourishment of the adrenal glands
	reno	CF	kidney	
	trop	R	nourishment	
	ic	S	pertaining to	
cretinism (krē′ tĭn-ĭzm)	cretin	R	cretin	A congenital deficiency in secretion of the thyroid hormones T_3 and T_4
	ism	S	condition of	

(Terminology—continued)

Term		Word Parts		Definition
diabetes (dī″ ă-bē′ tēz)	dia betes	P S	through to go	A disease characterized by excessive discharge of urine
dwarfism (dwar′ fizm)	dwarf ism	R S	small condition of	A condition of being abnormally small
endocrine (ĕn′ dō-krĭn)	endo crine	P R	within to secrete	A ductless gland that produces an internal secretion
endocrinologist (ĕn″ dō-krĭn-ŏl′ ō-gĭst)	endo crino log ist	P CF R S	within to secrete study of one who specializes	One who specializes in the study of the endocrine glands
endocrinology (ĕn″ dō-krĭn-ŏl′ ō-jē)	endo crino logy	P CF S	within to secrete study of	The study of the endocrine glands
endocrinopathy (ĕn″ dō-krĭn-ŏp′ ă-thē)	endo crino pathy	P CF S	within to secrete disease	A disease of an endocrine gland or glands
endocrino- therapy (ĕn″ dō-krĭn″ ō-thĕr′ ă-pē)	endo crino therapy	P CF S	within to secrete treatment	Treatment with endocrine preparations
euthyroid (ū-thī′ royd)	eu thyr oid	P R S	good, normal thyroid, shield resemble	Normal activity of the thyroid gland
exocrine (ĕks′ ō-krĭn)	exo crine	P R	out, away from to secrete	External secretion of a gland
exophthalmic (ĕks″ ŏf-thăl′ mĭk)	ex ophthalm ic	P R S	out, away from eye pertaining to	Pertaining to an abnormal protrusion of the eye
galactorrhea (gă-lăk″ tō-rĭ′ ă)	galacto rrhea	CF S	milk flow, discharge	Excessive secretion of milk after cessation of nursing
gigantism (jī′ găn-tĭzm)	gigant ism	R S	giant condition of	A condition of being abnormally large
glandular (glăn′ dū-lăr)	glandul ar	R S	little acorn pertaining to	Pertaining to a gland

(Terminology—continued)

Term	Word Parts			Definition
glucocorticoid (glū″ kō-kŏrt′ ĭ-koyd)	gluco	CF	sweet, sugar	A general classification of the adrenal cortical hormones
	cortic	R	cortex	
	oid	S	resemble	
hirsutism (hŭr′ sūt-ĭzm)	hirsut	R	hairy	An adnormal condition characterized by excessive growth of hair, especially in women
	ism	S	condition of	
hypergonadism (hī″ pĕr-gō′ năd-ĭzm)	hyper	P	excessive	A condition of excessive secretion of the sex glands
	gonad	R	seed	
	ism	S	condition of	
hyperinsulinism (hī″ pĕr-ĭn′ sū-lĭn-ĭzm)	hyper	P	excessive	A condition of excessive amounts of insulin in the blood
	insulin	R	insulin	
	ism	S	condition of	
hyperkalemia (hī″ pĕr-kă-lē′ mĭ-ă)	hyper	P	excessive	A condition of excessive amounts of potassium in the blood
	kal	R	potassium (K)	
	emia	S	blood condition	
hyperthyroidism (hī″ pĕr-thī′ royd-ĭzm)	hyper	P	excessive	A condition caused by excessive secretion of the thyroid gland
	thyr	R	thyroid, shield	
	oid	S	resemble	
	ism	S	condition of	
hypocrinism (hī″ pō-krī′ nĭzm)	hypo	P	deficient	A condition caused by deficient secretion of any gland
	crin	R	to secrete	
	ism	S	condition of	
hypogonadism (hī″ pō-gō′ năd-ĭzm)	hypo	P	deficient	A condition caused by deficient internal secretion of the gonads
	gonad	R	seed	
	ism	S	condition of	
hypoparathyroid-ism (hī″ pō-păr″ ă-thī′ royd-ĭzm)	hypo	P	deficient	Deficient internal secretion of the parathyroid glands
	para	P	beside	
	thyr	R	thyroid, shield	
	oid	S	resemble	
	ism	S	condition of	
hypophysis (hī-pŏf′ ĭ-sĭs)	hypo	P	deficient, under	Any undergrowth; the pituitary body
	physis	S	growth	
hypothyroidism (hī″ pō-thī′ royd-ĭzm)	hypo	P	deficient	Deficient secretion of the thyroid gland
	thyr	R	thyroid, shield	
	oid	S	resemble	
	ism	S	condition of	

(Terminology—continued)

Term	Word Parts			Definition
insulinogenic (ĭn″ sū-lĭn″ ō-jěn′ ĭk)	insulino genic	CF S	insulin formation produce	The formation or production of insulin
insulinoid (ĭn′ sū-lĭn-oyd″)	insulin oid	R S	insulin resemble	Resembling insulin
insuloma (ĭn′ sū-lō″ mǎ)	insul oma	R S	insulin tumor	A tumor of the islets of Langerhans
lethargic (lě-thar′ jĭk)	letharg ic	R S	drowsiness pertaining to	Pertaining to drowsiness, sluggish
myxedema (mĭks″ ě-dē′ mǎ)	myx edema	R S	mucus swelling	A condition of mucus swelling resulting from hypofunction of the thyroid gland
pancreatic (păn″ krē-ăt′ ĭk)	pan creat ic	P R S	all flesh pertaining to	Pertaining to the pancreas
parathyroid (păr″ ă-thī′ royd)	para thyr oid	P R S	beside thyroid, shield resemble	An endocrine gland located beside the thyroid gland
pineal (pĭn′ ē-ăl)	pine al	R S	pine cone pertaining to	An endocrine gland that is shaped like a small pine cone
pinealectomy (pĭn″ ē-ăl-ĕk′ tō-mē)	pineal ectomy	R S	pineal body excision	Surgical excision of the pineal body
pinealoma (pĭn″ ē-ă-lō′ mǎ)	pineal oma	R S	pineal body tumor	A tumor of the pineal body
pituitarism (pĭt-ū′ ĭ-tă-rĭzm)	pituitar ism	R S	phlegm condition	Any condition of the pituitary gland
pituitary (pĭ-tū′ ĭ-tăr″ ē)	pituitar y	R S	phlegm pertaining to	Pertaining to phlegm; the pituitary body or gland, the hypophysis
progeria (prō-jē′ rĭ-ă)	pro ger ia	P R S	before old age condition	A condition of premature old age occurring in childhood
thymectomy (thī-měk′ tō-mē)	thym ectomy	R S	thymus excision	Surgical excision of the thymus gland
thymitis (thī-mī′ tĭs)	thym itis	R S	thymus inflammation	Inflammation of the thymus gland

(Terminology—continued)

Term	Word Parts			Definition
thymopexy (thī′ mō-pĕks″ ē)	thymo pexy	CF S	thymus fixation	Surgical fixation of an enlarged thymus in a new position
thyroid (thī′ royd)	thyr oid	R S	thyroid, shield resemble	Resembling a shield; one of the endocrine glands
thyroidectomy (thī″ royd-ĕk′ tō-mē)	thyr oid ectomy	R S S	thyroid, shield resemble excision	Surgical excision of the thyroid gland
thyroiditis (thī″ royd′ī′ tĭs)	thyr oid itis	R S S	thyroid, shield resemble inflammation	Inflammation of the thyroid gland
thyroptosis (thī″ rŏp-tō′ sĭs)	thyro ptosis	CF S	thyroid, shield drooping	Downward drooping of the thyroid into the thorax
thyrosis (thī-rō′ sĭs)	thyr osis	R S	thyroid, shield condition of	Any condition of abnormal functioning of the thyroid
thyrotherapy (thī″ rō-thĕr′ ă-pē)	thyro therapy	CF S	thyroid, shield treatment	Pertaining to the treatment using thyroid gland extracts
thyrotome (thī″ rō-tōm)	thyro tome	CF S	thyroid, shield instrument to cut	An instrument used to cut the thyroid cartilage
thyrotoxicosis (thī″ rō-tŏks″ ĭ-kō′ sĭs)	thyro toxic osis	CF R S	thyroid, shield poison condition of	A poisonous condition of the thyroid gland caused by hyperactivity
virilism (vĭr′ ĭl-ĭzm)	viril ism	R S	masculine condition of	The condition of masculinity developed in a woman

Vocabulary Words

Vocabulary words are terms that have not been divided into component parts. They are common words or specialized terms associated with the subject of this chapter. These words are provided to enhance your medical vocabulary.

Word	Definition
aldosterone (ăl-dŏs′ tĕr-ōn)	A mineralocorticoid hormone secreted by the adrenal cortex that helps regulate metabolism of sodium, chloride, and potassium
androgen (ăn′ drō-jĕn)	Hormones that produce or stimulate the development of male characteristics. The two major androgens are testosterone and androsterone
catecholamines (kăt″ ĕ-kōl′ ăm-ēns)	Biochemical substances, epinephrine, norepinephrine, and dopamine
cortisone (kŏr′ tĭ-sōn)	A glucocorticoid hormone that is isolated from the adrenal cortex; used as an anti-inflammatory agent
dopamine (dō′ pă-mēn)	An intermediate substance in the synthesis of norepinephrine; used in the treatment of shock as it acts to elevate blood pressure and increase urinary output
epinephrine (ĕp″ ĭ-nĕf′ rĭn)	A hormone produced by the adrenal medulla; used as a vasoconstrictor, as a cardiac stimulant, to relax bronchospasm, and to relieve allergic symptoms; also called adrenaline, Adrenalin
estrogen (ĕs′ trō-jĕn)	Hormones produced by the ovaries, including estradiol, estrone, and estriol; female sex hormones important in the development of secondary sex characteristics and regulation of the menstrual cycle
hormone (hor′ mōn)	A chemical substance produced by the endocrine glands
hydrocortisone (hĭ″ drō-kŏr′ tĭ-sōn)	A glucocorticoid hormone produced by the adrenal cortex; used as an anti-inflammatory agent
insulin (in′ sū-lĭn)	A hormone produced by the beta cells of the islets of Langerhans of the pancreas; essential for the metabolism of carbohydrates and fats; used in the management of diabetes mellitus
iodine (ī′ ō-dīn)	A trace mineral that aids in the development and functioning of the thyroid gland
norepinephrine (nŏr-ĕp″ ĭ-nĕf′ rĭn)	A hormone produced by the adrenal medulla; used as a vasoconstrictor of peripheral blood vessels in acute hypotensive states
oxytocin (ŏk″ sĭ-tō′ sĭn)	A hormone produced by the pituitary gland that stimulates uterine contraction during childbirth and stimulates the release of milk during nursing
progesterone (prō-jĕs′ tĕr-ōn)	A hormone produced by the corpus luteum of the ovary, the adrenal cortex, or the placenta; released during the second half of the menstrual cycle

(Vocabulary—continued)

Word	Definition
somatotropin (sō-măt′ ō-trō″ pĭn)	Growth stimulating hormone produced by the anterior lobe of the pituitary gland
steroids (stĕr′ oydz)	A group of chemical substances that includes hormones, vitamins, sterols, cardiac glycosides, and certain drugs
testosterone (tĕs-tŏs′ tĕr-ōn)	A hormone produced by the testes; male sex hormone important in the development of secondary sex characteristics and masculinization
thyroxine (thī-rŏks′ ēn)	A hormone produced by the thyroid gland; important in growth and development and regulation of the body's metabolic rate and metabolism of carbohydrates, fats, and proteins
vasopressin (văs″ ō-prĕs′ ĭn)	A hormone produced by the hypothalamus and stored in the posterior lobe of the pituitary gland; also called antidiuretic hormone, ADH

ABBREVIATIONS

ACTH	adrenocorticotropic hormone	**MIF**	melanocyte-stimulating hormone release-inhibiting factor
ADA	American Diabetes Association	**MSH**	melanocyte-stimulating hormone
ADH	antidiuretic hormone	**NIDDM**	noninsulin-dependent diabetes mellitus
BG, bG	blood glucose		
BMR	basal metabolic rate	**PBI**	protein-bound iodine
CRF	corticotropin-releasing factor	**PIF**	prolactin release-inhibiting factor
DI	diabetes insipidus	**PRF**	prolactin-releasing factor
DM	diabetes mellitus	**PTH**	parathormone
FBS	fasting blood sugar	**RAIU**	radioactive iodine uptake
FSH	follicle-stimulating hormone	**RIA**	radioimmunoassay
GH	growth hormone	**SMBG**	self-monitoring of blood glucose
GHb	glycosylated hemoglobin		
GHRF	glycosylated hemoglobin-releasing factor	**STH**	somatotropin hormone
		T_3	triiodothyronine
GnRF	gonadotropin-releasing factor	T_3RU	triiodothyronine resin uptake
GTT	glucose tolerance test	T_4	thyroxine
IDDM	insulin-dependent diabetes mellitus	**TFS**	thyroid function studies
		TSH	thyroid-stimulating hormone
K	potassium		
LH	luteinizing hormone	**VMA**	vanillylmandelic acid
LTH	lactogenic hormone	**VP**	vasopressin

Drug Highlights

Drugs that are generally used for endocrine system diseases and disorders include thyroid hormones, antithyroid hormones, insulin, and oral hypoglycemic agents.

Thyroid Hormones

Increase metabolic rate, cardiac output, oxygen consumption, body temperature, respiratory rate, blood volume, and carbohydrate, fat and protein metabolism, and influence growth and development at cellular level. Thyroid hormones are used as supplements or replacement therapy in hypothyroidism, myxedema, and cretinism.

Examples: Levothroid and Synthroid (levothyroxine sodium), Cytomel (liothyronine sodium), Euthroid and Thyrolar (liotrix), and thyroid, USP.

Antithyroid Hormones

Inhibit the synthesis of thyroid hormones by decreasing iodine use in manufacture of thyroglobin and iodothyronine. They do not inactivate or inhibit thyroxine or triiodothyronine. They are used in the treatment of hyperthyroidism.

Example: Tapazole (methimazole), potassium iodide solution, Lugol's solution (strong iodine solution), and Iodotope I-131 (sodium iodide).

Insulin

Stimulates carbohydrate metabolism by increasing the movement of glucose and other monosaccharides into cells. It also influences fat and carbohydrate metabolism in the liver and adipose cells. It decreases blood sugar, phosphate, and potassium, and increases blood pyruvate and lactate. *Insulin* is used in the treatment of insulin-dependent-diabetes mellitus (Type I IDDM), noninsulin-dependent diabetes mellitus (Type II NIDDM) when other regimens are not effective, and to treat ketoacidosis.

Insulin Preparations

Insulin is given by subcutaneous injection and is available in rapid-acting, intermediate-acting, and long-acting preparations.

Rapid-Acting

Examples: Regular Iletin I, Regular Insulin, Novolin R, Humulin R, Velosulin, Semilente Iletin I, and Semilente Insulin.
Onset of Action 0.5 hour   Appearance—clear

Intermediate-Acting

Examples: NPH Iletin I, NPH Insulin, Novolin N, Humulin N, Lente Iletin I, Lente Insulin, and Novolin L.
Onset of Action 1-1.5 hours   Appearance—cloudy

Long-Acting

Examples: Protamine, Zinc and Iletin I, Ultralente, and Ultralente Iletin I.
Onset of Action 4-8 hours   Appearance—cloudy

Oral Hypoglycemic Agents

Are agents of the sulfonylurea class and are used to stimulate insulin secretion from pancreatic cells in non-insulin-dependent diabetics with some pancreatic function.

Examples: Dymelor (acetohexamide), Diabinese (chlorpropamide), Glucotrol (glipizide), DiaBeta and Micronase (glyburide), Tolinase (tolazamide), and Orinase (tolbutamide).

Communication Enrichment

This segment is provided for those who wish to enhance their ability to communicate in either English or Spanish.

RELATED TERMS

English	Spanish
adrenal	adrenal (ă-*drĕ*-năl)
diabetes	diabetes (dĭ-ă-*bĕ*-tĕs)
endocrine system	sistema endocrino (sĭs-*tĕ*-mă ĕn-dō-crĭ-nō)
gland	glándula (glăn-*dŭ*-lă)
goiter	bocio (*bŏ*-sĭ-ō)
insulin	insulina (ĭn-sŭ-*lĭ*-nă)
pancreas	pancreas (păn-*krĕ*-ăs)
parathyroids	paratiroides (pă-*ră*-tĭ-rō-ĭ-dĕs)
pituitary	pituitario (pĭ-tŭ-ĭ-*tă*-rĭ-ō)
thyroid	tiroides (tĭ-rō-ĭ-*dĕs*)
adrenalin	adrenalina (ă-*drĕ*-nă-lĭ-nă)
hormone	hormona (ōr-mō-nă)
iodine	iodo (ĭ-ō-dō)
acidosis	acidismo (*ă*-sĭ-dĭs-mō)
extremity	extremidad (ĕx-trĕ-*mĭ*-dăd)
soften	ablandar (*ă*-blăn-dăr)
harden	endurecer (ĕn-*dŭ*-rĕ-sĕr)
small	pequeño (pĕ-*kĕ*-ñō)
large	grande (*grănd*-ĕ)

English	Spanish
giant	gigante (hǐ-*găn*-tě)
thyroidectomy	tiroidectomía (tǐ-rō-ǐ-děc-tō-mǐ-ă)
thyroxine	tiroxina (tǐ-rōx-*sǐ*-nă)
hairy	peludo (pě-*lŭ*-dō)
sweet	dulce (*dŭl*-sě)
excessive	excesivo (ěx-sě-*sǐ*-vō)
seed	semilla (*sě*-mǐ-jă)
potassium	potasio (pō-*tă*-sǐ-ō)
deficient	deficiente (dě-fǐ-sǐ-*ěn*-tě)
phlegm	flema (*flě*-mă)
masculine	masculino (*măs*-kŭ-lǐ-nō)
within	dentro (*děn*-trō)

DIAGNOSTIC AND LABORATORY TESTS

Test	Description
catecholamines (kăt″ ě-kōl′ ă-mēns)	A test performed on urine to determine the amount of epinephrine and norepinephrine present. These adrenal hormones increase in times of stress.
corticotropin, corticotropin-releasing factor (CRF) (kor″ tǐ-kō-trō′ pin)	A test performed on blood plasma to determine the amount of corticotropin present. Increased levels may indicate stress, adrenal cortical hypofunction, and/or pituitary tumors. Decreased levels may indicate adrenal neoplasms and/or Cushing's syndrome.
fasting blood sugar (FBS) (făs-tǐng blod shoog′ ar)	A test performed on blood to determine the level of sugar in the bloodstream. Increased levels may indicate diabetes mellitus, diabetic acidosis, and many other conditions. Decreased levels may indicate hypoglycemia, hyperinsulinism, and many other conditions.
glucose tolerance test (GTT) (gloo′ kōs tŏl′ ěr-ăns test)	A blood sugar test performed at specified intervals after the patient has been given a certain amount of glucose. Blood samples are drawn, and the blood glucose level of each sample is determined. It is more accurate than other blood sugar tests, and it is used to diagnose diabetes mellitus.

Test	Description
17-hydroxycorticosteroids (17-OHCS) (hĭ-drŏk″ sē-kor″ tĭ-kō-stĕr′ oyd)	A test performed on urine to identify adrenocorticosteroid hormones. It is used to determine adrenal cortical function.
17-ketosteroids (17-KS) (kē″ tō-stĕr′ oyd)	A test performed on urine to determine the amount of 17-KS present. 17-KS is the end product of androgens and is secreted from the adrenal glands and testes. It is used in the diagnosing of adrenal tumors.
protein-bound iodine (PBI) (prō′ tēn bound ī′ ō-dīn)	A test performed on serum to indicate the amount of iodine that is attached to serum protein. It may be used to indicate thyroid function.
radioactive iodine uptake (RAIU) (rā″ dē-ō-ăk′ tīv ī′ ō-dīn ŭp′ tāk)	A test to measure the ability of the thyroid gland to concentrate ingested iodine. Increased level may indicate hyperthyroidism, cirrhosis, and/or thyroiditis. Decreased level may indicate hypothyroidism.
thyroid scan (thī′ royd skăn)	A test to detect tumors of the thyroid gland. The patient is given radioactive iodine 131, which localizes in the thyroid gland, and the gland is then visualized with a scanner device.
thyroxine (T$_4$) (thī-rōks′ ĭn)	A test performed on blood serum to determine the amount of thyroxine present. Increased levels may indicate hyperthyroidism. Decreased levels may indicate hypothyroidism.
triiodothyronine uptake (T$_3$) (trī″ ī-ō″ dō-thī′ rō-nĭn ŭp′ tāk)	A test performed on blood serum to determine the amount of triiodothyronine present. Increased levels may indicate thyrotoxicosis, toxic adenoma, and/or Hashimoto's struma. Decreased levels may indicate starvation, severe infection, and severe trauma.
total calcium (tōt′ l kăl′ sē-ŭm)	A test performed on blood serum to determine the amount of calcium present. Increased levels may indicate hyperparathyroidism. Decreased levels may indicate hypoparathyroidism.
ultrasonography (ŭl-tră-sŏn-ŏg′ ră-fē)	The use of high-frequency sound waves to visualize the structure being studied. May be used to visualize the pancreas, thyroid, and any other gland. It is used as a screening test or as a diagnostic tool.

Learning Exercises

Anatomy and Physiology

Write your answers to the following questions. Do not refer back to the text.

1. Name the primary glands of the endocrine system.

   a. _____   b. _____

   c. _____   d. _____

   e. _____   f. _____

   g. _____   h. _____

2. Name the secondary glands of the endocrine system.

   a. _____   b. _____

   c. _____

3. State the vital function of the endocrine system. _____
   _____

4. Define hormone. _____

5. State the vital role of the hypothalamus in regulating endocrine functions.

   _____
   _____
   _____

6. Why is the pituitary gland known as the master gland of the body? _____
   _____

7. Name the hormones secreted by the adenohypophysis.

   a. _____   b. _____

   c. _____   d. _____

   e. _____   f. _____

   g. _____

8. Name the hormones secreted by the neurohypophysis.

   a. _____   b. _____

9. The pineal gland secretes the hormones _____ and
   _____.

10. State the vital role of the thyroid gland. _____
    _____

11. Name the hormones stored and secreted by the thyroid gland.

    a. _____   b. _____

    c. _____

12. Parathormone is essential for the maintenance of a normal level of _____
    _____ and also plays a role in the metabolism of _____.

13. Insulin is essential for the maintenance of a normal level of _____
    _____.

14. The adrenal cortex secretes a group of hormones known as the _____, the _____, and the _____.

15. Name four functions of cortisol.

    a. _____   b. _____

    c. _____   d. _____

16. Name four functions of corticosterone.

    a. _____   b. _____

    c. _____   d. _____

17. _____ is the principal mineralocorticoid secreted by the adrenal cortex.

18. Define androgen. _____
    _____

19. Name the three main catecholamines synthesized, secreted, and stored by the adrenal medulla.

    a. _____   b. _____

    c. _____

20. Name three functions of the hormone epinephrine.

    a. _____

    b. _____

    c. _____

21. The ovaries produce the hormones _____ and _____ .

22. The testes produce the hormone _____.

23. Name the two hormones secreted by the thymus.

    a. _____   b. _____

24. Name the four hormones secreted by the gastrointestinal mucosa.

    a. _____   b. _____

    c. _____   d. _____

Word Parts

1. In the spaces provided, write the definitions of these prefixes, roots, combining forms, and suffixes. Do not refer to the listings of terminology words. Leave blank those terms you cannot define.

2. After completing as many as you can, refer back to the terminology word listings to check your work. For each word missed or left blank, write the term and its definition several times on the margins of these pages or on a separate sheet of paper.

3. To maximize the learning process, it is to your advantage to do the following exercises as directed. To refer to the terminology listings before completing these exercises invalidates the learning process.

PREFIXES

Give the definitions of the following prefixes:

1. ad- _____ 2. dia- _____

3. endo- _____ 4. eu- _____

5. ex- _____ 6. exo- _____

7. hyper- _____ 8. hypo- _____

9. pan- _____ 10. para- _____

11. pro- _____

ROOTS AND COMBINING FORMS

Give the definitions of the following roots and combining forms:

1. acid _____ 2. acro _____

3. aden _____ 4. adeno _____

5. cortic _____ 6. creat _____

7. cretin _____ 8. crin _____

9. crine _____ 10. crino _____

11. dwarf _____ 12. galacto _____

13. ger _____ 14. gigant _____

15. glandul _____ 16. gluco _____

17. gonad _____ 18. hirsut _____

19. insul _____ 20. insulin _____

21. insulino _____ 22. kal _____

23. letharg _____ 24. log _____

25. myx _____ 26. ophthalm _____

27. pine _____ 28. pineal _____

29. pituitar _____ 30. ren _____

31. reno _____ 32. scler _____

33. thym _____ 34. thymo _____

35. thyr _____ 36. thyro _____

37. toxic _____ 38. trop _____

39. viril _____

SUFFIXES

Give the definitions of the following suffixes:

1. -al _____ 2. -algia _____

3. -ar _____ 4. -betes _____

5. -ectomy _____ 6. -edema _____

7. -emia _____ 8. -genic _____

9. -ia _____   10. -ic _____

11. -ism _____   12. -ist _____

13. -itis _____   14. -logy _____

15. -malacia _____   16. -megaly _____

17. -oid _____   18. -oma _____

19. -osis _____   20. -pathy _____

21. -pexy _____   22. -physis _____

23. -ptosis _____   24. -rrhea _____

25. -therapy _____   26. -tome _____

27. -y _____

Identifying Medical Terms

In the spaces provided, write the medical terms for the following meanings:

1. _____ Any disease condition of a gland

2. _____ A congenital deficiency in secretion of the thyroid hormone

3. _____ A disease characterized by excessive discharge of urine

4. _____ The study of the endocrine system

5. _____ Normal activity of the thyroid gland

6. _____ External secretion of a gland

7. _____ A condition of being abnormally large

8. _____ A general classification of the adrenal cortex hormones

9. _____ An excessive amount of potassium in the blood

10. _____ Deficient secretion of any gland

11. _____ Deficient internal secretion of the gonads

12. _____ Pertaining to drowsiness; sluggishness

13. _____ A tumor of the pineal body

14. _____ Inflammation of the thymus

Spelling

In the spaces provided, write the correct spelling of these misspelled terms:

1. adensclrosis _____   2. crtinism _____

3. exopthalmic _____   4. hypthyoidism _____

5. myexdema _____   6. pinael   _____

7. pitutary _____   8. thyoid   _____

9. thyrtome _____   10. virlism   _____

Review Questions

Matching

Select the appropriate lettered meaning for each numbered line.

_____ 1. aldosterone

_____ 2. androgen

_____ 3. catecholamines

_____ 4. cortisone

_____ 5. dopamine

_____ 6. epinephrine

_____ 7. insulin

_____ 8. iodine

_____ 9. thyroxine

_____ 10. vasopressin

a. Also called antidiuretic hormone, ADH

b. Biochemical substances, epinephrine, nor-epinephrine, and dopamine

c. A hormone essential for the metabolism of carbo-hydrates and fats

d. A hormone produced by the thyroid gland

e. The principal mineralocorticoid secreted by the adrenal cortex

f. Hormones that produce or stimulate the develop-ment of male characteristics

g. A glucocorticoid hormone used as an anti-inflammatory agent

h. An intermediate substance in the synthesis of norepinephrine

i. Also called adrenaline, Adrenalin

j. A trace mineral that aids in the development and functioning of the thyroid gland

k. A hormone produced by the testes

Abbreviations

Place the correct word, phrase, or abbreviation in the space provided.

_____ 1. basal metabolic rate

_____ 2. diabetes mellitus

_____ 3. FBS

_____ 4. GTT

_____ 5. protein-bound iodine

_____ 6. PTH

_____ 7. RIA

_____ 8. somatotropin hormone

_____ 9. TFS

_____ 10. VP

Diagnostic and Laboratory Tests

Select the best answer to each multiple choice question. Circle the letter of your choice.

1. A test performed on urine to determine the amount of epinephrine and norepinephrine present.

    a. catecholamines

    b. corticotropin

    c. protein-bound iodine

    d. total calcium

2. Increased levels may indicate diabetes mellitus, diabetes acidosis, and many other conditions.

    a. protein-bound iodine

    b. total calcium

    c. fasting blood sugar

    d. thyroid scan

3. A test used to detect tumors of the thyroid gland.

    a. thyroxine

    b. total calcium

    c. thyroid scan

    d. protein-bound iodine

4. A blood sugar test performed at specific intervals after the patient has been given a certain amount of glucose.

    a. fasting blood sugar

    b. glucose tolerance test

    c. protein-bound iodine

    d. corticotropin

5. A test used in the diagnosing of adrenal tumors.

    a. 17-HCS

    b. 17-OHCS

    c. 17-KS

    d. 17-HDL

12 *n* The Nervous System

The nervous system is usually described as having two interconnected divisions: the CNS or central nervous system and the PNS or peripheral nervous system. The CNS includes the brain and spinal cord. The PNS consists of the network of nerves and neural tissues branching throughout the body from 12 pairs of cranial nerves and 31 pairs of spinal nerves.

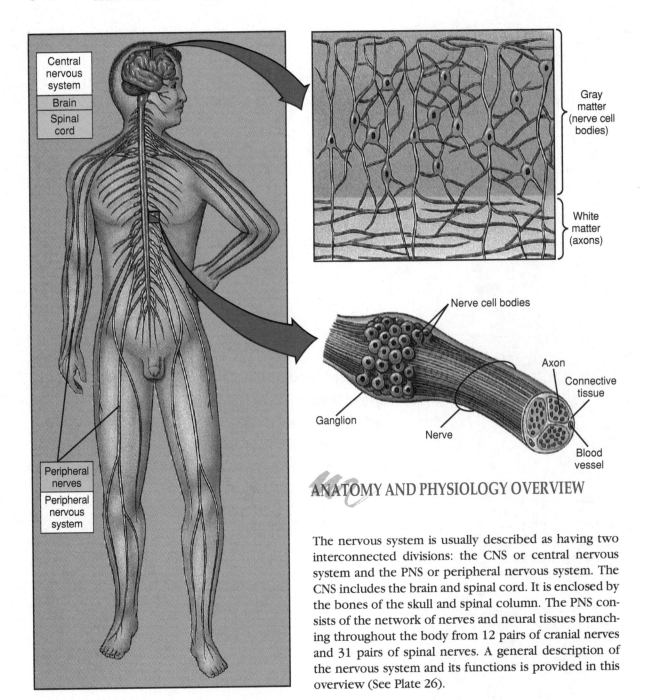

Central
nervous
system

Brain

Spinal
cord

Gray
matter
(nerve cell
bodies)

White
matter
(axons)

Nerve cell bodies

Axon

Connective
tissue

Ganglion

Nerve

Blood
vessel

Peripheral
nerves

Peripheral
nervous
system

ANATOMY AND PHYSIOLOGY OVERVIEW

The nervous system is usually described as having two interconnected divisions: the CNS or central nervous system and the PNS or peripheral nervous system. The CNS includes the brain and spinal cord. It is enclosed by the bones of the skull and spinal column. The PNS consists of the network of nerves and neural tissues branching throughout the body from 12 pairs of cranial nerves and 31 pairs of spinal nerves. A general description of the nervous system and its functions is provided in this overview (See Plate 26).

THE NERVOUS SYSTEM	
Organ	**Primary Functions**
Central Nervous System (CNS)	Control center for nervous system: processes information, provides short-term control over activities of other systems
Brain	Performs complex integrative functions, controls voluntary activities
Spinal cord	Relays information to the brain and performs less complex integrative functions: directs many simple involuntary activities
Peripheral Nervous System (PNS)	Links CNS with other systems and with sense organs

Tissues of the Nervous System

There are two principal tissue types in the nervous system. These tissues are made up of neurons or nerve cells and their supporting tissues, collectively called neuroglia. Neurons are the structural and functional units of the nervous system. These cells are specialized conductors of impulses that enable the body to interact with its internal and external environments. There are several types of neurons, three of which are described below.

MOTOR NEURONS

Motor neurons cause contractions in muscles and secretions from glands and organs. They also act to inhibit the actions of glands and organs, thereby controlling most of the body's functions. Motor neurons may be described as being efferent processes as they transmit impulses away from the neural cell body to the muscles or organs to be innervated. Motor neurons consist of a nucleated cell body with protoplasmic processes extending away from it in several directions. These processes are known as the axon and dendrites. Most axons are long and are covered with a fatty substance, the myelin sheath, that acts as an insulator and increases the transmission velocity of the nerve fiber it surrounds. Axons may be as long as several feet and reach from the cell body to the area to be activated. Dendrites resemble the branches of a tree, are short, or unsheathed, and transmit impulses to the cell body. Neurons usually have several dendrites and only one axon (Fig. 12-1).

SENSORY NEURONS

Sensory neurons differ in structure from motor neurons because they do not have true dendrites. The processes transmitting sensory information to the cell bodies of these neurons are called peripheral processes, are sheathed, and resemble axons. They are attached to sensory receptors and transmit impulses to the central nervous system. In turn, the CNS may stimulate motor neurons in response to this sensory information. Sensory neurons are sometimes referred to as afferent nerves as they carry impulses to the cell body and the central nervous system.

INTERNEURONS

Interneurons are sometimes called central or associative neurons and are located entirely within the central nervous system. They function to mediate impulses between sensory and motor neurons.

Nerve Fibers, Nerves, and Tracts

The terms **nerve fiber, nerve,** and **tract** are used to describe neuronal processes conducting impulses from one location to another. Each term is defined.

NERVE FIBER

A single elongated process, usually a long axon or a peripheral process from a sensory neuron, is called a nerve fiber. Each peripheral nerve fiber is wrapped by a protective membrane called a sheath. There are two types of sheaths, myelinated (thick) and unmyelinated (thin), formed by accessory cells. Some nerve fibers have only the unmyelinated sheath or neurilemma composed of Schwann cells. Myelinated fibers have an inner sheath of myelin, a thick fatty substance, and an outer sheath, the neurilemma. Nerve fibers of the central nervous system (within the brain and spinal cord) do not contain Schwann cells, which are necessary for the regeneration of a damaged nerve fiber. Therefore, damage to fibers of the CNS is permanent, whereas damage to a peripheral nerve may be reversible.

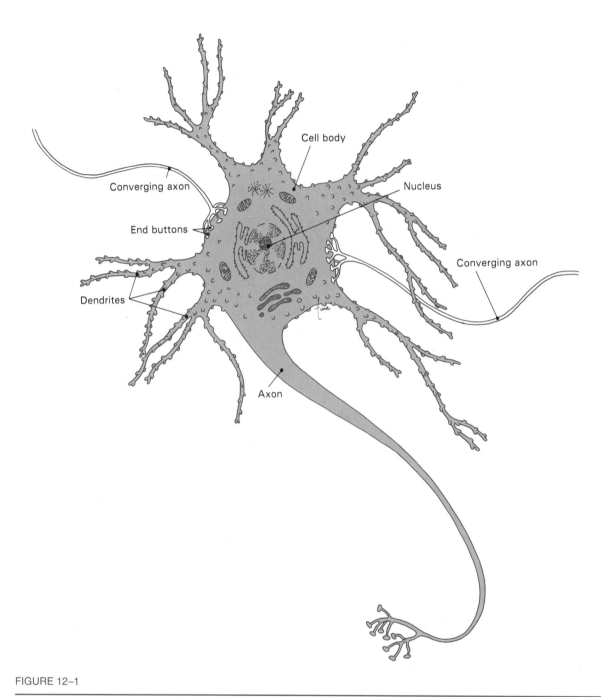

FIGURE 12–1

A neuron with two converging axons. (*Adapted from Evans WF. Anatomy and Physiology, 3rd ed. Englewood Cliffs, NJ: Prentice-Hall, 1983, with permission.*)

NERVE

A nerve is a bundle of nerve fibers, located outside the brain and spinal cord, that connects to various parts of the body. Nerves are usually described as being afferent (conducting to the CNS) or efferent (conducting to muscles, organs, and glands). Some nerves contain a mixture of afferent and efferent fibers and are called mixed nerves. Nerves are also referred to as sensory (afferent) and motor (efferent).

TRACTS

Groups of nerve fibers within the central nervous system are sometimes referred to as tracts when they have the same origin, function, and termination. The spinal cord contains afferent sensory tracts ascending to the brain and efferent motor tracts descending from the brain. The brain itself contains numerous tracts, the largest of which is the corpus callosum joining the left and right hemispheres.

Transmission of Nerve Impulses

Stimulation of a nerve occurs at a receptor. Sensory receptors are of different types, ranging from the simplest, which are free nerve endings for pain, to the most complex, as in the retina of the eye for vision. Receptors are generally specialized to specific types of stimulation such as heat, cold, light, pressure, or pain and react by initiating a chemical change or impulse. The transmission of an impulse by a nerve fiber is based on the all-or-none principle. This means that no transmission occurs until the stimulus reaches a set minimum strength, which may vary with different receptors. Once the minimum stimulus or threshold is reached, a maximum impulse is produced. A stimulation that is stronger than the minimum needed does not produce a larger impulse. Impulses travel from receptors, through dendrites or peripheral processes, to the neural cell bodies and on to an axon that terminates in several specialized knob-like branch endings. At this point, called a synapse, the impulse is transmitted, with the help of certain chemical agents, across a space separating the axon's end knobs from the dendrites of the next neuron or from a motor end plate attached to a muscle. This space is called a synaptic cleft, and the chemical agents released are called neurotransmitters. They are discharged into the synaptic cleft and alter the permeability of the postsynaptic membrane in which the cleft is located. This alteration may have an excitatory effect or, in some cases, an inhibitory effect, depending on the chemical reaction that occurs when the neurotransmitter crosses the synaptic cleft.

The Central Nervous System (CNS)

Consisting of the brain and spinal cord, the central nervous system receives impulses from throughout the body, processes the information, and responds with an appropriate action. This activity may be at the conscious or unconscious level, depending on the source of the sensory stimulus. Both the brain and spinal cord can be divided into gray and white matter. The gray matter consists of unsheathed cell bodies and true dendrites. The white matter is composed of myelinated nerve fibers. In the spinal cord, the arrangement of white and gray matter results in an H-shaped core of gray cell bodies surrounded by tracts of nerve fibers interconnected to the brain. The reverse is generally true of the brain where the surface layer or cortex is gray matter and most of the internal structures are white matter.

THE BRAIN

The nervous tissue of the brain consists of millions of nerve cells and fibers. It is the largest mass of nervous tissue in the body weighing about 1380 g in the male and 1250 g in the female. When fully developed, the brain fills the cranial cavity and is enclosed by three membranes known collectively as the meninges. From the outside in, these are the dura mater, arachnoid, and pia mater. The major substructures or divisions of the brain are the cerebrum, diencephalon, midbrain, cerebellum, pons, medulla oblongata, and the reticular formation (Fig. 12-2 and Table 12-1).

The Cerebrum

Representing seven eighths of the brain's total weight, the cerebrum contains never centers governing all sensory and motor activity. It is divided by the longitudinal fissure into two

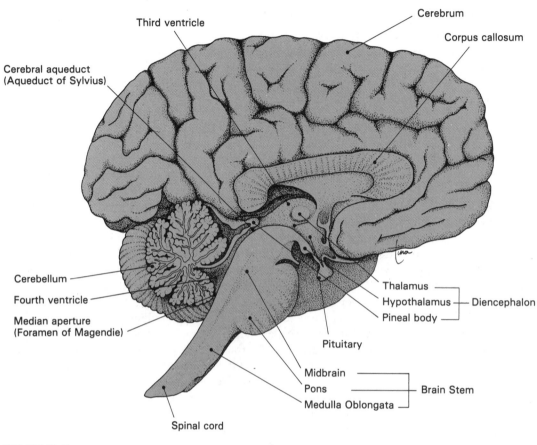

FIGURE 12–2

The major divisions of the brain. (*Adapted from Evans WF.* Anatomy and Physiology, *3rd ed. Englewood Cliffs, NJ: Prentice-Hall, 1983, with permission.*)

TABLE 12–1. MAJOR DIVISIONS/SUBDIVISIONS OF THE BRAIN AND FUNCTIONS

Division/ Subdivision	Function
Cerebrum	Governs all sensory and motor acitivity
Frontal lobe	Brain's major motor area
Parietal lobe	Also called the somesthetic area-sensory input for all parts of the body (temperature, pressure, touch, muscle control)
Temporal lobe	Auditory and language input
Occipital lobe	Primary sensory area for vision
Diencephalon (second portion of the brain)	
Thalamus	Relay center for all sensory impulses (except olfactory); emotional behavior (emotions, alert and/or arousal). Also relays motor impulses from cerebellum and the basal ganglia to motor areas of the cortex
Hypothalamus	Principal regulator of autonomic activity that is associated with behavior and emotional expression. Regulation of body temperature, water balance, sugar and fat metabolism, other metabolic activities, sleep-cycle control, appetite, and sexual arousal
Brain stem	
Midbrain	Two-way conduction pathway; relay for visual (seeing) and auditory (hearing) impulses
Pons	Two-way conduction pathway between regions of the body and areas of the brain; influences respiration
Medulla oblongata	Regulation and control of breathing, swallowing, coughing, sneezing, and vomiting, arterial blood pressure, control over the circulation of blood
Reticular formation	Exerts control over or influences wakefulness, sleep, and certain reflex activities of the spinal nerves
Cerebellum	Important part in the coordination of voluntary movement; muscle coordination; maintenance of posture and equilibrium

cerebral hemispheres, the right and left, that are joined by large fiber tracts (the corpus callosum) that allow information to pass from one hemisphere to the other. The surface or cortex of each hemisphere is arranged in folds creating bulges and shallow furrows. Each bulge is called a gyrus or convolution. A furrow is known as a sulcus. This surface is composed of gray, unmyelinated cell bodies and is known as the cerebral cortex. The cortex has been divided into lobes as a means of identifying certain locations. These lobes correspond to the overlying bones of the skull and are the frontal lobe, parietal lobe, temporal lobe, and occipital lobe. Another reference system for locating areas of the cerebral cortex is by way of fissures and sulci. As noted earlier, the cerebrum is divided by a deep longitudinal fissure. Each hemisphere, thus created, contains six major sulci. The two most often used as reference points are the lateral and central sulci. The lateral sulcus lies below the frontal and parietal lobes and forms the upper border of the temporal lobe. The central sulcus runs from the longitudinal fissure to the lateral sulcus and separates the frontal lobe from the parietal lobe. The occipital lobe is the lower rear part of the cerebrum beneath the parietal lobe and posterior to the temporal lobe (Fig. 12-3).

Electrical stimulation of the various areas of the cortex during neurosurgery has identified specialized cell activity within the different lobes. The frontal lobe has been identified as the brain's major motor area. The parietal lobe contains centers for sensory input from all parts of the body and is known as the somesthetic area. Temperature, pressure, touch, and an awareness of muscle control are some of the sensory activities centered in this area. The temporal lobe contains centers for auditory and language input, and the occipital lobe is considered to be the primary sensory area for vision. Throughout the cortex are areas known to integrate and store information. These memory or association areas comprise more than three fourths of the cerebral cortex. Below the cortex are masses of nerve fibers, the white matter, that interconnect areas within the brain and lead to the spinal cord. Four paired masses of gray matter, the dorsal ganglia, have been found embedded within the white fibers. The dorsal ganglia function in the control of motor activity and an injury or a disease in this area can result in a loss of motor control.

FIGURE 12–3

A drawing of the brain showing its lobes, principal sulci, and the locations of certain sensory and motor areas. (*Adapted from Evans WF. Anatomy and Physiology, 3rd ed. Englewood Cliffs, NJ: Prentice-Hall, 1983, with permission.*)

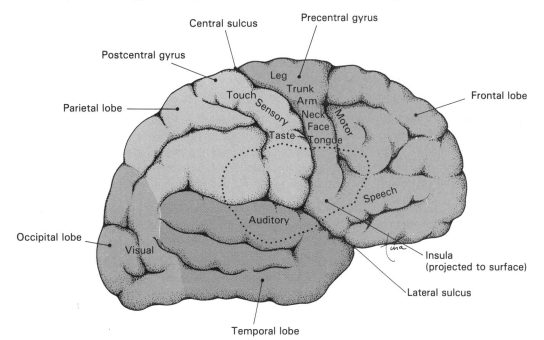

The Diencephalon

The word **diencephalon** means "second portion of the brain" and refers to the thalamus and hypothalamus.

The Thalamus. The thalamus is the largest of the two divisions of the diencephalon and is actually two large masses of gray cell bodies joined by a third or intermediate mass. The thalamus serves as a relay center for all sensory impulses (except olfactory) being transmitted to the sensory areas of the cortex. Besides its sensory function, the thalamus also relays motor impulses from the cerebellum and the basal ganglia to motor areas of the cortex. Some impulses related to emotional behavior are also passed from the hypothalamus, through the thalamus, to the cerebral cortex.

The Hypothalamus. The hypothalamus lies beneath the thalamus and is a principal regulator of autonomic nervous activity that is associated with behavior and emotional expression. It also produces neurosecretions for the control of water balance, sugar and fat metabolism, regulation of body temperature, and other metabolic activities. Additionally, the hypothalamus produces hormones for the posterior pituitary gland and exerts control over secretions from both the anterior and posterior pituitary. The pituitary gland is attached to the hypothalamus by a narrow stalk, the infundibulum.

The Midbrain

Located between the forebrain, which has just been described, and the hindbrain, the midbrain contains a number of large afferent and efferent pathways connecting major motor areas of the fore- and hindbrain. Also found in the midbrain are four small masses of gray cells known collectively as the corpora quadrigemina. The upper two, called the superior colliculi, are associated with visual reflexes such as the tracking movements of the eyes. The lower two, or inferior colliculi, are involved with the sense of hearing.

The Hindbrain

The hindbrain consists of the cerebellum, the pons, the medulla oblongata, and the recticular formation.

The Cerebellum. The largest part of the hindbrain is the cerebellum. It occupies a space in the back of the skull, inferior to the cerebrum and dorsal to the pons and medulla oblongata. The cerebellum is oval in shape and divided into lobes by deep fissures. The surface of the cerebellum has a cortex of gray cell bodies, and its interior contains nerve fibers, white matter, connecting it to every part of the central nervous system. The cerebellum plays an important part in the coordination of voluntary movement.

The Pons. The pons is a broad band of white matter located anterior to the cerebellum and between the midbrain and the medulla oblongata. The pons contains fiber tracts linking the cerebellum and medulla to higher cortical areas.

The Medulla Oblongata. That part of the brain stem that connects the pons and the rest of the brain to the spinal cord is called the medulla oblongata. All the afferent and efferent tracts from the spinal cord either pass through or terminate in the medulla oblongata. The medulla also contains nerve centers instrumental to the regulation and control of breathing, swallowing, coughing, sneezing, and vomiting. Other centers in the medulla regulate arterial blood pressure, thereby exerting control over the circulation of blood.

The Reticular Formation. The reticular formation is a diffuse network, consisting of small groups of cell bodies and their processes, located in the area of the brain stem. The reticular formation exerts control over or influences wakefulness, sleep, and certain reflex activities of the spinal nerves.

THE SPINAL CORD

As previously mentioned, the spinal cord has an H-shaped gray area of cell bodies encircled by an outer region of white matter. The white matter consists of nerve tracts and fibers providing sensory input to the brain and conducting motor impulses from the brain to spinal neurons. Other fibers connect nerve cells within the spinal cord with other areas of the cord. The spinal cord is about 44 cm long and extends down the vertebral canal from the medulla to terminate near the junction of the first and second lumbar vertebrae. The functions of the spinal cord are to conduct sensory impulses to the brain, to conduct motor impulses from the brain, and to serve as a reflex center for impulses entering and leaving the spinal cord without involvement of the brain (Fig. 12–4 and Plate 7).

THE CEREBROSPINAL FLUID

The brain and spinal cord are surrounded by cerebrospinal fluid. This colorless fluid is produced by the choroid plexuses within the ventricles of the brain. There are four cavities or ventricles within the brain that are interconnected and are continuous with a small central canal that extends through the length of the spinal cord. Cerebrospinal fluid circulates through the ventricles, the central canal, and the subarachnoid space. This is a thin space between the arachnoid membrane and the pia mater, which is the membrane covering the surface of the brain and spinal cord. Cerebrospinal fluid is removed from circulation by the arachnoid villi, which are small projections of the arachnoid membrane that penetrate the tough outer membrane, the dura mater. The arachnoid villi allow the fluid to drain into the superior sagittal sinus. The normal adult will have between 120 and 150 mL of cerebrospinal fluid in circulation. The fluid serves to cushion the brain and cord from shocks that might cause injury. It also helps to support the brain by allowing it to float within the supporting liquid. It also contains neurotransmitters such as monoamines, acetylcholine, and neuropeptides.

The Peripheral Nervous System (PNS)

The network of nerves branching throughout the body from the brain and spinal cord is known as the peripheral nervous system. There are 12 pairs of cranial nerves that attach to the brain and 31 pairs of spinal nerves connected to the spinal cord.

THE CRANIAL NERVES

The nerves described below attach to the brain and provide sensory input, motor control, or a combination of these functions. They are arranged symmetrically, 12 to each side of the brain, and generally are named for the area or function they serve (Fig. 12–5 and Table 12–2).

The Olfactory Nerve (I)
The olfactory nerve provides sensory input only and carries impulses for smell to the brain. The cell bodies of these nerve fibers are located in the nasal mucous membrane and serve as receptors for the sense of smell.

The Optic Nerve (II)
The optic nerve provides sensory input only and carries impulses for vision to the brain. The rods and cones of the eyes are receptors and transmit images through the cells of the retina to processes that form the optic nerve. The optic nerves from each eye unite after entering the cranial cavity to form the optic chiasm from which tracts, carrying images from both eyes, connect to the brain.

The Oculomotor Nerve (III)
The oculomotor nerve conducts motor impulses to four of the six external muscles of the eye and to the muscle that raises the eyelid. The cell bodies of motor nerves are located in the brain.

The Trochlear Nerve (IV)
The trochlear nerve conducts motor impulses to control the superior oblique muscle of the eyeball.

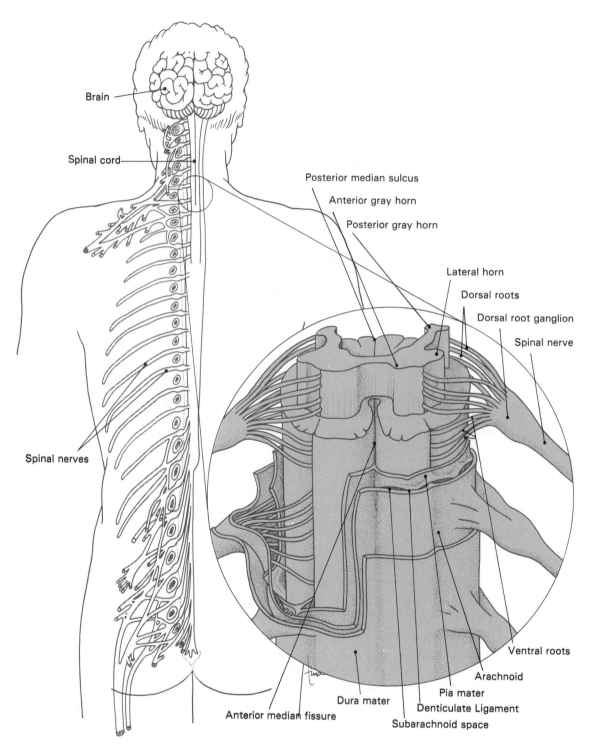

FIGURE 12–4

The brain, spinal cord, and spinal nerves with an exploded view of a spinal nerve. (*Adapted from Evans WF. Anatomy and Physiology, 3rd ed. Englewood Cliffs, NJ: Prentice-Hall, 1983, with permission.*)

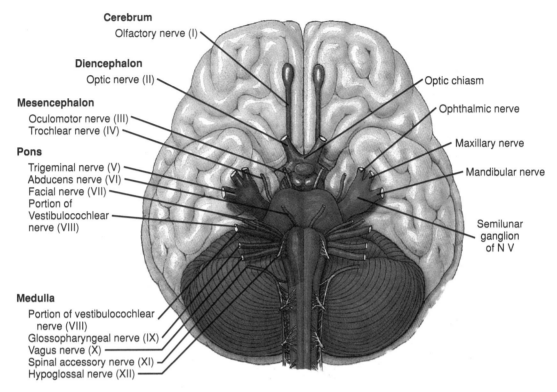

Cerebrum
Olfactory nerve (I)

Diencephalon
Optic nerve (II)

Mesencephalon
Oculomotor nerve (III)
Trochlear nerve (IV)

Pons
Trigeminal nerve (V)
Abducens nerve (VI)
Facial nerve (VII)
Portion of
Vestibulocochlear
nerve (VIII)

Medulla
Portion of vestibulocochlear
nerve (VIII)
Glossopharyngeal nerve (IX)
Vagus nerve (X)
Spinal accessory nerve (XI)
Hypoglossal nerve (XII)

Optic chiasm
Ophthalmic nerve
Maxillary nerve
Mandibular nerve
Semilunar
ganglion
of N V

FIGURE 12–5

Origins of the cranial nerves. On the left half of this inferior view of the brain, note the relationships between the cranial nerves and specific regions of the brain. On the right, the brain surface is shown as it appears on gross dissection. (*From Martini F. Fundamentals of Anatomy and Physiology, 2nd ed. Englewood Cliffs, NJ: Prentice-Hall, 1992, with permission.*)

The Trigeminal Nerve (V)

The trigeminal nerve has both sensory and motor fibers. Its fibers form three sensory divisions, the ophthalmic, maxillary, and mandibular. These fibers provide sensory input from the face, nose, mouth, forehead, and top of the head. The mandibular division also contains motor fibers to the muscles of the jaw.

TABLE 12–2. CRANIAL NERVES AND FUNCTIONS

Nerve/Number	Function
Olfactory (I)	Sense of smell
Optic (II)	Vision
Oculomotor (III)	Motor impulses to four of the six external muscles of the eye and to the muscle that raises the eyelid
Trochlear (IV)	Motor impulses to control the superior oblique muscle of the eyeball
Trigeminal (V)	Provide sensory input from the face, nose, mouth, forehead, and top of the head; motor fibers to the muscles of the jaw (chewing)
Abducens (VI)	Conducts motor impulses to the lateral rectus muscle of the eyeball
Facial (VII)	Controls the muscles of the face and scalp; control the lacrimal glands of the eye and the submandibular and sublingual salivary glands; input from the tongue for the sense of taste
Acoustic (VIII)	Input for hearing and equilibrium
Glossopharyngeal (IX)	General sense of taste; swallowing; control secretion of saliva
Vagus (X)	Controls muscles of the pharynx and larynx and of the thoracic and abdominal organs; swallowing, voice production, slowing of heartbeat, acceleration of peristalsis
Accessory (XI)	Control of the trapezius and sternocleidomastoid muscles, permitting movement of the head and shoulders
Hypoglossal (XII)	Control of the tongue; tongue movements

The Abducens Nerve (VI)

The abducens nerve conducts motor impulses to the lateral rectus muscle of the eyeball.

The Facial Nerve (VII)

The facial nerve has both sensory and motor fibers. Its motor fibers control the muscles of the face and scalp, thereby providing for facial expression. It also provides efferent fibers to control the lacrimal glands of the eyes as well as the submandibular and sublingual salivary glands. Sensory fibers of the facial nerve provide input from the forward two thirds of the tongue for the sense of taste.

The Acoustic Nerve (VIII)

Sometimes called the vestibulocochlear nerve, the acoustic nerve provides sensory input for hearing and equilibrium. Fibers of the cochlea division connect with receptors in the cochlea of the ear for hearing. Fibers of the vestibular division connect to receptors in the semicircular canals and vestibule located in the ear for the sense of equilibrium.

The Glossopharyngeal Nerve (IX)

The glossopharyngeal nerve has both sensory and motor fibers. The sensory fibers provide for the general sense of taste and attach to the back of the tongue and pharynx. Motor fibers innervate the stylopharyngeus muscle and are important to the act of the swallowing. Other efferent fibers control the secretion of saliva from the parotid gland.

The Vagus Nerve (X)

The vagus nerve contains both sensory and motor fibers and is the longest of the cranial nerves. The motor fibers control muscles of the pharynx and larynx. The sensory fibers provide input from the autonomic control of most of the organs in the thoracic and abdominal cavities.

The Accessory Nerve (XI)

The accessory nerve conducts motor impulses for the control of the trapezius and sternocleidomastoid muscles, permitting movement of the head and shoulders.

The Hypoglossal Nerve (XII)

The hypoglossal nerve conducts motor impulses for control of the muscles of the tongue.

THE SPINAL NERVES

There are 31 pairs of spinal nerves distributed along the length of the spinal cord and emerging from the vertebral canal on either side through the intervertebral foramina. At the point of attachment, each nerve is divided into two roots (see Fig. 12-4 and Plate 7). The dorsal or sensory root is composed of afferent fibers carrying impulses to the cord, and the ventral root contains motor fibers carrying efferent impulses to muscles and organs. The cell bodies of the motor fibers lie in the gray matter of the spinal cord. The cell bodies for the sensory fibers are clustered just outside the spinal cord in small enlargements on each dorsal root. These enlargements are called the spinal ganglia. Named for the region of the vertebral column from which they exit, there are 8 pairs of cervical spinal nerves, 12 pairs of thoracic spinal nerves, 5 pairs of lumbar spinal nerves, 5 pairs of sacral spinal nerves, and 1 pair of coccygeal spinal nerves. A short distance from the cord, the fibers of the two roots unite to form a spinal nerve. Having formed a single nerve composed of afferent and efferent fibers, each spinal nerve then branches into several smaller nerves. The two primary branches from each spinal nerve are the dorsal and ventral rami. The dorsal rami (branches) carry motor and sensory fibers to the muscles and skin of the back and serve an area from the back of the head to the coccyx. The ventral rami, serving a much larger area, carry both motor and sensory fibers to the muscles and organs of the body, including the arms, legs, feet, and hands. The following describes the origin and purpose of the ventral branches of the 31 pairs of spinal nerves.

The ventral fibers from the first four cervical nerves form a network of interlaced nerve fibers called a plexus, which gives rise to peripheral nerves. Located in the neck, the cervical plexus innervates the muscles and skin of the neck and back of the head. The phrenic nerve, serving the diaphragm, also arises from the cervical plexus. Ventral fibers of cervical nerves 4 through 8 and the first thoracic nerve interlace to form the brachial plexus. Located in the area of the shoulder, the peripheral nerves from the brachial plexus innervate the shoulder, arm, forearm, wrist, and hand. The ventral rami of thoracic nerves 1 through 12 form the intercostal (between the ribs) nerves and the subcostal (below the ribs) nerves. Fibers of these nerves serve the muscles and skin of the thorax and upper abdomen. Ventral fibers of the first three and most of the fourth lumbar nerves interlace to form the lumbar plexus. Peripheral nerves from the lumbar plexus serve the muscles of the thigh and leg and the skin of the hip, scrotum, thigh, and leg. The ventral rami of the fourth and fifth lumbar together with those of the five sacral nerves interlace to form the sacral plexus. Peripheral nerves from the sacral plexus innervate the skin and muscles of the leg, foot, and external genitalia. Part of the fifth sacral and the entire coccygeal nerve are of limited importance and innervate the coccygeus muscle and the skin over the coccyx.

The Autonomic Nervous System (ANS)

Actually a part of the peripheral nervous system, the autonomic nervous system controls involuntary bodily functions such as sweating, secretions of glands, arterial blood pressure, smooth muscle tissue, and the heart. The autonomic nervous system is primarily composed of efferent fibers from certain cranial and spinal nerves and can be functionally divided into two divisions, the sympathetic and parasympathetic. These two divisions counteract each other's activity to keep the body in a state of homeostasis.

THE SYMPATHETIC DIVISION

Branches from the ventral roots of the 12 thoracic and the first 3 lumbar spinal nerves form the first part of the sympathetic division. The cell bodies of these nerve fibers are located in the gray matter of the spinal cord. Just outside the spinal cord, axons of these nerve cells leave the spinal nerves and enter almost immediately into masses of nerve cell bodies, the sympathetic ganglia, which form a chain that runs next to the vertebral column. This chain of about 23 ganglia runs from the base of the head to the coccyx and is known as the sympathetic trunk. Within the ganglia of the sympathetic trunk, fibers from the spinal nerves synapse with ganglionic nerve cell bodies. These ganglionic neurons produce long axons that reach to the parts of the body to be innervated. This arrangement, characteristic of autonomic nerves, creates a two-neuron chain as opposed to single-neuron control of regular motor nerves (Fig. 12-6).

Because of the arrangement whereby sympathetic fibers from spinal nerves synapse with many cell bodies in the sympathetic ganglia, they tend to produce widespread innervation when activated. This condition has been described as preparing the individual for "fight or flight." On the other hand, fibers from the parasympathetic division have only the two-neuron chain and do not interact with as many cell bodies; therefore, their transmissions result in localized responses.

THE PARASYMPATHETIC DIVISION

Very long fibers branching from cranial nerves 3, 7, 9, and 10 along with long fibers of sacral nerves 2, 3, and 4 form the first stage of the parasympathetic division. Cell bodies for these long fibers are located in the brain and spinal cord. These long fibers extend to ganglia located close by the organs to be innervated. Fibers of cranial and sacral nerves synapse with ganglionic cell bodies, which then conduct impulses over short axons to the gland, smooth muscle tissue, or organ to be innervated. Fibers from the cranial nerves serve the iris and ciliary muscles of the eye, lacrimal glands, and salivary glands through four ganglia located in the head. Cranial nerve fibers extend via the vagus nerve to ganglia serving the thoracic, abdominal, and pelvic viscera. The fibers of the sacral spinal nerves form the pel-

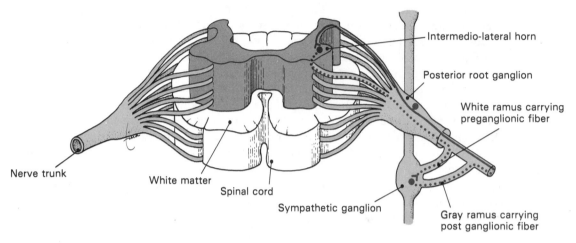

FIGURE 12–6

Origin of the sympathetic neurons of the autonomic nervous system. (*Adapted from Evans WF.* Anatomy and Physiology, *3rd ed. Englewood Cliffs, NJ: Prentice-Hall, 1983, with permission.*)

vic nerve, which branches to synapse with small ganglia near or within the organs to be innervated. The cell bodies of these ganglia serve the lower colon, rectum, bladder, and reproductive organs. The hypothalamus is instrumental in the control of parasympathetic and sympathetic activity and is discussed elsewhere in this chapter and in the chapter on The Endocrine System.

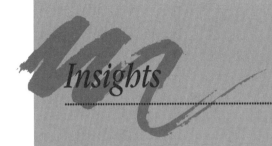

STRESS AND ANXIETY

There seems to be a lump in your throat. Your stomach feels as though it is tied in knots and your heart is beating rapidly. Your fingers are cold as ice, but your palms are sweaty. You know these signs of stress and anxiety, because you have had them before. Stress may be defined as the physical and/or psychological forces that are experienced by an individual. According to the Occupational Health and Safety News, US Chamber of Commerce, US Department of Human Services, and the National Institute of Drug Abuse an estimated 14% of all occupational disease claims were stress related with a cost of approximately 34 billion dollars.

Symptoms of Anxiety

Physical:

fast heart rate	nausea
palpitations	dyspepsia
shortness of breath	diarrhea
hot flashes	cold, sweaty, tremulous hands
chills	smothering sensation
dry mouth	frequent urination
dizziness	lump in throat
lightheadedness	band-like pressure about the head

Tension:

restlessness	trembling, twitching, or feeling shaky
fatigue	

Emotional:

irritability	extreme feeling of worry
keyed-up feeling	inability to concentrate
problems with sleeping	

Stress is implicated in immune system dysfunction, cancer, hypertension, heart disease, and ulcers. An agent or condition that is capable of causing stress is called a stressor. There are many conditions that can be stressors and these will vary with each individual. Finances, health problems, birth, death of a loved one, school, peer pressure, relationships, crime, and things beyond one's control are only a few conditions that may be stressors. It is believed that a certain amount of stress helps the body maintain homeostasis, a state of balance. When stress becomes more powerful than an individual can handle, certain physical symptoms appear.

The body responds to stressful situations the same way as it responds to physical danger. It automatically prepares one for combat or retreat. This is known as the "fight-or-flight" response

(Insights continues on next page)

that is produced when the hypothalamus flashes signals through the nervous and endocrine systems. The anterior pituitary gland secretes the hormone adrenocorticotropic (ACTH) into the bloodstream, thereby stimulating the adrenal glands. During this alarm reaction, the adrenal medulla releases epinephrine (adrenaline; Adrenalin) and norepinephrine directly into the bloodstream.

Epinephrine elevates the systolic blood pressure; increases the heart rate and cardiac output; increases glycogenolysis, thereby hastening the release of glucose from the liver. It is through this action that the blood sugar level is elevated and the body is supplied with a "spurt-of-energy"; it also dilates the bronchial tubes and the pupils. Norepinephrine acts as a vasoconstrictor and elevates the systolic blood pressure.

As stress continues perspiration increases and the palms become moist. Blood flow is slowed to the extremities and the fingers and toes feel "cold." The digestive process is slowed down and under prolonged stress hydrochloric acid within the stomach begins to eat away at the stomach lining. Muscles tense up and breathing may become rapid and then shallow.

Anxiety may be defined as a feeling of uneasiness, apprehension, worry, or dread. It is an involuntary or reflex reaction of the body to stress. When its negative effects cause a change in one's behavior or performance and it continues for a long period of time, then persistent underlying anxiety may be diagnosed.

It is important to recognize the symptoms of stress and anxiety, and then to find out what is causing the symptoms. Once this is done, the stressor or stressors may be eliminated or the individual must learn to cope with the situation. Developing coping skills is a technique that one can learn. Find out what works for you, such as taking a warm bath/shower, talking to a friend, taking a walk, reading a book.

You have heard the saying "laughter is the best medicine" and to relieve stress and anxiety, it certainly can work wonders. Try it. Just laugh out loud and see how you feel.

One afternoon my husband and I were walking downtown and we passed a "Pins and Needles" Alteration Shop. He said to me, "a her shouldn't have any trouble finding a 'hem' in that shop."

To me, taking a patient's body temperature using the tympanic thermometer is funny. "I would like to take your temperature, so I am going to place this instrument in your ear." "You're going to take my temperature where?"

Terminology with Surgical Procedures & Pathology

Term	Word Parts			Definition
acrophobia (ăk″ rō-fō′ bĭ-ă)	acro phobia	CF S	extremity fear	An abnormal fear of high places
akinesia (ă″ kĭ-nē′ zĭ-ă)	a kinesia	P S	lack of motion	A loss or lack of the power of voluntary motion
amentia (ă-měn′ shē-ah)	a ment ia	P R S	lack of mind condition	A congenital condition of mental retardation; also called dementia
amnesia (ăm-nē′ zĭ-ă)	a mnes ia	P R S	lack of memory condition	A condition in which there is a loss or lack of memory
analgesia (ăn″ ăl-jē′ zĭ-ă)	an algesia	P S	lack of pain	A lack of the sense of pain
anencephaly (ăn″ ĕn-sĕf′ ăl-ē)	an encephal y	P R S	lack of brain condition	A congenital condition in which there is a lack of development of the brain
anesthesia (ăn″ ĕs-thē′ zĭ-ă)	an esthesia	P S	lack of feeling	A loss or lack of the sense of feeling
anesthesiologist (ăn″ ĕs-thē″ zĭ-ŏl′ ō-jĭst)	an esthesio log ist	P CF R S	lack of feeling study of one who specializes	A physician who specializes in the science of anesthesia
aphagia (ă-fā′ jĭ-ă)	a phagia	P S	lack of to eat	A loss or lack of the ability to eat or swallow
aphasia (ă-fā′ zĭ-ă)	a phasia	P S	lack of to speak	A loss or lack of the ability to speak
apraxia (ă-prăks′ ĭ-ă)	a praxia	P S	lack of action	A loss or lack of the ability to use objects properly
arachnitis (ă″ răk-nī′ tĭs)	arachn itis	R S	spider inflammation	Inflammation of the arachnoid membrane
asthenia (ăs-thē′ nĭ-ă)	a sthenia	P S	lack of strength	A loss or lack of strength
astrocyte (ăs′ trō-sīt)	astro cyte	P S	star-shaped cell	A star-shaped neuroglial cell with many branching processes

(Terminology—continued)

Term	Word Parts			Definition
astrocytoma (ăs″ trō-sī-tō′ mă)	astro cyt oma	P R S	star-shaped cell tumor	A tumor composed of astrocytes
ataxia (ă-tăks′ ĭ-ă)	a taxia	P S	lack of order	A loss or lack of muscular coordination
atelencephalia (ăt-ĕl″ ĕn-sĭ-fā′ lĭ-ă)	atel encephal ia	R R S	imperfect brain condition	A congenital condition of imperfect development of the brain
atelomyelia (ăt″ ĕ-lō-mī-ē′ lĭ-ă)	atelo myel ia	CF R S	imperfect spinal cord condition	A condition of imperfect development of the spinal cord
bradykinesia (brăd″ ĭ-kĭ-nē′ sĭ-ă)	brady kinesia	P S	slow motion	An abnormal slowness of motion
bradylalia (brăd″ ĭ-lā′ lĭ-ă)	brady lalia	P S	slow to talk	An abnormal slowness of speech
cephalalgia (sĕf″ ă-lăl′ jĭ-ă)	cephal algia	R S	head pain	Head pain; headache
cephalohemo-meter (sĕf″ ă-lō-hē-mōm′ ĕ-tĕr)	cephalo hemo meter	CF CF S	head blood instrument to measure	An instrument used to measure the intracranial blood pressure
cerebellar (sĕr″ ĕ-bĕl′ ăr)	cerebell ar	R S	little brain pertaining to	Pertaining to the cerebellum
cerebellospinal (sĕr″ ĕ-bĕl″ ō-spī′ năl)	cerebello spin al	CF R S	little brain a thorn, spine pertaining to	Pertaining to the cerebellum and spinal cord
cerebromalacia (sĕr″ ĕ-brō″ mă-lā′ shĭ-ă)	cerebro malacia	CF S	cerebrum softening	A softening of the cerebrum
cerebrospinal (sĕr″ ĕ-brō-spī′ năl)	cerebro spin al	CF R S	cerebrum a thorn, spine pertaining to	Pertaining to the cerebrum and the spinal cord
cordotomy (kŏr-dŏt′ ō-mē)	cordo tomy	CF S	cord incision	Surgical incision into the spinal cord, the anterolateral tracts, for relief of pain
craniectomy (krā″ nĭ-ĕk′ tō-mē)	crani ectomy	R S	skull excision	Surgical excision of a portion of the skull

(Terminology—continued)

Term	Word Parts			Definition
craniocele (krā′ nĭ-ō-sēl)	cranio cele	CF S	skull hernia	Herniation of the brain substances through the skull
cranioplasty (krā′ nĭ-ō-plăs″ tē)	cranio plasty	CF S	skull surgical repair	Surgical repair of the skull
craniotomy (krā″ nĭ-ŏt′ ō-mē)	cranio tomy	CF S	skull incision	Surgical incision of the skull
diplegia (dĭ-plē′ jĭ-ă)	di(s) plegia	P S	two stroke, paralysis	Paralysis of identical parts on both sides of the body
diskectomy (dĭs-kĕk′ tō-mē)	disk ectomy	R S	a disk excision	Surgical excision of an intervertebral disk
dyslexia (dĭs-lĕks′ ĭ-ă)	dys lexia	P S	difficult diction	A condition in which an individual has difficulty in comprehending the written language
dysphasia (dĭs-fā′ zĭ-ă)	dys phasia	P S	difficult speak	Impairment of speech caused by a brain lesion
dysthymia (dĭs-thī′ mē-ă)	dys thym ia	P R S	difficult mind, emotion condition	A condition of mental disorder or disease
egocentric (ē″ gō-sĕn′ trĭk)	ego centr ic	CF R S	I, self center pertaining to	Pertaining to being self-centered
electroencephalo-graph (ē-lĕk″ trō-ĕn-sĕf′ ă-lō-grăf)	electro encephalo graph	CF CF S	electricity brain to write	An instrument used to record the electrical activity of the brain
electromyo-graphy (ē-lĕk″ trō-mī-ŏg′ ră-fē)	electro myo graphy	CF CF S	electricity muscle recording	The recording of the contraction of a skeletal muscle as a result of electrical stimulation; used in diagnosing disorders of nerves supplying muscles
encephalitis (ĕn-sĕf″ ă-lī′ tĭs)	encephal itis	R S	brain inflammation	Inflammation of the brain
encephalocele (ĕn-sĕf′ ă-lō-sēl)	encephalo cele	CF S	brain hernia	Herniation of the brain via a congenital or traumatic opening of the skull

(Terminology—continued)

Term	Word Parts			Definition
encephalomalacia (ĕn-sĕf″ ă-lō-mă-lā′ sĭ-ă)	encephalo malacia	CF S	brain softening	A softening of the brain
encephalopathy (ĕn-sĕf′ ă-lŏp′ ă-thē)	encephalo pathy	CF S	brain disease	Pertaining to any disease of the brain
epidural (ĕp″ ĭ-dū′ răl)	epi dur al	P R S	upon dura, hard pertaining to	Pertaining to situated upon the dura mater
foraminotomy (fō-răm″ ĭ-nŏt′ ō-mē)	foramino tomy	CF S	foramen incision	Surgical incision into the intervertebral foramen
ganglionectomy (gang″ lĭ-ō-nĕk′ tō-mē)	ganglion ectomy	R S	knot excision	Surgical excision of a ganglion (a mass of nerve tissue outside the brain and spinal cord)
glioma (glī-ō′ mă)	gli oma	R S	glue tumor	A tumor composed of neuroglial tissue
hemianopsia (hĕm″ ĭ-ă-nŏp′ sĭ-ă)	hemi an opsia	P P S	half lack of eye, vision	A condition of blindness of half the field of vision in one or both eyes
hemiparesis (hĕm″ ĭ-păr′ ĕ-sĭs)	hemi paresis	P S	half weakness	Slight paralysis that affects one side of the body
hemiplegia (hĕm″ ĭ-plē′ jĭ-ă)	hemi plegia	P S	half stroke, paralysis	Paralysis that affects one half of the body
hydrocephalus (hī″ drō-sĕf′ ă-lŭs)	hydro cephal us	P R S	water head pertaining to	Pertaining to an increased amount of cerebrospinal fluid within the brain
hyperesthesia (hī″ pĕr-ĕs-thē′ zĭ-ă)	hyper esthesia	P S	excessive feeling	Excessive feelings of sensory stimuli, such as pain, touch, or sound
hyperkinesis (hī″ pĕr-kĭn-ē′ sĭs)	hyper kinesis	P S	excessive motion	Excessive muscular movement and motion; inability to be still; also known as hyperactivity
hypermnesia (hī″ pĕrm-nē′ zĭ-ă)	hyper mnesia	P S	excessive memory	A state of excellent memory for names, dates, and details; may occur with psychosis, during neurosurgical procedures, or with brain injuries

(Terminology—continued)

Term	Word Parts			Definition
hypnology (hĭp-nŏl′ ō-jē)	hypno logy	CF S	sleep study of	The scientific study of sleep
hypnosis (hĭp-nō′ sĭs)	hypn osis	R S	sleep condition of	An artificially induced condition of sleep
infratentorial (ĭn″ frăh-tĕn-tō′ rĕ-ăl)	infra tentori al	P CF S	below tentorium, tent pertaining to	Pertaining to below the tentorium of the cerebellum
intracranial (ĭn″ trăh-krā′ nĕ-ăl)	intra crani al	P R S	within skull pertaining to	Pertaining to within the skull
laminectomy (lăm″ ĭ-nĕk′ tō-mē)	lamin ectomy	R S	thin plate excision	Surgical excision of a vertebral posterior arch
lobotomy (lō-bŏt′ ō-mē)	lobo tomy	CF S	lobe incision	Surgical incision into the prefrontal or frontal lobe of the brain
logomania (lŏg″ ō-mā′ nĭ-ă)	logo mania	CF S	word madness	An excessive, repetitious, continuous flow of speech seen in monomania, a form of mental illness
macrocephalia (măk″ rō-sĕ-fā′ lĭ-ă)	macro cephal ia	CF R S	large head condition	An abnormal condition in which the head is large
meningioma (mĕn-ĭn″ jĭ-ō′ mă)	meningi oma	CF S	membrane tumor	A tumor of the meninges that originates in the arachnoidal tissue
meningitis (mĕn″ ĭn-jī′ tĭs)	mening itis	R S	membrane inflammation	Inflammation of the meninges of the spinal cord or brain
meningocele (mĕn-ĭn-gō-sēl)	meningo cele	CF S	membrane hernia	Congenital herniation of the skull or spinal column in which the meninges protrude through an opening
meningoence-phalitis (mĕn-ĭn″ gō-ĕn-sĕf″ ă-lī ′ tĭs)	meningo encephal itis	CF R S	membrane brain inflammation	Inflammation of the brain and its meninges
meningomyelo-cele (mĕn-ĭn″ gō-mī-ĕl′ ō-sēl)	meningo myelo cele	CF CF S	membrane spinal cord hernia	Congenital herniation of the spinal cord and meninges through a defect in the vertebral column

(Terminology—continued)

Term	Word Parts			Definition
meningopathy (měn″ ĭn-gŏp′ă-thē)	meningo pathy	CF S	membrane disease	Any disease of the meninges
microcephalus (mī″ krō-sĕf′ ă-lŭs)	micro cephal us	P R S	small head pertaining to	Pertaining to an individual with a very small head
myelitis (mī″ ĕ-lī′ tĭs)	myel itis	R S	spinal cord inflammation	Inflammation of the spinal cord
myelodysplasia (mī″ ĕl-ō-dĭs-plā′ zĭ-ă)	myelo dys plasia	CF P S	spinal cord difficult formation	Difficult or defective formation of the spinal cord
myelography (mī″ ĕ-lŏg′ ră-fē)	myelo graphy	CF S	spinal cord recording	An x-ray recording of the spinal cord after injection of a radiopaque medium into the spinal canal
myelophthisis (mī″ ĕ-lŏf′ thĭ-sĭs)	myelo phthisis	CF S	spinal cord a wasting	Atrophy or a wasting away of the spinal cord
myelotome (mī-ĕl′ ō-tōm)	myelo tome	CF S	spinal cord instrument to cut	An instrument used to cut or dissect the spinal cord
neuralgia (nū-răl′ jĭ-ă)	neur algia	R S	nerve pain	Pain in a nerve or nerves
neurasthenia (nū″ răs-thē′ nĭ-ă)	neur asthenia	R S	nerve weakness	Nervous weakness, exhaustion, prostration common after depressed states
neurectomy (nū-rĕk′ tō-mē)	neur ectomy	R S	nerve excision	Surgical excision of a nerve
neurilemma (nū′ rĭ-lĕm″ mă)	neuri lemma	CF S	nerve a sheath, husk, rind	A thin membranous sheath that envelops a nerve fiber; also called sheath of Schwann or neurolemma
neuritis (nū-rī′ tĭs)	neur itis	R S	nerve inflammation	Inflammation of a nerve
neuroblast (nū′ rō-blăst)	neuro blast	CF S	nerve germ cell	The germ cell from which nervous tissue is formed
neuroblastoma (nū″ rō-blăs-tō′ mă)	neuro blast oma	CF S S	nerve germ cell tumor	A malignant tumor composed chiefly of neuroblast; occurs mostly in infants and children

(Terminology—continued)

Term	Word Parts			Definition
neurocyte (nū′ rō-sīt)	neuro	CF	nerve	A nerve cell, a neuron
	cyte	S	cell	
neuroglia (nū-rŏg′ lĭ-ă)	neuro	CF	nerve	The supporting elements of the nervous system (astrocytes, oligodendrocytes, and macroglia)
	glia	S	glue	
neurologist (nū-rŏl′ ō-jĭst)	neuro	CF	nerve	One who specializes in the study of the nervous system
	log	R	study of	
	ist	S	one who specializes	
neurology (nū-rŏl′ ō-jē)	neuro	CF	nerve	The study of the nervous system
	logy	S	study of	
neurolysis (nū-rŏl′ ĭs-ĭs)	neuro	CF	nerve	Destruction of nerve tissue
	lysis	S	destruction	
neuroma (nū-rō′ mă)	neur	R	nerve	A tumor of nerve cells and nerve fibers
	oma	S	tumor	
neuromyelitis (nū″ rō-mĭ″ ĕl-ī′ tĭs)	neuro	CF	nerve	Inflammation of the nerves and spinal cord
	myel	R	spinal cord	
	itis	S	inflammation	
neuropathy (nū-rŏp′ ă-thē)	neuro	CF	nerve	Any nerve disease
	pathy	S	disease	
neuroplasty (nū′ rō-plăs″ tē)	neuro	CF	nerve	Surgical repair of a nerve or nerves
	plasty	S	surgical repair	
neurorrhaphy (nū-rōr′ ă-fē)	neuro	CF	nerve	Suture of the ends of a severed nerve
	rrhaphy	S	suture	
neurosclerosis (nū″ rō-sklĕ-rō′ sĭs)	neuro	CF	nerve	A condition of hardening of nerve tissue
	scler	R	hardening	
	osis	S	condition of	
neurosis (nū-rō′ sĭs)	neur	R	nerve	An emotional condition or disorder
	osis	S	condition of	
neurotomy (nū-rŏt′ ō-mē)	neuro	CF	nerve	Surgical incision or dissection of a nerve
	tomy	S	incision	
neurotripsy (nū′ rō-trĭp″ sē)	neuro	CF	nerve	Surgical crushing of a nerve
	tripsy	S	crushing	
oligodendroglioma (ŏl″ ĭ-gō-dĕn″ drō-glī-ō′ mă)	oligo	P	little	A malignant tumor derived and composed of oligodendroglia
	dendro	CF	tree	
	gli	R	glue	
	oma	S	tumor	

(Terminology—continued)

Term	Word Parts			Definition
papilledema (păp″ ĭl-ĕ-dē′ mă)	papill edema	R S	papilla swelling	Swelling of the optical disk, usually caused by increased intracranial pressure; also called choked disk
paranoia (păr″ ă-noy′ ă)	para noia	P S	beside mind	A mental disorder
paraplegia (păr″ ă-plē′ jĭ-ă)	para plegia	P S	beside stroke, paralysis	Paralysis of both legs and, in some cases, the lower portion of the body
paresthesia (păr″ ĕs-thē′ zĭ-ă)	par esthesia	P S	beside feeling	An abnormal sensation, feeling of numbness, prickling or tingling
phagomania (făg″ ō-mā′ nĭ-ă)	phago mania	CF S	to eat madness	A madness for food
pheochromocy-toma (fē-ō-krō″ mō-sī-tō′ mă)	pheo chromo cyt oma	CF CF R S	dusky color cell tumor	A chromaffin cell tumor of the adrenal medulla or of the sympathetic nervous system
pneumoenceph-alography (nū″ mō-ĕn-sĕf″ ă-lŏg′ ră-fē)	pneumo encephalo graphy	CF CF S	air brain recording	X-ray examination of the ventricles and subarachnoid spaces of the brain after injection of air via a lumbar puncture
poliomyelitis (pōl″ ĭ-ō-mī″ ĕl-ī′ tĭs)	polio myel itis	CF R S	gray spinal cord inflammation	Inflammation of the gray matter of the spinal cord
polyneuritis (pŏl″ ē nū-rī′ tĭs)	poly neur itis	P R S	many nerve inflammation	Inflammation of many nerves
psychologist (sī-kŏl′ ō-jĭst)	psycho log ist	CF R S	mind study of one who specializes	One who specializes in the study of the mind
psychology (sī-kŏl′ ō-jē)	psycho logy	CF S	mind study of	The study of the mind
psychosis (sī-kō′ sĭs)	psych osis	R S	mind condition of	An abnormal condition of the mind
psychosomatic (sī″ kō-sō-măt′ ĭk)	psycho somat ic	CF R S	mind body pertaining to	Pertaining to the interrelationship of the mind and the body

(Terminology—continued)

Term	Word Parts			Definition
pyromania (pī″ rō-mā′ nĭ-ă)	pyro	P	fire	A madness for fire
	mania	S	madness	
quadriplegia (kwŏd″ rĭ plē′ jĭ-ă)	quadri	CF	four	Paralysis of all four extremities
	plegia	S	stroke, paralysis	
rachiomyelitis (rā″ kĭ-ō-mī″ ĕ-lī′ tĭs)	rachio	CF	spine	Inflammation of the spinal cord
	myel	R	spinal cord	
	itis	S	inflammation	
radicotomy (răd″ i-kŏt′ ō-mē)	radico	CF	root	A division or section of spinal nerve roots; also called rhizotomy
	tomy	S	incision	
radiculitis (ră-dĭk″ ū-lī′ tĭs)	radicul	R	root	Inflammation of spinal nerve roots
	itis	S	inflammation	
somnambulism (sŏm-năm′ bū-lĭzm)	somn	R	sleep	A condition of sleepwalking
	ambul	R	to walk	
	ism	S	condition of	
spondylosyndesis (spŏn″ dĭ-lō-sĭn′ dĕ-sĭs)	spondylo	CF	vertebra	A surgical procedure to bind vertebra after removal of a herniated disk; also called spinal fusion
	syn	P	together	
	desis	S	binding	
subdural (sŭb-dū′ răl)	sub	P	below	Pertaining to below the dura mater
	dur	R	dura, hard	
	al	S	pertaining to	
supratentorial (sū″ pră-tĕn-tō′ rĭ-ăl)	supra	P	above	Pertaining to above the tentorium
	tentori	R	tentorium, tent	
	al	S	pertaining to	
sympathectomy (sĭm″ pă-thĕk′ tō-mē)	sympath	R	sympathy	Surgical excision of a portion of the sympathetic nervous system
	ectomy	S	excision	
sympathomimetic (sĭm″ pă-thō-mĭm-ĕt′ ĭk)	sympatho	CF	sympathy	Imitating effects of the sympathetic nervous system
	mimetic	S	imitating	
trephination (trĕf″ ĭn-ā′ shŭn)	trephinat	R	a bore	The process of using a cylindrical saw to cut a circular piece of bone out of the skull
	ion	S	process	

(Terminology—continued)

Term	Word Parts			Definition
vagotomy (vă-gŏt′ ō-mē)	vago	CF	vagus, wandering	Surgical incision of the vagus nerve
	tomy	S	incision	
ventriculocister- **nostomy** (věn-trĭk″ū-lō-sĭs″těr- nōs′ tō-mē)	ventriculo	CF	little belly	Surgical creation of an opening between the third ventricle and the interpeduncular cistern for drainage of cerebrospinal fluid
	cisterno	CF	reservoir, cavity	
	stomy	S	new opening	
ventriculogram (věn-trĭk′ ū-lō-grăm)	ventriculo	CF	little belly	An x-ray record of the cerebral ventricles
	gram	S	mark, record	
ventriculometry (věn-trĭk″ ū-lōm′ ě trē)	ventriculo	CF	little belly	Measurement of intracranial pressure
	metry	S	measurement	

Vocabulary Words

Vocabulary words are terms that have not been divided into component parts. They are common words or specialized terms associated with the subject of this chapter. These words are provided to enhance your medical vocabulary.

Word	Definition
acetylcholine **(ACh)** (ăs″ ě-tĭl-kō′ lēn)	A cholinergic neurotransmitter that occurs in various tissues and organs of the body. It is thought to play an important role in the transmission of nerve impulses at synapses and myoneural junctions
agoraphobia (ăg″ ō-ră-fō′ bĭ ă)	Abnormal fear of being alone in public places; an anxiety syndrome and panic disorder
akathisia (ăk″ ă-thĭ′ zĭ ă)	The inability to remain still, motor restlessness, and anxiety
Alzheimer's **disease** (ahlts′ hĭ-merz dĭ-zēz′)	A severe form of senile dementia that may be due to some defect in the neurotransmitter system. There is cortical destruction that causes variable degrees of confusion, memory loss, and other cognitive defects
amyotrophic **lateral sclerosis** **(ALS)** (ă-mī″ ō-trŏf′ ĭk lăt′ ěr-ăl sklě-rō′ sĭs)	Muscular weakness, atrophy, with spasticity caused by degeneration of motor neurons of the spinal cord, medulla, and cortex; also called Lou Gehrig's disease
anorexia nervosa (ăn″ ō-rěks′ ĭ-ă ner-vō′ să)	A complex psychological disorder in which the individual refuses to eat or has an aberrant eating pattern

(Vocabulary—continued)

Word	Definition
apoplexy (ăp′ ō-plĕk″ sē)	A sudden loss of consciousness caused by an embolus, a thrombus, or rupture of an artery in the brain; also called a stroke or CVA (cerebrovascular accident)
autism (ŏ′ tĭzm)	A mental disorder in which the individual is self-absorbed, inaccessible, unable to relate to others, and has language disturbances. A syndrome usually beginning in infancy and becoming apparent in the first or second year of life
biogenic amines (bī″ ō-jĕn′ ĭk ăm′ ēns)	Chemical substances (neurotransmitters) that alter cerebral and vascular functions; epinephrine, norepinephrine, acetylcholine, dopamine, and serotonin
bulimia (bū-lĭm′ ĭ-ă)	A condition of episodic binge eating with or without self-induced vomiting
chemonucleo- lysis (kĕm″ ō-nŭ-klē-ŏl′ ĭ-sĭs)	A method of dissolving a herniated nucleus pulposis by injection of a chemolytic agent
chorea (kō-rē′ ă)	A condition of rapid, jerky involuntary muscular movements of the limbs or face
coma (kō′ mă)	An unconscious state or stupor from which the patient cannot be aroused
concussion (brain) (kŏn-kŭsh′ ŭn)	A loss of consciousness, temporary or prolonged, caused by a blow to the head
delirium (dē-lĭr′ ĭ-ŭm)	A state of mental confusion marked by illusions, hallucinations, excitement, restlessness, delusions, and speech incoherence
dorsal cord stimulation (DCS) (dōr-săl kōrd stĭm′ ū-lā′ shŭn)	A procedure used to relieve pain of the spinal cord by electric stimulation
endorphins (ĕn-dor′ fĭns)	Chemical substances produced in the brain that act as natural analgesics (opiates)
enkephalins (ĕn-kĕf′ ă-lĭns)	Chemical substances produced in the brain that act as natural analgesics (opiates). They bind to opiate receptor sites involved in pain perception
epilepsy (ĕp′ ĭ-lĕp″ sē)	A disorder of cerebral function resulting from abnormal electrical activity or malfunctioning of the chemical substances of the brain
evoked potentials (ē-vōkd′ pō-tĕn′ shăls)	Changes in electrical activity of the nervous system that are elicited by a physical stimulus or psychological event. They are used for evaluation of sensory function, localization of brain lesions, and evaluation of higher nervous function

(Vocabulary—continued)

Word	Definition
herpes zoster (hĕr′ pēz zŏs′ tĕr)	An acute viral disease characterized by painful vesicular eruptions along the segment of the spinal or cranial nerves; also called shingles
lyssa (līs′ să)	An acute infectious disease of the central nervous system transmitted to humans through the bite of a rabid animal; also called rabies, hydrophobia
multiple sclerosis (mŭl′ tĭ-pl sklē′ -rō′ sĭs)	A chronic disease of the central nervous system. Plaques occur in the brain and spinal cord causing tremor, weakness, incoordination, paresthesia, and disturbances in vision and speech
myasthenia gravis (mĭ-ăs-thē′ nĭ-ă gră′ vĭs)	A chronic disease caused by a defect in the myoneural conduction system. It is characterized by progressive muscular weakness, primarily of the face and neck. Secondarily, it may involve the muscles of the trunk and extremities
narcolepsy (nar′ kō-lĕp″ sē)	A chronic condition in which there are recurrent attacks of uncontrollable drowsiness and sleep
nerve transposition (nerv trăns″ pō-zĭ′ shŭn)	The surgical process of dissecting and transposing the ulnar nerve
neuroleptic (nŭ″ rō-lĕp′ tĭk)	Medicine that produces psychomotor slowing, emotional quieting, and extrapyramidal effects; also called antipsychotic and major tranquilizer
neuropeptide (nŭ″ rō-pĕp′ tīd)	Biochemical units of emotion
neurotransmitter (nŭ″ rō-trăns′ mĭt-ĕr)	Substances within neurons and the cerebrospinal fluid that allow nerve cells to communicate with one another
nucleotome (nŭ″ klē-ō-tōm)	An instrument (probe) used to remove fluid from a herniated, slipped, or ruptured disk
palsy (pawl′ zē)	A loss of sensation or an impairment of motor function; also called paralysis. There are many types of palsy
paresis (păr′ ē-sĭs)	A slight, partial, or incomplete paralysis
Parkinson's disease (păr′ kĭn-sŭnz dĭ-zēz′)	A chronic disease of the nervous system. It is characterized by a loss of equilibrium and by salivation, frustration, nausea, dryness of the mouth, and muscular tremors; also called paralysis agitans, shaking palsy
paroxysm (păr′ ŏk-sĭzm)	A sudden recurrence of the symptoms of a disease, an exacerbation; also means a spasm or seizure

(Vocabulary—continued)

Word	Definition
percutaneous diskectomy (pĕr″ kū-tā′ nē-ŭs dĭs-kĕk′ tō-mē)	A surgical procedure that can be done on an outpatient basis for slipped or herniated disks. With the use of fluoroscopy, the surgeon inserts a nucleotome into the middle of the affected spinal disk and removes the thick, sticky nucleus of the disk. This allows the disk to soften and contract, thereby relieving the pressure on the spinal nerve that caused the severe pain of the low back and leg
plethysmography (plē″ thĭz-mŏg′ ră-fē)	A noninvasive neurovascular examination technique
receptor (rē-sĕp′ tōr)	A sensory nerve ending that receives and relays responses to stimuli
Reye's syndrome (rīz sĭn′ drōm)	An acute disease that causes edema of the brain and increased intracranial pressure, hypoglycemia, and fatty infiltration of the liver and other vital organs. Occurs in children and has a relation to aspirin administration. May be viral in origin
rhizotomy (rī-zŏt′ ō-mē)	Surgical incision and sectioning of a nerve root
sciatica (sī-ăt′ ĭ-kă)	Severe pain along the course of the sciatic nerve
sleep (slēp)	A state of rest for the body and mind. There are two distinct types: REM for rapid eye movement, sometimes called dream sleep, and NREM for no rapid eye movement
syncope (sĭn′ kŭ-pē)	A temporary loss of consciousness caused by a lack of blood supply to the brain; also called fainting
tactile (tăk′ tĭl)	Pertaining to the sense of touch
Tay-Sachs disease (tā săks′ dĭ-zēz′)	An inherited disease that predominantly affects Jewish children of Ashkenazi origin. It is a progressive disease marked by degeneration of brain tissue
transcutaneous electrical nerve stimulations (TENS) (trăns-kū-tā′ nē-ŭs nerv stĭm′ ū-lā′ shŭn)	The use of mild electrical stimulation to interfere with the transmission of painful stimuli. It has proved useful in relieving pain in some patients
ventriculostomy (vĕn-trĭk″ ū-lŏs′ tō-mē)	The surgical creation of an opening between the third ventricle and the interpeduncular cistern for the relief of hydrocephalus

ABBREVIATIONS

ACh	acetylcholine	**HNP**	herniated nucleus pulposus
AD	Alzheimer's disease	**ICP**	intracranial pressure
ALS	amyotrophic lateral sclerosis	**IVC**	intraventricular catheter
		LP	lumbar puncture
ANS	autonomic nervous system	**MR**	mental retardation
CBS	chronic brain syndrome	**MS**	multiple sclerosis
CNS	central nervous system	**NCV**	nerve conduction velocity
CP	cerebral palsy	**PEG**	pneumoencephalography
CSF	cerebrospinal fluid	**PET**	positron emission tomography
CT	computerized tomography		
CVA	cerebrovascular accident	**PNS**	peripheral nervous system
DCS	dorsal cord stimulation	**TENS**	transcutaneous electrical nerve stimulation
EEG	electroencephalogram		
EST	electric shock therapy	**TIA**	transient ischemic attack
HDS	herniated disk syndrome	**TNS**	transcutaneous nerve stimulation

Drug Highlights

Drugs that are generally used for nervous system diseases and disorders include analgesics, analgesic-antipyretics, sedatives and hypnotics, antiparkinsonism drugs, anticonvulsants, and anesthetics.

Analgesics	Inhibit ascending pain pathways in the central nervous system. They increase pain threshold and alter pain perception.
Narcotic	*Examples: codeine phosphate, codeine sulfate, Dilaudid (hydromorphone HCl), Demerol (meperidine HCl), Darvon-N (propoxyphene napsylate), and morphine sulfate.*
Non-narcotic	*Examples: Stadol (butorphanol tartrate), Levoprome (methotrimeprazine), and Nubain (nalbuphine HCl).*
Analgesics-Antipyretics	Act to relieve pain (analgesic effect) and reduce fever (antipyretic effect).
	Examples: Tylenol (acetaminophen), Bayer aspirin, ibuprofen (Advil, Motrin, Nuprin), Naprosyn (naproxen), and Zomax (zomepirac sodium).
Sedatives and Hypnotics	Depress the central nervous system by interfering with the transmission of nerve impulses. Depending upon the dosage, barbiturates, benzodiazepines, and certain other drugs can produce either a sedative or a hypnotic effect. When used as a sedative, the dosage is designed to produce a calming effect without causing sleep. Used as a hypnotic, the dosage is sufficient to cause sleep.

Barbiturates	*Examples: Amytal (amobarbital), Buticaps (butabarbital sodium), Nembutal (pentobarbital), Seconal (secobarbital), and Luminal (phenobarbital).*
Nonbarbiturates	*Examples: Noctec (chloral hydrate), Placidyl (ethchlorvynol), Dalmane (flurazepam HCl), Restoril (temazepam), and Halcion (triazolam).*
Antiparkinsonism Drugs	Exert an inhibitory effect upon the parasympathetic nervous system. They prolong the action of dopamine by blocking its uptake into presynaptic neurons in the central nervous system.
	Examples: Symmetrel (amantadine HCl), Dopar (levodopa), Artane (trihexyphenidyl HCl), and Cogentin (benztropine mesylate).
Anticonvulsants	Inhibits the spread of seizure activity in the motor cortex.
	Examples: Dilantin (phenytoin), Tridione (trimethadione), Depakene (valproic acid), Mesantoin (mephenytoin), and Diamox (acetazolamide).
Anesthetics	Interfere with the conduction of nerve impulses and are used to produce loss of sensation, muscle relaxation, and/or complete loss of consciousness. Block nerve transmission in the area to which they are applied.
Local	Block nerve transmission in the area to which they are applied.
	Examples: Solarcaine (benzocaine), Nupercaine (dibucaine), Novocaine (procaine HCl), Xylocaine (lidocaine HCl), and Tronothane (pramoxine HCl).
General	Affect the central nervous system and produce either partial or complete loss of consciousness. They also produce analgesia, skeletal muscle relaxation, and reduction of reflex activity.
	Examples: Pentothal (thiopental sodium), Fluothane (halothane), Penthrane (methoxyflurane), and nitrous oxide.

Communication Enrichment

This segment is provided for those who wish to enhance their ability to communicate in either English or Spanish.

RELATED TERMS

English	Spanish
anxiety	ansiedad (ăn-*sĭ*-ĕ-dăd)
confused	confundido (cōn-*fŭn*-*dĭ*-dō)
conscious	consciente (cōns-sĭ-*ĕn*-tĕ)
consciousness, loss of	perdida de consciencia (pĕr-*dĭ*-dă dĕ cōns-sĭ-*ĕn*-sĭ-ă)
convulsion	convulsión (cōn-*vŭl*-sĭ-ōn)
coordination, loss of	perdida de coordinación (pĕr-*dĭ*-dă dĕ cōōr-dĭ-nă-sĭ-ōn)
cranial nerves	nervio craneal (*nĕr*-vĭ-ō *kră*-nĕ-ăl)
depression	depresión (*dĕ*-prĕ-sĭ-ōn)
disorientation	desorientación (dĕ-sō-rĭ-*ĕn*-tă-sĭ-ōn)
emotional problems	problemas emocionales (prō-*blĕ*-măs ĕ-mō-sĭ-ō-nă-lĕs)
fainting	desmayo (dĕs-*mă*-yō)
headache	dolor de cabeza (dō-*lōr* dĕ *kă*-bĕ-ză)
insomnia	insomnio (ĭn-*sōm*-nĭ-ō)
loss of memory	perdida de memoria (pĕr-*dĭ*-dă dĕ mĕ-*mō*-rĭ-ă)
nervous	nervioso (nĕr-vĭ-*ō*-sō)
nervous system	sistema nervioso (sĭs-*tĕ*-mă nĕr-vĭ-ō-sō)
paralysis	parálisis (pă-*ră*-lĭ-sĭs)
polio	polio (*pō*-lĭ-ō)
psychiatric problem	problema psiquiatrico (prō-*blĕ*-mă sĭ-*kĭă*-trĭ-kō)

English	Spanish
sensation, loss of	perdida de sensación (pĕr-*dĭ*-dă dĕ sĕn-*să*-sĭ-ōn)
stress	tensión (tĕn-sĭ-ōn)
stroke	latido (*lă*-tĭ-dō)
tremor	temblor (tĕm-*blōr*)
unconscious	inconsciente (ĭn-cōns-sĭ-ĕn-tĕ)
confuse	confundir (*cōn*-fūn-dĭr)
nerve	nervio (*nĕr*-vĭ-ō)
knowledge	conocimiento (cō-*nō*-cĭ-mĭ-ĕn-tō)
cranium	cráneo (*kră*-nĕ-ō)
craniotomy	craneotomia (*kră*-nĕ-ō-tō-mĭ-ă)
nerve cell	neurona (nĕ-ū-*rō*-mă)
nerve fiber	fibra nerviosa (*fĭ*-bră *nĕr*-vĭ-ō-să)
concussion	concusión (cōn-*kū*-sĭ-ōn)
epilepsy	epilepsia (ĕ-pĭ-*lĕp*-sĭ-ă)
sleep	sueño (sū-*ĕ*-ñō)
fight	lucha (*lū*-chă)
flight	vuelo (*vū*-ĕ-lō)
"fight or flight"	"vuelo o lucha" (vū-ĕ-lō ō lū-chă)
hypnosis	hipnosis (*ĭp*-nō-sĭs)
neurology	neurología (nĕ-ū-rō-*lō*-hĭ-ă)
psychology	psicología (sĭ-kō-*lō*-hĭ-ă)

DIAGNOSTIC AND LABORATORY TESTS

Test	Description
cerebral angiography (sĕr′ ĕ-brăl ăn″ jĭ-ŏg′ ră-fē)	The process of making an x-ray record of the cerebral arterial system. A radiopaque substance is injected into an artery of the arm or neck, and x-ray films of the head are taken. Cerebral aneurysms, tumors, or ruptured blood vessels may be visualized
cerebrospinal fluid (CSF) analysis (sĕr″ ĕ-brō-spī′ năl floo′ ĭd ă-năl′ ĭ-sĭs)	Examination of spinal fluid for color, pressure, pH, and the level of protein, glucose, and leukocytes. Abnormal results may indicate hemorrhage, a tumor, and various disease processes
computed tomography (CT) (kŏm-pū′ tĕd tō-mŏg″ ră-fē)	A diagnostic procedure used to study the structure of the brain. Computerized three-dimensional x-ray images allow the radiologist to differentiate between intracranial tumors, cysts, edema, and hemorrhage
echoencephalography (ĕk″ ō-ĕn-sĕf′ ă-lŏg′ ră-fē)	The process of using ultrasound to determine the presence of a centrally located mass in the brain
electroencephalography (EEG) (ē-lĕk-trō-ĕn-sĕf′ ă-lŏg′ ră-fē)	The process of determining the electrical activity of the brain via an electroencephalograph. Abnormal results may indicate epilepsy, brain tumor, infection, abscess, hemorrhage, and/or coma. Also brain "death" may be determined by an EEG
lumbar puncture (lŭm′ băr pŭnk′ chūr)	Insertion of a needle into the lumbar subarachnoid space for removal of spinal fluid. The fluid is examined for color, pressure, and the level of protein, chloride, glucose, and leukocytes
myelogram (mī′ ĕ-lō-grăm)	The x-ray of the spinal canal after the injection of a radiopaque dye. Useful in diagnosing spinal lesions, cysts, herniated disks, tumors, and nerve root damage
neurological examination (nū″-rō-lōj′ ĭ-kăl ĕks-ăm″ ĭ-nā′ shŭn)	Assessment of a patient's vision, hearing, sense of taste, smell, touch and pain, position, temperature, gait, muscle strength, coordination, and reflex action. Used to determine a patient's neurological status
positron emission tomography (PET) (pŏz′ ĭ-trŏn ē-mĭsh′ ŭn tō-mŏg″ ră-fē)	A computer-based nuclear imaging procedure that can produce three-dimensional pictures of actual organ functioning. Useful in locating a brain lesion, in identifying blood flow and oxygen metabolism in stroke patients, in showing metabolic changes in Alzheimer's disease, and in studying biochemical changes associated with mental illness
ultrasonography, brain (ŭl-tră-sŏn-ŏg′ ră-fē, brān)	The use of high-frequency sound waves to record echoes on an oscilloscope and film. Used as screening test or diagnostic tool

Learning Exercises

Anatomy and Physiology

Write your answers to the following questions. Do not refer back to the text.

1. Name the two interconnected divisions of the nervous system.

   a. _____ b. _____

2. _____ are the structural and functional units of the nervous system.

3. State the three actions of motor neurons.

   a. _____

   b. _____

   c. _____

4. Describe an axon. _____

5. Describe a dendrite. _____

6. State an action of sensory nerves. _____
   _____

7. _____ function to mediate impulses between sensory and motor neurons.

8. Define the following terms:

   a. Nerve fiber _____

   b. Nerve _____

   c. Tracts _____

9. The central nervous system consists of the _____ and the
   _____ _____.

10. State three functions of the central nervous system.

    a. _____ b. _____

    c. _____

11. Name the three meninges enclosing the brain.

    a. _____ b. _____ c. _____

12. Name the seven major divisions of the brain.

    a. _____ b. _____

    c. _____ d. _____

    e. _____ f. _____

    g. _____

13. The _____ _____ has been identified as the brain's major motor area.

14. The parietal lobe is also known as the _____ _____.

15. The temporal lobe contains centers for _____ and _____ input.

16. The occipital lobe is the primary area for _____.

17. State the functions of the thalamus.

a. _____ b. _____

18. State three functions of the hypothalamus.

a. _____ b. _____

c. _____

19. The cerebellum plays an important part in the _____ of _____.

20. State five functions of the medulla oblongata.

a. _____ b. _____

c. _____ d. _____

e. _____

21. State the three functions of the spinal cord.

a. _____ b. _____

c. _____

22. The normal adult will have between _____ and _____ mL of cerebrospinal fluid in circulation.

23. Name the 12 pairs of cranial nerves.

a. _____ b. _____ c. _____

d. _____ e. _____ f. _____

g. _____ h. _____ i. _____

j. _____ k. _____ l. _____

24. Name the four plexus that are formed from the spinal nerves.

a. _____ b. _____

c. _____ d. _____

25. State four functions of the autonomic nervous system.

a. _____ b. _____

c. _____ d. _____

26. Name the two divisions of the autonomic nervous system.

a. _____ b. _____

Word Parts

1. In the spaces provided, write the definitions of these prefixes, roots, combining forms, and suffixes. Do not refer to the listings of terminology words. Leave blank those terms you cannot define.

2. After completing as many as you can, refer back to the terminology word listings to check your work. For each word missed or left blank, write the term and its

definition several times on the margins of these pages or on a separate sheet of paper.
3. To maximize the learning process, it is to your advantage to do the following exercises as directed. To refer to the terminology listings before completing these exercises invalidates the learning process.

PREFIXES

Give the definitions of the following prefixes:

1. a- _____   2. an- _____
3. astro- _____   4. brady- _____
5. di(s) _____   6. dys- _____
7. epi- _____   8. hemi- _____
9. hydro- _____   10. hyper- _____
11. infra- _____   12. intra- _____
13. mirco- _____   14. oligo- _____
15. par- _____   16. para- _____
17. poly- _____   18. pyro- _____
19. sub- _____   20. supra- _____
21. syn- _____

ROOTS AND COMBINING FORMS

Give the definitions of the following roots and combining forms:

1. acro _____   2. ambul _____
3. arachn _____   4. atel _____
5. atelo _____   6. centr _____
7. cephal _____   8. cephalo _____
9. cerebell _____   10. cerebello _____
11. cerebro _____   12. chromo _____
13. cisterno _____   14. cordo _____
15. crani _____   16. cranio _____
17. cyt _____   18. dendro _____
19. disk _____   20. dur _____
21. ego _____   22. electro _____
23. encephal _____   24. encephalo _____
25. esthesio _____   26. foramino _____
27. ganglion _____   28. gli _____
29. hemo _____   30. hypn _____
31. hypno _____   32. lamin _____
33. lobo _____   34. log _____

35. logo _____   36. macro _____

37. mening _____   38. meningi _____

39. meningo _____   40. ment _____

41. mnes _____   42. myel _____

43. myelo _____   44. myo _____

45. neur _____   46. neuri _____

47. neuro _____   48. papill _____

49. phago _____   50. pheo _____

51. pneumo _____   52. polio _____

53. psych _____   54. psycho _____

55. quadri _____   56. rachio _____

57. radico _____   58. radicul _____

59. scler _____   60. spin _____

61. spondylo _____   62. somat _____

63. somn _____   64. sympath _____

65. sympatho _____   66. tentori _____

67. thym _____   68. trephinat _____

69. vago _____   70. ventriculo _____

SUFFIXES

Give the definitions of the following suffixes:

1. -al _____   2. -algesia _____

3. -algia _____   4. -ar _____

5. -asthenia _____   6. -blast _____

7. -cele _____   8. -cyte _____

9. -desis _____   10. -ectomy _____

11. -edema _____   12. -esthesia _____

13. -glia _____   14. -gram _____

15. -graph _____   16. -graphy _____

17. -ia _____   18. -ic _____

19. -ion _____   20. -ism _____

21. -ist _____   22. -itis _____

23. -kinesia _____   24. -kinesis _____

25. -lalia _____   26. -lemma _____

27. -lexia _____   28. -logy _____

29. -lysis _____   30. -malacia _____

31. -mania _____   32. -meter _____

33. -metry _____   34. -mimetic _____

35. -mnesia _____   36. -noia _____

37. -oma _____   38. -opsia _____

39. -osis _____   40. -paresis _____

41. -pathy _____   42. -phagia _____

43. -phasia _____   44. -phobia _____

45. -phthisis _____ 46. -plasia _____

47. -plasty _____   48. -plegia _____

49. -praxia _____   50. -rrhaphy _____

51. -sthenia _____ 52. -stomy _____

53. -taxia _____   54. -tome _____

55. -tomy _____   56. -tripsy _____

57. -us _____   58. -y _____

Identifying Medical Terms

In the spaces provided, write the medical terms for the following meanings:

1. _____ A condition in which there is a loss or lack of memory

2. _____ A lack of the sense of pain

3. _____ A loss or lack of the ability to eat or swallow

4. _____ Inflammation of the arachnoid membrane

5. _____ A loss or lack of muscular coordination

6. _____ Head pain; headache

7. _____ Pertaining to the cerebellum

8. _____ Surgical excision of a portion of the skull

9. _____ A condition in which an individual has difficulty in comprehending the written language

10. _____ Inflammation of the brain

11. _____ Pertaining to situated on the dura mater

12. _____ Paralysis that affects one side of the body

13. _____ The scientific study of sleep

14. _____ An abnormal condition in which the head is large

15. _____ Inflammation of the meninges of the spinal cord or brain

16. _____ Any disease of the meninges

17. _____ An instrument used to cut or dissect the spinal cord

18. _____ Pain in a nerve or nerves

19. _____ Inflammation of a nerve

20. _____ A nerve cell, a neuron

21. _____ The study of the nervous system

22. _____ A tumor of nerve cells and nerve fibers

23. _____ Surgical repair of a nerve or nerves

24. _____ An emotional condition or disorder

25. _____ A madness for food

26. _____ Inflammation of many nerves

27. _____ The study of the mind

28. _____ Inflammation of spinal nerve roots

29. _____ Surgical incision of the vagus nerve

30. _____ Measurement of intracranial pressure

Spelling

In the spaces provided, write the correct spelling of these misspelled terms.

1. anestesia _____   2. atelomylia _____

3. cerebospinal _____   4. cranitomy _____

5. encephaocele _____   6. meningoma _____

7. meningmyelcele _____   8. neurpathy _____

9. polomyelitis _____   10. ventriulogram _____

Review Questions

Matching

Select the appropriate lettered meaning for each numbered line.

_____ 1. acetylcholine

_____ 2. Alzheimer's disease

_____ 3. apoplexy

_____ 4. endorphins

_____ 5. epilepsy

_____ 6. palsy

_____ 7. percutaneous diskectomy

_____ 8. neuropeptide

_____ 9. nucleotome

_____ 10. sciatica

a. An instrument used to remove fluid from a herniated, slipped, or ruptured disk

b. Chemical substances produced in the brain that act as natural analgesics

c. A stroke

d. A severe form of senile dementia

e. A disorder of cerebral function resulting from abnormal electrical activity or malfunctioning of the chemical substances of the brain

f. Biochemical units of emotion

g. A cholinergic neurotransmitter that occurs in various tissues and organs of the body

h. A loss of sensation or an impairment of motor function

i. Severe pain along the course of the sciatic nerve

j. A surgical procedure that can be done on an outpatient basis for slipped disk

k. An anxiety syndrome and panic disorder

Abbreviations

Place the correct word, phrase, or abbreviation in the space provided.

_____ 1. Alzheimer's disease

_____ 2. amyotrophic lateral sclerosis

_____ 3. CNS

_____ 4. CP

_____ 5. computerized tomography

_____ 6. herniated disk syndrome

_____ 7. ICP

_____ 8. LP

_____ 9. MS

_____ 10. positron emission tomography

Diagnostic and Laboratory Tests

Select the best answer to each multiple choice question. Circle the letter of your choice.

1. A diagnostic procedure used to study the structure of the brain.

    a. computed tomography

    b. echoencephalography

    c. electroencephalography

    d. myelogram

2. The process of using ultrasound to determine the presence of a centrally located mass in the brain.

    a. computed tomography

    b. echoencephalography

    c. electroencephalography

    d. myelogram

3. The x-ray of the spinal canal after the injection of a radiopaque dye.

    a. cerebral angiography

    b. computed tomography

    c. myelogram

    d. ultrasonography

4. A computer-based nuclear imaging procedure that can produce three-dimensional pictures of actual organ functioning.

    a. electroencephalography

    b. myelogram

    c. ultrasonography

    d. positron emission tomography

5. The use of high-frequency sound waves to record echoes on an oscilloscope and film.

    a. electroencephalography

    b. myelogram

    c. ultrasonography

    d. positron emission tomography

13 The Ear

The ear is the site of hearing and equilibrium. It contains specially designed anatomical structures that receive sound vibrations, are sensitive to the force of gravity, and react to the movement of the head. These anatomical structures are connected to sensory areas of the brain by specialized fibers from the eighth cranial nerve. The eighth cranial nerve is also known as the acoustic or auditory nerve. The ear is generally described as having three distinct divisions: the external ear, the middle ear, and the inner ear.

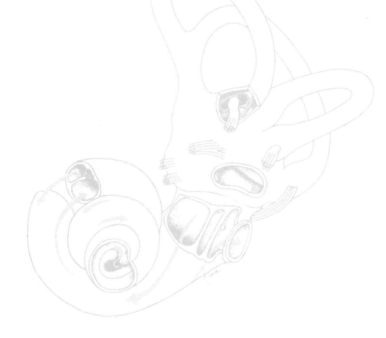

HARD ON YOUR HEARING

Noise at 85 decibels 8 hours a day will eventually cause hearing loss. Risk doubles with each 5-decibel increase. Are you harming your hearing?

Firecracker at 10 feet	*160 decibels*
Rock concert	*125 decibels*
Stereo headset, volume at six	*115 decibels*
Subway	*100 decibels*
Car horn	*100 decibels*
Garbage disposal	*95 decibels*
City traffic	*90 decibels*
Vacuum cleaner	*85 decibels*

ANATOMY AND PHYSIOLOGY OVERVIEW

The ear is the site of hearing and equilibrium. It contains specially designed anatomical structures that receive sound vibrations, are sensitive to the force of gravity, and react to the movements of the head. These anatomical structures are connected to sensory areas of the brain by specialized fibers from the eighth cranial nerve. The ear is generally described as having three distinct divisions: the external ear, the middle ear, and the inner ear. The following is a listing of the major components of the ear and some of their functions.

The External Ear

The external ear is the appendage on the side of the head consisting of the auricle, the external acoustic meatus or auditory canal, and the tympanic membrane or eardrum. The auricle collects sound waves that then pass through the auditory canal to vibrate the tympanic membrane that separates the external ear from the middle ear. The auditory canal is an S-shaped tubular structure about 2.5 cm long. Numerous glands line the canal and secrete cerumen or earwax to lubricate and protect the ear (Fig. 13–1 and Plate 6).

The Middle Ear

Beyond the tympanic membrane is a tiny cavity in the temporal bone of the skull. This cavity contains three small bones or ossicles instrumental to the hearing process. These ossicles are the malleus, incus, and stapes. Sometimes referred to as the hammer, anvil, and stirrup because of their shapes, these bones mechanically transmit sound vibrations from the tympanic membrane, to which the malleus is attached, through the incus to the stapes, which attaches to a thin membrane covering a small opening, the oval window, that marks

FIGURE 13–1

The auditory apparatus and its anatomical relationships. (*Adapted from Evans WF. Anatomy and Physiology, 3rd ed. Englewood Cliffs, NJ: Prentice-Hall, 1983, with permission.*)

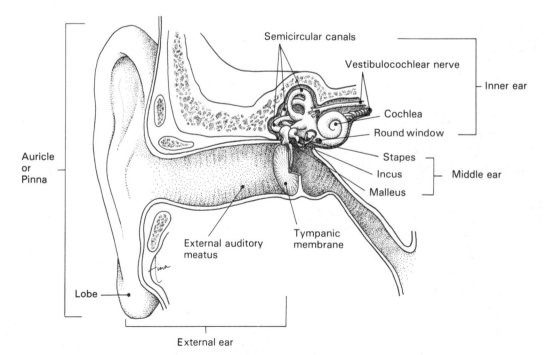

the beginning of the inner ear. During transmission, tympanic vibrations may be amplified as much as 22 times their original force.

The cavity of the middle ear has five openings, one covered by the tympanic membrane, another to the auditory or eustachian tube, a third to the mastoid cells, and two openings to the inner ear, the oval and round windows (Fig. 13–1). The cavity is lined by mucous membrane that is continuous with that found in the mastoid air cells, the eustachian tube, and the throat. The spread of infection from the throat along this membrane to the middle ear is called otitis media. The continued spread of infection to the mastoid air cells is called mastoiditis.

Three functions have been attributed to the middle ear:

1. It transmits sound vibrations.
2. It equalizes external/internal air pressure on the tympanic membrane.
3. It exerts control over potentially damaging or disruptive loud sounds through reflex contractions of the stapedius and tensor tympani muscles, which are attached to the stapes and the malleus, respectively.

The Inner Ear

The inner ear consists of a membranous labyrinth or maze located within a bony labyrinth. These structures are called labyrinths because of their complicated shapes. The bony labyrinth, located in the temporal bone, consists of the cochlea, vestibule, and three semicircular canals. Within the bony labyrinth, but separated from it by a fluid called perilymph, is the membranous labyrinth. It has much the same shape as the bony labyrinth and has three distinct divisions: the cochlear duct inside the cochlea, the semicircular ducts within the semicircular canals, and two sac-like structures, the utricle and saccule, located in the vestibule. Nerve endings in the form of hair cells located in various parts of the inner ear serve as receptors for the senses of hearing and equilibrium.

THE COCHLEA

The cochlea is a spiral-shaped bony structure containing the cochlear duct and so named because it resembles a snail shell. The spiral cavity of the bony cochlea is partitioned into three tube-like channels that run the entire length of the spiral. Two membranes form these tube-like areas. The basilar membrane forms the lower channel or scala tympani, and the vestibular membrane (Reissor's membrane) forms the upper channel, which is called the scala vestibuli. Between the two scala is a space, the cochlear duct, formed by the vestibular membrane on top and the basilar membrane as a floor. Located on the basilar membrane is the organ of Corti containing hair cell sensory receptors for the sense of hearing. A pale fluid, perilymph, fills the scala vestibuli and scala tympani. A different fluid, endolymph, fills the cochlear duct (Fig. 13–2).

The Hearing Process in the Inner Ear

The scala vestibuli and scala tympani open to the middle ear through the oval and round windows, respectively. The stapes fits into the round window and causes vibration of the perilymph, which, in turn, vibrates the basilar membrane and endolymph of the cochlear duct, thereby exciting the nerve endings contained on the organ of Corti. These nerve endings transmit the sounds, via the eighth cranial nerve, to the auditory areas of the brain. The sound waves, having excited the fluid of the cochlear duct, then pass on to the perilymph of the scala tympani and are dissipated against the membrane covering the round window.

THE VESTIBULE

The vestibule is a bony structure located between the cochlea and the three semicircular canals. The bony vestibule contains the utricle and saccule, membranous pouches contain-

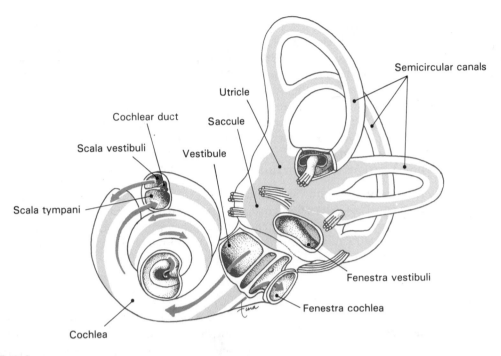

FIGURE 13–2

The cochlea. (*Adapted from Evans WF. Anatomy and Physiology, 3rd ed. Englewood Cliffs, NJ: Prentice-Hall, 1983, with permission.*)

ing perilymph. The utricle communicates with the semicircular canals and contains hair cell sensory receptors connected to fibers from the eighth cranial nerve. These hair cells react to the forces of gravity and movement and are a part of the sense of equilibrium.

THE SEMICIRCULAR CANALS

Located at right angles to each other, there are the superior, posterior, and inferior semicircular canals. Within the bony canals are the membranous semicircular ducts containing endolymph. At the base of each canal is an enlargement called an ampulla containing nerve endings in the form of hair cells. Changes in the position of the head causes the fluid in the canals to move against these sensory receptors, which, in turn, report such movement to the brain through fibers leading to the eighth cranial nerve. Dizziness and motion sickness are associated with rapid or erratic movement and the resulting sensory sensation in these areas.

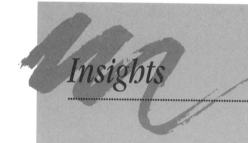
Insights

THERMOSCAN INSTANT THERMOMETER
(See Fig. 13–3)

Infrared tympanic (ear) thermometry (IRT) is based on the detection of infrared radiation (heat). Any material object emanates electromagnetic waves from its surface. The cooler the object, the less energy these waves carry. The hotter the object, the more energy the waves carry. The energy of the radiation emanating from our bodies is below the longest waves we can see, which are red; hence the term infrared meaning below red.

The use of the eardrum as the location to measure temperature is based on clinical studies that show the tympanic membrane and its surrounding tissue to be an accurate indicator of true

Proper Technique for Taking Ear Temps

1. To ensure optical clarity, make sure the probe tip window is clean and intact and a new probe cover is installed before each temperature is taken. Press the Thermoscan Pro-1 Instant Thermometer probe straight down into the cover box. You'll see and feel the cover slip securely into place, automatically putting it in the operating mode. When "ready" appears on the display, the unit is ready to take a temperature.
2. If the patient is lying down: Position the patient flat on his or her back. Turn the head 90 degrees for easy access to the ear. If the patient is sitting or standing: Simply ask them to hold their head still as you take the temperature. For a child: Have a helper hold the child on his or her lap, facing you. Turn the child's head to the side and stabilize it against the helper's chest.
3. Ear canals vary from person to person. Temperatures in the ear canal vary, with the warmest spot at the tympanic membrane. Most people have a bend in their canal that obstructs the view of the tympanic membrane. To get an accurate reading, straighten the ear canal by tugging the ear as you would for a standard otoscope exam. If you are right handed, hold unit in right hand and take temperature in patient's right ear, standing slightly behind patient. Left handers should hold unit in left hand and take temperature in left ear. Using your free hand, grasp the ear pinna, then pull back and up. (For babies under 12 months, pull straight back.) You are now ready to insert the probe.
4. Aim the probe slightly forward of the opposite ear. Use a slight rocking motion to insert the probe as far as possible and seal the ear canal. Press and hold the activation button for 1 full second, then release. Remove the probe from the ear, read temperature and discard cover. Record your results on the patient's chart.

If a temperature seems too low, repeat the procedure. Studies have shown that actual temperatures in the ear canal vary from person to person, temperature to temperature and ear to ear.

(Insights continues on next page)

core body temperature. The reason is that the eardrum shares blood supply and is in close proximity with the hypothalamus, the body thermostat.

Operation of the Thermoscan thermometer is similar to that of a photographic camera: it takes a snapshot of infrared heat and registers it on a sensitive surface. A gold-plated wave guide covered by a protective membrane is used instead of a lens, and an infrared sensor is used instead of photographic film. The use of a shutter resembles that of a camera.

The heart of the device is a dynamic (pyroelectric) sensor unique to Thermoscan. Use of the pyroelectric sensor allows the unit to retain high levels of accuracy as well as ease of operation and handling.

To measure a person's temperature, the HM-1's probe is positioned in the ear canal to get a view of the tympanic membrane and surrounding tissue. With the probe snugly in place, the operator then depresses the activation button, which quickly opens the shutter, allowing the infrared radiation emanating from the tympanum to pass onto the pyroelectric sensor. The resulting signal from the sensor is converted into digital form by an A/D (analog-to-digital) converter. A microprocessor calculates the temperature, then digitally displays it in either oral or rectal equivalents. The process takes just 1 second. The Thermoscan HM-1 operates on one 9-volt battery that takes a minimum of 300 temperatures before requiring replacement.

FIGURE 13–3

The Thermoscan Instant Thermometer. *(Courtesy of Thermoscan, Inc., San Diego, CA.)*

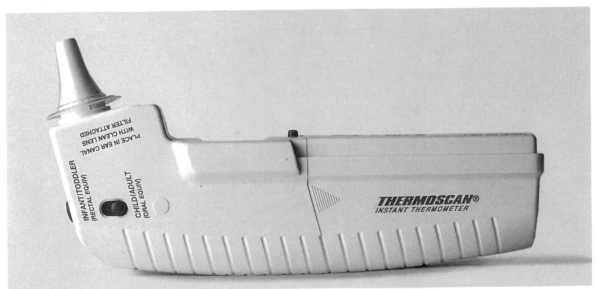

Terminology with Surgical Procedures & Pathology

Term	Word Parts			Definition
acoustic (ă-koos′ tĭk)	acoust	R	hearing	Pertaining to the sense of hearing
	ic	S	pertaining to	
audiogram (ŏ′ dĭ-ō-grăm″)	audio	CF	to hear	A record of hearing by audiometry
	gram	S	a mark, record	
audiologist (ŏ″ dĭ-ŏl′ ō-jĭst)	audio	CF	to hear	One who specializes in disorders of hearing
	log	R	study of	
	ist	S	one who specializes	
audiology (ŏ″ dĭ-ŏl′ ō-jĭ)	audio	CF	to hear	The study of hearing disorders
	logy	S	study of	
audiometer (ŏ″ dĭ-ŏm′ ĕ-tĕr)	audio	CF	to hear	An instrument used to measure hearing
	meter	S	instrument to measure	
audiometry (ŏ″ dĭ-ŏm′ ĕ-trē)	audio	CF	to hear	Measurement of the hearing sense
	metry	S	measurement	
audiphone (ŏ′ dĭ-fōn)	audi	CF	to hear	An instrument that conveys sound to the auditory nerve through teeth or bone
	phone	R	voice	
auditory (ŏ′ dĭ-tō″ rē)	auditor	R	hearing	Pertaining to the sense of hearing
	y	S	pertaining to	
aural (ŏ′ răl)	aur	R	the ear	Pertaining to the ear
	al	S	pertaining to	
cholesteatoma (kō″ lē-stē″ ă-tō′ mă)	chole	CF	gall or bile	A tumor-like mass filled with epithelial cells and cholesterol
	steat	R	fat	
	oma	S	tumor	
electrocochleography (ē-lĕk″ trō-kŏk″ lē-ŏg′ ră-fē)	electro	CF	electricity	A recording of the electrical activity produced when the cochlea is stimulated
	cochleo	CF	land snail	
	graphy	S	recording	
endaural (ĕn′ dŏ″ ral)	end	P	within	Pertaining to within the ear
	aur	R	ear	
	al	S	pertaining to	
endolymph (ĕn′ dō-lĭmf)	endo	P	within	The clear fluid contained within the labyrinth of the ear
	lymph	S	serum, clear fluid	

(Terminology—continued)

Term	Word Parts			Definition
labyrinthectomy (lăb″ ĭ-rĭn-thĕk′ tō-mē)	labyrinth ectomy	R S	maze excision	Surgical excision of the labyrinth
labyrinthitis (lăb″ ĭ-rĭn-thī′ tĭs)	labyrinth itis	R S	maze inflammation	Inflammation of the labyrinth
labyrinthotomy (lăb″ ĭ-rĭn-thŏt′ ō-mē)	labyrintho tomy	CF S	maze incision	Incision of the labyrinth
mastoidalgia (măs″ toyd-ăl′ jĭ-ā)	mast oid algia	R S S	breast form pain	Pain in the mastoid
mastoiditis (măs″ toyd-ī′ tĭs)	mast oid itis	R S S	breast form inflammation	Inflammation of the mastoid
myringectomy (mĭr-ĭn-jĕk′ tō-mē)	myring ectomy	R S	drum membrane excision	Surgical excision of the tympanic membrane
myringoplasty (mĭr-ĭn′ gō-plăst″ ē)	myringo plasty	CF S	drum membrane surgical repair	Surgical repair of the tympanic membrane
myringoscope (mĭr-ĭn′ gō-skōp)	myringo scope	CF S	drum membrane instrument	An instrument used to examine the eardrum
myringotome (mĭ-rĭn′ gō-tōm)	myringo tome	CF S	drum membrane instrument to cut	An instrument used for cutting the eardrum
otic (ō′ tĭk)	ot ic	R S	ear pertaining to	Pertaining to the ear
otitis (ō-tī′ tĭs)	ot itis	R S	ear inflammation	Inflammation of the ear
otodynia (ō″ tō-dĭn′ ĭ-ā)	oto dynia	CF S	ear pain	Pain in the ear, earache
otolaryngologist (ō″ tō-lar″ ĭn-gŏl″ ō-jĭst)	oto laryngo log ist	CF CF R S	ear larynx study of one who specializes	One who specializes in the study of the ear and larynx

(Terminology—continued)

Term	Word Parts			Definition
otolaryngology (ō″ tō-lar″ ĭn-gŏl′ ō-jē)	oto	CF	ear	The study of the ear and larynx
	laryngo	CF	larynx	
	logy	S	study of	
otolith (ō′ tō-lĭth)	oto	CF	ear	Ear stone
	lith	S	stone	
otomycosis (ō″ tō-mī-kō′ sĭs)	oto	CF	ear	A fungus condition of the ear
	myc	R	fungus	
	osis	S	condition of	
otoneurology (ō″ tō-nū-rŏl′ ō-jē)	oto	CF	ear	The study of ear conditions with nerve complications
	neuro	CF	nerve	
	logy	S	study of	
otopharyngeal (ō″ tō-far-ĭn′ jē-āl)	oto	CF	ear	Pertaining to the ear and pharynx
	pharynge	CF	pharynx	
	al	S	pertaining to	
otoplasty (ō′ tō-plăs″ tē)	oto	CF	ear	Surgical repair of the ear
	plasty	S	surgical repair	
otopyorrhea (ō″ tō-pī″ ō-rē′ ă)	oto	CF	ear	Flow of pus from the ear
	pyo	CF	pus	
	rrhea	S	flow	
otorhinolaryng- ology (ō″ tō-rī″ nō-lăr″ ĭn-gŏl′ ō-jē)	oto	CF	ear	The study of the ear, nose, and larynx
	rhino	CF	nose	
	laryngo	CF	larynx	
	logy	S	study of	
otosclerosis (ō″ tō-sklē-rō′ sĭs)	oto	CF	ear	A hardening condition of the ear characterized by progressive deafness
	scler	R	hardening	
	osis	S	condition of	
otoscope (ō′ tō-skōp)	oto	CF	ear	An instrument used to examine the ear
	scope	S	instrument	
perilymph (pĕr′ ĭ-lĭmf)	peri	P	around	Serum fluid of the inner ear
	lymph	S	serum, pale fluid	
presbycusis (prĕz″ bĭ-kū′ sĭs)	presby	R	old	Impairment of hearing in old age
	cusis	S	hearing	
stapedectomy (stā″ pē-dĕk′ tō-mē)	staped	R	stirrup	Surgical excision of the stapes in the ear
	ectomy	S	excision	
tinnitus (tĭn-ī′ tŭs)	tinnit	R	a jingling	A ringing or jingling sound in the ear
	us	S	pertaining to	

(Terminology—continued)

Term	Word Parts			Definition
tympanectomy (tĭm″ păn-ĕk′ tō-mē)	tympan ectomy	R S	drum excision	Surgical excision of the tympanic membrane
tympanic (tĭm-păn′ ĭk)	tympan ic	R S	drum pertaining to	Pertaining to the eardrum
tympanitis (tĭm-păn-ī′ tĭs)	tympan itis	R S	drum inflammation	Inflammation of the eardrum

Vocabulary Words

Vocabulary words are terms that have not been divided into component parts. They are common words or specialized terms associated with the subject of this chapter. These words are provided to enhance your medical vocabulary.

Word	Definition
auricle (ŏ′ rĭ-kl)	The external portion of the ear, known as the flap of the ear; the pinna (pin′ na)
binaural (bīn-aw′ răl)	Pertaining to both ears
cerumen (sē-roo′ měn)	Earwax, the yellowish substance secreted by the glands in the canal of the external ear
cochlea (kŏk′ lē-ă)	A portion of the inner ear shaped like a snail shell; contains the organ of hearing sometimes referred to as the organ of Corti
deafness (dĕf′ nĕs)	Complete or partial loss of the ability to hear
ear (ēr)	Organ of hearing and equilibrium
equilibrium (ē″ kwĭ-lĭb′ rē-ŭm)	A state of balance. In the inner ear, the semicircular canals are the site of the organs of balance
eustachian tube (yoo-stā′ shən tūb)	A narrow tube between the middle ear and the throat that serves to equalize pressure on both sides of the eardrum
fenestration (fĕn″ ĕs-trā′ shŭn)	Surgical operation in which a new opening is made in the labyrinth of the inner ear for restoration of hearing
incus (ing′ kŭs)	The anvil, the middle of the three ossicles
labyrinth (lăb′ ĭ-rĭnth)	The inner ear; made up of the vestibule, cochlea, and semicircular canals

(Vocabulary—continued)

Word	Definition
malleus (măl′ ē-ŭs)	The hammer, the largest of the three ossicles
Meniere's disease (mān″ ē-ārz)	A disease of the inner ear (labyrinth) that presents a group of symptoms that reoccur. In acute attacks, bedrest is recommended. Vertigo and dizziness are the classic symptoms, and the patient experiences nausea, tinnitus, and a sensation of fullness or pressure in the ears. Deafness can occur
monaural (mŏn-aw′ răl)	Pertaining to one ear
myringotomy (mĭr-ĭn-gŏt′ ō-mē)	Surgical incision of the tympanic membrane. It is used to remove unwanted fluids from the ear
ossicle (ŏs′ ĭ-kl)	Small bone. Any one of the three bones of the middle ear: the malleus, the incus, or the stapes
oval window (ō′ văl wĭn′ dō)	Membrane in the middle ear into which fits the footplate of the stapes
Rinne test (rĭn′ nē test)	A hearing test made with a tuning fork to compare bone conduction hearing with air conduction
stapes (stā′ pēz)	The stirrup, the innermost of the ossicles
tympanoplasty (tĭm″ păn-ō-plăs′ tē)	Surgical repair of the tympanic membrane
utricle (ū′ trĭk-l)	A small, sac-like structure of the labyrinth of the inner ear
vertigo (ver′ tĭ-gō)	A feeling of dizziness, lightheadedness, caused by a disturbance of the equilibrium organs in the labyrinth

ABBREVIATIONS

AC	air conduction	**EENT**	eyes, ears, nose, throat
AD	auris dexter (right ear)	**ETF**	eustachian tube function
AS	auris sinistra (left ear)	**HD**	hearing distance
AU	auris unitas (both ears)	**OM**	otitis media
BC	bone conduction	**Oto**	otology
CPS	cycles per second	**PE tube**	polyethylene tube
db, dB	decibel	**SOM**	serous otitis media
ENG	electronystagmography	**UCHD**	usual childhood diseases
ENT	ear, nose, and throat		

Drug Highlights

Drugs that are generally used for ear diseases and disorders include antibiotics and those used for vertigo.

Antibiotics
Used to treat infectious diseases. They may be natural or synthetic substances that inhibit the growth of or destroy microorganisms, especially bacteria.

Penicillins
Act by interfering with bacterial cell wall synthesis among newly formed bacterial cells. Penicillins are contraindicated in patients who are known to be allergic or hypersensitive to any of its varieties, or to any of the cephalosporins.

Examples: penicillin G, ampicillin, penicillin V, piperacillin, and amoxicillin.

Cephalosporins
Are chemically and pharmacologically related to the penicillins. They act by inhibiting bacterial cell wall synthesis, thereby promoting the death of the developing microorganisms. Hypersensitivity to cephalosporins and/or penicillins may result in an allergic reaction.

Examples: Ancef (cefazolin sodium), Mandol (cefamandole nafate), Precef (ceforanide), Ceclor (cefaclor), Keflex (cephalexin), and Suprax (cefixime).

Tetracyclines
Primarily bacteriostatic, and are active against a wide range of gram-negative and gram-positive microorganisms. They inhibit protein synthesis in the bacterial cell. Contraindicated in children 8 years of age and younger. These drugs cause permanent discoloration of tooth enamel.

Examples: oxytetracycline (Terramycin, Oxymycin), tetracycline hydrochloride (Achromycin, Sumycin, Tetracyn), and Minocin (minocycline).

Erythromycin
Works by inhibiting protein synthesis in susceptible bacteria. These drugs may be used for patients who are allergic to penicillin.

Examples: E-Mycin, Ilotycin, Ilosone, E.E.S., Pediamycin, and Erypar.

Drugs Used in Vertigo
Vertigo is an illusion of movement. It may be caused by a lesion or other process affecting the brain, the eighth cranial nerve, or the labyrinthine system of the ear. Drugs that are used for vertigo may include anticholinergics, antihistamines, and antidopamines.

Examples: Dramamine (dimenhydrinate), Benadryl (diphenhydramine), Antivert (meclizine), and Torecan (thiethylperazine maleate).

Communication Enrichment

This segment is provided for those who wish to enhance their ability to communicate in either English or Spanish.

RELATED TERMS

English	Spanish
balance, loss of	pérdida de equilibrio (*pĕr*-dĭ-dă dĕ ĕ-kĭ-lĭ-brĭ-ō)
deaf	sordo (*sōr*-dō)
dizziness	vértigo (*vĕr*-tĭ-gō)
drops	gotas (*gō*-tăs)
earache	dolor de oído (dō-*lōr* dĕ o-ē-dō)
ear	oído (o-ē-dō)
hear; listen	oír; escuchar (ō-*ĭr*; ĕs-kū-*chăr*)
hearing, difficulty in	dificultad de escuchar (*dĭ*-fi-cūl-tăd dĕ ĕs-kū-*chăr*)
hearing, loss of	pérdida de oído (*pĕr*-dĭ-dă dĕ o-ē-dō)
infection	infección (*ĭn*-fĕk-sĭ-ōn)
inflammation	inflamación (ĭn-flă-*mă*-sĭ-ōn)
loud	fuerte (*fū*-ĕr-tĕ)
left	izquierdo (iz-kū-*ĕr*-dō)
right	derecho (dĕ-*rĕ*-chō)
deafness	sordera (sōr-*dĕ*-ră)
wax	cera (*sĕ*-ra)
hearing	oir (ō-*ĭr*)
buzz, hum	zumbido (zūm-*bĭ*-dō)
temperature	temperatura (tĕm-pĕ-ră-*tū*-ră)

English	Spanish
thermometer	termómetro (tĕr-*mō*-mĕ-trō)
equilibrium	equilibrio (ĕ-kĭ-lĭ-brĭ-ō)
air	aire (ă-ĭ-rĕ)
both	ambos (*ăm*-bōs)
nose	nariz (*nă*-rĭz)
throat	garganta (găr-*găn*-tă)
eye	ojo (*ō*-hō)
middle	medio (*me*-dĭ-ō)
inner	interior (ĭn-*tĕ*-rĭ-ōr)
vibration	vibración (vĭ-*bră*-sĭ-ōn)
external	externo (ĕx-*tĕr*-nō)
internal	interno (ĭn-*tĕr*-nō)
ring	timbre (*ŭm*-brĕ)

DIAGNOSTIC AND LABORATORY TESTS

Test	Description
auditory evoked response (aw′ dĭ-tō″ rē ĕ-vōkd′ rē-spŏns)	The response to auditory stimuli (sound) that can be measured independent of the patient's subjective response. By using an electroencephalograph, the intensity of sound and presence of response can be determined. This test is useful for testing the hearing of children who are too young for standard tests, autistic, hyperkinetic, and/or retarded
electronystagmography (ē-lĕk″ trō-nĭs″ tăg-mŏg′ ră-fē)	A recording of eye movement in response to specific stimuli, such as sound. It is used to determine the presence and location of a lesion in the vestibule of the ear, to help diagnose unilateral hearing loss of unknown origin, and to help identify the cause of vertigo, tinnitus, and dizziness
falling test (fă′ lĭng test)	A test to observe the patient for marked swaying or falling. With eyes open, the patient is asked to stand on one foot, stand heel to toe, and then to walk forward. The patient is asked to repeat each of the above with the eyes closed. Marked swaying or falling may indicate vestibular and cerebellar dysfunction

Test	Description
past-pointing test (păst-poynt′ ĭng test)	The patient is instructed to reach out and touch the examiner's index finger, which is held at shoulder level, then to lower the arm, close the eyes, and touch the finger again. The test is repeated using the finger of the examiner's opposite hand. The degree and direction of past-pointing is observed
otoscopy (ō-tŏs′ kō-pē)	Visual examination of the external auditory canal and the tympanic membrane via an otoscope
tuning fork test (tūn′ ĭng fork test)	A method of testing hearing by the use of a tuning fork. Two types of hearing loss (conductive and perceptive) may be distinguished through the use of this test
tympanometry (tĭm″ păn-nŏm′ ĕ-trē)	Measurement of the movement of the tympanic membrane and pressure in the middle ear. It is used for detecting middle ear disorders

Learning Exercises

Anatomy and Physiology

Write your answers to the following questions. Do not refer back to the text.

1. The ear is the site of the senses of _____ and _____.

2. Name the three divisions of the ear.

   a. _____   b. _____

   c. _____

3. The external ear consists of the _____ , the _____ , and the _____.

4. Which structure of the external ear collects sound waves? _____

5. State the two functions of cerumen.

   a. _____   b. _____

6. Name the three ossicles of the middle ear.

   a. _____   b. _____

   c. _____

7. State the function of the ossicles. _____
   _____

8. State the three functions of the middle ear.

   a. _____   b. _____

   c. _____

9. The bony labyrinth of the inner ear consists of the _____ ,
   _____ , and the _____.

10. Name the three divisions of the membranous labyrinth.

    a. _____   b. _____

    c. _____

11. Located on the basilar membrane is the _____ , containing hair cell sensory receptors for the sense of hearing.

12. The _____ is a bony structure located between the cochlea and the three semicircular canals.

13. The auditory nerve is also known as the _____ .

14. The hair cells located in each ampulla of the semicircular canals sense changes in _____ and report this information to the brain.

15. Name the two types of fluid found in the ear.

    a. _____   b. _____

Word Parts

1. In the spaces provided, write the definitions of these prefixes, roots, combining forms, and suffixes. Do not refer to the listings of terminology words. Leave blank those terms you cannot define.
2. After completing as many as you can, refer back to the terminology word listings to check your work. For each word missed or left blank, write the term and its definition several times on the margins of these pages or on a separate sheet of paper.
3. To maximize the learning process, it is to your advantage to do the following exercises as directed. To refer to the terminology listings before completing these exercises invalidates the learning process.

PREFIXES

Give the definitions of the following prefixes:

1. end- _____ 2. endo- _____

3. peri- _____

ROOTS AND COMBINING FORMS

Give the definitions of the following roots and combining forms:

1. acoust _____ 2. audi _____

3. audio _____ 4. auditor _____

5. aur _____ 6. chole _____

7. cochleo _____ 8. electro _____

9. labyrinth _____ 10. labyrintho _____

11. laryngo _____ 12. log _____

13. mast _____ 14. myc _____

15. myring _____ 16. myringo _____

17. neuro _____ 18. ot _____

19. oto _____ 20. pharynge _____

21. phone _____ 22. presby _____

23. pyo _____ 24. rhino _____

25. scler _____ 26. staped _____

27. steat _____ 28. tinnit _____

29. tympan _____

SUFFIXES

Give the definitions of the following suffixes:

1. -al _____ 2. -algia _____

3. -cusis _____ 4. -dynia _____

5. -ectomy _____ 6. -gram _____

7. -graphy _____ 8. -ic _____

9. -ist _____   10. -itis _____

11. -lith _____   12. -logy _____

13. -lymph _____   14. -meter _____

15. -metry _____   16. -oid _____

17. -oma _____   18. -osis _____

19. -plasty _____   20. -rrhea _____

21. -scope _____   22. -tome _____

23. -tomy _____   24. -us _____

25. -y _____

Identifying Medical Terms

In the spaces provided, write the medical terms for the following meanings:

1. _____ One who specializes in disorders of hearing

2. _____ Measurement of the hearing sense

3. _____ Pertaining to the sense of hearing

4. _____ Pertaining to within the ear

5. _____ Inflammation of the labyrinth

6. _____ Surgical repair of the tympanic membrane

7. _____ An instrument used for cutting the eardrum

8. _____ Pain in the ear, earache

9. _____ The study of the ear and larynx

10. _____ Pertaining to the ear and pharynx

11. _____ An instrument used to examine the ear

12. _____ Serum fluid of the inner ear

13. _____ Surgical excision of the stapes of the ear

14. _____ Surgical excision of the tympanic membrane

15. _____ A ringing or jingling sound in the ear

Spelling

In the spaces provided, write the correct spelling of these misspelled terms:

1. acostic _____   2. audilogy _____

3. cholestoma _____   4. electrochleography _____

5. labrinthitis _____   6. myringplasty _____

7. otomcosis _____   8. otosterosis _____

9. typanic _____   10. typanitis _____

Review Questions

Matching

Select the appropriate lettered meaning for each numbered line.

_____ 1. auricle

_____ 2. binaural

_____ 3. cerumen

_____ 4. equilibrium

_____ 5. fenestration

_____ 6. labyrinth

_____ 7. myringotomy

_____ 8. ossicle

_____ 9. tympanoplasty

_____ 10. vertigo

a. A state of balance

b. The inner ear

c. Small bone

d. Surgical repair of the tympanic membrane

e. Pertaining to both ears

f. A feeling of dizziness

g. Surgical operation in which a new opening is made in the labyrinth

h. The external portion of the ear

i. Earwax

j. Surgical incision of the tympanic membrane

k. Organ of hearing

Abbreviations

Place the correct word, phrase, or abbreviation in the space provided.

_____ 1. air conduction

_____ 2. right ear

_____ 3. AS

_____ 4. both ears

_____ 5. ENT

_____ 6. EENT

_____ 7. hearing distance

_____ 8. otology

_____ 9. SOM

_____ 10. usual childhood diseases

Diagnostic and Laboratory Tests

Select the best answer to each multiple choice question. Circle the letter of your choice.

1. The response to auditory stimuli that can be measured independent of the patient's subjective response.

    a. auditory evoked response

    b. electronystagmography

    c. falling test

    d. otoscopy

2. A recording of eye movement in response to specific stimuli.

    a. auditory evoked response

    b. electronystagmography

    c. falling test

    d. otoscopy

3. A test to observe the patient for marked swaying.

    a. auditory evoked response

    b. electronystagmography

    c. falling test

    d. past-pointing test

4. The visual examination of the external auditory canal and the tympanic membrane.

    a. tuning fork test

    b. tympanometry

    c. electronystagmography

    d. otoscopy

5. The measurement of the movement of the tympanic membrane.

    a. tuning fork tests

    b. tympanometry

    c. otoscopy

    d. past-pointing test

14

The Eye

The eye is composed of special anatomical structures that work together to facilitate sight. Light passes through the cornea, pupil, lens, and the vitreous body to stimulate sensory receptors (rods and cones) on the retina or innermost layer of the eye. Vision is made possible through the coordinated actions of nerves that control the movement of the eyeball, the amount of light admitted by the pupil, the focusing of that light on the retina by the lens, and the transmission of the resulting sensory impulses to the brain by the optic nerve.

WHAT'S YOUR RISK OF DEVELOPING GLAUCOMA?

Three million people have glaucoma, and thousands more may be at risk of developing glaucoma. You don't have to be one of them. Know the following factors and see an ophthalmologist on a regular basis.

Risk Factors:
- *Over 60 years of age*
- *African ancestry*
- *Someone in family has glaucoma or diabetes*
- *Previous serious eye injury*
- *Taking steroid medication*

ANATOMY AND PHYSIOLOGY OVERVIEW

In this overview of the anatomy and physiology of the eye, a general description is offered as an aid to those learning the terminology associated with the functions of the eye.

The eye is composed of special anatomical structures that work together to facilitate sight. Light passes through the cornea, pupil, lens, and the vitreous body to stimulate sensory receptors (rods and cones) on the retina or innermost layer of the eye. Vision is made possible through the coordinated actions of nerves that control the movement of the eyeball, the amount of light admitted by the pupil, the focusing of that light on the retina by the lens, and the transmission of the resulting sensory impulses to the brain by the optic nerve. Listed below in outline form are the major components of the eye and some of their functions.

External Structures

The orbit, the muscles of the eye, the eyelids, the conjunctiva, and the lacrimal apparatus make up the external structures of the eye.

THE ORBIT

The orbit is a cone-shaped cavity in the front of the skull that contains the eyeball. Formed by the combination of several bones, this cavity is lined with fatty tissue that cushions the eyeball and has several openings of foramina through which blood vessels and nerves pass. The largest of these is the optic foramen for the optic nerve and ophthalmic artery.

THE MUSCLES OF THE EYE

Connecting the eyeball to the orbital cavity are six short muscles that provide it with support and rotary movement. Of the six, four are straight (rectus) muscles and two are slanted (oblique) muscles.

THE EYELIDS

Each eye has a pair of eyelids that protect the eyeball from intense light, foreign particles, and impact. Known as the superior and inferior palpebrae, those movable "curtains" join to form a canthus or angle at either corner of the eye. The slit between the eyelids is called the palpebral fissure, through which light reaches the inner eye. The edges of the eyelids contain cilia or eyelashes and sebaceous glands, which secrete an oily substance onto the eyelids.

THE CONJUNCTIVA

Lining the underside of each eyelid and reflected onto the anterior portion of the eyeball is a mucous membrane known as the conjunctiva. This membrane acts as a protective covering for the exposed surface of the eyeball.

THE LACRIMAL APPARATUS

Included in the lacrimal apparatus are those structures that produce, store, and remove the tears that cleanse and lubricate the eye. These structures are the lacrimal gland, its ducts, the lacrimal canaliculi, the lacrimal sac, and the nasolacrimal duct, which empties into the nasal cavity (Fig. 14-1). A brief explanation of these structures and their functions follows.

The Lacrimal Gland

Located above the outer corner of the eye, the lacrimal gland secretes tears through approximately 12 ducts onto the surface of the conjunctiva of the upper lid. This fluid washes across the anterior surface of the eye and is collected by the lacrimal canaliculi.

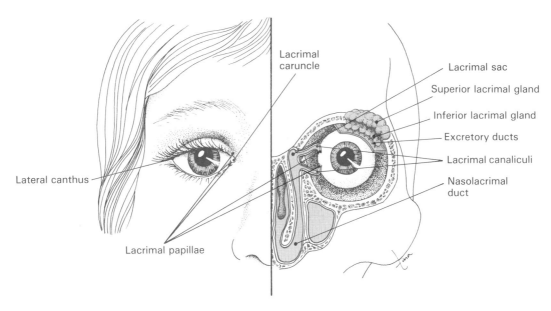

FIGURE 14–1

The lacrimal apparatus and its anatomical relations. (*Adapted from Evans WF. Anatomy and Physiology, 3rd ed. Englewood Cliffs, NJ: Prentice-Hall, 1983, with permission.*)

The Lacrimal Canaliculi

The lacrimal canaliculi are the two ducts (superior and inferior) at the inner corner of the eye that collect tears and drain into the lacrimal sac.

The Lacrimal Sac

The enlargement of the upper portion of the lacrimal duct is known as the lacrimal sac. Tears secreted by the lacrimal glands are pulled into this sac and subsequently forced into the nasolacrimal duct by the blinking action of the eyelids. The sac is dilated and pulls in fluid as the muscles associated with blinking close the lids. The sac constricts, forcing the fluid down the nasolacrimal duct, as the lids are opened.

The Nasolacrimal Duct

The passageway draining lacrimal fluid into the nose is known as the nasolacrimal duct. The lacrimal sac is the enlarged upper portion of this duct.

Internal Structures

The eyeball, its various structures, and the nerve fibers connecting it to the brain make up the internal eye (Fig. 14–2 and Plate 5).

THE EYEBALL

The eyeball is the organ of vision. It is globe shaped and divided into two cavities. The space in front of the lens, called the ocular cavity, is further divided by the iris into anterior and posterior chambers, both filled with a watery fluid known as the aqueous humor. Behind the lens is a much larger cavity filled with a jelly-like material, the vitreous humor, which maintains the eyeball's spherical shape. The three layers forming the outer, middle, and inner surfaces of the eyeball are discussed, along with the lens and its functions.

The Outer Layer

The eyeball's outer layer is composed of the sclera or white of the eye and the cornea or anterior transparent portion of the eye's fibrous outer surface. The curved surface of the

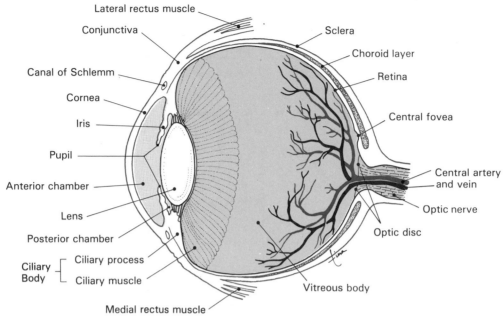

Lateral rectus muscle
Conjunctiva
Sclera
Canal of Schlemm
Choroid layer
Cornea
Retina
Iris
Central fovea
Pupil
Anterior chamber
Central artery and vein
Lens
Optic nerve
Posterior chamber
Optic disc
Ciliary Body {
Ciliary process
Ciliary muscle
Vitreous body
Medial rectus muscle

FIGURE 14–2

The structure of the eyeball. (*Adapted from Evans WF.* Anatomy and Physiology, *3rd ed. Englewood Cliffs, NJ: Prentice-Hall, 1983, with permission.*)

cornea is important in that it bends light rays and helps to focus them on the surface of the retina.

The Middle Layer

Known as the uvea, the middle layer of the eyeball, lying just below the sclera, consists of the iris, the ciliary body, and the choroid or pigmented vascular membrane that prevents internal reflection of light.

The Ciliary Body. The ciliary body is a thickened portion of the vascular membrane to which the iris is attached. Smooth muscle forming a part of the ciliary body governs the convexity of the lens. The ciliary body secretes nutrient fluids (the aqueous humor) that nourish the cornea, the lens, and the surrounding tissues.

The Iris. The iris is a colored membrane attached to the ciliary body and suspended between the lens and the cornea in the aqueous humor. It has a circular opening in its center, the pupil, and two muscles that contract or dilate to regulate the amount of light admitted by the pupil.

The Inner Layer

The innermost layer, or retina, contains photoreceptive cells that translate light waves focused on its surface into nerve impulses. The photosensitive cells of the retina are the rods and cones. Most of the approximately 6 million cone cells are grouped into a small area called the macula lutea. In the center of the macula lutea is a small depression, the fovea centralis, containing only cone cells, which is the central focusing point within the eye. The eye contains approximately 120 million rods that are sensitive to dim light. They contain rhodopsin, a pigment necessary for night vision. The point at which nerve fibers from the retina converge to form the optic nerve is known as the optic disk. At this point, fibers of the optic nerve extend, through the optic chiasm, to the thalamus and on to the visual cortical areas of the brain. The absence of rods and cones in the area of the optic disk creates a blind spot in the visual field.

The Lens

A colorless crystalline body, biconvex in shape and enclosed in a transparent capsule, the lens is suspended by ligaments just behind the iris. Contraction and relaxation of the ciliary muscle control the tension of the suspensory ligaments to change the shape of the lens. The function of the lens is to sharpen the focus of light on the retina. This process, called accommodation, is reflexive in nature and combines changes in the size of the pupil, the curvature of the lens, and the convergence of the optic axes to keep the image in the same place on both retinae. Accommodation occurs for both near and distant vision.

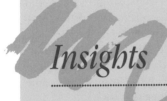

Insights

CATARACT(s)—The No-Stitch Surgery

Approximately 1 million people will have cataract surgery during a given year. It is the most frequently performed operation in people who are 65 years of age and older. With the No-Stitch (phacoemulsification) surgery, there is over a 95% success rate and the patient is able to return to normal activities in a short time. This type of surgery is generally performed under local anesthesia and on an outpatient basis. If the medical condition of the patient so indicates, he or she will be hospitalized for the surgery.

The eye is composed of special anatomical structures that work together to facilitate sight. Light passes through the cornea, pupil, lens, and the vitreous body to stimulate sensory receptors (rods and cones) on the retina. Vision is made possible through the coordinated actions of nerves that control the movement of the eyeball, the amount of light admitted by the pupil, the focusing of that light on the retina by the lens, and the transmission of the resulting sensory impulses to the brain by the optic nerve. As long as the lenses are clear, a sharp image can be formed. With cataract(s), the lens become cloudy, therefore the image cannot get through as easily and it becomes faint and hazy. This condition usually develops over several years.

Benefits of No-Stitch Surgery

- Minimal trauma for the eye
- Fast recovery
- Quick vision improvement
- Outpatient instead of hospitalization (for most patients)
- Surgery takes about 20–40 minutes
- Use of a local instead of a general anesthetic

Risks of Surgery

- Loss of vision
- Hemorrhage
- Infection
- Edema
- Retinal detachment
- Intraocular lens displacement
- Corneal clouding
- Formation of secondary membranes
- Chronic inflammation
- Astigmatism
- Glare
- Drooping eye lid

Contraindications for Intraocular Lens Implantation

- Recurrent uveitis
- Proliferative diabetic retinopathy
- Neovascular glaucoma

(Insights continues on next page)

Signs and Symptoms: The most common symptom of a cataract is blurred vision. Some people complain of a film over their vision, or feel like their glasses are dirty all of the time. Some patients see halos around lights or double vision. As the cataract(s) progress, driving, reading, and close work becomes impossible. Eventually the patient can only tell the difference between light and dark.

Causes: Most cataract(s) are a natural part of the aging process and are present to some degree in most people who are over 65. Other forms of cataract(s) may be congenital, caused by infection, injury, exposure to radiation, ultraviolet radiation, long-term adrenocorticotropic hormone (ACTH) therapy, and as a complication of diabetes.

Diagnosis is accomplished by having a complete eye exam and the magnitude of the cataract(s) determines the priority of treatment, which is surgery. There is no medical treatment for cataract(s).

Before surgery, the patient should have a complete history and physical examination. The benefits and possible risks should be explained, and the patient is asked to sign a consent form.

Surgical Procedure: Phacoemulsification is the process of using an ultrasonic device to disintegrate the cataract, which is then aspirated and removed. Think of the cataract as if it were inside a grape. The skin of the grape surrounds the jelly-like substance of the grape and it has to be opened to squeeze out the grape's contents. The natural lens of the eye that developed the cataract is surrounded by a thin tissue called a capsule. To remove the cataract, the capsule must be partially opened so a small 3–4 mm incision is made (capsulotomy). Next the tip of an ultrasonic instrument is inserted and the removal of the cataract begins. The tip of the instrument is vibrating at approximately 40,000 cycles per second and this ultrasonic action fragments the cataract while the center of the instrument gently vacuums away the cataract. Soon all that remains is a soft tissue known as the cortex, which is also vacuumed from the eye using a second type of instrument called an irrigation and aspiration unit. The posterior capsule (capsular bag) is left in place and serves as a platform for the placement of the intraocular lens. Next the intraocular lens (IOL) is folded in half and inserted through the original small incision. The small incision seals itself and needs No-Stitch.

Patient Education: After surgery, the patient is advised not to lift any heavy objects, run, jog, or ride a horse. The patient should avoid sleeping on the operative side, rubbing the eye(s), squeezing the eyelids shut, straining at bowel movement, getting soap in the eye(s), sexual relations, driving (if possible), coughing, sneezing, vomiting, and bending head down below waist.

Advise the patient to report any unusual symptoms such as pain, changes in vision, persistent headache, and discharge from eye(s) to his or her physician.

Terminology with Surgical Procedures & Pathology

Term		Word Parts		Definition
amblyopia (ăm″blĭ-ō′pĭ-ă)	ambly	R	dull	Dullness of vision
	opia	S	vision	
ametropia (ă″mĕ-trō′pĭ-ă)	ametr	R	dispropor-tionate	A defect in the refractive powers of the eye in which images fail to come to focus on the retina
	opia	S	eye, vision	
anisocoria (ăn-ī″sō-kŏ′rĭă)	aniso	CF	unequal	A condition in which the pupils are unequal
	cor	R	pupil	
	ia	S	condition	
aphakia (ă-fā′kĭ-ă)	a	P	lack of, without	A condition in which the crystalline lens is absent
	phak	R	lentil, lens	
	ia	S	condition	
astigmatism (ă-stĭg′mă-tĭzm)	a	P	lack of, without	A defect in the refractive powers of the eye in which a ray of light is not focused on the retina but is spread over an area
	stigmat	R	point	
	ism	S	condition of	
bifocal (bī-fō′kăl)	bi	P	two	Pertaining to having two foci, as in bifocal glasses
	foc	R	focus	
	al	S	pertaining to	
blepharitis (blĕf″ăr-ī-′tĭs)	blephar	R	eyelid	Inflammation of the edges of the eyelids
	itis	S	inflammation	
blepharoptosis (blĕf″ ă-rō-tō′ sĭs)	blepharo	CF	eyelid	A drooping of the upper eyelid(s)
	ptosis	S	prolapse, drooping	
choroiditis (kō″royd-ī′tĭs)	choroid	R	choroid	Inflammation of the vascular coat of the eye
	itis	S	inflammation	
choroidoretinitis (kō″royd-ō-rĕt″ ĭn-ī′tĭs)	choroido	CF	choroid	Inflammation of the choroid and retina
	retin	R	retina	
	itis	S	inflammation	
corneal (kŏr′nēəl)	corne	R	cornea	Pertaining to the cornea
	al	S	pertaining to	
cycloplegia (sī″klō-plē′jĭ-ă)	cyclo	CF	ciliary body	Paralysis of the ciliary muscle
	plegia	S	stroke, paralysis	

(Terminology—continued)

Term	Word Parts			Definition
dacryocystitis (dăk″rĭ-ō-sĭs-tī′tĭs)	dacryo	CF	tear	Inflammation of the tear sac(s)
	cyst	R	sac	
	itis	S	inflammation	
dacryoma (dăk‴rĭ-ō′mă)	dacry	R	tear	A tumor-like swelling caused by obstruction of the tear duct(s)
	oma	S	tumor	
diplopia (dĭp-lō′pĭ-ă)	dipl	P	double	Double vision
	opia	S	eye, vision	
ectropion (ĕk-trō′pĭ-ŏn)	ec	P	out	A process of turning outward, as the edge of an eyelid(s)
	trop	R	turn	
	ion	S	process	
electroretinogram (ē-lĕk″trō-rĕt′ĭ-nō-grăm)	electro	CF	electricity	A record of the electrical response of the retina to light stimulation
	retino	CF	retina	
	gram	S	mark, record	
emmetropia (ĕm″ĕ-trō′pĭ-ă)	em	P	in	Normal or perfect vision
	metr	R	measure	
	opia	S	eye, vision	
esotropia (ĕs″ō-trō′pĭ-ă)	eso	P	inward	A condition in which the eye or eyes turn inward; crossed eyes
	trop	R	turn	
	ia	S	condition	
gonioscope (gō′nĭ-ō-skōp)	gonio	CF	angle	An instrument used to examine the angle of the anterior chamber of the eye
	scope	S	instrument	
hyperopia (hī″pĕr-ō′pĭ-ă)	hyper	P	beyond	A defect in vision in which parallel rays come to a focus beyond the retina; farsightedness
	opia	S	eye, vision	
intraocular (ĭn″trăh-ŏk′ū-lăr)	intra	P	within	Pertaining to within the eye
	ocul	R	eye	
	ar	S	pertaining to	
iridectomy (ĭr″ĭ-dĕk′tō-mē)	irid	R	iris	Surgical excision of a portion of the iris
	ectomy	S	excision	
iridocyclitis (ĭr″ĭd-ō-sī-klī′tĭs)	irido	CF	iris	Inflammation of the iris and ciliary body
	cycl	R	ciliary body	
	itis	S	inflammation	
iridodesis (ĭr″ĭ-dŏd′ĕ-sĭs)	irido	CF	iris	Surgical binding of part of the iris to form an artificial one
	desis	S	binding	
iridomalacia (ĭr″ĭd-ō-mă-lā′shĭ-ă)	irido	CF	iris	A softening of the iris
	malacia	S	softening	

(Terminology—continued)

Term	Word Parts			Definition
iridotasis (ĭr″ ĭ-dŏt′ ă-sĭs)	irido tasis	CF S	iris stretching	A stretching of the iris in treatment of glaucoma
keratitis (kĕr″ ă-tī′ tĭs)	kerat itis	R S	cornea inflammation	Inflammation of the cornea
keratometer (kĕr″ ă-tŏm′ ĕ-tĕr)	kerato meter	CF S	cornea instrument to measure	An instrument used to measure the curve of the cornea
keratoplasty (kĕr′ ă-tō-plăs″ tē)	kerato plasty	CF S	cornea surgical repair	Surgical repair of the cornea
lacrimal (lăk′ rĭm-ăl)	lacrim al	R S	tear pertaining to	Pertaining to tears
myopia (mī-ō′ pĭ-ă)	my opia	R S	to shut eye, vision	A defect in vision in which parallel rays come to a focus in front of the retina; nearsightedness
nyctalopia (nĭk″tă-lō′ pĭ-ă)	nyctal opia	R S	blind eye, vision	A condition in which the individual has difficulty seeing at night; night blindness
ocular (ŏk′ ū-lar)	ocul ar	R S	eye pertaining to	Pertaining to the eye
ophthalmologist (ŏf″ thăl-mŏl′ ō-jĭst)	ophthalmo log ist	CF R S	eye study of one who specializes	One who specializes in the study of the eye
ophthalmology (ŏf″ thăl-mŏl′ ō-jē)	ophthalmo logy	CF S	eye study of	The study of the eye
ophthalmopathy (of″ thăl-mŏp′ ă-thē)	ophthalmo pathy	CF S	eye disease	Any eye disease
ophthalmoscope (ŏf″ thăl′ mō-skōp)	ophthalmo scope	CF S	eye instrument	An instrument used to examine the interior of the eye
optic (op′ tĭk)	opt ic	R S	eye pertaining to	Pertaining to the eye
optomyometer (ŏp″ tō-mī-ŏm′ ĕt-ĕr)	opto myo meter	CF CF S	eye muscle instrument to measure	An instrument used to measure the strength of the muscles of the eye

(Terminology—continued)

Term	Word Parts			Definition
phacolysis (făk-ŏl″ ĭ-sĭs)	phaco lysis	CF S	lens destruction, to separate	Surgical destruction and removal of the crystalline lens in the treatment of cataract
phacosclerosis (făk″ ō-sklĕr-ō′ sĭs)	phaco scler osis	CF R S	lens hardening condition of	A condition of hardening of the crystalline lens
photophobia (fō″ tō-fō′ bĭ-ă)	photo phobia	CF S	light fear	Unusual intolerance of light
presbyopia (prĕz″ bĭ-ō′ pĭ-ă)	presby opia	R S	old eye, vision	A defect in vision in which parallel rays come to a focus beyond the retina; occurs normally with aging; farsightedness
pupillary (pū′ pĭ-lĕr-ē)	pupill ary	R S	pupil pertaining to	Pertaining to the pupil
retinal (rĕt′ ĭ-năl)	retin al	R S	retina pertaining to	Pertaining to the retina
retinitis (rĕt″ĭ-nī′ tĭs)	retin itis	R S	retina inflammation	Inflammation of the retina
retinoblastoma (rĕt″ ĭ-nō-blăs-tō′ mă)	retino blast oma	CF S S	retina germ cell tumor	A malignant tumor arising from the germ cell of the retina
retinopathy (rĕt″ ĭn-ŏp′ ă-thē)	retino pathy	CF S	retina disease	Any disease of the retina
scleritis (sklē-rī′ tĭs)	scler itis	R S	sclera inflammation	Inflammation of the sclera
tonography (tō-nŏg′ ră-fē)	tono graphy	CF S	tone recording	Recording of intraocular pressure used in detecting glaucoma
tonometer (tŏn-ŏm′ ĕ-tĕr)	tono meter	CF S	tone instrument to measure	An instrument used to measure intraocular pressure
trifocal (trĭ-fō′ căl)	tri foc al	P R S	three focus pertaining to	Pertaining to having three foci
uveal (ū′ vē-ăl)	uve al	R S	uvea pertaining to	Pertaining to the second or vascular coat of the eye

(Terminology—continued)

Term	Word Parts			Definition
uveitis (ū-vē-ī′ tĭs)	uve	R	uvea	Inflammation of the uvea
	itis	S	inflammation	
xenophthalmia (zĕn″ ŏf-thăl′ mē-ă)	xen	R	foreign material	Inflamed eye condition caused by foreign material
	ophthalm	R	eye	
	ia	S	condition	
xerophthalmia (zē-rŏf-thăl′ mĭ-ă)	xer	R	dry	An eye condition in which there is dryness of the conjunctiva
	ophthalm	R	eye	
	ia	S	condition	

Vocabulary Words

Vocabulary words are terms that have not been divided into component parts. They are common words or specialized terms associated with the subject of this chapter. These words are provided to enhance your medical vocabulary.

Word	Definition
accommodation (ă-kŏm″ ō-dā′shŭn)	The process whereby the eyes make adjustments for seeing objects at various distances
anomaloscope (ă-nŏm′ a-lō-skōp)	Instrument used for detecting color blindness
cataract (kăt″ə răkt′)	An opacity of the crystalline lens or its capsule; most often occurs in adults past middle age
chalazion (kă-lā′ zĭ-ŏn)	A small, hard, painless cyst of a Meibomian gland (one of the sebaceous follicles of the eyelids)
conjunctivitis (kŏn-jŭnk″ tĭ-vī′tĭs)	Inflammation of the conjunctiva caused by allergy, trauma, chemical injury, bacterial, viral, or rickettsial infection. The type called "pinkeye" is infectious and contagious
corneal transplant (kŏr′ nē-ăl trăns′ plănt)	The surgical process of transferring the cornea from a donor to a patient
cryosurgery (krī″ ō-sur′ jur-ē)	A type of surgery that uses extreme cold for destruction of tissue or for production of well-demarcated areas of cell injury; may be used in the removal of cataracts and in the repair of retinal detachment
entropion (ĕn-trō-pē-ŏn)	The turning inward of the margin of the lower eyelid
enucleation (ē-nū″ klē-ā′ shŭn)	A process of removing an entire part or mass without rupture, as the eyeball from its orbit

(Vocabulary—continued)

Word	Definition
epiphora (ĕ-pĭf′ō-ră)	The abnormal downpour of tears caused by excessive secretion or obstruction of a lacrimal duct
exotropia (ĕks″ō-trō′ pē-ă)	The turning outward of one or both eyes
glaucoma (glaw-kō′ mă)	A disease characterized by increased intraocular pressure, which results in atrophy of the optic nerve and blindness
hemianopia (hĕm″ē-ă-nō′ pē-ă)	The inability (blindness) to see half the field of vision
keratoconjuncti-vitis (kĕr″ ă-tō-kŏn-jŭnk ″ tĭ-vī′ tĭs)	Inflammation of the cornea and the conjunctiva
laser (lā′ zĕr)	An acronym for **l**ight **a**mplification by **s**timulated **e**mission of **r**adiation
laser trabeculoplasty (tră-bĕk′ ū-lō-plăs″ tē)	The use of a laser to reduce intraocular pressure; may be used to treat glaucoma
microlens (mī′ krō-lĕns)	A small, thin corneal contact lens
miotic (mī-ŏt′ ĭk)	Pertaining to an agent that causes the pupil to contract
mydriatic (mĭd″ rĭ-ăt′ ĭk)	Pertaining to an agent that causes the pupil to dilate
nystagmus (nĭs-tăg′ mŭs)	An involuntary, constant, rhythmic movement of the eyeball
optician (ŏp-tĭsh′ ăn)	One who specializes in the making of optical products and accessories. This person is not a physician
optometrist (ŏp-tŏm′ ĕ-trĭst)	One who specializes in examining the eyes for refractive errors and providing appropriate corrective lenses. This person is not a physician but is trained and licensed as a Doctor of Optometry (O.D.)
orthoptics (or-thŏp′ tĭks)	The study and treatment of defective binocular vision resulting from defects in ocular musculature; also a technique of eye exercises for correcting defective binocular vision
phacoemulsifi-cation (făk″ ō-ē′ mŭl′ sĭ-fĭ-kā″ shŭn)	The process of using ultrasound to disintegrate a cataract. A needle is inserted through a small incision, and the disintegrated cataract is aspirated

(Vocabulary—continued)

Word	Definition
photocoagulation (fō″ tō-kō-ăg″ ū-lā′ shŭn)	The process of altering proteins in tissue by the use of light energy such as the laser beam; used in the treatment of retinal detachment, retinal bleeding, or intraocular tumors
pterygium (tĕr-ĭj′ ĭ-ŭm)	An abnormal triangular fold of membrane that extends from the conjunctiva to the cornea
radial keratotomy (rā′ dē-ăl kĕr-ă′ tŏt′ ō-mē)	A surgical procedure that may be performed to correct near-sightedness (myopia). Delicate spoke-like incisions are made in the cornea to flatten it, thereby shortening the eyeball so that light reaches the retina. Not all patients have their vision improved, and complications could lead to blindness
retrolental fibroplasia (RLF) (rĕt″ rō-lĕn-tăl fĭ-brō-plā-sē-ă)	A disease of the retinal vessels present in premature infants; may be caused by excessive use of oxygen in the incubator. Retinal detachment and blindness may occur
Snellen chart (snĕl′ ĕn chart)	A chart for testing visual acuity. It is printed with lines of black letters that are graduated in size from smallest, on the bottom to largest on the top (Fig. 14–3)
strabismus (stră-bĭz′ mŭs)	A disorder of the eye in which the optic axes cannot be directed to the same object; also called a squint
sty(e) (stī)	Inflammation of one or more of the sebaceous glands of the eyelid; also called a hordeolum
trachoma (tră-kō′ mă)	A chronic contagious disease of the conjunctiva and cornea. The disease affects millions of people, mostly in Asia and Africa, but is also seen in the southwestern part of the United States
trichiasis (trĭk-ī′ ăs-ĭs)	A condition of ingrowing eyelids that rub against the cornea causing a constant irritation to the eyeball

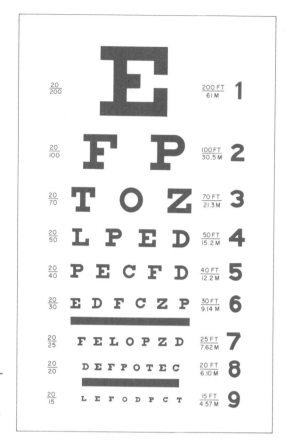

FIGURE 14–3

The Snellen test chart for visual acuity. Individuals with normal vision can read line 8 of the full-sized chart at 20 ft. (*Adapted from Evans WF.* Anatomy and Physiology, *3rd ed. Englewood Cliffs, NJ: Prentice-Hall, 1983, with permission.*)

ABBREVIATIONS

Acc	accomodation		**MY**	myopia
ALT	argon laser trabeculoplasty		**NVA**	near visual acuity
D	diopter		**OD**	oculus dexter (right eye)
DVA	distance visual acuity		**OS**	oculus sinister (left eye)
ECCE	extracapsular cataract extraction		**OU**	ocului unitas (both eyes)
EM	emmetropia		**PERLA**	pupils equal, react to light and accommodation
EOM	extraocular movement; extraocular muscles		**RE**	right eye
			REM	rapid eye movement
HT	hypermetropia (hyperopia)		**SMD**	senile macular degeneration
ICCE	intracapsular cataract cryoextraction		**ST**	esotropia
			VA	visual acuity
IOL	intraocular lens		**VF**	visual field
IOP	intraocular pressure		**XT**	exotropia
L & A	light and accommodation		**+**	plus or convex
LE	left eye		**−**	minus or concave
LTP	laser trabeculoplasty			

Drug Highlights

Drugs that are generally used for the eye include those that are used for glaucoma, during diagnostic examination of the eye, and in intraocular surgery. Antibiotics, antifungal, and antiviral drugs are used in the treatment of eye infections.

Drugs Used to Treat Glaucoma

Either increase the outflow of aqueous humor, decrease its production, or produce both of these actions. These drugs may be diuretics, cholinergics, and/or cholinesterase inhibitors.

Diuretics

Examples: Diamox (acetazolamide), Daranide (dichlorphenamide), Glycerol (glycerin), Osmitrol (mannitol), and Ureaphil (urea).

Cholinergics

Examples: Miochol (acetylcholine chloride) and Carbacel (carbachol).

Cholinesterase Inhibitors

Examples: Humorsol (demecarium bromide), Phospholine Iodide (echothiophate), Floropryl (isoflurophate), and Eserine Sulfate (physostigmine sulfate).

Mydriatics

Agents that are used to produce dilation of the pupil (mydriasis) may be anticholinergics or sympathomimetics.

Anticholinergics

Produce dilation of the pupil and interfere with the ability of the eye to focus properly (cycloplegia). They are used primarily as an aid in refraction, during internal examination of the eye, in intraocular surgery, and in the treatment of anterior uveitis and secondary glaucomas.

Examples: Atropisol (atropine sulfate), Cyclogyl (cyclopentolate HCl), Homatrocel (homatropine HBr), Hyoscine (scopolamine HBr), and Mydriacyl (tropicamide).

Sympathomimetics

Produced mydriasis without cycloplegia. Pupil dilation is obtained as the drug causes contraction of the dilator muscle of the iris. They also affect intraocular pressure by decreasing production of aqueous humor while increasing its outflow from the eye.

Examples: Propine (dipivefrin), Paredrine (hydroxyamphetamine HBr), Naphcon (naphazoline HCl), and Murine, Visine (tetrahydrozoline HCl).

Antibiotics

Used to treat infectious diseases. Those that are used for the eye may be in the form of an ointment, cream, or solution.

Examples: Aureomycin ophthalmic (chlortetracycline hydrochloride) ointment 1%, erythromycin, bacitracin, tetracycline HCl, chloramphenicol, and polymyxin B sulfate.

Antifungal Agent

Natacyn (natamycin) is used in treating fungal infections of the eye, such as blepharitis, conjunctivitis, and keratitis.

Antiviral Agents

Stoxil, Herplex (idoxuridine) is a potent antiviral agent used in the treatment of keratitis caused by the herpes simplex virus. *Vira-A (vidarabine) and Viroptic (trifluridine)* are also used to treat viral infections of the eye and are effective in the treatment of herpes simplex infections.

Communication Enrichment

This segment is provided for those who wish to enhance their ability to communicate in either English or Spanish.

RELATED TERMS

English	Spanish
blind	ciego (sĭ-ĕ-gō)
blindness	ceguedad (sĕ-gĕ-dăd)
cloudy vision	visión nublada (vĭ-sĭ-ōn nū-blă-dă)
double vision	visión doble (vĭ-sĭ-ōn dō-blĕ)
cataract	catarata (că-tă-ră-tă)
conjunctiva	conjuntiva (cōn-hūn-tĭ-vă)
contact lens	lente de contacto (lĕn-tĕ dĕ cōn-tăc-tō)
for distance	para distancia (pă-ră dĭs-tăn-sĭ-ă)
for close-up	para de cerca (pă-ră dĕ sĕr-kă)
for reading	para leer (pă-ră lĕ-ĕr)
all the time	todo el tiempo (tō-dō ĕl tĭ-ĕm-pō)
since when	¿desde cuándo? (dĕs-dĕ kwan-dō)
eyebrow	ceja (sĕ-hă)
eyelash	pestaña (pĕs-tan-yă)
eyelid	párpado (păr-pă-do)
eye	ojo (ō-hō)
eyeglasses	anteojos; espejuelos (ăn-tĕ-ō-hō; ĕs-pĕ-hū-ĕ-lōs)
glaucoma	glaucoma (glă-ū-cō-mă)
pupil	pupila (pū-pĭ-lă)

English	Spanish
vision	visión *(vĭ-sĭ-ōn)*
loss of	pérdida de visión *(pĕr-dĭ-dă dĕ vĭ-sĭ-ōn)*
problems	problemas *(prō-blĕ-măs)*
test	examen *(ex-să-mĕn)*
laser	láser *(lă-sĕr)*
view	paisaje *(pă-ĭ-să-hĕ)*
conjunctivitis	conjuntivitis *(con-hūn-tĭ-vĭ-tĭs)*
near	cerca *(sĕr-kă)*
far	lejos *(lĕ-hōs)*
see	ver *(vĕr)*
sight	vista *(vĭs-tă)*
cornea	córnea *(cōr-nĕ-ă)*
lens	lente *(lĕn-tĕ)*
optic	óptico *(ōp-tĭ-kō)*
orbit	órbita *(ōr-bĭ-tă)*
iris	iris *(ĭ-rĭs)*
tear	lágrima *(lă-grĭ-ma)*

DIAGNOSTIC AND LABORATORY TESTS

Test	Description
color vision tests (kul′ or vĭzh′ ŭn test)	The use of polychromatic plates or an anomaloscope to assess the ability to recognize differences in color
exophthalmometry (ĕk″ sŏf-thăl-mŏm′ ĕ-trē)	Measurement of the forward protrusion of the eye via an exophthalmometer; used to evaluate an increase or decrease in exophthalmos
gonioscopy (gō″ nē-ŏs′ kō-pē)	Examination of the anterior chamber of the eye via a gonioscope; used for determining ocular motility and rotation

Test	Description
keratometry (kĕr″ ă-tŏm′ ĕ-trē)	Measurement of the cornea via a keratometer
ocular ultrasonography (ŏk′ ū lăr ŭl-tră-sŏn-ŏg′ ră-fē)	The use of high-frequency sound waves (via a small probe placed on the eye) to measure for intraocular lenses and to detect orbital and periorbital lesions; also used to measure the length of the eye and the curvature of the cornea in preparation for surgery
ophthalmoscopy (ŏf-thăl-mŏs′ kō-pē)	Examination of the interior of the eyes via an ophthalmoscope; used to identify changes in the blood vessels in the eye and to diagnose systemic diseases
tonometry (tōn-ŏm′ ĕ-trē)	Measurement of the intraocular pressure of the eye via a tonometer; used to screen for and detect glaucoma
visual acuity (vĭzh′ ū-ăl ă-kū′ ĭ-tē)	Measurement of the acuteness or sharpness of vision. A Snellen eye chart may be used, and the patient reads letters of various sizes from a distance of 20 ft. Normal vision is 20/20

Learning Exercises

Anatomy and Physiology

Write your answers to the following questions. Do not refer back to the text.

1. The external structures of the eye are the _____ , _____ , _____ , _____ , and the _____ _____ .

2. The orbit is lined with _____ _____ , which cushions the eyeball.

3. The optic foramen is an opening for the _____ _____ and _____ _____ .

4. State the functions of the muscles of the eye.

    a. _____

    b. _____

5. Each eye has a pair of eyelids that function to protect the eyeball from _____ _____ , _____ _____ , and _____ .

6. Describe the conjunctiva and state its function. _____ _____

7. Define lacrimal apparatus. _____ _____

8. The internal structures of the eye are the _____ , _____ , and the _____ _____ .

9. The eyeball is the organ of _____ .

10. The point at which nerve fibers from the retina converge to form the optic nerve is known as the _____ _____ .

11. Define accommodation. _____ _____

12. Match the following terms and definitions by placing the correct letter on the line provided.

    _____ 1. Aqueous humor   a. White of the eye

    _____ 2. Vitreous humor   b. Colored membrane attached to the ciliary body

    _____ 3. Iris   c. Watery fluid

    _____ 4. Sclera   d. Opening in the center of the iris

    _____ 5. Uvea   e. Jelly-like material

    _____ 6. Pupil   f. Middle layer of the eyeball

    _____ 7. Retina   g. Anterior transparent portion of the eyeball

    _____ 8. Rods and cones   h. Innermost layer of the eyeball

    _____ 9. Lens   i. Photoreceptive cells

    _____ 10. Cornea   j. Colorless crystalline body

Word Parts

1. In the spaces provided, write the definitions for the following prefixes, roots, combining forms, and suffixes. Do not refer to the listings of terminology words. Leave blank those terms you cannot define.
2. After completing as many as you can, refer back to the terminology word listings to check your work. For each word missed or left blank, write the term and its definition several times on the margins of these pages or on a separate sheet of paper.
3. To maximize the learning process, it is to your advantage to do the following exercises as directed. To refer to the terminology listings before completing these exercises invalidates the learning process.

PREFIXES

Give the definitions of the following prefixes:

1. a- _____   2. bi- _____

3. dipl- _____   4. ec- _____

5. em- _____   6. eso- _____

7. hyper- _____   8. intra- _____

9. tri- _____

ROOTS AND COMBINING FORMS

Give the definitions of the following roots and combining forms:

1. ambly _____   2. ametr _____

3. aniso _____   4. blephar _____

5. blepharo _____   6. choroid _____

7. choroido _____   8. cor _____

9. corne _____   10. cycl _____

11. cyclo _____   12. cyst _____

13. dacry _____   14. dacryo _____

15. electro _____   16. foc _____

17. gonio _____   18. irid _____

19. irido _____   20. kerat _____

21. kerato _____   22. lacrim _____

23. log _____   24. metr _____

25. my _____   26. myo _____

27. nyctal _____   28. ocul _____

29. ophthalm _____   30. ophthalmo _____

31. opt _____   32. opto _____

33. phaco _____   34. phak _____

35. photo _____   36. presby _____

37. pupill	_____	38. retin	_____
39. retino	_____	40. scler	_____
41. stigmat	_____	42. tono	_____
43. trop	_____	44. uve	_____
45. xen	_____	46. xer	_____

SUFFIXES

Give the definitions of the following suffixes:

1. -al	_____	2. -ar	_____
3. -ary	_____	4. -blast	_____
5. -desis	_____	6. -ectomy	_____
7. -gram	_____	8. -graphy	_____
9. -ia	_____	10. -ic	_____
11. -ion	_____	12. -ism	_____
13. -ist	_____	14. -itis	_____
15. -logy	_____	16. -lysis	_____
17. -malacia	_____	18. -meter	_____
19. -oma	_____	20. -opia	_____
21. -osis	_____	22. -pathy	_____
23. -phobia	_____	24. -plasty	_____
25. -plegia	_____	26. -ptosis	_____
27. -scope	_____	28. -tasis	_____

Identifying Medical Terms

In the spaces provided, write the medical terms for the following meanings:

1. _____ Dullness of vision

2. _____ Pertaining to having two foci

3. _____ A drooping of the upper eyelid

4. _____ Pertaining to the cornea

5. _____ A tumor-like swelling caused by obstruction of the tear duct

6. _____ Double vision

7. _____ Normal or perfect vision

8. _____ Pertaining to within the eye

9. _____ A softening of the iris

10. _____ Inflammation of the cornea

11. _____ Surgical repair of the cornea

12. _____ Pertaining to tears

13. _____ Pertaining to the eye

14. _____ Any eye disease

15. _____ Unusual intolerance of light

Spelling

In the spaces provided, write the correct spelling of these misspelled terms:

1. atigmatism _____ 2. cyloplegia _____

3. irdectomy _____ 4. opthalmologist _____

5. pacosclerosis _____ 6. pupilary _____

7. retinblastoma _____ 8. sleritis _____

9. tonmeter _____ 10. ueal _____

Review Questions

Matching

Select the appropriate lettered meaning for each numbered line.

_____ 1. anomaloscope

_____ 2. entropion

_____ 3. epiphora

_____ 4. hemianopia

_____ 5. phacoemulsification

_____ 6. photocoagulation

_____ 7. radial keratotomy

_____ 8. retrolental fibroplasia

_____ 9. strabismus

_____ 10. sty(e)

a. A squint

b. A disease of the retinal vessels present in premature infants

c. The process of using ultrasound to disintegrate a cataract

d. The use of a laser to treat retinal detachment and/or retinal bleeding

e. An instrument used for detecting color blindness

f. The turning inward of the margin of the lower eyelid

g. A surgical procedure that may be performed to correct myopia

h. The inability to see half the field of vision

i. A hordeolum

j. The abnormal downpour of tears

k. A disease characterized by increased intraocular pressure

Abbreviations

Place the correct word, phrase, or abbreviation in the space provided.

_____ 1. distance visual acuity

_____ 2. EM

_____ 3. HT

_____ 4. intraocular lens

_____ 5. light and accommodation

_____ 6. MY

_____ 7. OD

_____ 8. left eye

_____ 9. both eyes

_____ 10. XT

Diagnostic and Laboratory Tests

Select the best answer to each multiple choice question. Circle the letter of your choice.

1. The measurement of the forward protrusion of the eye.

   a. gonioscopy

   b. keratometry

   c. exophthalmometry

   d. tonometry

2. The meaurement of the cornea.

   a. gonioscopy

   b. keratometry

   c. exophthalmometry

   d. tonometry

3. Used to identify changes in the blood vessels in the eye and to diagnose systemic diseases.

   a. exophthalmometry

   b. gonioscopy

   c. ophthalmoscopy

   d. tonometry

4. The measurement of the intraocular pressure of the eye.

   a. exophthalmometry

   b. gonioscopy

   c. ophthalmoscopy

   d. tonometry

5. The measurement of the acuteness or sharpness of vision.

   a. color vision tests

   b. ultrasonography

   c. tonometry

   d. visual acuity

15

The Female Reproductive System

The female reproductive system consists of the ovaries, fallopian tubes, uterus, vagina, vulva, and breasts. The ovaries are the primary sex organs of the female and their activity is primarily controlled by the anterior lobe of the pituitary gland. The ovaries produce ova (the female reproductive cells) and hormones. In an average, normal woman more than 400 ova may be produced during her reproductive years.

PROTECT YOURSELF

Most frequently used contraceptives cited by 4000 women ages 18-50

Pill	*86%*
Barrier Method	*76%*
(condom/diaphragm)	
Sterilization	*34%*
Natural Planning	*25%*
IUD	*14%*
DepoProvera	*2%*
Norplant	*1%*
None	*5%*

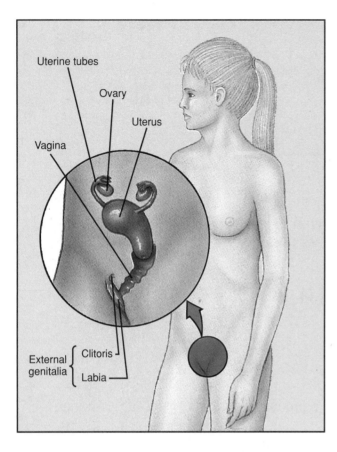

ANATOMY AND PHYSIOLOGY OVERVIEW

The female reproductive system consists of the left and right ovaries, which are the female's primary sex organs, and the following accessory sex organs: two fallopian tubes, the uterus, the vagina, the vulva, and two breasts. The vital function of the female reproductive system is to perpetuate the species through sexual or germ cell reproduction (See Plate 27).

THE REPRODUCTIVE SYSTEM OF THE FEMALE

Organ	Primary Functions
Ovaries	Produce eggs; endocrine function included in Chapter 11
Uterine Tubes	Deliver egg(s) or embryo(s) to uterus; site of normal fertilization
Uterus	Site of embryonic development and diffusion between maternal and embryonic bloodstreams
Vagina	Site of sperm deposition; birth canal at delivery; provides passage of fluids at menses
External Genitalia	
Clitoris	Erectile organ, produces pleasurable sensations during sexual act
Labia	Contain glands that lubricate entrance to vagina
Mammary Glands	Produce milk that nourishes newborn infant

The Uterus

The uterus is a muscular, hollow, pear-shaped organ having three identifiable areas: the body or upper portion, the isthmus or central area, and the cervix, which is the lower cylindrical portion or neck. The fundus is the bulging surface of the body of the uterus extending from the internal os (mouth) of the cervix upward above the fallopian tubes. The uterus is suspended in the anterior part of the pelvic cavity, halfway between the sacrum and the symphysis pubis, above the bladder, and in front of the rectum. A number of ligaments support the uterus and hold it in position. There are two broad ligaments, two round ligaments, two uterosacral ligaments, and the ligaments that are attached to the bladder. The normal position of the uterus is with the cervix pointing toward the lower end of the sacrum and the fundus toward the suprapubic region. An average, normal uterus is about 8 cm long, 5 cm wide, and 2.5 cm thick (Fig. 15-1).

THE UTERINE WALL

The wall of the uterus consists of three layers: the peritoneal or outer layer, the myometrium or muscular middle layer, and the endometrium, which is the mucous membrane lining the inner surface of the uterus. The endometrium is composed of columnar epithelium and connective tissue and is supplied with blood by both straight and spiral arteries. It undergoes marked changes in response to hormonal stimulation during the menstrual cycle. These changes are discussed in the last section of this overview.

FUNCTIONS OF THE UTERUS

There are three primary functions associated with the uterus:

1. It is the organ of the cyclic discharge of a bloody fluid from the uterus and the changes that occur to its endometrium.
2. It functions as a place for the protection and nourishment of the fetus during pregnancy.
3. During labor, the muscular uterine wall contracts rhythmically and powerfully to expel the fetus from the uterus.

ABNORMAL POSITIONS OF THE UTERUS

The uterus may become malpositioned because of weakness of any of its supporting ligaments. Trauma, disease processes of the uterus, or multiple pregnancies may contribute to the weakening of the supporting ligaments. The following terms describe some of the abnormal positions of the uterus:

Anteflexion. The process of bending forward of the uterus at its body and neck

Retroflexion. The process of bending the body of the uterus backward at an angle with the cervix usually unchanged from its normal position

Anteversion. The process of turning the fundus forward toward the pubis, with the cervix tilted up toward the sacrum

Retroversion. The process of turning the uterus backward, with the cervix pointing forward toward the symphysis pubis

The Fallopian Tubes

Also called the uterine tubes or oviducts, the fallopian tubes extend laterally from either side of the uterus and end near each ovary. An average, normal fallopian tube is about 11.5 cm long and 6 mm wide. Its wall is composed of three layers: the serosa or outermost layer, composed of connective tissue; the muscular layer, containing inner circular and outer lon-

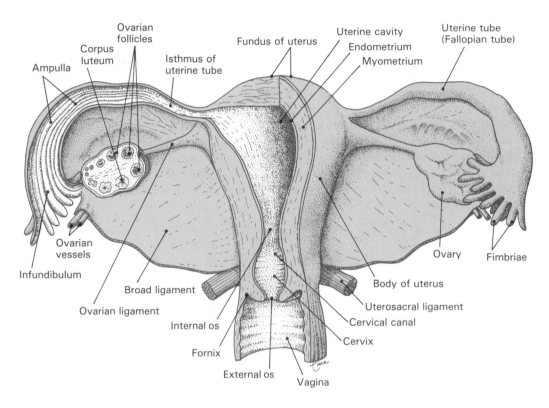

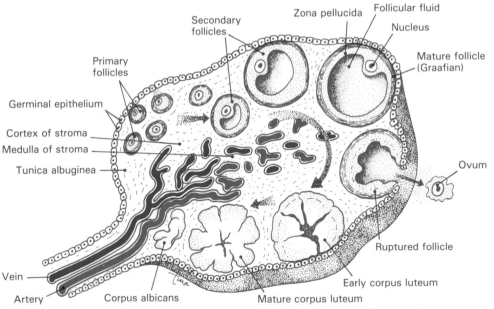

FIGURE 15–1

Details of the uterus, ovary, and associated structures with an exploded view of a mammalian ovary showing successive stages of graafian follicle and ovum development. Begin with primary follicles and follow clockwise to the final stage, corpus albicans. (*Adapted from Evans WF. Anatomy and Physiology, 3rd ed. Englewood Cliffs, NJ: Prentice-Hall, 1983, with permission.*)

gitudinal layers of smooth muscle; and the mucosa or inner layer, consisting of simple columnar epithelium.

ANATOMICAL FEATURES OF THE FALLOPIAN TUBES

The isthmus is the constricted portion of the tube nearest the uterus (see Fig. 15-1). From the isthmus, the tube continues laterally and widens to form a section called the ampulla. Beyond the ampulla, the tube continues to expand and ends as a funnel-shaped opening. This end of the tube is called the infundibulum, and its opening is the ostium. Surrounding each ostium are fimbriae or finger-like processes that work to propel the discharged ovum into the tube, where ciliary action aids in moving it toward the uterus. Should the ovum become impregnated by a spermatozoon while in the tube, the process of fertilization occurs.

FUNCTIONS OF THE FALLOPIAN TUBES

The two basic functions of the fallopian tubes are as follows:

1. Each tube serves as a duct for the conveyance of the ovum from the ovary to the uterus.
2. The tubes serve as ducts for the conveyance of spermatozoa from the uterus toward each ovary.

The Ovaries

Located on either side of the uterus, the ovaries are almond-shaped organs attached to the uterus by the ovarian ligament and lie close to the fimbriae of the fallopian tubes. The anterior border of each ovary is connected to the posterior layer of the broad ligament by the mesovarium. Each ovary is attached to the side of the pelvis by the suspensory ligaments. An average, normal ovary is about 4 cm long, 2 cm wide, and 1.5 cm thick.

MICROSCOPIC ANATOMY

Each ovary consists of two distinct areas: the cortex or outer layer and the medulla or inner portion. The cortex contains small secretory sacs or follicles in three stages of development. These stages are known as primary, growing, and graafian, which is the follicles' mature stage. The ovarian medulla contains connective tissue, nerves, blood and lymphatic vessels, and some smooth muscle tissue in the region of the hilus (see Fig. 15-1).

FUNCTION OF THE OVARIES

The functional activity of the ovary is primarily controlled by the anterior lobe of the pituitary gland, which produces the gonadotropic hormones FSH and LH. These abbreviations are for follicle-stimulating hormone, instrumental in the development of the ovarian follicles, and luteinizing hormone, which stimulates the development of the corpus luteum, a small yellow mass of cells that develops within a ruptured ovarian follicle.

Two functions have been identified for the ovary: the production of ova or female reproductive cells and the production of hormones.

The Production of Ova
Each month a graafian follicle ruptures on the ovarian cortex, and an ovum (singular of ova) discharges into the pelvic cavity where it enters the fallopian tube. This process is known as ovulation. In an average, normal woman more than 400 ova may be produced during her reproductive years (see Fig. 15-1).

The Production of Hormones
The ovary is also an endocrine gland, producing estrogen and progesterone. Estrogen is the female sex hormone secreted by the follicles. Progesterone is a steroid hormone secreted

by the corpus luteum. These hormones are essential in promoting growth, development, and maintenance of the female secondary sex organs and characteristics. They also prepare the uterus for pregnancy, promote development of the mammary glands, and play a vital role in a woman's emotional well-being and sexual drive.

The Vagina

The vagina is a musculomembranous tube extending from the vestibule to the uterus. It is 10 to 15 cm in length and is situated between the bladder and the rectum. It is lined by mucous membrane made up of squamous epithelium. A fold of mucous membrane, the hymen, partially covers the external opening of the vagina (Fig. 15–2 and Plate 11).

FUNCTIONS OF THE VAGINA

The vagina has three basic functions:

1. It is the female organ of copulation. The vagina receives the seminal fluid from the male penis.
2. It serves as a passageway for the discharge of menstruation.
3. It serves as a passageway for the birth of the fetus.

The Vulva

The vulva consists of the following five organs that comprise the external female genitalia (see Fig. 15–2 and Plate 11):

FIGURE 15–2

Sagittal section through the female pelvis, showing organs of the reproductive system. (*Adapted from Evans WF. Anatomy and Physiology, 3rd ed. Englewood Cliffs, NJ: Prentice-Hall, 1983, with permission.*)

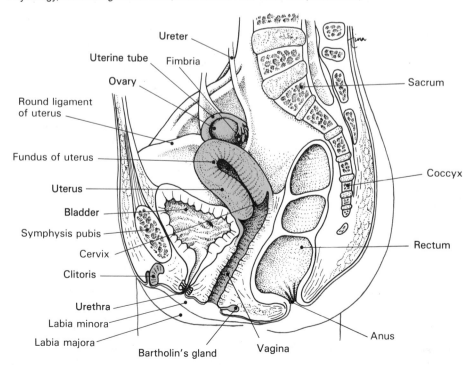

Mons Pubis. A pad of fatty tissue of triangular shape and, after puberty, covered with pubic hair. It may be referred to as the mons veneris or "mound of Venus," and is the rounded area over the symphysis pubis

Labia Majora. The two folds of adipose tissue, which are large lip-like structures, lying on either side of the vaginal opening

Labia Minora. Two thin folds of skin that lie within the labia majora and enclose the vestibule

Vestibule. The cleft between the labia minora. It is approximately 4 to 5 cm long and 2 cm wide. Four major structures open into it: the urethra, the vagina, and two excretory ducts of the Bartholin glands

Clitoris. A small organ consisting of sensitive erectile tissue that is homologous to the penis of the male

Between the vulva and the anus is an external region known as the perineum. It is composed of muscle covered with skin. During the second stage of labor, a decision is made by the attending physician as to the need to perform an episiotomy, a surgical procedure to prevent tearing of the perineum and to facilitate delivery of the fetus.

The Breast

The breasts or mammary glands are compound alveolar structures consisting of 15 to 20 glandular tissue lobes separated by septa of connective tissue. Most women have two breasts that lie anterior to the pectoral muscles and curve outward from the lateral margins of the sternum to the anterior border of the axilla. The size of the breast may greatly vary according to age, heredity, and adipose (fatty) tissue present. The areola is the dark, pigmented area found in the skin over each breast, and the nipple is the elevated area in the center of the areola. During pregnancy, the areola changes from its pinkish color to a dark brown or reddish color. The areola is supplied with a row of small sebaceous glands that secrete an oily substance to keep it resilient. The lactiferous glands consist of 20 to 24 glands in the areola of the nipple and, during lactation, secrete and convey milk to a suckling infant (Fig. 15–3). The hormone prolactin, which is produced by the anterior lobe of the pituitary, stimulates the mammary glands to produce milk after childbirth. Other hormones playing a role in milk production are insulin and glucocorticoids. Colostrum, a thin yellowish secretion, is the "first milk" and contains mainly serum and white blood cells. Suckling stimulates the production of oxytocin by the posterior lobe of the pituitary gland. It acts on the mammary glands to stimulate the release of milk and stimulates the uterus to contract during parturition.

BREAST-FEEDING

Among the natural advantages of breast-feeding are the following:

1. It provides an ideal food for most newborn babies.
2. The milk provides essential nutrients for growth and development.
3. The milk is virtually free from harmful bacteria.

After the first 2 weeks, the nursing mother may produce 1 or more pints of milk per day. Milk production may be affected by emotions, food, fluids, physical health, and medications. The nursing mother will usually have a supply of milk for her suckling infant for a period of 6 to 9 months. The nursing process is usually a satisfying experience for both mother and infant. For the mother, the nursing causes contractions of the muscles of the uterus, which aid in its rapid return to normal size. For the infant, breast milk is a natural substance that provides almost everything needed for the first months of life.

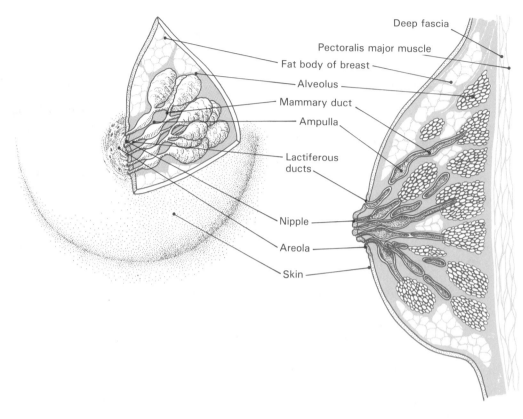

FIGURE 15–3

The breast. (*Adapted from Evans WF.* Anatomy and Physiology, *3rd ed. Englewood Cliffs, NJ: Prentice-Hall, 1983, with permission.*)

The Menstrual Cycle

The onset of the menstrual cycle occurs at the age of puberty and its cessation is at menopause. It is a periodic recurrent series of changes occurring in the uterus, ovaries, vagina, and breasts approximately every 28 days. The menstrual cycle is divided into four phases, each of which is described for you.

MENSTRUATION PHASE

The menstruation phase is characterized by the discharge of a bloody fluid from the uterus accompanied by a shedding of the endometrium. This phase averages 4 to 5 days and is considered to be the first to the fifth days of the cycle.

PROLIFERATION PHASE

The proliferation phase is characterized by the stimulation of estrogen, the thickening and vascularization of the endometrium, along with the maturing of the ovarian follicle. This phase begins about the fifth day and ends at the time of rupture of the graafian follicle—about 14 days before the onset of menstruation.

LUTEAL OR SECRETORY PHASE

The luteal phase is characterized by continued thickening of the endometrium, by the glands within the endometrium becoming tortuous, and by the appearance of coiled arteries in its tissues. The endometrium becomes edematous, and the stroma becomes compact.

During this phase, the corpus luteum in the ovary is developing and secreting progesterone. The progesterone level is highest during this phase as the estrogen level decreases. This phase lasts about 10 to 14 days.

PREMENSTRUAL OR ISCHEMIC PHASE

During the premenstrual phase, the coiled arteries become constricted, the endometrium becomes anemic and begins to shrink, and the corpus luteum decreases in functional activity. This phase lasts about 2 days and ends with the occurrence of menstruation. Premenstrual syndrome is a condition that affects certain women and may cause distressful symptoms such as constipation, diarrhea, nausea, anorexia, appetite cravings, headache, backache, muscular aches, edema, insomnia, clumsiness, malaise, irritability, indecisiveness, mental confusion, and depression. These symptoms may occur 2 weeks before the onset of menstruation. Although the exact cause of this syndrome has not been determined, it may be due to the amount of prostaglandin produced, a deficient or excessive amount of estrogen or progesterone, or an interrelationship between these factors.

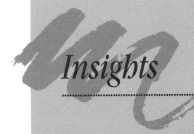
Insights

BIRTH CONTROL

According to the Association of Reproductive Health Professional's survey, four out of five American women ages 18 to 50 are sexually active. Of these, nine out of ten, were interested in becoming more educated about various methods of birth control.

In the United States, there are numerous methods that may be used for birth control and some of these are birth control pills, condoms, a diaphragm, foams, jellies, natural planning, an IUD (intrauterine device), a cervical cap, a contraceptive sponge, a vasectomy, and female sterilization. New methods of birth control that have been approved by the Food and Drug Administration (FDA) include the Norplant System, DEPO-PROVERA contraceptive injection, and the female condom (Reality).

"Case-In-Point"

According to a national survey of men, that was published in an issue of Family Planning Perspectives, nearly all men ages 20–39 in the United States are sexually experienced.

- Twenty-three percent have had 20 or more partners in their lifetimes, yet only 25% say they used a condom in the past 4 weeks.
- Single men (45%) are twice as likely as married men (18%) to use a condom.
- Twenty-seven percent of men say they are embarrassed to buy condoms.

The Norplant System—The Norplant System consists of six thin capsules that contain levonorgestrel (a progestin). The capsules are made of a soft flexible material and are placed in a fan-like pattern just under the skin, on the inside surface of the upper arm.

Contraceptive action that is 99% effective begins within hours and last up to 5 years. The capsules must be removed at the end of 5 years and the contraceptive effect stops within 24 hours.

Prior to the placement of the Norplant System, a complete medical history and physical examination are performed. It is recommended that the capsules be inserted within 7 days after the onset of menses, during menses, or immediately following an abortion. The patient who chooses this method should be carefully evaluated on a regular basis and the physician should inform her about warnings and possible side effects.

Reported side effects of the Norplant System include prolonged menstrual bleeding, unexpected bleeding, spotting between periods, no bleeding at all for several months, and/or a combination of these. There are other side effects that may occur and the patient should report any unusual symptoms to her physician.

(Insights continues on next page.)

DEPO-PROVERA—DEPO-PROVERA is a contraceptive injection (medroxyprogesterone acetate) and when administered at the recommended dose to women every 3 months, it inhibits the secretion of gonadotropins, which, in turn, prevents follicular maturation and ovulation and results in endometrial thinning. These actions produce its contraceptive effect, which is 99% effective. DEPO-PROVERA is given as an intramuscular injection in the dorsogluteal area or in the deltoid muscle.

Before the initiation of this type of contraception, the patient should have a complete medical history and physical examination performed. The physician should inform the patient of precautions, warnings, adverse reactions, and possible side effects. Because DEPO-PROVERA is a long-acting birth control method, it takes some time after the last injection for its effect to wear off.

The Female Condom (Reality)—The FDA approved the use of Reality in 1993. It affords women some protection against sexually transmitted diseases, including AIDS, as well as pregnancy. The female condom in tests had a 26% failure rate in preventing pregnancy, and the FDA stresses that male latex condoms are better safeguards against pregnancy and disease.

Reality is a prelubricated polyurethane sheath that has flexible polyurethane rings on each end, one of which is inserted into the vagina like a diaphragm. One of its two flexible rings holds the device in place, fitting over the cervix, and the other ring forms the external edge and remains outside the vagina. It shields the entire vaginal and urethral area from the shaft and base of the penis. It provides women with an opportunity to protect themselves when their sexual partner refuses to use a male condom.

Terminology with Surgical Procedures & Pathology

Term	Word Parts			Definition
abortion (ă-bōr′ shŭn)	abort ion	R S	to miscarry process	The process of miscarrying
amenorrhea (ă-měn″ ō-rē′ ă)	a meno rrhea	P CF S	lack of month flow	A lack of the monthly flow or menstruation
amniocentesis (ăm″ nĭ-ō-sĕn-tē′ sĭs)	amnio centesis	CF S	lamb surgical puncture	Surgical puncture of the amniotic sac to obtain a sample of amniotic fluid
amniotome (ăm′ nĭ-ō-tōm)	amnio tome	CF S	lamb instrument to cut	An instrument used to cut fetal membranes
anovular (ăn-ŏv′ ū-lăr)	an ovul ar	P R S	lack of ovary pertaining to	Pertaining to the lack of production and discharge of an ovum
antenatal (ăn″ tē-nā′ tal)	ante nat al	P R S	before birth pertaining to	Pertaining to before birth
ante partum (ăn′ tē pär′ tŭm)	ante partum	P R	before labor	The time before the onset of labor
bartholinitis (bar″ tō-lĭn-ī′ tĭs)	bartholin itis	R S	Bartholin's glands inflammation	Inflammation of Bartholin's glands
catamenia (kăt ă-mē′ nĭ-ă)	cata men ia	P R S	down month condition	The condition of monthly discharge of blood from the uterus
cervicitis (sĕr-vĭ-sī′ tĭs)	cervic itis	R S	cervix inflammation	Inflammation of the uterine cervix
colpoperineo-plasty (kŏl″ pō-pĕr″ĭn-ē′ ō-plăs″tē)	colpo perineo plasty	CF CF S	vagina perineum surgical repair	Surgical repair of the vagina and perineum
colporrhaphy (kŏl-pōr′ ă-fē)	colpo rrhaphy	CF S	vagina suture	Suture of the vagina
colposcope (kŏl′ pō-skōp)	colpo scope	CF S	vagina instrument	An instrument used to examine the vagina and cervix by means of a magnifying lens

(Terminology—continued)

Term	Word Parts			Definition
conception (kŏn-sĕp′ shŭn)	con cept ion	P R S	together receive process	Process of the union of the male's sperm and the female's ovum; fertilization
contraception (kŏn″ tră-sĕp′ shŭn)	contra cept ion	P R S	against receive process	Process of preventing conception
culdocentesis (kŭl″ dō-sĕn-tē′ sĭs)	culdo centesis	CF S	cul-de-sac surgical puncture	Surgical puncture of the cul-de-sac for removal of fluid
cystocele (sĭs′ tō-sēl)	cysto cele	CF S	bladder hernia	A hernia of the bladder that protrudes into the vagina
dysmenorrhea (dĭs″ mĕn-ō-rē′ ă)	dys meno rrhea	P CF S	difficult, painful month flow	Difficult or painful monthly flow
dyspareunia (dĭs′ pă-rū′ nĭ-ă)	dys par eunia	P P R	difficult, painful beside a bed	Difficult or painful sexual intercourse
dystocia (dĭs-tō′ sĭ-ă)	dys toc ia	P R S	difficult, painful birth condition	The condition of a difficult and painful childbirth
endometriosis (ĕn″ dō-mĕ″ trĭ-ō′ sĭs)	endo metri osis	P CF S	within uterus condition of	A condition in which endometrial tissue occurs in various sites in the abdominal or pelvic cavity
episiotomy (ĕ-pĭs″ ĭ-ŏt′ ō-mē)	episio tomy	CF S	vulva, pudenda incision	Incision of the perineum to prevent tearing of the perineum and to facilitate delivery
eutocia (ū-tō′ sĭ-ă)	eu toc ia	P R S	good, normal birth condition	The condition of a good, normal childbirth
fibroma (fĭ-brō′ mă)	fibr oma	R S	fibrous tissue tumor	A fibrous tissue tumor
genitalia (jĕn-ĭ-tāl′ ĭ-ă)	genital ia	R S	belonging to birth condition	The male or female reproductive organs

(Terminology—continued)

Term	Word Parts			Definition
gynecologist (gī″ nĕ-kŏl′ ō-jĭst)	gyneco log ist	CF R S	female study of one who specializes	One who specializes in the study of the female
gynecology (gī″ nĕ-kŏl′ ō-jē)	gyneco logy	CF S	female study of	The study of the female
hematosalpinx (hē″ mă-tō-săl′ pĭnks)	hemato salpinx	CF R	blood tube	A collection of blood in the fallopian tube that may be associated with tubal pregnancy
hymenectomy (hī″ mĕn-ĕk′ tō-mē)	hymen ectomy	R S	hymen excision	Surgical excision of the hymen
hysterectomy (hĭs″ tĕr-ĕk′ tō-mē)	hyster ectomy	R S	womb, uterus excision	Surgical excision of the uterus
hysterotomy (hĭs″ tĕr-ŏt′ ō-mē)	hystero tomy	CF S	womb, uterus incision	Incision into the uterus; also called a cesarean section
intrauterine (ĭn′ tră-ū′ tĕr-ĭn)	intra uter ine	P R S	within uterus pertaining to	Pertaining to within the uterus
mammography (măm-ŏg′ ră-fē)	mammo graphy	CF S	breast recording	Process of obtaining pictures of the breast by the use of roentgen gays
mammoplasty (măm′ ō-plăs″ tē)	mammo plasty	CF S	breast surgical repair	Surgical repair of the breast
mastectomy (măs-tĕk′ tō-mē)	mast ectomy	R S	breast excision	Surgical excision of the breast
mastitis (măs-tī′ tĭs)	mast itis	R S	breast inflammation	Inflammation of the breast
menopause (mĕn′ ō-pawz)	meno pause	CF R	month cessation	Cessation of the monthly flow; also called climacteric
menorrhagia (mĕn″ ō-rā′ jĭ-ă)	meno rrhagia	CF S	month to burst forth	Excessive bursting forth of blood at the time of the monthly flow
menorrhea (mĕn″ ō-rē′ ă)	meno rrhea	CF S	month flow	A normal monthly flow
multipara (mŭl-tĭp′ ă-ră)	multi para	P R	many to bear	A woman who has borne more than one child

(Terminology—continued)

Term	Word Parts			Definition
myometritis (mī″ ō-mē-trī′ tĭs)	myo metr itis	CF R S	muscle womb, uterus inflammation	Inflammation of the muscular wall of the uterus
neonatal (nē″ ō-nā′ tăl)	neo nat al	P R S	new birth pertaining to	Pertaining to the first 4 weeks after birth
nullipara (nŭl-ĭp′ ă-ră)	nulli para	P R	none to bear	A woman who has borne no offspring
oligomenorrhea (ŏl″ ĭ-gō-měn″ ō-rē′ ă)	oligo meno rrhea	P CF S	scanty month flow	A scanty monthly flow
oogenesis (ō″ ō-jěn′ ě-sĭs)	oo genesis	CF S	ovum, egg formation, produce	Formation of the ovum
oophorectomy (ō″ ŏf-ō-rěk′ tō-mē)	oophor ectomy	R S	ovary excision	Surgical excision of an ovary
oophoritis (ō″ ŏf-ō-rī′ tĭs)	oophor itis	R S	ovary inflammation	Inflammation of an ovary
panhysterectomy (păn″ hĭs-těr-ěk′ tō-mē)	pan hyster ectomy	P R S	all womb, uterus excision	Surgical excision of the entire uterus
pelvimetry (pěl-vĭm′ ět-rē)	pelvi metry	CF S	pelvis measurement	Measurement of the pelvis to determine its capacity and diameter
perinatalogy (pěr″ ĭ-nă-tŏl′ ō-jē)	peri nata logy	P CF S	around birth study of	Study of the fetus and infant from 20–29 weeks of gestation to 1–4 weeks after birth
postcoital (pōst-kō′ ĭt-ăl)	post coit al	P R S	after a coming together pertaining to	Pertaining to after sexual intercourse
postpartum (pōst păr′ tŭm)	post partum	P R	after labor	Pertaining to after childbirth
prenatal (prē-nā′ tl)	pre nat al	P R S	before birth pertaining to	Pertaining to before birth
primipara (prī-mĭp′ ă-ră)	primi para	P R	first to bear	A woman who is bearing her first child

(Terminology—continued)

Term	Word Parts			Definition
pseudocyesis	pseudo	P	false	A false pregnancy
(sū″ dŏ-sī-ē′ sĭs)	cyesis	S	pregnancy	
pyometritis	pyo	CF	pus	Purulent (pus) inflammation
(pī″ ŏ-mē-trī′ tĭs)	metr	R	womb, uterus	of the uterus
	itis	S	inflammation	
pyosalpinx	pyo	CF	pus	Accumulation of pus in the
(pī″ ō-săl′ pĭnks)	salpinx	R	tube	fallopian tube
rectovaginal	recto	CF	rectum	Pertaining to the rectum and
(rĕk″ tō-văj′ ĭ-năl)	vagin	R	vagina	vagina
	al	S	pertaining to	
retroversion	retro	P	backward	The process of being turned
(rĕt″ rō-vur′ shŭn)	vers	R	turning	backward, such as the
	ion	S	process	displacement of the uterus
				with the cervix pointed
				forward
salpingectomy	salping	R	tube	Surgical excision of a fallopian
(săl″ pĭn-jĕk′ tō-mē)	ectomy	S	excision	tube
salpingitis	salping	R	tube	Inflammation of a fallopian
(săl″ pĭn-jī′ tĭs)	itis	S	inflammation	tube
salpingo-oophor-ectomy	salpingo	CF	tube	Surgical excision of an ovary
	oophor	R	ovary	and a fallopian tube
(săl′ pĭng″ gō-ō″ ŏf-ō-rĕk′ tō-mē)	ectomy	S	excision	
trimester	tri	P	three	A period of 3 months
(trī-mĕs′ tĕr)	mester	R	month	
vaginitis	vagin	R	vagina	Inflammation of the vagina
(văj″ ĭn-ī′ tĭs)	itis	S	inflammation	
venereal	venere	R	sexual intercourse	Pertaining to or resulting from
(vē-nē′ rē-ăl)				sexual intercourse
	al	S	pertaining to	

Vocabulary Words

Vocabulary words are terms that have not been divided into component parts. They are common words or specialized terms associated with the subject of this chapter. These words are provided to enhance your medical vocabulary.

Word	Definition
amniocentesis (ăm″ nĭ-ō-sĕn-tē′ sĭs)	A surgical puncture of the amniotic sac to obtain amniotic fluid from which it can be determined if the fetus has Down syndrome, neural tube defects, Tay-Sach's disease, or other genetic defects
biotics (bī-ŏt′ ĭks)	The science of living organisms and the sum of knowledge regarding the life process
blastocyst (blăs′ tō-sĭst)	An embryonic cell mass that attaches to the uterus wall and is a stage in the development of a mammalian embryo
decidua (dē-sĭd′ ū-ă)	The endometrium or mucous membrane of the pregnant uterus that envelops the impregnated ovum
diagnostic ultrasound (dī″ ăg-nŏs′ tĭk ŭl′ tră-sŏund)	The use of extremely high-frequency sound waves for the purpose of diagnosing genetic defects and hydrocephalic conditions in the unborn fetus
Doppler ultrasound (däp′ lər ŭl′ trăh-sŏund)	A procedure using an audio transformation of high-frequency sounds to monitor the fetal heartbeat
fetus (fē′ tŭs)	The developing young in the uterus from the third month to birth
gamete intrafallopian transfer (GIFT) (găm′ ēt ĭn″ tră-fă-lō′ pē-ăn)	A procedure that places the sperm (spermatozoa) and eggs (oocytes) directly in the fimbriated end of the fallopian tube via a laparoscope
genetics (jĕn-ĕt′ ĭks)	The science of biology that studies the phenomenon of heredity and the laws governing it
hysteroscope (hĭs′ tĕr-ō-skōp)	An instrument used in the biopsy of uterine tissue before 12 weeks of gestation. This tissue is then analyzed for chromosome arrangement, DNA sequence, and genetic defects
laser ablation (lā′ zĕr ăb-lā′ shŭn)	A procedure that uses a laser to destroy the uterine lining. A biopsy is performed before the procedure to make sure no cancer is present. This procedure may be used for disabling menstrual bleeding. It does cause sterility
laser laparoscopy (lā′ zĕr lăp-ăr-ŏs′ kō-pē)	A procedure that uses a long, telescope-like instrument equipped with a laser, lights, and a tiny video camera. It may be used to explore the abdominal area and to treat ectopic pregnancy

(Vocabulary—continued)

Word	Definition
laser lumpectomy (lā-zĕr lŭm-pĕk′ tō-mē)	The use of a contact Yag laser to remove a tumor from the breast. It appears to cause less pain for the patient and discharge time from the hospital is sooner
lumpectomy (lŭm-pĕk′ tō-mē)	The surgical removal of a tumor from the breast. In this procedure, no other tissue or lymph nodes are removed, only the tumor; usually not considered for large tumors, although the latest strategy involves shrinking large tumors with chemotherapy so that they become small enough to be removed by this method
menarche (mĕn-ar′ kē)	The beginning of the monthly flow; menses
mittelschmerz (mĭt′ ĕl-shmārts)	Abdominal pain that occurs midway between the menstrual periods at ovulation
morula (mor′ ū-lă)	A solid mass of cells resulting from cell division after fertilization of an ovum
nonstress test (nŏn′ strĕs tĕst)	A diagnostic procedure, often done in a physician's office, wherein a monitor is placed on the mother's abdomen and fetal heartbeats are recorded. The fetal heartbeats should accelerate if the fetus moves
ovulation (ŏv″ ū-lā′ shăn)	The process in which an ovum is discharged form the cortex of the ovary
ovum transfer (ō′ vum trăns′ fer)	A method of fertilization for women who cannot conceive children. A donor ovum is impregnated within the donor's body by artificial insemination and later transferred to the recipient female
"parking" (părk′ ĭng)	A surgical procedure in which the fallopian tube is detached from the ovary. An incision is made into the peritoneum and the tube is sewn into it. This is a reversible sterilization procedure
parturition (par″ tū-rĭsh′ ŭn)	The act of giving birth; also known as childbirth or delivery
pudendal (pū-dĕn′ dăl)	Pertaining to the external female genitalia
puerperium (pū″ ĕr-pē′ rĭ-ŭm)	The 4 to 6 weeks after childbirth when the female generative organs usually return to a normal state
quickening (kwĭk′ ĕn-ĭng)	The first movement of the fetus felt in the uterus, occurring during the 16th to 20th week of pregnancy
secundines (sĕk′ ŭn-dīnz)	The afterbirth consisting of the placenta, umbilical cord, and fetal membranes

(Vocabulary—continued)

Word	Definition
sonogram (sŏ′ nŏ-grăm)	A procedure using high-frequency sound waves to display a visual echo image of the fetus; used to determine size of the fetus and to diagnose genetic defects
surrogate mother (sur′ ŏ-gāt mŭth′ ēr)	A female who contracts to bear a child for another. Pregnancy may occur as a result of artificial insemination
"test-tube baby" (tĕs′ tūb bā′ bē)	An *in vitro* fertilization technique whereby the ovum is fertilized outside the body and later implanted in the host female
toxic shock syndrome (tŏk′ sĭk shŏk sĭn′ drōm)	A poisonous *Staphylococcus aureus* infection that may strike young, menstruating women
uterine adnexa (ū′ tĕr-ĭn ăd-nĕk′ sah)	The ovaries and fallopian tubes
zygote (zī′ gōt)	The fertilized ovum. The zygote is produced by the union of two gametes

ABBREVIATIONS

AB	abortion	**grav I**	pregnancy one
AFP	alpha-fetoprotein	**Gyn**	gynecology
AH	abdominal hysterectomy	**HCG**	human chorionic
BBT	basal body temperature		gonadotropin
C-section	cesarean section	**HRT**	hormone replacement
CS	cesarean section		therapy
CVS	chorionic villus sampling	**HSG**	hysterosalpingography
D&C	dilation (dilatation) and	**IUD**	intrauterine device
	curettage	**LH**	luteinizing hormone
DES	diethylstilbestrol	**LMP**	last menstrual period
DUB	dysfunctional uterine	**MH**	marital history
	bleeding	**OB**	obstetrics
EDC	expected date of	**PAP**	Papanicolaou (smear)
	confinement	**PID**	pelvic inflammatory disease
FSH	follicle-stimulating	**PMP**	previous menstrual period
	hormone	**PMS**	premenstrual syndrome
GIFT	gamete intrafallopian	**TSS**	toxic shock syndrome
	transfer	**UC**	uterine contractions

Drug Highlights

Drugs that are generally used for the female reproductive system include hormones, contraceptives, and those used during labor and delivery.

Female Hormones

Estrogens
Are used for a variety of conditions. They may be used in the treatment of amenorrhea, dysfunctional bleeding, hirsutism, and in palliative therapy for breast cancer in women and prostatic cancer in men. They are also used as replacement therapy in the treatment of uncomfortable symptoms that are related to menopause. In this instance, it is believed that estrogen replacement therapy is useful in preventing osteoporosis and possibly heart disease.

Examples: TACE (chlorotrianisene), Premarin (conjugated estrogens, USP), DES (diethylstilbestrol), Estrace (estradiol), Theelin (estrone), and ESTRADERM (estradiol) Transdermal System.

Progestogens/
Progestins
Synthetic preparations of progesterone. They are used to prevent uterine bleeding, and is combined with estrogen for treatment of amenorrhea. They may be used in cases of infertility and threatened or habitual miscarriage. Progesterone is responsible for changes in the uterine endometrium during the second half of the menstrual cycle, development of maternal placenta after implantation, and development of mammary glands.

Examples: Provera (medroxyprogesterone acetate), Norlutin (norethindrone), Norlutate (norethindrone acetate), and Gesterol (progesterone).

Contraceptives

Oral
Nearly 100% effective when used as directed. These pills contain mixtures of estrogen and progestin in various levels of strength. The estrogen in the pill inhibits ovulation and the progestin inhibits pituitary secretion of luteinizing hormone (LH), causes changes in the cervical mucus that renders it unfavorable to penetration by sperm, and alters the nature of the endometrium.

Examples: Ortho-Novum 10/11–21, Triphasil-21, Micronor, Enovid-E 21, Ovulen-28, Brevicon 21-day, Demulen 1/50–21, and Lo/Ovral-21.

The Norplant
System
Consists of six thin capsules that contain levonorgestrel (a progestin). The capsules are made of a soft flexible material and are placed in a fan-like pattern just under the skin on the inside surface of the upper arm. They have a 99% effective contraceptive action that begins within hours after placement and lasts up to 5 years.

Uterine Stimulants

Oxytocic agents (uterine stimulants) may be used in obstetrics to induce labor at term. They are also used to control postpartum hemorrhage and to induce therapeutic abortion.

Examples: Ergotate Maleate (ergonovine maleate) and Pitocin (oxytocin).

Uterine Relaxants   May be administered to delay labor until the fetus has gained sufficient maturity as to be likely to survive outside the uterus.

Examples: Ethanol (ethyl alcohol) and Yutopar (ritodrine HCl).

Communication Enrichment

This segment is provided for those who wish to enhance their ability to communicate in either English or Spanish.

RELATED TERMS

English	Spanish
abortion	aborto (ă-*bōr*-tō)
breast examination	examen de pecho (ex-*să*-měn dě *pě*-chō)
breasts	pechos; senos (*pe*-chōs; *sě*-nōs)
cesarean	cesarea (sě-*să*-rě-ă)
contraception	contracepción (cōn-tră-*cěp*-sǐ-ōn)
Do you use?	¿usa? (¿*ū*-să?)
the pill	la píldora (lă pǐl-*dō*-ră)
the diaphragm	el diafragma (ěl *dǐ*-ă-frăg-mă)
an IUD	un dispositivo ultra intrauterino (ūn dǐs-*pō*-sǐ-*tǐ*-vō *ūl*-tră *ū*-tě-rǐ-nō)
foam	espuma (ěs-*pū*-mă)
condoms	preservativos (condones) (*prě*-sěr-vă-tǐ-vōs; cōn-*dō*-něs)
the rhythm method	el método de ritmo (ěl *mě*-tō-dō dě *rǐt*-mō)
the method of withdrawal	el método de retirar (ěl *mě*-tō-dō dě *rě*-tǐ-răr)
abstinence	abstinencia (ăbs-tǐ-*něn*-sǐ-ă)
injection	inyección (ín-jěc-sǐ-*ōn*)
cramps	calambres (că-*lăm*-brěs)

English	Spanish
delivery	parto (*pă*r-tō)
episiotomy	episiotomia (ĕ-*pĭ*-sĭ-ō-tō-mĭ-ă)
intercourse	acto sexual; cópula (ăk-*tō sĕx*-sū-ăl; *cō*-pū-lă)
lump	protuberancia (prō-tū-bĕ-*răn*-sĭ-ă)
marital status	estado civil (ĕs-*tă*-dō *sĭ*-vĭl)
menopause	menopausia (mĕ-nō-*pă*-ū-sĭ-ă)
menstrual history	historia menstrual (ĭs-*tō*-rĭ-ă *mĕns*-trū-ăl)
multiple births	nacimientos múltiples (*nă*-sĭ-mĭ-ĕn-tōs *mūl*-tĭ-plĕs)
nipple	pezón (pĕ-*zōn*)
ovary	ovario (ō-*vă*-rĭ-ō)
Pap smear	papanicolao (*pă*-pă-nĭ-kō-lă-ō)
pelvic examination	examen de la pelvis (ĕx-*să*-mĕn dĕ lă pĕlvĭs)
period	periódo (pĕ-rĭ-ō-dō)
placenta	placenta (plă-*cĕn*-tă)
pregnancy	embarazo; preñez (ĕm-bă-*ră*-zō; prĕn-*yĕz*)
pregnant	embarazada (ĕm-bă-ră-*să*-dă)
premature	prematuro (prĕ-mă-*tū*-rō)
sanitary napkin	toalla sanitaria (tō-*ă*-jă săn-nĭ-*tă*-rĭ-ă)
uterus	útero (*ū*-tĕ-rō)
vagina	vagina (vă-*hĭ*-nă)
womb	matriz (*mă*-trĭz)

DIAGNOSTIC AND LABORATORY TESTS

Test	Description
amniotic fluid analysis (ăm-nē-ŏt′ ĭk floo′ ĭd ă-năl′ ĭ-sĭs)	A procedure that involves the removal of amniotic fluid via a large needle. Ultrasound is used to give the location of the fetus, and then the needle is inserted into a suprapubic site of the mother. Abnormal results can indicate spina bifida, Down's syndrome, hemophilia, hemolytic disease, and/or poor fetal maturity
breast examination (brest ĕks-ăm″ ĭ-nā′ shŭn)	Visual inspection and manual examination of the breast for changes in contour, symmetry, "dimpling" of skin, retraction of the nipple(s), and for the presence of lumps
chorionic villus sampling (CVS) (kō-rē-ŏn′ ĭk vĭl′ ŭs sam′ plĭng)	A procedure that involves the insertion of a catheter into the cervix and into the outer portion of the membranes surrounding the fetus. A sample of the chorionic villi can be examined for the chromosomal abnormalities and biochemical disorders. This procedure can be done 8 weeks into pregnancy
colposcopy (kŏl-pŏs′ kō-pē)	Visual examination of the vagina and cervix via a colposcope. Abnormal results may indicate cervical or vaginal erosion, tumors, and dysplasia
culdoscopy (kŭl-dŏs′ kō-pē)	Visual examination of the viscera of the female pelvis via a culdoscope. May be used in suspected ectopic pregnancy and unexplained pelvic pain, and to check for pelvic masses
estrogens (es′ trō-jĕns)	A urine test or blood serum test to determine the level of estrone, estradiol, and estriol
human chorionic gonadotropin (HCG) (hū′ măn kō-rē-ŏn′ ĭk gŏn″ ă-dō- trō′ pĭn)	A urine test or blood serum test to determine the presence of HCG. A positive result may indicate pregnancy
hysterosalpingography (hĭs″ tĕr-ō-săl″ pĭn-gŏg′ ră-fē)	X-ray of the uterus and fallopian tubes after the injection of a radiopaque substance. Size and structure of the uterus and fallopian tubes can be evaluated. Uterine tumors, fibroids, tubal pregnancy, and tubal occlusion may be observed
laparoscopy (lăp-ăr-ŏs′ kō-pē)	Visual examination of the abdominal cavity via a laparoscope. Used to examine the ovaries and fallopian tubes
mammography (măm-ŏg′ ră-fē)	The process of obtaining pictures of the breast by use of x-rays. This procedure is able to locate breast tumors before they grow to 1 cm. It is the most effective means of detecting early breast cancers

Test	Description
Papanicolaou (PAP smear) (păp′ ăh-nĭk″ ō-lă′ oo)	A test used to detect cancer of the cervix and vagina. The cervical and vaginal cells are fixed on two separate slides and examined by a pathologist. Results are reported as Class I: absence of abnormal cells; Class II: abnormal cells, no malignancy; Class III: suggestive of malignancy; Class IV: strongly suggestive of malignancy; and Class V: conclusive of malignancy
pregnanediol (prĕg″ nān-dī-ŏl)	A urine test that determines menstrual disorders or possible abortion
wet mat or wet-prep (wĕt măt or wĕt-prĕp)	Examination of vaginal discharge for the presence of bacteria and yeast. A vaginal smear is placed on a microscopic slide, wet with normal saline, and then viewed under a microscope by the physician

Learning Exercises

Anatomy and Physiology

Write your answers to the following questions. Do not refer back to the text

1. List the primary and accessory sex organs of the female reproductive system.

    a. _____   b. _____

    c. _____   d. _____

    e. _____   f. _____

2. State the vital function of the female reproductive system. _____
    _____

3. Name the three identifiable areas of the uterus.

    a. _____   b. _____

    c. _____

4. Define fundus. _____
    _____

5. Name the ligaments that support the uterus and hold it in position.

    a. _____   b. _____

    c. _____   d. _____

6. Name the three layers of the uterine wall.

    a. _____   b. _____

    c. _____

7. State the three primary functions associated with the uterus.

    a. _____

    b. _____

    c. _____

8. Define the following terms:

    a. Anteflexion _____
    _____

    b. Retroflexion _____
    _____

    c. Anteversion _____
    _____

    d. Retroversion _____
    _____

9. The fallopian tubes are also called the _____ _____
    or _____ .

10. Name the three layers of the fallopian tubes.

    a. _____   b. _____

    c. _____

11. Define fimbriae. _____
    _____

12. Should the ovum become impregnated by a spermatozoon while in the fallopian tube, the process of _____ occurs.

13. State two functions of the fallopian tubes.

    a. _____

    b. _____

14. Describe the ovaries. _____
    _____

15. Name the three stages of an ovarian follicle.

    a. _____   b. _____

    c. _____

16. The functional activity of the ovary is controlled by the _____ .

17. State the two functions of the ovary.

    a. _____   b. _____

18. The vagina is a _____ tube extending from the _____ to the uterus.

19. State the three functions of the vagina.

    a. _____   b. _____

    c. _____

20. Name the organs that comprise the external female genitalia.

    a. _____   b. _____

    c. _____   d. _____

    e. _____

21. Between the vulva and the anus is an external region known as the _____
    _____ .

22. Define episiotomy. _____
    _____

23. The breasts or _____ _____ are compound alveolar structures.

24. The _____ is the dark pigmented area found in the skin over each breast and the _____ is the elevated area in its center.

25. Name the three hormones that play a role in milk production.

    a. _____   b. _____

    c. _____

26. Define colostrum. _____
    _____

27. Name the four phases of the menstrual cycle.

    a. _____   b. _____

    c. _____   d. _____

28. Define premenstrual syndrome. _____
    _____
    _____

Word Parts

1. In the spaces provided, write the definitions of these prefixes, roots, combining forms, and suffixes. Do not refer to the listings of terminology words. Leave blank those terms you cannot define.
2. After completing as many as you can, refer back to the terminology word listings to check your work. For each word missed or left blank, write the term and its definition several times on the margins of these pages or on a separate sheet of paper.
3. To maximize the learning process, it is to your advantage to do the following exercises as directed. To refer to the terminology listings before completing these exercises invalidates the learning process.

PREFIXES

Give the definitions of the following prefixes:

1. a-	_____	2. an-	_____
3. ante-	_____	4. cata-	_____
5. con-	_____	6. contra-	_____
7. dys-	_____	8. endo-	_____
9. eu-	_____	10. intra-	_____
11. multi-	_____	12. neo-	_____
13. nulli-	_____	14. oligo-	_____
15. pan-	_____	16. par-	_____
17. peri-	_____	18. post-	_____
19. pre-	_____	20. primi-	_____
21. pseudo-	_____	22. retro-	_____
23. tri-	_____		

ROOTS AND COMBINING FORMS

Give the definition of the following roots and combining forms:

1. abort	_____	2. amnio	_____
3. bartholin	_____	4. cept	_____
5. cervic	_____	6. coit	_____
7. colpo	_____	8. culdo	_____
9. cysto	_____	10. episio	_____
11. eunia	_____	12. fibr	_____
13. genital	_____	14. gyneco	_____
15. hemato	_____	16. hymen	_____

17. hyster _____   18. hystero _____

19. log _____   20. mammo _____

21. mast _____   22. men _____

23. meno _____   24. mester _____

25. metr _____   26. metri _____

27. myo _____   28. nat _____

29. nata _____   30. oo _____

31. oophor _____   32. ovul _____

33. para _____   34. partum _____

35. pause _____   36. pelvi _____

37. perineo _____   38. pyo _____

39. recto _____   40. salping _____

41. salpingo _____   42. salpinx _____

43. toc _____   44. uter _____

45. vagin _____   46. venere _____

47. vers _____

SUFFIXES

Give the definitions of the following suffixes:

1. -al _____   2. -ar _____

3. -cele _____   4. -centesis _____

5. -cyesis _____   6. -ectomy _____

7. -genesis _____   8. -graphy _____

9. -ia _____   10. -ine _____

11. -ion _____   12. -ist _____

13. -itis _____   14. -logy _____

15. -metry _____   16. -oma _____

17. -osis _____   18. -plasty _____

19. -rrhagia _____   20. -rrhaphy _____

21. -rrhea _____   22. -scope _____

23. -tome _____   24. -tomy _____

Identifying Medical Terms

In the spaces provided, write the medical terms for the following meanings:

1. _____ The process of miscarrying

2. _____ An instrument used to cut fetal membranes

3. _____ The time before the onset of labor

4. _____ Inflammation of the uterine cervix

5. _____ Suture of the vagina

6. _____ A difficult or painful monthly flow

7. _____ A good, normal childbirth

8. _____ A fibrous tissue tumor

9. _____ The study of the female

10. _____ Surgical excision of the hymen

11. _____ Surgical repair of the breast

12. _____ A normal monthly flow

13. _____ Pertaining to the first 4 weeks after birth

14. _____ Formation of the ovum

15. _____ Pertaining to after childbirth

Spelling

In the spaces provided, write the correct spelling of these misspelled terms:

1. amiocentesis _____   2. bartolinitis _____

3. dytocia _____   4. epsiotomy _____

5. hystrotomy _____   6. menorhagia _____

7. oophritis _____   8. salpinitis _____

9. vajinitis _____   10. veneral _____

Review Questions

Matching

Select the appropriate lettered meaning for each numbered line.

_____ 1. gamete intrafal-
          lopian transfer

_____ 2. laser ablation

_____ 3. lumpectomy

_____ 4. menarche

_____ 5. mittelschmerz

_____ 6. morula

_____ 7. ovulation

_____ 8. parturition

_____ 9. pudendal

_____ 10. quickening

a. A solid mass of cells resulting from cell division after fertilization of an ovum

b. Pertaining to the external female genitalia

c. The beginning of the monthly flow; menses

d. Surgical removal of a tumor from the breast

e. Abdominal pain that occurs midway between the menstrual periods at ovulation

f. A procedure that places the sperm and eggs directly in the fimbriated end of the fallopian tube

g. The process in which an ovum is discharged from the cortex of the ovary

h. The act of giving birth

i. The first movement of the fetus felt in the uterus, occurring during the 16th to 20th week of pregnancy

j. A procedure that uses a laser to destroy the uterine lining

k. The fertilized ovum

Abbreviations

Place the correct word, phrase, or abbreviation in the space provided.

_____ 1. AB

_____ 2. alpha-fetoprotein

_____ 3. AH

_____ 4. cesarean section

_____ 5. DES

_____ 6. expected date of confinement

_____ 7. grav I

_____ 8. Gyn

_____ 9. intrauterine device

_____ 10. pelvic inflammatory disease

Diagnostic and Laboratory Tests

Select the best answer to each multiple choice question. Circle the letter of your choice.

1. A procedure that involves the insertion of a catheter into the cervix and into the outer portion of the membranes surrounding the fetus.

    a. amniotic fluid analysis

    b. chorionic villus sampling

    c. colposcopy

    d. culdoscopy

2. A positive result may indicate pregnancy.

    a. colposcopy

    b. culdoscopy

    c. HCG

    d. laparoscopy

3. X-ray of the uterus and fallopian tubes after the injection of a radiopaque substance.

    a. hysterosalpingography

    b. laparoscopy

    c. culdoscopy

    d. mammography

4. Used to examine the ovaries and fallopian tubes.

    a. colposcopy

    b. culdoscopy

    c. laparoscopy

    d. mammography

5. The process of obtaining pictures of the breast by use of x-rays.

    a. colposcopy

    b. culdoscopy

    c. laparoscopy

    d. mammography

16

The Male Reproductive System

The male reproductive system consists of the testes, various ducts, the urethra, and the accessory glands: bulbourethral, prostrate, and the seminal vesicles. The supporting structures and accessory sex organs are the scrotum and the penis.

The testes are two ovoid-shaped organs located in the scrotum. Within the testes are small tubes called the seminiferous tubules. It is within these tubes that spermatozoa are formed. An average, normal male produces approximately 200 million sperm each day.

HULK OR HOAX

Anabolic steroids (testosterone) may be abused by individuals who seek to increase muscle mass, strength, and overall athletic ability. This form of use is illegal. Signs of possible abuse may include:

Flu-like symptoms
Gastrointestinal distress
Headaches
Muscle aches
Dizziness
Bruises

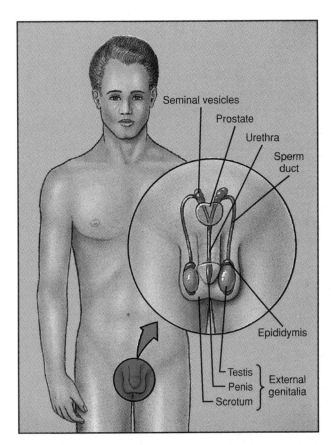

ANATOMY AND PHYSIOLOGY OVERVIEW

The male reproductive system consists of the testes, various ducts, the urethra, and the following accessory glands: bulbourethral, prostate, and the seminal vesicles. The supporting structures and accessory sex organs are the scrotum and the penis (Fig. 16–1 and Plate 27). The vital function of the male reproductive system is to provide the sperm cells necessary to fertilize the ovum thereby perpetuating the species. The following is a general overview of the organs and functions of this system.

THE REPRODUCTIVE SYSTEM OF THE MALE

Organ	Primary Functions
Testes	Produce sperm (see Fig. 16–3)
Accessory Organs	
Epididymis	Site of sperm maturation
Ductus deferens (sperm duct)	Conducts sperm between epididymis and prostate
Seminal vesicles	Secrete fluid that makes up much of the volume of semen
Prostate	Secretes buffers and fluid
External Genitalia	
Penis	Erectile organ used to deposit sperm in the vagina of a female
Scrotum	Surrounds the testes

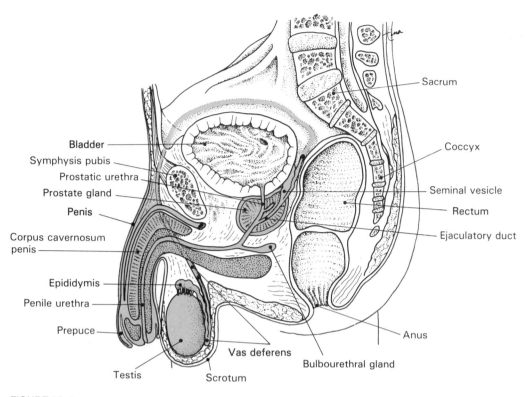

Bladder
Symphysis pubis
Prostatic urethra
Prostate gland
Penis
Corpus cavernosum penis
Epididymis
Penile urethra
Prepuce
Testis
Vas deferens
Scrotum
Bulbourethral gland
Anus
Ejaculatory duct
Rectum
Seminal vesicle
Coccyx
Sacrum

FIGURE 16–1

Sagittal section through the male pelvis, showing organs of the reproductive system. *(Adapted from Evans WF. Anatomy and Physiology, 3rd ed. Englewood Cliffs, NJ: Prentice-Hall, 1983, with permission.)*

External Organs

In the male, the scrotum and the penis are the external organs of reproduction.

THE SCROTUM

The scrotum is a pouch-like structure located behind the penis. It is suspended from the perineal region and is divided by a septum into two sacs, each containing one of the testes along with its connecting tube called the epididymis. Within the tissues of the scrotum are fibers of smooth muscle that contract in the absence of sufficient heat, giving the scrotum a wrinkled appearance. This contractile action brings the testes closer to the perineum where they can absorb sufficient body heat to maintain the viability of the spermatozoa. Under normal conditions, the walls of the scrotum are generally free of wrinkles, and it hangs loosely between the thighs (Fig. 16–1 and Plate 10).

THE PENIS

The penis is the external male sex organ and is composed of erectile tissue covered with skin. The size and shape of the penis varies with an average erect penis being 15 to 20 cm in length. The penis has three longitudinal columns of erectile tissue that are capable of significant enlargement when engorged with blood, as is the case during sexual stimulation. Two of these columns, located side by side, form the greater part of the penis. These columns are known as the corpora cavernosa penis. The third longitudinal column, the corpus spongiosum, has the same function as the first two columns but is transversed by the penile portion of the urethra and tends to be more elastic when in an erectile state. The corpus spongiosum, at its distal end, expands to form the glans penis. The glans penis is the cone-shaped head of the penis and is the site of the urethral orifice. It is covered with loose skin folds called the foreskin or prepuce. The foreskin contains glands that secrete a lubricating fluid called smegma. The foreskin may be removed by a surgical procedure known as circumcision (Fig. 16-2).

The erectile state in the penis results when sexual stimulation causes large quantities of blood from dilated arteries supplying the penis to fill the cavernous spaces in the erectile

FIGURE 16-2

Section through the bladder, prostate gland, and penis. *(Adapted from Evans WF. Anatomy and Physiology, 3rd ed. Englewood Cliffs, NJ: Prentice-Hall, 1983, with permission.)*

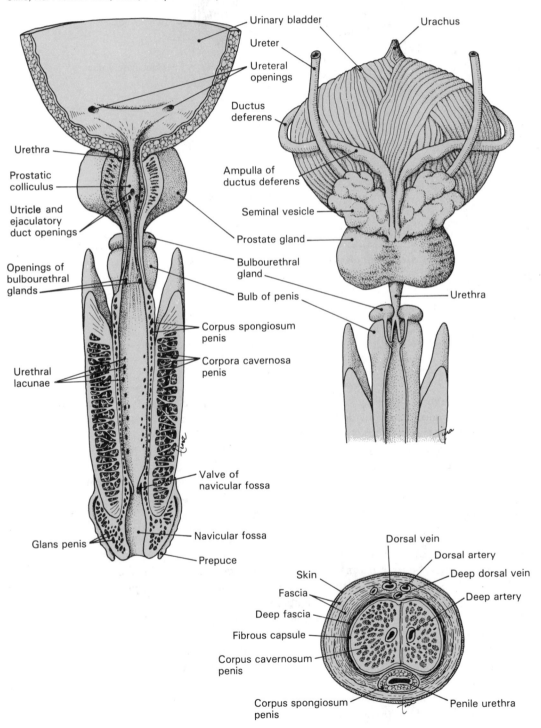

tissue. When the arteries constrict, the pressure on the veins in the area is reduced, thus allowing more blood to leave the penis than enters, and the penis returns to its normal state. The functions of the penis are to serve as the male organ of copulation and as the site of the orifice for the elimination of urine and semen from the body.

The Testes

As mentioned earlier, the male has two ovoid-shaped organs, the testes, located in the scrotum. Each testis is about 4 cm long and 2.5 cm wide. The interior of each testis is divided into about 250 wedge-shaped lobes by fibrous tissues. Coiled within each lobe are one to three small tubes called the seminiferous tubules. These tubules are the site of the development of male reproductive cells, the spermatozoa. Cells within the testes also produce the male sex hormone, testosterone, which is responsible for the development of secondary male characteristics during puberty. Testosterone is essential for normal growth and development of the male accessory sex organs. It plays a vital role in the erection process of the penis, and thus, is necessary for the reproductive act, copulation. Additionally, it affects the growth of hair on the face, muscular development, and vocal timbre. The seminiferous tubules form a plexus or network called the rete testis from which 15 to 20 small ducts, the efferent ductules, leave the testis and open into the epididymis (Fig. 16–1 and Plate 10).

The Epididymis

Each testis is connected by efferent ductules to an epididymis, which is a coiled tube lying on the posterior aspect of the testis. The epididymis is between 13 and 20 feet in length but is coiled into a space less than 2 inches (5 cm) long and ends in the ductus deferens. Each epididymis functions as a storage site for the maturation of sperm (Fig. 16–3) and as the first part of the duct system through which sperm pass on their journey to the urethra (see Fig. 16–1 and Plate 10).

The Ductus Deferens or Vas Deferens

The ductus deferens is a slim muscular tube, about 45 cm in length, and is a continuation of the epididymis. It has been described as the excretory duct of the testis and extends from a point adjacent to the testis to enter the abdomen through the inguinal canal. It is later joined by the duct from the seminal vesicle. Between the testis and the part of the abdomen known as the internal inguinal ring, the ductus deferens is contained within a structure known as the spermatic cord. The spermatic cord also contains arteries, veins, lymphatic vessels, and nerves (see Fig. 16–2).

The Seminal Vesicles

There are two seminal vesicles, each connected by a narrow duct to a ductus deferens, which then forms a short tube, the ejaculatory duct, that penetrates the base of the prostate gland and opens into the prostatic portion of the urethra. The seminal vesicles produce a slightly alkaline fluid that becomes a part of the seminal fluid or semen (see Fig. 16–2).

The Prostate Gland

The prostate gland is about 4 cm wide and weighs about 20 g. It is composed of glandular, connective, and muscular tissue and lies behind the urinary bladder. It surrounds the first 2.5 cm of the urethra and secretes an alkaline fluid that aids in maintaining the viability of spermatozoa. Enlargement of the prostate (benign prostatic hypertrophy) is a condition

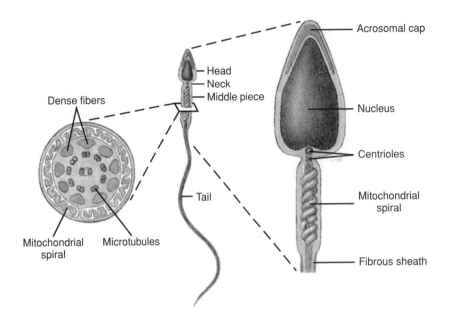

FIGURE 16-3

Spermatozoon structure. The basic structure of a single spermatozoon as seen with the electron microscope is compared with diagrammatic views highlighting aspects of internal organization. (SEM, ×8750). (*From Martini F.* Fundamentals of Anatomy and Physiology, *2nd ed. Englewood Cliffs, NJ: Prentice-Hall, 1992, with permission.*)

that sometimes occurs in older men. In this condition, the prostate obstructs the urethra and causes interference with the normal passage of urine. When this occurs, a prostatectomy is usually performed to remove a part of the gland. The prostate gland may also be a site for cancer in older men (see Fig. 16-2).

The Bulbourethral or Cowper's Glands

The bulbourethral glands are two small pea-sized glands located below the prostate and on either side of the urethra. A duct about 2.5 cm long connects them with the wall of the urethra. The bulbourethral glands produce a mucous secretion before ejaculation, which becomes a part of the semen (see Fig. 16-2).

The Urethra

The male urethra is approximately 20 cm long and is divided into three sections: prostatic, membranous, and penile. It extends from the urinary bladder to the external urethral orifice at the head of the penis. It serves the function of transmitting urine and semen out of the body (see Fig. 16-2).

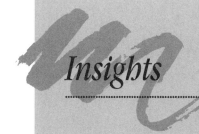

Insights

ENLARGEMENT OF THE PROSTATE GLAND
(Benign Prostatic Hypertrophy BPH)

The prostate gland is about 4 centimeters wide and weighs about 20 grams. It is composed of glandular, connective, and muscular tissue and lies behind the urinary bladder. It surrounds the first 2.5 centimeters of the urethra and secretes an alkaline fluid that aids in maintaining the viability of spermatozoa.

Benign Prostatic Hypertrophy

Enlargement of the prostate gland may occur in men who are 50 years of age and older. As the prostate enlarges, it compresses the urethra, thereby restricting the normal flow of urine. This restriction generally causes a number of symptoms and can be referred to as prostatism. Prostatism is any condition of the prostate gland that interferes with the flow of urine from the bladder.
Symptoms usually include:

- a weak or hard-to-start urine stream
- a feeling that the bladder is not empty
- a need to urinate often, especially at night
- a feeling of urgency (a sudden need to urinate)
- abdominal straining, a decrease in size and force of the urinary stream
- interruption of the stream
- acute urinary retention
- recurrent urinary infections

Treatment for benign prostatic hypertrophy may include surgery, medication, and/or balloon dilation of the urethra.

Surgery—Transurethral resection of the prostate (TURP or TUR) is the most common form of surgery used for benign prostatic hypertrophy. During this procedure, an endoscopic instrument that has ocular and surgical capabilities is introduced directly through the urethra to the prostate and small pieces of the prostate gland are removed by using an electrical cutting loop.

Medication—Proscar (finasteride), an oral medication, may be prescribed by a physician to help relieve the symptoms of BPH. It lowers the levels of dihydrotestosterone (DHT), which is a major factor in enlargement of the prostate. Lowering of DHT leads to shrinkage of the enlarged prostate gland in most men. Although this can lead to gradual improvement in urine flow and symptoms, it does not work for all cases. Sometimes the prostate may shrink without improvement in symptoms and it may take 6 months or more to determine if it is working for an individual. Side

(Insights continues on next page.)

effects may include impotence and less desire for sex. Proscar can alter the Prostate-Specific Antigen test (PSA) that is used to screen for prostate cancer.

Balloon Dilation—During this procedure, a balloon catheter is placed in the distal urethra and inflated by injecting a dilute contrast media at high pressure. The balloon is left in place for approximately 10 minutes and then the pressure is released.

By age 60, four out of five men may have an enlarged prostate, and suffer urinary difficulties. By age 75, one in eleven men may develop prostate cancer. Approximately 165,000 new cases of prostate cancer occurs each year with a death toll of 34,000 lives.

It is recommended that men ages 40 and up, should have a digital rectal exam each year and that men ages 50 and over, should have a Prostate-Specific Antigen (PSA) blood test each year. Those men who are at high-risk should have the exam and blood test at an earlier age.

Laboratory experiments have indicated that Proscar may prevent prostate cancer by blocking chemical processes in which testosterone is converted into a more potent hormone, dihydro-testosterone. The National Cancer Institute (NCI) began clinical trials of Proscar for the prevention of prostate cancer in 1993 in 222 sites nationwide. This trial will last for 7 years and involves 18,000 men ages 55 and older, who are in good health and have no evidence of prostate cancer.

Terminology with Surgical Procedures & Pathology

Term	Word Parts			Definition
anorchism (ăn-ōr′ kĭzm)	an	P	lack of	A condition in which there is a lack of one or both testes
	orch	R	testicle	
	ism	S	condition of	
aspermatism (ă-spĕr′ mă-tĭzm)	a	P	lack of	A condition in which there is a lack of secretion of the male seed
	spermat	R	seed	
	ism	S	condition of	
azoospermia (ă-zō″ ō-spĕr′ mē-ă)	a	P	lack of	A condition in which there is a lack of spermatozoa in the semen
	zoo	CF	animal	
	sperm	R	seed	
	ia	S	condition	
balanitis (băl″ ă-nī′ tĭs)	balan	R	glans	Inflammation of the glans penis
	itis	S	inflammation	
circumcision (sĕr″ kŭm-sĭ′ shŭn)	circum	P	around	The surgical process of removing the foreskin of the penis
	cis	R	to cut	
	ion	S	process	
cryptorchism (krĭpt-ōr′ kĭzm)	crypt	R	hidden	A condition in which the testis fails to descend into the scrotum
	orch	R	testicle	
	ism	S	condition of	
epididymectomy (ĕp″ ĭ-dĭd″ ĭ-mĕk′ tō-mē)	epi	P	upon	Surgical excision of the epididymis
	didym	R	testis	
	ectomy	S	excision	
epididymitis (ĕp″ ĭ-dĭd″ ĭ-mī′ tĭs)	epi	P	upon	Inflammation of the epididymis
	didym	R	testis	
	itis	S	inflammation	
epispadias (ĕp″ ĭ-spā′ dĭ-ăs)	epi	P	upon	A congenital defect in which the urethra opens on the dorsum of the penis
	spadias	R	a rent, an opening	
hydrocele (hī′ drō-sēl)	hydro	P	water	A collection of serous fluid in a sac-like cavity; specifically the tunica vaginalis testis
	cele	S	hernia	
hypospadias (hī″ pō-spă′ dĭ-ăs)	hypo	P	under	A congenital defect in which the urethra opens on the underside of the penis
	spadias	R	a rent, an opening	
oligospermia (ŏl″ ĭ-gō-spĕr′ mĭ-ă)	oligo	P	scanty	A condition in which there is a scanty amount of spermatozoa in the semen
	sperm	R	seed	
	ia	S	condition	

(Terminology—continued)

Term	Word Parts			Definition
orchidectomy (or″ kĭ-dĕk′ tō-mē)	orchid	R	testicle	Surgical excision of a testicle
	ectomy	S	excision	
orchidopexy (or′ kĭd-ō-pēk″ sē)	orchido	CF	testicle	Surgical fixation of a testicle
	pexy	S	fixation	
orchidoplasty (or′ kĭd-ō-plăs″ tē)	orchido	CF	testicle	Surgical repair of a testicle
	plasty	S	surgical repair	
orchidotomy (or″ kĭd-ŏt′ ō-mē)	orchido	CF	testicle	Incision into a testicle
	tomy	S	incision	
orchitis (or-kī′ tĭs)	orch	R	testicle	Inflammation of a testicle
	itis	S	inflammation	
parenchyma (păr-ĕn′ kĭ-mă)	par	P	beside	The essential cells of a gland or organ that are concerned with its function
	enchyma	R	to pour	
penitis (pē-nī′ tĭs)	pen	R	penis	Inflammation of the penis
	itis	S	inflammation	
phimosis (fĭ-mō′ sĭs)	phim	R	a muzzle	A condition of narrowing of the opening of the prepuce wherein the foreskin cannot be drawn back over the glans penis
	osis	S	condition of	
prostatalgia (prŏs″ tă-tăl′ jĭ-ă)	prostat	R	prostate	Pain in the prostate
	algia	S	pain	
prostatectomy (prŏs″ tă-tĕk′ tō-mē)	prostat	R	prostate	Surgical excision of the prostate
	ectomy	S	excision	
prostatitis (prŏs″ tă-tī′ tĭs)	prostat	R	prostate	Inflammation of the prostate
	itis	S	inflammation	
prostatocystitis (prŏs″ tă-tō-sĭs-tī′ tĭs)	prostato	CF	prostate	Inflammation of the prostate and bladder
	cyst	R	bladder	
	itis	S	inflammation	
prostatomegaly (prŏs″ tă-tō-mĕg′ ă-lē)	prostato	CF	prostate	Enlargement of the prostate
	megaly	S	enlargement	
spermatoblast (spĕr-măt′ ō-blăst)	spermato	CF	seed, sperm	The sperm germ cell
	blast	S	immature cell, germ cell	
spermatocyst (spĕr-măt′ ō-sĭst)	spermato	CF	seed, sperm	A cyst of the epididymis that contains spermatozoa
	cyst	R	sac, bladder	

(Terminology—continued)

Term	Word Parts			Definition
spermatogenesis (spĕr″ măt-ō-jĕn′ ĕ-sĭs)	spermato genesis	CF S	seed, sperm formation, produce	Formation of spermatozoa
spermatozoon (spĕr″ măt-ō-zō′ ŏn)	spermato zoon	CF R	seed, sperm life	The male sex cell. The plural form is spermatozoa
spermaturia (spĕr″ mă-tū′ rĭ-ă)	spermat uria	R S	seed, sperm urine	Discharge of semen with the urine
spermicide (spĕr′ mĭ-sīd)	spermi cide	CF S	sperm to kill	An agent that kills sperm
testicular (tĕs-tĭk′ ū-lar)	testicul ar	R S	testicle pertaining to	Pertaining to a testicle
varicocele (văr′ ĭ-kō-sēl)	varico cele	CF S	twisted vein hernia	An enlargement and twisting of the veins of the spermatic cord
vasectomy (văs-ĕk′ tō-mē)	vas ectomy	R S	vessel excision	Surgical excision of the vas deferens
vesiculitis (vĕ-sĭk″ ū-lī′ tĭs)	vesicul itis	R S	vesicle inflammation	Inflammation of a vesicle; in particular, the seminal vesicle

Vocabulary Words

Vocabulary words are terms that have not been divided into component parts. They are common words or specialized terms associated with the subject of this chapter. These words are provided to enhance your medical vocabulary.

Word	Definition
artificial insemination (ăr″ tĭ-fĭsh′ ăl ĭn-sĕm″ ĭn-ā′ shŭn)	The process of artificial placement of semen into the vagina so that conception may take place
capacitation (kăh-păs″ ĭ-tā′ shŭn)	The process by which spermatozoa are conditioned to fertilize an ovum in the female genital tract
castrate (kăs′ trāt)	To remove the testicles or ovaries; to geld, to spay
cloning (klōn′ ing)	The process of creating a genetic duplicate of an individual organism through asexual reproduction
coitus (kō′ ĭ-tŭs)	Sexual intercourse between a man and a woman

(Vocabulary—continued)

Word	Definition
condom (kŏn′ dŭm)	A thin, flexible protective sheath, usually rubber, worn over the penis during copulation to help prevent impregnation or venereal disease
condyloma (kŏn″ dĭ-lō′ mă)	A wart-like growth of the skin; most often seen on the external genitalia and is either viral or syphilitic in origin
ejaculation (ē-jăk″ ū-lā′ shŭn)	The process of expulsion of seminal fluid from the male urethra
Ericsson sperm separation method (er′ ik-son sperm sĕp″ ă-rā′ shŭn mĕth′ od	A process of separating the Y-chromosome sperm from the X-chromosome sperm. A sperm sample is taken and placed in a tube of albumin. Those that survive are Y-chromosome sperm, which make male babies. Women inseminated with these sperm have a 75 to 80% chance of producing a male child
eugenics (ū-jĕn′ ĭks)	The study and control of the bringing forth of offspring as a means of improving genetic characteristics of future generations
eunuch (ū′ nŭk)	A male who has been castrated, i.e., had his testicles removed
gamete (găm′ ēt)	A mature reproductive cell of the male or female; a spermatozoon or ovum
gonorrhea (gŏn″ ŏ-rē′ ă)	A highly contagious venereal disease of the genital mucous membrane of either sex; the infection transmitted by the gonococcus *Neisseria gonorrhoeae*
gossypol (gŏs′ sĕ-pŏl)	An extract of cottonseed oil that acts as a spermicide and may inhibit or prevent herpes simplex virus infection
gynecomastia (jī″ nĕ-kō-măs′ tĭ-ă)	A condition of excessive development of the mammary glands in the male
herpes genitalis (hĕr′ pēz jĕn-ĭ-tăl′ ĭs)	A highly contagious venereal disease of the genitalia of either sex; caused by herpes simplex virus-2 (HSV-2)
heterosexual (hĕt″ ĕr-ō-sĕk′ shū-ăl)	Pertaining to the opposite sex; refers to an individual who has a sexual preference for the opposite sex
homosexual (hō″ mō-sĕks′ ū-ăl)	Pertaining to the same sex; refers to an individual who has a sexual preference for the same sex
infertility (ĭn″ fĕr-tĭl′ ĭ-tē)	The inability to produce a viable offspring
mitosis (mī-tō′ sĭs)	The ordinary condition of cell division

(Vocabulary—continued)

Word	Definition
prepuce (prē′ pūs)	The foreskin over the glans penis in the male
puberty (pū′ ber-tē)	The stage of development in the male and female when secondary sex characteristics begin to develop and become functionally capable of reproduction
semen (sē′ měn)	The fluid transporting medium for spermatozoa discharged during ejaculation
syphilis (sĭf′ ĭ-lĭs)	A chronic infectious venereal disease caused by *Treponema pallidum*, which is transmitted sexually
trisomy (trī′ sōm-ē)	A genetic condition of having three chromosomes instead of two. The condition causes various birth defects

ABBREVIATIONS

AIH	artificial insemination homologous	**PSA**	prostate-specific antigen
BPH	benign prostatic hypertrophy	**SPP**	suprapubic prostatectomy
		STDs	sexually transmitted diseases
FTA-ABS	fluorescent treponemal antibody absorption	**STS**	serologic test for syphilis
		TPA	*Treponema pallidum* agglutination
Gc	gonorrhea	**TUR**	transurethral resection
HLA	human leukocyte antigen	**UG**	urogenital
HPV	human papilloma virus	**VD**	venereal disease
HSV-2	herpes simplex virus-2	**VDRL**	venereal disease research laboratory
NPT	nocturnal penile tumescence	**WR**	Wassermann reaction

Drug Highlights

Drugs that are generally used for the male reproductive system include androgenic hormones. Testosterone is the most important androgen and adequate secretions of this hormone are necessary to maintain normal male sex characteristics, the male libido, and sexual potency.

Testosterone

Is responsible for growth, development, and maintenance of the male reproductive system, and secondary sex characteristics.

Therapeutic Use

As replacement therapy in primary hypogonadism, and to stimulate puberty in carefully selected males. It may be used to relieve male menopause symptoms due to androgen deficiency. It may also be used to help stimulate sperm production in oligospermia and in impotence due to androgen deficiency. In the female, it may be used when there is advanced inoperable metastatic breast cancer who are 1 to 5 years postmenopausal and to prevent postpartum breast pain and engorgement in the non-nursing mother.

Examples: Halotestin (fluoxymesterone), Metandren (methyltestosterone), Andro (testosterone enanthate in oil), and Testex (testosterone propionate in oil).

Patient Teaching

Educate the patient to be aware of possible adverse reactions and report any of the following to the physician. *All patients:* nausea, vomiting, jaundice, edema. *Males:* frequent or persistent erection of the penis. Adolescent males: signs of premature epiphyseal closure. Should have bone development checked every 6 months. *Females:* hoarseness, acne, changes in menstrual periods, growth of hair on face and/or body.

Special Considerations

In diabetic patients, the effects of testosterone may decrease blood glucose and insulin requirements.

Testosterone may decrease the anticoagulant requirements of patients receiving oral anticoagulants. These patients require close monitoring when testosterone therapy is begun and then when it is stopped.

Anabolic steroids (testosterone) may be abused by individuals who seek to increase muscle mass, strength, and overall athletic ability. This form of use is illegal and signs of abuse may include flu-like symptoms, headaches, muscle aches, dizziness, bruises, needle marks, increased bleeding (nosebleeds, petechiae, gums, conjunctiva), enlarged spleen, liver, and/or prostate, edema, and in the female increased facial hair, menstrual irregularities, and enlarged clitoris.

Communication Enrichment

This segment is provided for those who wish to enhance their ability to communicate in either English or Spanish.

RELATED TERMS

English	Spanish
AIDS (Acquired Immunodeficiency Syndrome)	SIDA (Síndrome de Immunodeficiencia Adquirida) (sĭ-*dă* [sĭn-*drō*-mĕ dĕ ĭmm-*mū*-nō-dĕ-fĭ-cĭ-ĕn-cĭ-ă *ăd*-kĭ-rĭ-dă])
bisexual	bisexual (bĭ-*sĕx*-sū-ăl)
chlamydiae	chlamydiae (klă-*mĭ*-dĭ-ă)
circumcision	circuncisión (sĭr-*cūn*-sĭ-ōn)
condom	condon (*cōn*-dōn)
ejaculation	eyaculación (ĕ-yă-kū-lă-sĭ-*ōn*)
ejaculate	eyacular (ĕ-yă-kū-*lăr*)
erection	erección (ĕ-rĕk-sĭ-*ōn*)
genitals	genitales (hĕ-nĭ-*tă*-lĕs)
gonorrhea	gonorrea (gō-*nō*-rĕ-ă)
herpes	herpe (*ĕr*-pĕ)
heterosexual	heterosexual (ĕ-tĕ-rō-sĕx-sū-ăl)
homosexual	homosexual (ō-mō-sĕx-sū-ăl)
impotence	impotencia (ĭm-pō-*tĕn*-sĭ-ă)
masturbate	masturbarse (*măs*-tūr-băr-sĕ)
masturbation	masturbación (*măs*-tūr-bă-sĭ-ōn)
penis	pene (*pĕ*-nĕ)

English	Spanish
prostate	prostático; prostata (prōs-*ta*-tĭ-kō; prōs-*tă*-tă)
prostatectomy	prostatectomia (prōs-*tă*-tĕk-tō-mĭ-ă)
prostate gland	glándula prostática (*glăn*-dū-lă prōs-*tă*-tĭ-ka)
reproduction	reproducción (rĕ-prō-dūk-sĭ-*ōn*)
reproductive system	sistema reproductivo (sĭs-*tĕ*-mă rĕ-prō-*dūk*-tĭ-vō)
semen	semen (*sĕ*-mĕn)
sexual desires	deseos sexual (dĕ-*sĕ*-ōs *sĕx*-sū-ăl)
sexual relations	relaciones sexual (re-*lă*-sĭ-ō-nĕs *sĕx*-sū-ăl)
sterile	estéril (ĕs-*tĕ*-rĭl)
syphilis	sífilis (*sĭ*-fí-lĭs)
testicle	testículo (tĕs-*tĭ*-kū-lō)
underwear	ropa interior (*rō*-pă ĭn-*tĕ*-rĭ-ōr)
venereal	venéreo (vĕ-*nĕ*-rĕ-ō)
veneral infection	enfermedad venérea (ĕn-*fĕr*-mĕ-dăd vĕ-*nĕ*-rĕ-ă)

DIAGNOSTIC AND LABORATORY TESTS

Test	Description
fluorescent treponemal antibody absorption (floo-ō-rĕs′ ĕnt trĕp″ ō-nē′ măl ăn′ tĭ-bŏd″ ē ăb-sorp′ shŭn)	A test performed on blood serum to determine the presence of *Treponema pallidum*. Used to detect syphilis
paternity (pă-tĕr′ nĭ-tē)	A test to determine whether a certain man could be the father of a specific child. The test can only indicate who is not the father. Types of tests that may be used are blood type, human leukocyte antigen (HLA), white blood cell, enzyme and protein, and genetic. The blood type of the child and accused father are analyzed for compatibility. For example, a parent with type O blood cannot be the parent of a child with type AB blood. The HLA looks at the body's tissue compatibility system, and the white blood cell test looks at chemical markers (antigens) on the surface of the white blood cells. Enzyme and protein looks at red blood cell enzymes, and a new genetic test is being developed that uses molecular and protein biology to look at family-related patterns among genes
prostate-specific antigen (PSA) immunoassay (prŏs′ tāt-spĕ-sĭf′ ĭk ăn′ tĭ-jĕn ĭm″ ū-nō-ăs′ sā)	A blood test that measures concentrations of a special type of protein known as prostate-specific antigen. Increased level indicates prostate disease or possibly prostate cancer
semen (sē′ mĕn)	A test performed on semen that looks at the volume, pH, sperm count, sperm motility, and morphology. Used to evaluate infertility in men
testosterone toxicology (tĕs-tŏs′ tĕr-ōn tŏks″ ĭ-kŏl′ ō-jē)	A test performed on blood serum to identify the level of testosterone. Increased level may indicate benign prostatic hypertrophy. Decreased level may indicate hypogonadism, testicular hypofunction, hypopituitarism, and/or orchidectomy
venereal disease research laboratory (vē-nē′ rē-ăl dĭ-zēz rē′ sĕrch lăb′ ră-tor″ ē)	A test performed on blood serum to determine the presence of *Treponema pallidum*. Used to detect syphilis

SEXUALLY TRANSMITTED DISEASES (STDs)

Sexually transmitted diseases can occur in men, women, and children. They are passed from person to person through sexual contact or from mother to child. The following is a summary of the most common sexually transmitted diseases:

Disease	Cause	Symptoms	Treatment
Chlamydia (klă-mĭd′ ē-ă)	*Chlamydia trachomatis* (bacterium)	**MAY BE ASYMPTOMATIC OR** **MALE:** Mucopurulent discharge from penis, burning, itching in genital area, dysuria, swollen testes. Can lead to sterility **FEMALE:** Mucopurulent discharge from vagina, cystitis, pelvic pain, cervicitis. Can lead to pelvic inflammatory disease (PID) and sterility **NEWBORN:** Eye infection, pneumonia. Can cause death	Antibiotics—tetracycline or erythromycin
Genital warts (jĕn′ ĭ-tăl wörts)	Human papilloma virus (HPV)	**MALE:** Cauliflower-like growths on the penis and perianal area **FEMALE:** Cauliflower-like growths around vagina and perianal area	Laser surgery, chemotherapy, cryosurgery, cauterization
Gonorrhea (gŏn″ ŏ-rē′ ă)	*Neisseria gonorrhoeae* (bacterium)	**MALE:** Purulent urethral discharge, dysuria, urinary frequency **FEMALE:** Purulent vaginal discharge, dysuria, urinary frequency, abnormal menstrual bleeding, abdominal tenderness. Can lead to PID and sterility **NEWBORN:** Gonorrheal ophthalmia neonatorum, purulent eye discharge. Can cause blindness	Antibiotics—penicillin or tetracycline
Herpes genitalis (hĕr′ pēz jĕn-ĭ-tāl′ ĭs)	Herpes simplex virus-2 (HSV-2)	**ACTIVE PHASE MALE:** Fluid-filled vesicles (blisters) on penis. Rupture causes acute pain and itching **FEMALE:** Blisters in and around vagina **NEWBORN:** Can be infected during vaginal delivery. Severe infection, physical and mental damage	**NO CURE:** Antiviral drug acyclovir (Zovirax) may be used to relieve symptoms during acute phase

Disease	Cause	Symptoms	Treatment
		GENERALIZED: "Flu-like" symptoms, fever, headache, malaise, anorexia, muscle pain	
Syphilis (sĭf′ ĭ-lĭs)	*Treponema pallidum* (bacterium)	**PRIMARY**—1st stage Chancre at point of infection. **Male**—penis, anus, rectum. **Female**—vagina, cervix. **Both**—lips, tongue, fingers, or nipples	Antibotics—penicillin, tetracycline, or erythromycin
		SECONDARY—2nd stage "Flu-like" symptoms with a skin rash over moist, fatty areas of the body. Alopecia	
		TERTIARY—latent-3rd stage No symptoms—damage to internal organs	
		NEWBORN: Congenital syphilis—may have a heart defect, bone deformity, or other deformities	
Trichomoniasis (trĭk″ ō-mō-nĭ′ ă-sĭs)	*Trichomonas* (parasitic protozoa)	**MALE:** Usually asymptomatic. Can lead to cystitis, urethritis, prostatitis	Metronidazole (Flagyl)
		FEMALE: White frothy vaginal discharge, burning and itching of vulva. Can lead to cystitis, urethritis, vaginitis	

Learning Exercises

Anatomy and Physiology

Write your answers to the following questions. Do not refer back to the text.

1. List the primary and accessory glands of the male reproductive system.

   a. _____   b. _____

   c. _____   d. _____

   e. _____   f. _____

2. Name the supporting structure and accessory sex organs of the male reproductive system.

   a. _____   b. _____

3. State the vital function of the male reproductive system. _____
   _____

4. Describe the scrotum. _____
   _____

5. The _____ _____ _____ and the
   _____ _____ are names of the three longitudinal
   columns of erectile tissue in the penis.

6. The average erect penis measures _____ to _____
   cm in length.

7. The _____ _____ is the cone-shaped head of the
   penis.

8. Define prepuce. _____
   _____

9. Define smegma. _____

10. State two functions of the penis.

    a. _____   b. _____

11. Describe the testes. _____
    _____
    _____

12. _____ _____ are the site of the development of spermatozoa.

13. List five effects of testosterone regarding male development.

    a. _____   b. _____

    c. _____   d. _____

    e. _____

14. Name the plexus that the seminiferous tubules form. _____

15. Describe the epididymis. _____
    _____

16. State two functions of the epididymis.

    a. _____   b. _____

17. The excretory duct of the testes is known by two names, _____ _____ or _____ _____ .

18. The spermatic cord contains five types of structures and connects the testes with organs in the abdomen. Name these five structures.

   a. _____   b. _____

   c. _____   d. _____

   e. _____

19. State the function of the seminal vesicles. _____ _____

20. Describe the prostate gland. _____ _____

21. Define the condition known as benign prostatic hypertrophy. _____ _____

22. The two small pea-sized glands located below the prostate and on either side of the urethra are known as the _____ glands or as _____ glands.

23. Name the three sections of the male urethra.

   a. _____   b. _____

   c. _____

24. State a function of the male urethra. _____

25. The male urethra is approximately _____ cm long.

Word Parts

1. In the spaces provided, write the definitions of these prefixes, roots, combining forms, and suffixes. Do not refer to the listings of terminology words. Leave blank those terms you cannot define.
2. After completing as many as you can, refer back to the terminology word listings to check your work. For each word missed or left blank, write the term and its definition several times on the margins of these pages or on a separate sheet of paper.
3. To maximize the learning process, it is to your advantage to do the following exercises as directed. To refer to the terminology listings before completing these exercises invalidates the learning process.

PREFIXES

Give the definitions of the following prefixes:

1. a-   _____   2. an-   _____

3. circum-   _____   4. epi-   _____

5. hydro-   _____   6. hypo-   _____

7. oligo-   _____   8. par-   _____

ROOTS AND COMBINING FORMS

Give the definitions of the following roots and combining forms:

1. balan _____   2. cis _____

3. crypt _____   4. cyst _____

5. didym _____   6. enchyma _____

7. orch _____   8. orchid _____

9. orchido _____   10. pen _____

11. phim _____   12. prostat _____

13. prostato _____   14. spadias _____

15. sperm _____   16. spermat _____

17. spermato _____   18. spermi _____

19. testicul _____   20. varico _____

21. vas _____   22. vesicul _____

23. zoo _____   24. zoon _____

SUFFIXES

Give the definitions of the following suffixes:

1. -algia _____   2. -ar _____

3. -blast _____   4. -cele _____

5. -cide _____   6. -ectomy _____

7. -genesis _____   8. -ia _____

9. -ion _____   10. -ism _____

11. -itis _____   12. -megaly _____

13. -osis _____   14. -pexy _____

15. -plasty _____   16. -tomy _____

17. -uria _____

Identifying Medical Terms

In the spaces provided, write the medical terms for the following meanings:

1. _____ Inflammation of the glans penis

2. _____ Surgical excision of the epididymis

3. _____ Surgical excision of a testicle

4. _____ Surgical repair of a testicle

5. _____ Pain in the prostate

6. _____ Inflammation of the prostate and bladder

7. _____ The sperm germ cell

8. _____ The male sex cell

9. _____ An agent that kills sperm

10. _____ Pertaining to a testicle

Spelling

In the spaces provided, write the correct spelling of these misspelled terms:

1. crptorchism _____   2. hyospadias _____

3. orchdotomy _____   4. prostatmegaly _____

5. spermauria _____

Review Questions

Matching

Select the appropriate lettered meaning for each numbered line.

_____ 1. circumcision

_____ 2. coitus

_____ 3. condom

_____ 4. gamete

_____ 5. genital warts

_____ 6. gonorrhea

_____ 7. infertility

_____ 8. prepuce

_____ 9. syphilis

_____ 10. trichomoniasis

a. Caused by the bacterium *Treponema pallidum*

b. A mature reproductive cell of the male or female

c. Sexual intercourse between a man and a woman

d. Caused by a parasitic protozoa

e. The surgical process of removing the foreskin of the penis

f. A thin, flexible protective sheath worn over the penis during copulation to help prevent impregnation or venereal disease

g. Caused by the human papilloma virus

h. The inability to produce a viable offspring

i. Causes purulent urethral discharge in the male and purulent vaginal discharge in the female

j. Caused by the bacterium *Chlamydia trachomatis*

k. The foreskin over the glans penis in the male

Abbreviations

Place the correct word, phrase, or abbreviation in the space provided.

_____ 1. benign prostatic hypertrophy

_____ 2. Gc

_____ 3. human papilloma virus

_____ 4. HSV-2

_____ 5. STDs

_____ 6. *Treponema pallidum* agglutination

_____ 7. TUR

_____ 8. UG

_____ 9. venereal disease

_____ 10. Wassermann reaction

Diagnostic and Laboratory Tests

Select the best answer to each multiple choice question. Circle the letter of your choice.

1. A test performed on blood serum to detect syphilis.

   a. paternity

   b. semen

   c. FTA-ABS

   d. HSV-2

2. A test to determine whether a certain man could be the father of a specific child.

   a. paternity

   b. semen

   c. FTA-ABS

   d. HSV-2

3. An increased level indicates prostate disease or possibly prostate cancer.

   a. fluorescent treponemal antibody

   b. prostate-specific antigen

   c. semen

   d. testosterone toxicology

4. Used to determine infertility in men.

   a. paternity

   b. prostate-specific antigen

   c. semen

   d. testosterone toxicology

5. An increased level may indicate benign prostatic hypertrophy.

   a. fluorescent treponemal antibody

   b. prostate-specific antigen

   c. testosterone toxicology

   d. venereal disease research

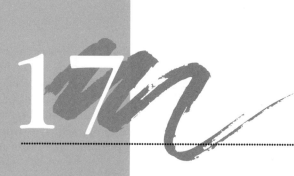

Oncology

Cancer was first identified around 400 BC during the time of Hippocrates and is a Latin term meaning crab. Early reports on cancer compared the disease to a crab because of its tendency to stretch out and spread like the crab's four pairs of legs.

Today, cancer refers to any malignant tumor. More than 200 different types of cancer have been identified; however, the majority of tumors can be classified into three main groups: carcinomas, sarcomas, and mixed cancers.

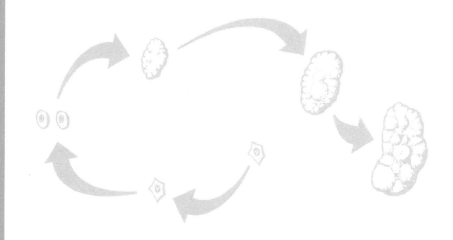

AN OVERVIEW OF CANCER

Cancer was first identified around 400 BC during the time of Hippocrates and is a Latin term meaning **a crab.** Early reports on cancer compared the disease to a crab because of its tendency to stretch out and spread like the crab's four pairs of legs. Today, cancer refers to any malignant tumor (neoplasm, oncoma). More than 200 different types of cancer have been identified; however, the majority of tumors can be classified into three main groups: carcinomas, which account for about 80% of cancers; sarcomas, which are the next largest group; and mixed cancers, which have characteristics of both carcinomas and sarcomas (see Classification of Cancer).

The incidence of cancer is now five times greater than it was 100 years ago. Cancer will strike one of every three Americans, according to recent statistics from the American Cancer Society. However, there is hope for those afflicted. Cancer has become one of the most curable of the major diseases in the United States, and those tumors that cannot be cured can be controlled through treatment, thereby giving the patient an extended life span. With early detection followed by immediate treatment, the cure rate for cancer is now one in every two. Highly advanced surgical techniques are being used to remove cancerous tissue, and it is usually possible to excise all the cancer cells when the malignancy is discovered in its earliest stages. Chemotherapy and radiation therapy are the other two principal means of treatment for patients with cancer. These treatments employ agents to kill cancerous cells that remain after surgery or in malignancies deemed inoperable. Other forms of treatment are under investigation as scientists continue their research into the causes of cancer. Although the exact cause or causes remain unknown, research has shown that some cancers can be prevented, especially those associated with environmental factors. Oncologists searching for the causes of cancer have identified numerous factors that play a role in the development of cancer. These factors are generally grouped under three main classifications: environmental, hereditary, and biological. Viruses have long been suspected of playing a role in the development of cancer; however, the human T-cell leukemia-lymphoma virus (HTLV) is the first known to cause cancer in humans. It has been found to be present in the cells of individuals with certain types of leukemia and lymphoma. Fortunately, not everyone affected by HTLV develops cancer. Scientists are studying the complex biological relation among viruses, genes, and the development of cancer with the hope of uncovering information leading to the prevention, control, and possible cure of cancer. The American Cancer Society has published the following list of safeguards against cancer, which encourages individuals to take specific steps to safeguard their health and aids in the early detection of cancer.

Site	Action
Breast	Monthly self-examination
Uterus	Pap test once a year
Lung	Don't smoke cigarettes
Skin	Avoid excess sun
Colon-rectum	Procto annually, especially after 40
Mouth	Exams regularly
Whole body	Annual health checkup

Classification of Cancer

The more than 200 types of cancer have been grouped into three main classifications: carcinomas, sarcomas, and mixed cancers.

CARCINOMAS

As mentioned earlier, carcinomas make up the great majority of all cancers and are malignant tumors of epithelial tissues. They are named according to the type of epithelial cell in which the malignancy occurs or the primary site of the tumor. For example, a cancer of squamous epithelium is a squamous carcinoma. Likewise, a cancer originating in the bronchus of the respiratory tract is a bronchogenic carcinoma. Epithelial tissue lines body surfaces including those of glands and organs; therefore, carcinomas make up the majority of the glandular cancers and are generally found in the breast, stomach, uterus, tongue, and skin.

SARCOMAS

Sarcomas are a less prevalent type of cancer that develops from embryonic cells of connective tissue such as muscle, fat, bone, and blood vessels. They are named by adding the suffix **sarcoma** to the prefix that identifies the tissue of origin. A cancer of the bone, for example, is an osteosarcoma.

MIXED CANCERS

Mixed cancers originate in cells capable of differentiating into epithelial or connective tissue or when malignancies occur concurrently in adjacent tissue types. For example, stomach cancer may be a mixed cancer when carcinoma originates in the epithelial lining of the stomach wall and a sarcoma arises in the adjacent muscular layer underlying the epithelium.

OTHER TYPES

Other types of cancer may be classified as leukemias, lymphomas, or melanomas. Leukemias are cancers of the blood-forming tissues. Lymphomas are cancers of lymphoid tissue, and melanomas are cancers of black moles.

Cell Differentiation

Normal cells reproduce themselves through an orderly process that assures growth, tissue repair, and cell reproduction or mitosis. Normal cells have a distinct appearance and a specialized function. In normal cell development, immature cells undergo normal changes as they mature and assume their specialized functions. This process is called differentiation. Knowledge of cell differentiation allows a pathologist or histologist, looking at a sample of tissue through a microscope, to identify the body area from which the tissue was removed. In cancer, there is an abnormal process wherein a cell or group of cells undergoes changes and no longer carries on normal cell functions. This failure of immature cells to develop specialized functions is called dedifferentiation. It is believed that this process involves a disturbance in the DNA of the affected cells. Malignant cells usually multiply rapidly, forming a mass of abnormal cells that enlarges, ulcerates, and sheds malignant cells to surrounding tissues. This process destroys the normal cells, with malignant cells taking their places. Microscopic analysis of a malignant cell reveals a loss of differentiation, anaplasia, nuclei of various sizes that are hyperchromatic, and cells in the process of rapid and disorderly division. Based on microscopic analysis, malignant tumors are further classified as grades I, II, III, or IV. The following describes each of the four grades of tumors in this system:

Grade I—the most differentiated and the least malignant tumors. Only a few cells are undergoing mitosis; however, some abnormality does exist

Grade II—moderately undifferentiated, more cells are undergoing mitosis, and the pattern is fairly irregular

Grade III—many cells are undifferentiated, and tissue origin may be difficult to recognize. Many cells are undergoing mitosis

Grade IV—the least differentiated and a high degree of malignancy

This system of grading tumors is used to report the prognosis of the disease and also to determine whether the tumor is likely to respond to radiation therapy.

The Invasive Process

Two ways in which malignant cells spread to body parts are by invasive growth (by active migration or direct extension) and metastasis.

INVASIVE GROWTH

Invasive growth is the spreading process of a malignant tumor into adjacent normal tissue. Young malignant cells divide at the periphery of the tumor and spread by active migration or direct extension. In active migration, the malignant cells break away from the neoplasm, invade surrounding tissue, divide, form secondary neoplasms, and then reunite with the primary tumor as growth continues. In direct extension, multiplication of malignant cells is rapid, and there is subsequent spreading into surrounding tissues via the interstitial spaces accompanied by engulfment and destruction of normal cells. As a tumor's mass enlarges, its weight is supported by connective fibers that attach to surrounding structures. Adjacent veins and lymph vessels are invaded by these fibers and become pathways for the spread of malignant cells.

METASTASIS

Metastasis is the process whereby cancer cells are spread from a primary site to distant secondary sites elsewhere in the body. This process usually occurs when malignant cells invade the bloodstream or lymph system and are transported to a secondary site where they become lodged and form a neoplasm. Malignant cells carried in the bloodstream may lodge in highly vascular organs such as the lungs or liver, and the development of a secondary neoplasm depends on the viability and the reception of the organ.

Staging

Further reporting of the development and spread of cancer cells may be made through the use of a system that evaluates the spread of the tumor. The staging system uses the letters T (tumor), N (node), and M (metastasis) to indicate spread and uses numerical subscripts to indicate degree of tumor involvement. For example, $T_2N_1M_0$ indicates a primary tumor at stage 2, abnormality of regional lymph nodes at stage 1, and no evidence of distant metastasis.

Characteristics of Neoplasms

Neoplasms or tumors, as they are commonly called, may be benign or malignant. The following characteristics will distinguish the differences between benign and malignant neoplasms:

Benign Tumors	Malignant Tumors
1. Grow slowly	1. Grow rapidly
2. Encapsulated	2. Not encapsulated
3. Cells resemble the normal cells from which they arose	3. Cells undergo permanent change, abnormal rapid proliferation
4. Grow by expansion and cause pressure on surrounding tissue	4. Invasive growth and metastasis
5. Remain localized	5. Spread via the bloodstream
6. Do not recur when surgically removed	6. May recur when surgically removed if invasive growth has occurred
7. Tissue destruction is minimal	7. Tissue destruction is extensive if invasive growth has occurred
8. No cachexia	8. Cancer cachexia (extreme weakness, fatigue, wasting, and malnutrition)
9. Usually not a threat to life	9. Threat to life unless detected early and properly treated

As malignant cells proliferate and begin the invasive process, the patient is unaware of the development of the cancer. In its early stages, cancer is said to be silent; however, cytological changes are occurring that could be detected if a tissue sample were taken and analyzed by a pathologist. With the proliferation of malignant cells and the continuation of the invasive process, tissues, organs, and surrounding structures become compressed, and ischemia may occur, causing necrosis, inflammation, ulceration, and bleeding. This bleeding is usually occult (hidden) and is not noted by the patient. The enlarging tumor eventually causes sufficient pressure on surrounding tissues and organs to create a feeling of numbness, tingling, and pain. Because the tumor itself does not have nerve endings, pain is not an early symptom of its development. Because of the "silent" development of cancer, the patient does not usually become aware of its symptoms until its systemic effects are evident. These systemic effects depend on the site and type of cancer but usually result in an imbalance in the patient's physiology, leading to subtle but noticeable changes that may warn of the disease.

The American Cancer Society lists seven warning signals of cancer. The first letters of each warning signal combine to spell the word CAUTION, and persons who develop any of the following symptoms should bring it to the attention of a physician immediately:

- Change in bowel or bladder habits
- A sore that does not heal
- Unusual bleeding or discharge
- Thickening or lump in breast or elsewhere
- Indigestion or difficulty in swallowing
- Obvious change in a wart or mole
- Nagging cough or hoarseness

Diagnosis

A variety of diagnostic tools and procedures is used to detect the possible presence of cancer. Principal among these are examination, visualization by endoscopy, laboratory analysis, biopsy, and diagnostic radiology.

EXAMINATION

An annual physical examination may be the best means of protecting one's state of health. The American Cancer Society publishes a cancer detection examination that recommends certain tests be included in an annual physical examination in addition to the medical history and usual tests.* These tests are listed below:

Skin—entire skin

Head and Neck—eyes; nose; mouth, under all dentures; vocal cords with mirror, if hoarseness

Chest—listen to heart and lungs; x-ray record of chest when indicated

Breast—palpation of breasts and under arms for any abnormalities; biopsy of lump in breast when indicated; instruct and encourage breast self-examination; ages 40–49 get a mammogram every 1 to 2 years, after age 49 every year

Abdomen—palpation for any abnormalities

Pelvis—pelvic examination, including a Pap test for all women

Colon and Rectum—digital examination of rectum; proctosigmoidoscopic examination; x-ray record of colon or intestinal tract when indicated

Prostate—digital examination of prostate; palpation of male testes; palpation of groin for enlarged lymph nodes; age 50 and over should have a Prostate-Specific Antigen (PSA) blood test each year

Blood—for leukemia or anemia

Urinalysis—for indication of bladder or kidney cancer

VISUALIZATION BY ENDOSCOPY

Endoscopy provides the physician with a direct view of certain portions of the body. The following is a list of endoscopic procedures used to assess specific locations within the body:

1. **Sigmoidoscopy.** The process of using a sigmoidoscope to examine the lower 10 inches of the large intestines
2. **Laryngoscopy.** The process of using a laryngoscope to examine the interior of the larynx
3. **Bronchoscopy.** The process of using a bronchoscope to examine the bronchi
4. **Gastroscopy.** The process of using a gastroscope to examine the interior of the stomach
5. **Cystoscopy.** The process of using a cystoscope to examine the bladder
6. **Colposcopy.** The process of using a colposcope to examine the cervix and vagina
7. **Proctoscopy.** The process of using a proctoscope to examine the anus and rectum
8. **Colonoscopy.** The process of using a colonoscope to examine the colon
9. **Laparoscopy.** The process of using a laparoscope to examine the abdomen

LABORATORY ANALYSIS

Laboratory analysis plays a key role in detecting specific types of cancer. The following are some of the laboratory tests used to diagnose cancer:

1. **Pap Smear/Test.** A cytological screening test developed by Dr. George Papanicolaou and used to detect the presence of abnormal or cancerous cells from the cervix and vagina

*This information was taken from American Cancer Society Professional Education publications.

2. **Hemoccult.** A strip test used to detect occult (hidden) blood. This test is commonly used to check for cancer of the colon
3. **Sputum Cytology Test.** Microscopic examination of sputum to detect abnormal or cancerous cells of the bronchi and lungs
4. **Blood Serum Test.** Analysis of blood serum provides useful information about certain proteins synthesized by cancer
5. **Abbot Lab's AFP-EIA Test.** An immunoassay test that uses alpha-fetoprotein to mark tumor cells when testing for cancer of the testicles
6. **Bone Marrow Study.** A test used to detect abnormal bone marrow cells, which may indicate leukemia
7. **Urine Assay Tests.** Tests providing useful information about catecholamines, which may indicate pheochromocytoma of the adrenal medulla
8. **Gravlee Jet Washer.** A device developed by Dr. Clark Gravlee to check for endometrial abnormalities as surface cells of the uterine cavity are studied under a microscope

BIOPSY

The surgical removal of a small piece of tissue for microscopic examination is known as biopsy. It is the method of providing the proof of cancer in the diagnosis of the disease. The following different types of biopsy may be used for tissue removal:

1. **Excisional Biopsy.** Surgical removal of a piece of tissue from the suspected body site
2. **Incisional Biopsy.** A surgical incision to remove a section or wedge of tissue from the suspected body site
3. **Needle Biopsy.** Puncture of a tumor for the removal of a core of tissue through the lumen of a needle
4. **Cone Biopsy.** Removal of a cone of tissue from the uterine cervix
5. **Sternal Biopsy.** Removal of a piece of bone marrow from the sternum
6. **Endoscopic Biopsy.** Removal of a piece of tissue through an endoscope
7. **Punch Biopsy.** Removal of a plug of tissue (epidermis, dermis, and subcutaneous tissue) from the skin

DIAGNOSTIC RADIOLOGY

Encompassing a wide range of tests and procedures, diagnostic radiology can reveal tumors that may not have been detected by other diagnostic procedures (See Chapter 18 on Radiology and Nuclear Medicine).

Treatment

The treatment of cancer may be any one or a combination of the following methods: surgery, chemotherapy, radiation therapy, or immunotherapy. The treatment of choice will depend on the type of cancer, its location, its invasive process, and the state of health of the patient.

SURGERY

Surgery may be the treatment of choice when the tumor is small and localized and the surrounding tissue is accessible for removal. The aim of surgery is the removal of all cancerous tissue plus some of the surrounding normal tissue. Surgery may also be used to alleviate some of the complications of cancer, such as the obstruction of an area caused by the enlargement of a tumor.

CHEMOTHERAPY

Chemotherapy may be the treatment of choice when the cancer is disseminated and cannot be surgically removed. It is also used when a tumor fails to respond to radiation therapy. Antineoplastic, anticancer drugs do injury to individual cells, interfere with their vital functions, and kill or destroy malignant cells. In rendering cancerous cells harmless, certain normal cells may also be destroyed. The normal cells with the greatest sensitivity to destruction are the hematopoietic cells, epithelial cells, and the hair follicles. The plan of treatment for patients undergoing chemotherapy is individualized. The aim of chemotherapy is to put the patient in remission so that life may continue without exacerbation of symptoms. The following are classifications of chemotherapeutic drugs used in the treatment of cancer.

Alkylating Agents

Alkylating agents are chemical compounds that cause chromosome breakage and prevent the formation of new DNA, thereby interfering with cell division. These agents are used in the treatment of leukemia, lymphoma, or disseminated malignancies. Nitrogen mustard, cyclophosphamide, melphalan, chlorambucil, busulfan, and thiotepa are some of the alkylating agents available.

Antimetabolites

Antimetabolites are substances that interfere with the metabolic process of the cell, thus preventing cell reproduction. They are used in the treatment of leukemia, disseminated solid tumors, and choriocarcinoma. Some of the antimetabolites used are methotrexate, 6-mercaptopurine, 5-fluorouracil, cytosine arabinoside, and thioguanine.

Vinca Alkaloids

The vinca alkaloids are compounds that interfere with cell division by interacting with the cell's miotic process. Alkaloids are used in the treatment of leukemia, lymphoma, Wilm's tumor, and neuroblastoma. Vincristine and vinblastine are alkaloids.

Antibiotics

Certain antibiotics have an antineoplastic effect and are used in the treatment of leukemia, Wilm's tumor, choriocarcinoma, and cancer of the testes. Actinomycin-D and mithramycin are such antibiotics.

Steroid Hormones

Steroid hormones are substances that alter the hormonal environment. Commonly used steroids and the cancers they treat include the following:

1. Androgen—breast cancer
2. Estrogen—prostate cancer
3. Progesterone—endometrial cancer
4. Adrenocortical hormones—leukemia

IMMUNOTHERAPY

Immunotherapy is the treatment of disease by stimulation of the body's immune system. It may be used as an adjuvant to other types of treatment. There are three types of immunotherapy: active specific, passive, and adoptive.

Active Immunotherapy

Active specific immunotherapy is the use of various agents to produce a specific host-immune response. The patient's own tumor cells, tumor antigens, oncogenic viruses, and bacterial products are a few of the agents that are being used to create an immune response of a specific nature.

Passive Immunotherapy

Passive immunotherapy is the use of serum or other products from an immunocompetent individual that are given to an immunodeficient individual to produce an immune response.

Adoptive Immunotherapy

Adoptive immunotherapy is the process of transferring a form of specific immune response from a donor to a recipient.

NEW FORMS OF TREATMENT

Differentiation Agents/Maturation Agents

This is a new classification of drugs that invade cancer cells and somehow cause them to mature into cells that are almost normal. They are being tested on humans and have demonstrated good activity against colon cancer.

Interleukin-2 (IL-2)

This is a genetically engineered immune-boosting drug that stimulates the patient's immune system to produce lymphokine-activated killer (LAK) cells that destroy some forms of tumor cells. It is used in the treatment of certain types of cancer.

Intraoperative Radiation Therapy

This is the delivery of tumoricidal doses of radiation directly onto a tumor bed while the surgical wound is still open. The surgeon and radiotherapist decide on the target area, and then the radiotherapist positions the sterile treatment cone in the incision. The treatment is usually for 15 to 30 min, and the incision is closed after the treatment is completed.

Photodynamic Therapy

This is the use of a red laser to kill cancerous cells. Hematoporphyrin derivative (Hpd), a light-sensitizing agent, is intravenously injected, and 3 days after the injection the physician uses the red laser. Normal cells eliminate Hpd and are not harmed during the treatment. Cancerous cells retain Hpd, and the red light kills them.

Recombinant Interferon Therapy

This is a genetically engineered immune system activator. It strengthens the body's immune system and helps it fight cancer cells. It is indicated for use in the treatment of hairy cell leukemia in people 18 years of age or older.

Tumor Necrosis Factor (TNF)

This is a lymphokine produced by macrophages (white blood cells). It triggers the macrophages to destroy malignant tumors. It is being tested in the treatment of low-grade lymphoma.

Whole Body Hyperthermia

This is the process of elevating the patient's body temperature to 108°F (42.2°C) to enhance the effect of radiation or chemotherapy. Cancer cells are sensitive to heat, so after radiation therapy, hyperthermia is employed to inhibit the cancer cells from repairing themselves. It is used before chemotherapy to increase the vulnerability of the cancer cells to the drug being used in the treatment process.

Prevention of Cancer

STOP SMOKING OR DON'T EVER START

Smoking is the most preventable cause of death in man. In the United States, tobacco use is responsible for more than one in six deaths. Cigarette smoking is responsible for 90% of lung cancer among men and 79% among women. Smoking accounts for about 30% of all cancer deaths. Those who smoke two or more packs of cigarettes a day have lung cancer mortality rates 15 to 25 times greater than nonsmokers. According to the World Health Organization, approximately 2.5 million people each year worldwide die as a result of smoking.

STOP USING SMOKELESS TOBACCO OR DON'T EVER START

There has been a resurgence in the use of all forms of smokeless tobacco. The greatest cause of concern centers on the increased use of "dipping snuff." In this practice, tobacco that has been processed into a coarse, moist powder is placed between the cheek and gum, and nicotine, along with a number of carcinogens, is absorbed through the oral mucosa. Use of chewing tobacco or snuff increases the risk of cancer of the mouth, larynx (voice box), pharynx (throat), and esophagus (food tube).

AVOID DIRECT SUNLIGHT AND/OR USE PROTECTIVE SUNSCREEN

Epidemiologic evidence shows that sun exposure is a major factor in the development of melanoma and that incidence increases for those living near the equator. Almost all of the more than 700,000 cases of basal and squamous cell skin cancer diagnosed each year in the United States are sun related (ultraviolet radiation).

AVOID IONIZING RADIATION AND/OR LIMIT EXPOSURE

Excessive exposure to ionizing radiation can increase cancer risk. Excessive radon exposure in homes, schools, and one's workplace may increase the risk of lung cancer, especially in cigarette smokers.

"EAT-RIGHT" NUTRITION AND DIET

More and more evidence shows that proper nutrition and diet can help prevent disease. One may reduce his or her cancer risk by:

1. Maintaining desirable weight. Individuals 40% or more overweight increase their risk of colon, breast, prostate, gallbladder, ovary, and uterus cancer.
2. Eat a variety of food.
3. Eat a variety of vegetables and fruits each day. The National Institute (NCI) suggest eating at least 5 servings of fruits and vegetables each day-"5 A Day For Better Health." Studies have shown that a daily consumption of vegetables and fruits may decrease the risk of lung, prostate, esophagus, colorectal, and stomach cancers.
4. Eat more foods that are high in fiber, such as whole grains, breads, pasta, vegetables, and fruits. High-fiber diets may reduce the risk of colon cancer.
5. Cut down on total fat intake. It is recommended that only 30% or less of one's daily intake be from fat. A high-fat diet may contribute to breast, colon, and prostate cancer.
6. If you drink, limit the consumption of alcohol to a minimum. The heavy use of alcohol, especially when accompanied by cigarette smoking or smokeless tobacco use, increases the risk of cancers of the mouth, larynx, pharynx (throat), esophagus, and liver.
7. Limit the consumption of salt-cured, smoked, and nitrite-cured foods. In areas of the world where salt-cured and smoked foods are eaten frequently, there is higher incidence of cancer of the esophagus and stomach.

AVOID OCCUPATIONAL HAZARDS

Exposure to several different industrial agents (nickel, chromate, asbestos, vinyl chloride, etc.) increases risk of various cancers. Risk of lung cancer from asbestos is greatly increased when combined with cigarette smoking.

FYI: The National Cancer Institute (NCI) and The American Cancer Society

The National Cancer Institute has designated several medical centers throughout the United States as Comprehensive Cancer Centers (CCCs). These centers develop comprehensive cancer programs and provide up-to-date regimens. For information on oncology you may call 800-4 CANCER or 800 422-6237.

The American Cancer Society is a voluntary organization dedicated to the control and eradication of cancer. National headquarters are in Atlanta, and there are 58 incorporated chartered Divisions: one in each state, in Puerto Rico, the District of Columbia and six metropolitan areas. For information you may call 800-ACS-2345 or write: American Cancer Society, Inc., 1599 Clifton Road, N. E., Atlanta, GA 30329-4251. The American Cancer Society is the nationwide, community-based, voluntary health organization dedicated to eliminating cancer as a major health problem by preventing cancer, saving lives from cancer, and diminishing suffering from cancer through research, education, and service.

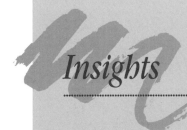

Insights

BREAST CANCER

This year approximately 182,000 women and approximately 1000 men will be diagnosed with breast cancer. It kills about 46,000 women a year, and is the leading cause of death in women between the ages of 32 and 52.

In cancer, there is an abnormal process wherein a cell or group of cells undergoes changes and no longer carries on normal cell functions. This failure of immature cells to develop specialized functions is called dedifferentiation. It is believed that this process involves a disturbance in the DNA of the affected cells. Malignant cells usually multiply rapidly, forming a mass of abnormal cells that enlarges, ulcerates, and sheds malignant cells to surrounding tissues. This process destroys the normal cells, with malignant cells taking their places, and often results in the formation of a tumor.

Know Your Breast and Your Risk Factors

More than 90% of all breast lumps are discovered by women themselves. The majority of these lumps are benign (noncancerous) but of those that are not, early detection and treatment are essential.

Your Breast:

Being Informed Could Save Your Life
Risk Factors in Order of Importance:

1. Family history—Increased risk when breast cancer occurs before menopause in mother, sister, or daughter especially if cancer occurs in both breasts.
2. Over age 50 and nullipara.
3. Having a first baby after age 30.
4. History of chronic breast disease, especially epithelial hyperplasia.
5. Exposure to ionizing radiation of more than 50 rad during adolescence.
6. Obesity.
7. Early menarche, late menopause.

Examine your breast every month
(BSE, Breast Self-Examination—see Fig. 17–1)
Appearance
Size, shape, symmetry
Tenderness, thickening, texture changes

(Insights continues on next page.)

If cancer is not detected and treated early, it will continue to grow, invade and destroy adjacent tissue and spread into surrounding lymph nodes. It can be carried by the lymph and/or blood to other areas of the body and once this process, known as metastasis, has occurred, the cancer is usually advanced and/or disseminated and the 5-year survival rate is low. Early detection of breast cancer is extremely important. The 5-year survival rate for women with localized, and properly treated breast cancer is 92%.

Approximately 50% of malignant tumors of the breast appear in the upper, outer quadrant and extend into the armpit. Eighteen percent of breast cancers occur in the nipple area, 11% in the lower outer quadrant, and 6% in the inner quadrant.

Signs and symptoms of breast cancer are generally insidious and may include:

- unusual secretions from the nipple
- changes in the nipple's appearance
- nontender, movable lump
- well-localized discomfort that may be described as a burning, stinging, or aching sensation
- dimpling or peau d'orange (orange-peel appearance) may be present over the area of cancer of the breast
- asymmetry and an elevation of the affected breast
- nipple retraction
- pain in the later stages

FYI: National Cancer Institute's Cancer Information Center 1–800–4-CANCER; American Cancer Society 1–800–227–2345; Breast Health Book: "Dr. Susan Love's Breast Book," Addison-Wesley Publishing Company; Susan Love, M.D., is the director of a high-profile new breast program at the University of California at Los Angeles and she is a breast-cancer surgeon who established the National Breast Coalition in 1991. A video-tape "Getting on with It" is available for those recovering from cancer. The tape is produced by Centocor, Inc, Malvern, Pa.

▼ WHY DO THE BREAST SELF-EXAM?

There are many good reasons for doing a breast self-exam each month. One reason is that it is easy to do and the more you do it, the better you will get at it. When you get to know how your breasts normally feel, you will quickly be able to feel any change, and early detection is the key to successful treatment and cure.

▼ WHEN TO DO BREAST SELF-EXAM

The best time to do breast self-exam is right after your period, when breasts are not tender or swollen. If you do not have regular periods or sometimes skip a month, do it on the same day every month.

▼ NOW, HOW TO DO BREAST SELF-EXAM

1. Lie down and put a pillow under your right shoulder. Place your right arm behind your head.

2. Use the finger pads of your three middle fingers on your left hand to feel for lumps or thickening. Your finger pads are the top third of each finger.

3. Press firmly enough to know how your breast feels. If you're not sure how hard to press, ask your health care provider. Or try to copy the way your health care provider uses the finger pads during a breast exam. Learn what your breast feels like most of the time. A firm ridge in the lower curve of each breast is normal.

4. Move around the breast in a set way. You can choose either the circle (A), the up and down line (B), or the wedge (C). Do it the same way every time. It will help you to make sure that you've gone over the entire breast area, and to remember how your breast feels.

▼ FOR ADDED SAFETY:

You should also check your breasts while standing in front of a mirror right after you do your breast self-exam each month. See if there are any changes in the way your breasts look: dimpling of the skin, changes in the nipple, or redness or swelling.

You might also want to do a breast self-exam while you're in the shower. Your soapy hands will glide over the wet skin making it easy to check how your breasts feel.

Remember: A breast self-exam could save your breast—and save your life. Most breast lumps are found by women themselves, but, in fact, most lumps in the breast are not cancer. Be safe, be sure.

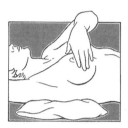
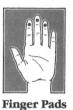

Finger Pads

5. Now examine your left breast using right hand finger pads.

6. If you find any changes, see your doctor right away.

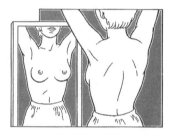

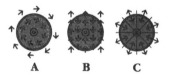

A   B   C

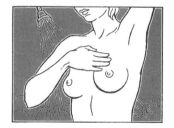

FIGURE 17–1

How to do breast self-examination. (*Courtesy of the American Cancer Society, Inc.*)

Terminology with Surgical Procedures & Pathology

Term	Word Parts			Definition
adenocarcinoma (ăd″ ĕ-nō-kăr″ sĭn-ō′ maă)	adeno carcin oma	CF R S	gland cancer tumor	A cancerous tumor of a gland
anaplasia (ăn″ ă-plā′ zĭ-ă)	ana plasia	P S	up formation	A characteristic of most cancerous cells in which there is a loss of differentiation
astrocytoma (ăs″ trō-sī-tō′ mă)	astro cyt oma	P R S	star-shaped cell tumor	A tumor composed of star-shaped neuroglial cells
carcinogen (kăr″ sĭn′ ō-jĕn)	carcino gen	CF S	cancer formation	Any agent or substance that incites or produces cancer
carcinoma (kăr″ sĭ-nō′ mă)	carcin oma	R S	cancer tumor	A cancerous tumor
chondrosarcoma (kŏn″ drō-săr-kō′ mă)	chondro sarc oma	CF R S	cartilage flesh tumor	A cancerous tumor derived from cartilage cells
choriocarcinoma (kō″ rĭ-ō-kăr″ sĭ-nō′ mă)	chorio carcin oma	CF R S	chorion cancer tumor	A cancerous tumor of the uterus or at the site of an ectopic pregnancy
fibrosarcoma (fī″ brō-săr-kō′ mă)	fibro sarc oma	CF R S	fiber flesh tumor	A cancerous tumor arising from collagen-producing fibroblasts
glioblastoma (glī′ ō-blăs-tō′ mă)	glio blast oma	CF S S	glue immature cell tumor	A cancerous tumor of the brain, usually of the cerebral hemispheres
glioma (glī-ō′ mă)	gli oma	R S	glue tumor	A cancerous tumor of the brain
hemangiosarcoma (hē-măn″ jĭ-ō-săr-kō′ mă)	hem angio sarc oma	R CF R S	blood vessel flesh tumor	A cancerous tumor originating from blood vessels
hypernephroma (hī″ pĕr-nĕ-frō′ mă)	hyper nephr oma	P R S	excessive kidney tumor	A cancerous tumor of the kidney
hyperplasia (hī″ pĕr-plā′ zĭ-ă)	hyper plasia	P S	excessive formation	Excessive formation and growth of normal cells

(Terminology—continued)

Term	Word Parts			Definition
immunotherapy (ĭm″ mū-nō-thĕr′ ă pē)	immuno therapy	CF S	safe treatment	Treatment of disease by active, passive, or adoptive immunity
leiomyosarcoma (lī″ ō-mī″ ō-săr-kō′ mă)	leio myo sarc oma	CF CF R S	smooth muscle flesh tumor	A cancerous tumor of smooth muscle tissue
leukemia (lū-kē′ mĭ-ă)	leuk emia	R S	white blood condition	A disease of the blood characterized by overproduction of leukocytes; cancer of the blood-forming tissues
leukoplakia (lū″ kō-plā′ kĭ-ă)	leuko plakia	CF S	white plate	White, thickened patches formed on the mucous membranes of the cheeks, gums, or tongue. These patches tend to become cancerous
liposarcoma (lĭp″ ō-săr-kō′ mă)	lipo sarc oma	CF R S	fat flesh tumor	A cancerous tumor of fat cells
lymphan-giosarcoma (lĭm-făn″ jē-ō-săr-kō′ mă)	lymph angio sarc oma	R CF R S	lymph vessel flesh tumor	A cancerous tumor of lymphatic vessels
lymphoma (lĭm-fō′ mă)	lymph oma	R S	lymph tumor	A cancerous tumor of the lymph nodes
lymphosarcoma (lĭm″ fō-săr-kō′ mă)	lympho sarc oma	CF R S	lymph flesh tumor	A cancerous disease of lymphatic tissue
medulloblastoma (mĕ-dŭl″ ō-blăs-tō′ mă)	medullo blast oma	CF S S	marrow immature cell tumor	A cancerous tumor of the brain, the fourth ventricle, and the cerebellum
melanoma (mĕl″ ă-nō′ mă)	melan oma	R S	black tumor	A cancerous black mole or tumor
meningioma (mĕn-ĭn″ jĭ-ō′ mă)	meningi oma	CF S	membrane tumor	A cancerous tumor arising in the arachnoidal tissue of the brain
mucositis (mū″ kō-sī′ tĭs)	mucos itis	R S	mucus inflammation	Inflammation of the oral mucosa caused by exposure to high-energy beams delivered by radiation therapy

(Terminology—continued)

Term	Word Parts			Definition
mycotoxin (mī″ kō-tŏk′ sĭn)	myco	CF	fungus	Pertaining to a fungus growing in food or animal feed that, if ingested, may cause cancer
	tox	R	poison	
	in	S	pertaining to	
myeloma (mī″ ĕ-lō′ mă)	myel	R	marrow	A tumor arising in the hemopoietic portion of the bone marrow
	oma	S	tumor	
myosarcoma (mī″ ō-săr-kō′ mă)	myo	CF	muscle	A cancerous tumor of muscle tissue
	sarc	R	flesh	
	oma	S	tumor	
neoplasm (nē′ ō-plăzm)	neo	P	new	A new thing formed, such as an abnormal growth or tumor
	plasm	S	a thing formed	
nephroblastoma (nĕf″ rō-blăs-tō′ mă)	nephro	CF	kidney	A cancerous tumor of the kidney; also called Wilm's tumor
	blast	S	immature cell	
	oma	S	tumor	
neuroblastoma (nū″ rō-blăs-tō′ mă)	neuro	CF	nerve	A cancerous tumor composed chiefly of neuroblasts; usually found in infants or young children
	blast	S	immature cell	
	oma	S	tumor	
oligodendro- glioma (ŏl″ ĭ-gō-dĕn″ drō-glī-ō′ mă)	oligo	P	little	A cancerous tumor composed chiefly of neuroglial cells and located in the cerebrum
	dendro	CF	tree	
	gli	R	glue	
	oma	S	tumor	
oncogenes (ŏng″ kō-jēnz′)	onco	CF	tumor	Cancer-causing genes
	genes	S	produce	
oncogenic (ŏng″ kō-jĕn′ ĭk)	onco	CF	tumor	The formation of tumors, especially cancerous tumors
	genic	S	formation, produce	
osteogenic sarcoma (ŏs″ tē-ō-jĕn′ ĭk săr-kō′ mă)	osteo	CF	bone	A cancerous tumor composed of osseous tissue
	genic	S	formation, produce	
	sarc	R	flesh	
	oma	S	tumor	
precancerous (prē-kăn′ sĕr-ŭs)	pre	P	before	Pertaining to the state of a growth or condition before the onset of cancer
	cancer	R	crab	
	ous	S	pertaining to	
reticulosarcoma (rĕ-tĭk″ ū-lō-săr-kō′ mă)	reticulo	CF	net	A cancerous tumor of the lymphatic system
	sarc	R	flesh	
	oma	S	tumor	

(Terminology—continued)

Term	Word Parts			Definition
retinoblastoma (rĕt″ ĭ-nō-blăs-tō′ mă)	retino blast oma	CF S S	retina immature cell tumor	A cancerous tumor of the retina
rhabdomyo-sarcoma (răb″ dō-mĭ″ ō-săr-kō′ mă)	rhabdo myo sarc oma	CF CF R S	rod muscle flesh tumor	A cancerous tumor arising in striated muscle tissue
sarcoma (săr-kō′ mă)	sarc oma	R S	flesh tumor	A cancerous tumor arising from connective tissue
sarcopoietic (săr″ kō-poy-ĕt′ ĭk)	sarco poietic	CF S	flesh formation	The formation of flesh or muscle
seminoma (sĕm″ ĭ-nō′ mă)	semin oma	R S	seed tumor	A cancerous tumor of the testis
teratoma (tĕr″ ă-tō′ mă)	terat oma	R S	monster tumor	A cancerous tumor of the ovary or testis; may contain embryonic tissues of hair, teeth, bone, or muscle
thymoma (thī-mō′ mă)	thym oma	R S	thymus tumor	A tumor of the thymus gland
trismus (trĭz′ mŭs)	trism us	R S	grating pertaining to	Pertaining to the inability to open the mouth fully; occurs in patients with oral cancer who undergo a combination of surgery and radiation therapy
xerostomia (zē″ rō-stō′ mē-ă)	xero stom ia	CF R S	dry mouth condition	A condition of dryness of the mouth; an oral change caused by radiation therapy or chemotherapy

Vocabulary Words

Vocabulary words are terms that have not been divided into component parts. They are common words or specialized terms associated with the subject of this chapter. These words are provided to enhance your medical vocabulary.

Word	Definition
Burkitt's lymphoma (bŭrk′ ĭtz lĭm-fō′ mă)	A malignant tumor, most commonly found in Africa, that affects children. The characteristic symptom is a massive, swollen jaw
dedifferentiation (dē-dĭf″ ĕr-ĕn″ shē-ā′ shŭn)	The process whereby normal cells lose their specialization (differentiation) and become malignant
deoxyribonucleic acid (dē-ŏk″ sĭ-rī″ bō-nū-klē′ ĭk ăs′ ĭd)	A complex protein of high molecular weight that is found in the nucleus of every cell. DNA controls all the cell's activities and contains the genetic material necessary for the organism's heredity
differentiation (dĭf″ ĕr-ĕn″ shē-ā″ shŭn)	The process whereby normal cells have a distinct appearance and specialized function
encapsulated (ĕn-kăp″ sū-lā′ tĕd)	Enclosed within a sheath or capsule
Ewing's sarcoma (ū′ ĭngz săr-kō′ mă)	A primary bone cancer occurring in the pelvic area or in one of the long bones
exacerbation (ĕks-ăs″ ĕr-bā′ shŭn)	The process of increasing the severity of symptoms. A time when the symptoms of a disease are most prevalent
fungating (fŭn′ gāt-ĭng)	The process of growing rapidly, like a fungus
Hodgkin's disease (hŏj′ kĭns dĭ-zēz′)	A form of lymphoma that occurs in young adults
human T-cell leukemia-lymphoma virus (HTLV) (hū′ măn tē′ sĕl lū-kē′ mĭ-ă lĭm-fō′ mă vī′ rŭs)	The first virus known to cause cancer in humans
immunosuppression (ĭm″ ū-nō-sŭ-prĕsh′ ŭn)	The process of preventing formation of the immune response

(Vocabulary—continued)

Word	Definition
infiltrative (ĭn′ fĭl-trā″ tĭve)	Pertaining to the process of extending or growing into normal tissue; invasive
in situ (ĭn sī′ too)	To stay within a site; refers to tumor cells that remain at a site and have not invaded adjacent tissue
interstitial (ĭn″ tĕr-stĭsh′ ăl)	Pertaining to between spaces
invasive (ĭn-vā′ sĭv)	The spreading process of a malignant tumor into normal tissue
Kaposi's sarcoma (kăp′ ō-sēz săr-kō′ mă)	A malignant neoplasm that causes violaceous vascular lesions and general lymphadenopathy
lesion (lē′ zhŭn)	A wound; an injury, altered tissue, or a single infected patch of skin
macrofollicular (măk″ rō-fō-lĭk′ ū-lăr)	A giant follicle lymphoma; occurs as a painless swelling of a lymph node but may be found in the spleen
malignant (mă-lĭg′ nănt)	Pertaining to a bad wandering; refers to the spreading process of cancer from one area of the body to another
metastasis (mĕ-tăs′ tă-sis)	The spreading process of cancer from a primary site to a secondary site
mutagen (mū′ tă-jĕn)	Any agent that causes a change in the genetic structure of an organism
mutation (mū-tā′ shŭn)	The process whereby the genetic structure is changed
Paget's disease (păj′ ĕts dĭ-zēz′)	An inflammatory bone disease that may precede the development of bone cancer
palliative (păl′ ĭ-ā-tĭv)	Pertaining to a form of treatment that will relieve or alleviate symptoms without curing
primary site (prī′ mă-rē sīt)	The original, initial, or principal site
proliferation (prō-lĭf″ ĕr-ā′ shŭn)	The process of rapid production; to grow by multiplying
remission (rē-mĭsh′ ŭn)	The process of lessening the severity of symptoms. A time when symptoms of a disease are at rest

(Vocabulary—continued)

Word	Definition
ribonucleic acid (RNA) (rī″ bō-nū′ klē′ ĭk ăs′ ĭd)	A nucleic acid found in all living cells that is responsible for protein synthesis. The three types are mRNA—messenger RNA, tRNA—transfer RNA, and rRNA—ribosomal RNA
scirrhus (skĭr′ ŭs)	A hard, cancerous tumor composed of connective tissue
secondary site (sĕk′ ăn-dĕr″ ē sīt)	The second site usually derived from the primary site
tamponade (cardiac) (tam′ pŏn-ād kăr′ dē-ăk)	A pathologic condition of the heart in which there is accumulation of excess fluid in the pericardium. It may be caused by advanced cancer of the lung or a tumor that has metastasized to the pericardium
tumor (tū′ mor)	An abnormal growth, swelling, or enlargement
violaceous (vī″-ō-lā′ shăs)	Pertaining to having a violet color
viral (vī′ răl)	Pertaining to a virus, which means poison in Latin. A virus is a minute organism that may be responsible for 50% of all diseases
Wilm's tumor (vĭlmz tū′ mor)	A cancerous tumor of the kidney occurring mainly in children

ABBREVIATIONS

Adeno-Ca	adenocarcinoma	**IL-2**	interleukin-2
AFP	alpha-fetoprotein	**LAK**	lymphokine-activated killer (cells)
Bx	biopsy		
CA	cancer	**Mets**	metastases
chem	chemotherapy	**RNA**	ribonucleic acid
DNA	deoxyribonucleic acid	**St**	stage (of disease)
HD	Hodgkin's disease	**TNF**	tumor necrosis factor
Hpd	hematoporphyrin derivative	**TNM**	tumor, node, metastasis
HTLV	human T-cell leukemia-lymphoma virus		

Communication Enrichment

This segment is provided for those who wish to enhance their ability to communicate in either English or Spanish.

SEVEN WARNING SIGNALS OF CANCER

SIETE SEÑALES CANSEROSAS
(sĭ-ĕ-tĕ sĕ-ñă-lĕs kăn-sĕ-rō-săs)

English	Spanish
CAUTION	CAUTELA (kă-ū-tĕ-lă)
Change in bowel or bladder habits	Cambio en movimentos fecales (kăm-bĭ-ō ĕn mō-vĭ-mĭ-ĕn-tōs fĕ-kă-lĕs)
A sore that does not heal	Ulcera que no se cura (ŭl-sĕ-ră kĕ nō sĕ cū-ră)
Unusual bleeding or discharge	Sangramiento inhabitual (săn-gră-mĭ-ĕn-tō ĭn-ă-bĭ-tū-ăl)
Thickening or lump in breast or elsewhere	Espesor o protuberancia en el seno o peson (ĕs-pe-sōr ō prō-tū-bĕ-răn-sĭ-ă ĕn ĕl sĕ-nō ō pĕ-zōn)
Indigestion or difficulty in swallowing	Indigestion o dificultad al tragar (ĭn-dĭ-hĕs-tĭ-ōn ō dĭ-fi-kŭl-tăd ăl tră-găr)
Obvious change in wart or mole	Cambio en una verruga (kăm-bĭ-ō ĕn ū-nă vĕ-rū-gă)
Nagging cough or hoarseness	Tos o ronquera persistente (tōs ō rōn-kĕ-ră pĕr-sĭs-tĕn-tĕ)

RELATED TERMS

English	Spanish
cancer	cancer (kăn-cĕr)
gland	glandula (glăn-dū-lă)
treatment	tratamiento (tră-tă-mĭ-ĕn-tō)
malignant	maligno (mă-lĭg-nō)
spread	extensión (ex-tĕn-sĭ-ōn)
remission	remiso; remision (rĕ-mĭ-sō; rĕ-mĭ-sĭ-ōn)

Learning Exercises

An Overview of Oncology

Write your answers to the following questions. Do not refer back to the text.

1. Name the three main classifications of cancer.

   a. _____   b. _____   c. _____

2. Define cell differentiation. _____
   _____

3. Define dedifferentiation. _____
   _____

4. Name three ways that malignant cells spread to body parts.

   a. _____   b. _____   c. _____

5. List the seven warning signals for cancer.

   a. _____   b. _____

   c. _____   d. _____

   e. _____   f. _____

   g. _____

6. Name four methods that may be used in the treatment of cancer.

   a. _____   b. _____

   c. _____   d. _____

Word Parts

1. In the spaces provided, write the definitions of these prefixes, roots, combining forms, and suffixes. Do not refer to the listings of terminology words. Leave blank those terms you cannot define.
2. After completing as many as you can, refer back to the terminology word listings to check your work. For each word missed or left blank, write the term and its definition several times on the margins of these pages or on a separate sheet of paper.
3. To maximize the learning process, it is to your advantage to do the following exercises as directed. To refer to the terminology listings before completing these exercises invalidates the learning process.

PREFIXES

Give the definitions of the following prefixes:

1. ana-   _____   2. astro-   _____

3. hyper-   _____   4. neo-   _____

5. oligo-   _____   6. pre-   _____

ROOTS AND COMBINING FORMS

Give the definitions of the following roots and combining forms:

1. adeno	_____	2. angio	_____
3. cancer	_____	4. carcin	_____
5. carcino	_____	6. chondro	_____
7. chorio	_____	8. cyt	_____
9. dendro	_____	10. fibro	_____
11. gli	_____	12. glio	_____
13. hem	_____	14. immuno	_____
15. leio	_____	16. leuk	_____
17. leuko	_____	18. lipo	_____
19. lymph	_____	20. lympho	_____
21. medullo	_____	22. melan	_____
23. meningi	_____	24. mucos	_____
25. myco	_____	26. myel	_____
27. myo	_____	28. nephr	_____
29. nephro	_____	30. neuro	_____
31. onco	_____	32. osteo	_____
33. reticulo	_____	34. retino	_____
35. rhabdo	_____	36. sarc	_____
37. sarco	_____	38. semin	_____
39. stom	_____	40. terat	_____
41. thym	_____	42. tox	_____
43. trism	_____	44. xero	_____

SUFFIXES

Give the definitions of the following suffixes:

1. -blast	_____	2. -emia	_____
3. -gen	_____	4. -genes	_____
5. -genic	_____	6. -ia	_____
7. -in	_____	8. -itis	_____
9. -oma	_____	10. -ous	_____
11. -plakia	_____	12. -plasia	_____
13. -plasm	_____	14. -poietic	_____
15. -therapy	_____	16. -us	_____

Identifying Medical Terms

In the spaces provided, write the medical terms for the following meanings:

1. _____ Any agent or substance that incites or produces cancer

2. _____ A cancerous tumor derived from cartilage cells

3. _____ A cancerous tumor of the brain

4. _____ A cancerous tumor of the kidney

5. _____ Cancer of the blood-forming tissues

6. _____ A cancerous tumor of lymphoid tissue

7. _____ A cancerous black mole or tumor

8. _____ A cancerous tumor of muscle tissue

9. _____ A cancerous tumor composed of osseous tissue

10. _____ A cancerous tumor arising from connective tissue

Spelling

In the spaces provided, write the correct spelling of these misspelled terms:

1. anplasia _____   2. fibrsarcoma _____

3. lymphsarcoma _____   4. myloma _____

5. oncgenic _____   6. semioma _____

Review Questions

Matching

Select the appropriate lettered meaning for each numbered line.

_____ 1. Hodgkin's disease

_____ 2. exacerbation

_____ 3. differentiation

_____ 4. in situ

_____ 5. interleukin-2

_____ 6. photodynamic therapy

_____ 7. recombinant interferon

_____ 8. tumor necrosis factor

_____ 9. Kaposi's sarcoma

_____ 10. malignant

a. The spreading process of cancer from one area of the body to another

b. A lymphokine produced by macrophages

c. A genetically engineered immune-boosting drug that stimulaties the patient's immune system

d. The process whereby normal cells have a distinct appearance and specialized function

e. A form of lymphoma that occurs in young adults

f. The use of a red laser to kill cancerous cells

g. To stay within a site

h. A malignant neoplasm that causes violaceous vascular lesions and general lymphadenopathy

i. The process of increasing the severity of symptoms

j. A genetically engineered immune system activator

k. Any agent that causes a change in the genetic structure of an organism

Abbreviations

Place the correct word, phrase, or abbreviation in the space provided.

_____ 1. adenocarcinoma

_____ 2. biopsy

_____ 3. CA

_____ 4. chem

_____ 5. deoxyribonucleic acid

_____ 6. IL-2

_____ 7. lymphokine-activated killer

_____ 8. Mets

_____ 9. TNF

_____ 10. tumor, node, metastases

18

Radiology and Nuclear Medicine

TECHNOLOGY IN DIAGNOSTICS

CT Scanners and Magnetic Resonance Imagers (MRI) have revolutionized diagnostic procedures for determining injury and disease. Prior to these new technologies, physicians had to open the body to look inside.

CT Scanners

- *Visually slice the body, providing a clear view of tissue and organs*

MRI

- *Uses magnetic fields and radio frequencies*
- *Used most frequently on the head and spine*
- *Provides unprecedented clarity*

Radiology is the study of x-rays, radioactive substances, radioactive isotopes, and ionizing radiation. Sometimes called roentgenology, this medical specialty was developed after the discovery of an unknown ray in 1895 by Wilhelm Konrad Roentgen, a German physicist, who called his discovery an x-ray.

Nuclear medicine uses atomic particles that emit electromagnetic radiation on disintegration. The radiant energy thus released is used for diagnostic, investigative, and therapeutic purposes. It may be administered externally from radiation machines such as the betatron and the linear accelerator or internally from small radionuclides implanted within the body near the site to be irradiated.

AN OVERVIEW OF RADIOLOGY AND NUCLEAR MEDICINE

Radiology

Radiology is the study of x-rays, radioactive substances, radioactive isotopes, and ionizing radiation. Sometimes called roentgenology, this medical specialty was developed after the discovery of an unknown ray in 1895 by Wilhelm Konrad Roentgen, a German physicist, who called his discovery an x-ray. An x-ray is produced by the collision of a stream of electrons against a target (usually an anode of one of the heavy metals) contained within a vacuum tube. This collision produces electromagnetic rays of short wavelengths and high energy. The physician who specializes in radiology, roentgen diagnosis, and roentgen therapy is called a radiologist. A roentgenologist is a physician who has specialized only in the use of x-rays for diagnosis and the treatment of disease.

CHARACTERISTICS OF X-RAYS

1. X-rays are an invisible form of radiant energy with short wavelengths traveling at 186,000 miles per second. They are able to penetrate and pass through opaque or solid substances such as the human body.
2. X-rays cause ionization of the substances through which they pass. Ionization is a process resulting in the gain or loss of one or more electrons in neutral atoms. The gain of an electron creates a negative electrical charge, whereas the loss of an electron results in a positively charged particle. These negatively or positively charged particles are called ions.
3. X-rays excite fluorescence in certain substances, thus allowing for the process known as fluoroscopy (Fig. 18–1). With this technique, internal structures show up as dark images on a glowing screen as x-rays pass through the area being examined. Fluoroscopy is conducted in a darkened room and allows the physician an opportunity to visualize internal structures that are in motion. It is also possible to take film records of the fluoroscopic examination for future study.
4. X-rays travel in a straight line, thus allowing the x-ray beam to be directed at a specific site during radiotherapy or to produce high-quality shadow images on film (radiographs).
5. X-rays are able to penetrate substances of different density with varying degrees of difficulty. In the body, x-rays pass through air in the lungs, fluids such as blood and lymph, fat around muscles, and calcium in bones with relative ease. Such substances are said to be radiolucent. Substances that obstruct the passage of radiant energy, such as lead or barium, are radiopaque. This characteristic allows x-rays to be used as a diagnostic tool. Control of the voltage applied to an x-ray tube, usually 80 to 120 kV, plus the length of exposure can produce precise radiographs (x-rays) of body structures of varying density. A radiopaque contrast medium, such as barium sulfate, can be introduced into radiolucent body areas to enhance certain x-ray images.
6. X-rays can destroy body cells. Radiation can be used in the treatment of malignant tumors. In these cases, the x-ray voltage is usually 1 to 2 MV and is administered by a radiotherapist using radiotherapy machines such as a linear accelerator or the betatron. Care must be exercised in the administration of radiotherapy, as x-rays can destroy healthy as well as abnormal tissue.

DANGERS AND SAFETY PRECAUTIONS

Because x-rays are invisible and produce no sound or smell, those working around and with them need to take certain precautions to avoid unnecessary exposure. Listed are some of the dangers known to be associated with x-rays and the safety precautions designed to prevent unnecessary exposure.

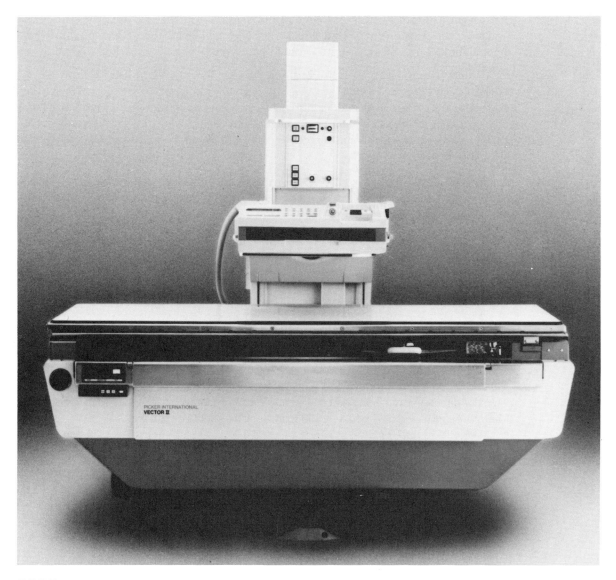

FIGURE 18–1

Vector II R/F table used for fluoroscopic examination of internal structures of the body. (*Courtesy of Picker International, Cleveland, Ohio.*)

Prolonged Exposure

Prolonged and continued exposure to x-rays can depress the hematopoietic system, which can cause leukopenia, leukemia, and damage to the gonads leading to sterility. Those involved with x-rays should spend only a fraction of a second per x-ray exposure. Personnel involved with radiation therapy should spend the minimal amount of time necessary when caring for patients receiving internal radiation therapy. The farther away one is from the source of radiation, the less the degree of exposure. One should know the guidelines for caring for patients receiving radiation therapy.

Secondary Radiation

X-rays can scatter or be diverted from their normal straight paths when they strike radiopaque objects. This scatter or secondary radiation tends to blur the desired x-ray image; therefore, a device known as a grid is positioned between the x-ray machine and the patient to absorb scatter before it reaches the x-ray film. The Potter-Bucky diaphragm, commonly known as the Bucky, is the most frequently used grid. It consists of alternating strips of lead and radiolucent material. The lead strips are arranged parallel to the stream of x-rays and are kept in motion by a mechanism to prevent them from becoming superimposed on the exposed film.

Safety Precautions

Not all scatter or secondary radiation is absorbed by a grid; therefore, those working in areas adjacent to x-ray equipment risk unintentional bombardment from this source unless proper safety precautions are observed. Generally, these safety precautions include the five described below.

Film Badge. A film badge is a device, usually pinned to the clothing, that is sensitive to ionizing radiation and monitors exposure to beta and gamma rays. A periodic analysis of the film badge reveals the amount of radiation the individual has received.

Lead Screen. Persons who operate x-ray machines do so from behind special screens equipped with a lead-treated window for viewing the patient.

Lead-Lined Room. X-ray equipment should be housed in an area featuring lead-lined walls, floors, and doors to prevent the escape of radiation from the room.

Protective Clothing. Lead-lined gloves and aprons are worn by personnel who hold or position patients for x-ray examination, especially if they hold a patient, such as a child, while an x-ray is being taken.

Gonad Shield. The reproductive organs are radiosensitive and must be protected by a lead shield while x-rays are being taken. X-rays can cause damage to the genetic material within the reproductive organs, which could lead to birth defects or cancer.

POSITIONS USED IN RADIOGRAPHY

Anteroposterior (AP) Position

In the anteroposterior position, the patient is placed with the anterior (front) part of the body facing the x-ray tube and the posterior (back) of the body facing the film. X-rays will pass through the body from the front to the back in reaching the film.

Posteroanterior (PA) Position

In the posteroanterior position, the patient is placed with the posterior (back) portion of the body facing the x-ray tube and the anterior (front) of the body facing the film. The x-rays will pass through the body from the back to the front to reach the film.

Lateral Position

In the lateral position, the x-ray beam passes from one side of the patient's body to the opposite side to reach the film. Placing the patient's right side next to the film and passing x-rays through the body from left to right is known as the right lateral (RL) position. Placing the patient's left side next to the film and passing x-rays through the body from right to left is known as the left lateral (LL) position.

Supine Position

In the supine position, the patient rests on the back, face upward, allowing the x-rays to pass through the body from the front to the back.

Prone Position

In the prone position, the patient is placed lying face down with the head to one side. The x-rays will pass from the back to the front side of the body.

Oblique Position

In the oblique position, the patient is placed so that the body or body part to be imaged is at an angle to the x-ray beam.

DIAGNOSTIC RADIOLOGY

Diagnostic radiology involves the use of x-rays, sound waves, radiopharmaceuticals, radiopaque media, and computers to provide the radiologist with images of internal body organs and processes. These images are used in identifying and locating tumors, fractures, hematomas, disease processes, and other abnormalities within the body, along with other information necessary to diagnose the patient's condition. In recent years, advances in the field of electronics have produced a variety of computer-assisted x-ray machines to enhance the images obtained by the radiologist. These sophisticated machines now make possible noninvasive procedures for the visualization of organs and processes that were previously not accessible or that required exploratory surgical procedures for examination. Of the computer-assisted radiology equipment now in general use, the computed tomography (CT) scanner and the magnetic resonance imaging (MRI) machine offer the greatest range of diagnostic potential. A brief description of each of these diagnostic tools is given below.

Computed Tomography

When first introduced, computed tomography was hailed as the most significant advance in diagnostic medicine since the discovery of x-rays. It combines an advanced x-ray scanning system with a powerful minicomputer and vastly improved imaging quality while making it possible to view parts of the body and abnormalities not previously open to radiography. The CT scanner combines tomography, the process of imaging structures by focusing on a specific body plane and blurring all details from other planes, with a microprocessor that provides high-speed analysis of the tissue variances scanned (Fig. 18–2).

Magnetic Resonance Imaging

MRI is a technique that offers greater safety, as it does not use x-rays, while providing images and data on body structures such as the heart, large blood vessels, brain and soft tissue. The MRI is a device that emits FM radio waves of a certain frequency that are directed at a specific body area that is contained within a magnetic field. After the radio waves are turned off, hydrogen nuclei in the patient emit weak radio waves or microwaves that are analyzed by a computer and transformed into cross-sectional pictures.

Other Imaging Techniques

Other diagnostic imaging techniques being used include thermography, in which detailed images of body parts are developed from data showing the degree of heat and cold present in areas being studied, and scintigraphy, which involves the production of two-dimensional images of tissue areas from the scintillations emitted by a radiopharmaceutical, internally administered, that concentrates in a targeted site.

Nuclear Medicine

Nuclear medicine uses atomic particles that emit electromagnetic radiation on disintegration. The radiant energy thus released is used for diagnostic, investigative, and therapeutic purposes. It may be administered externally from radiation machines such as the betratron and the linear accelerator or internally from small radionuclides implanted within the body near the site to be irradiated.

RADIATION THERAPY

The treatment of disease by the use of ionizing radiation may be called radiotherapy, x-ray therapy, cobalt treatment, or simply radiation therapy. In all cases, the aim of this treatment is to deliver a precise, calculated dose of radiation to diseased tissue, such as a tumor, while causing the least possible damage to surrounding normal tissue. **Radiation** can be defined as the process whereby energy is beamed from its source through space and matter to a selected target area. Substances that emit radiation are said to be radioactive. In radiation therapy, the radioactive substances used emit three types of rays: alpha, beta, and gamma.

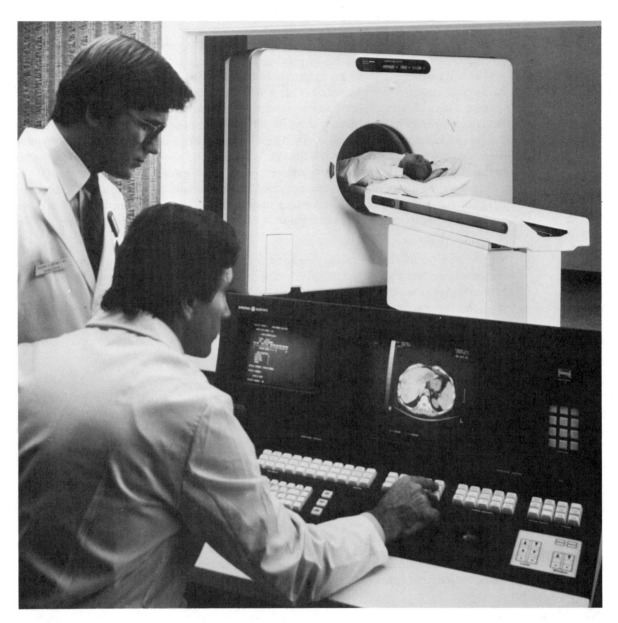

FIGURE 18–2

General Electric CT9800 computed tomography system, a computerized x-ray scanning system. (*Courtesy of General Electric Co., Medical Systems Group, Milwaukee, Wisconsin.*)

Alpha Rays

Alpha rays are the least penetrating of the three types and can be absorbed by a thin sheet of material. They consist of positively charged helium particles released by atomic disintegration of radioactive material.

Beta Rays

Beta rays are able to penetrate body tissues for a few millimeters and consist of negatively charged electrons released when atoms of radioactive substances undergo disintegration.

Gamma Rays

Gamma rays are electromagnetic waves emitted by atoms of radioactive elements as they undergo disintegration. They are similar to x-rays but originate from the element's nucleus, whereas x-rays derive from the element's orbit. Gamma rays are without mass or electrical charge and have great penetrating power. They can pass through most substances, including the body, but are absorbed by lead.

RADIOTHERAPY AND CANCER

Malignant cells are more sensitive to radiation than are normal cells. They seem less able to repair themselves; therefore, radiation is frequently used in the treatment of patients with cancer, either as a curative or palliative mode of therapy. Certain types of cancer cells can be destroyed by radiation therapy, thus preventing the unrestrained growth of such tumors. In other cancers, radiation has only a palliative effect, preventing cell growth, reducing pain, pressure, and bleeding, but not providing complete tumor destruction. Important factors that must be considered when determining the use of radiotherapy for the cancer patient include the following:

1. The tumor must be surrounded by normal tissue that can tolerate the radiation and then repair itself.
2. The tumor must not be widely spread. If the tumor has metastasized, radiation may be used as a palliative form of treatment.
3. The tumor must be moderately sensitive to radiation (a radiosensitive tumor).

Radiotherapy is often the treatment of choice for cancers of the skin, uterus, cervix, larynx, or those located within the oral cavity. With other types of cancer, radiotherapy is frequently used in combination with other forms of treatment including surgery and chemotherapy (Figs. 18-3 and 18-4).

TECHNIQUES OF RADIOTHERAPY

As mentioned earlier, there are two methods for the administration of radiation: external radiation therapy (ERT) and internal radiation therapy (IRT). The following is an overview of these two methods.

External Radiation Therapy (ERT)
With the ERT method, the patient receives calculated doses of radiation from a machine located at some distance from the site of the tumor. The patient is carefully prepared for treatment by a radiation therapist, sometimes assisted by the dosimetrist or a radiation physicist. The precise size and location of the tumor are determined, and the port, or point of entry for the radiation, is marked using a dye or tattoo. In formulating the treatment plan, a computer is used to calculate the radiation dosage that will be needed to effect maximal destruction of malignant cells and minimal damage to surrounding normal tissue. Special lead blockers or shields may be constructed by a radiation physicist to protect surrounding normal tissue from the harmful effects of radiation.

Internal Radiation Therapy (IRT)
The IRT method of treatment can have two forms of administration known as sealed and unsealed radiation therapy. Sealed radiation therapy involves the implantation of sealed containers of radioactive material near the tumor site within the body. Unsealed radiation therapy involves the introduction of a liquid containing a radioactive substance into the patient through the mouth, via the bloodstream, or by instillation into a body cavity.

Sealed Radiation Therapy. Radioactive material such as radium, cesium-137, cobalt-60, and iridium-192 is sealed in small gold containers called seeds or within molds, plaques, needles, or other devices designed to hold the radioactive substance near the malignancy. In some cases, the radiation source may be implanted within the diseased tissue. In other cases, special devices or applicators have been designed to hold the implant in position for the desired period of treatment.

Unsealed Radiation Therapy. Radioactive iodine-131, radioactive phosphorus-32, and radioactive gold-198 are some of the substances used in the unsealed form of internal radiation

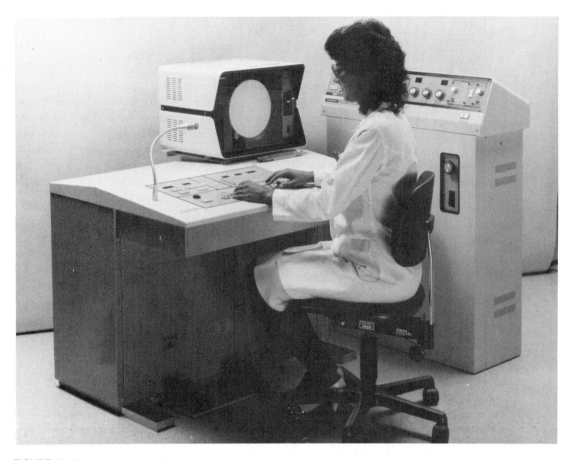

FIGURE 18–3

Toshiba diagnostic imaging system, LX-30A-AA-1. (*Courtesy of Toshiba Medical Systems, Tustin, California.*)

therapy. Phosphorus-32 may be intravenously administered for use in the treatment of leukemia or lymphoma. Gold-198 and/or phosphorus-32 may be placed in colloidal suspension and instilled in a body cavity for the palliative treatment of certain malignancies. Iodine-131 may be orally administered, usually in conjunction with a thyroidectomy.

SIDE EFFECTS OF RADIATION

Because radiotherapy unavoidably affects normal tissue while destroying malignant cells, patients usually experience some unpleasant side effects. The degree of severity associated with the side effects will depend on the individual, the cancer, its location, and the amount of radiation. The following is a listing of some side effects that may occur as a result of radiation therapy:

1. Anorexia
2. Nausea
3. Vomiting
4. Diarrhea
5. Malaise
6. Mild erythema
7. Edema
8. Ulcers
9. Alopecia
10. Taste blindness
11. Stomatitis
12. Mucositis
13. Xerostomia

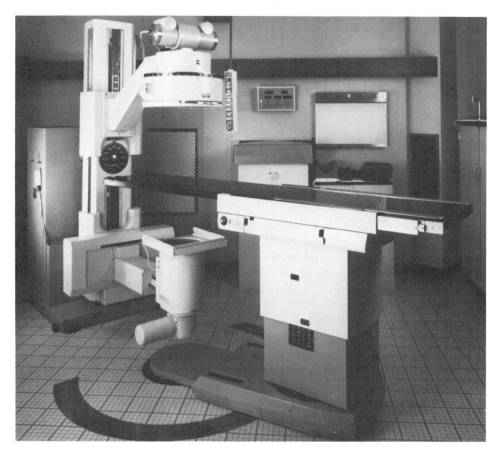

FIGURE 18–4

Toshiba diagnostic imaging system, LX-30A-AA-1. (*Courtesy of Toshiba Medical Systems, Tustin, California.*)

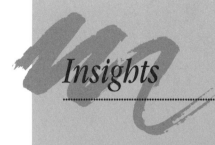

Insights

MAMMOGRAPHY

Mammography is the process of obtaining x-ray pictures of the breast. It is used as a screening tool for breast cancer and as a means to diagnose early breast cancer. It can detect a cancer the size of a grain of salt, 5 to 7 years before it can be detected by hand, and is also capable of detecting 85 to 90% of existing breast cancers.

A mammogram is the actual x-ray record (film) of the breast. A mammographer is an individual who is responsible for taking the x-ray and a radiologist is an individual who is responsible for making an accurate assessment of the film. It is recommended that the mammographer and radiologist be specifically trained in mammography and breast evaluation, and be certified by the American College of Radiology. To insure quality performance, the x-ray machine, processor, screens, and cassettes must be state-of-the-art equipment, and should be properly evaluated on a regular basis.

Screening Guidelines

The American Cancer Society and the National Cancer Institute endorse the following breast-cancer screening guidelines:

- Practice monthly breast self-examination (BSE).
- Between the ages 40 and 49, have your breasts examined by a health professional every year and get a mammogram every 1 or 2 years.
- After age 49, have a mammogram (along with a manual breast examination) every year.

Guidelines to help you prepare for a mammogram:

It is best to have a mammogram right after your menstrual cycle, as the breast will be less tender and less swollen. On the day of the test, do not use any deodorant, perfume, powders, oils, or ointments of any sort in the underarm area or on the breasts. These may cause shadows to appear on the mammogram.

Wear a skirt or slacks and a blouse that can be easily removed. You will have to remove all clothing from the waist up and put on a x-ray gown. Do not wear any jewelry around the neck.

If this is your first mammogram, ask your physician to explain the procedure of mammography to you before you go to the health facility where you will have the mammogram. The more knowledge you have about what is going to happen will generally lessen your fear and you will be better prepared for the procedure.

(Insights continues on next page)

The Procedure:

Once you reach the x-ray suite, you will be taken to a dressing area, where you are given an x-ray gown and instructed to remove all clothing and jewelry from the waist up. You should put the gown on so that it opens in the front.

You will then be taken to a room where the mammographer explains the procedure. If possible you will stand and remove one breast and place it on the x-ray device. The mammographer will position you by lifting your breast to a 90 degree angle to the chest wall. Your breast will be pulled forward onto the film holder, centrally with the nipple in profile. Your arm on the side being imaged should be relaxed and your shoulder is back out of the way. You will be asked to turn your head away from the side being imaged. Next, your breast will be compressed. Compression is used in combination with a specific shaped x-ray cone so that the more intense central portion of the x-ray beam penetrates the thicker base of the breast. (From experience, I can tell you that this is not painful, but it is most uncomfortable. The good thing is that it only lasts for a few seconds.) You will be asked to take a deep breath and to hold it and to be still, while the mammographer goes behind a lead screen and takes the picture. The same process will be followed for both breasts.

You will be asked to wait while the x-rays are being processed and if the pictures are satisfactory, then you may dress and leave. A radiologist will read the x-rays and send your physician a report, and then your physician will notify you of the findings.

The Male Patient Having a Mammogram

Approximately 1000 men a year are diagnosed with breast cancer. When a male is scheduled for a mammogram, he is most embarrassed, as breast cancer is a female disease, and not a man's. The male breast generally does not contain as much adipose tissue as the female; therefore it may be difficult to place the man's breast onto the film holder and obtain the proper amount of compression.

Terminology with Surgical Procedures & Pathology

Term	Word Parts			Definition
angiocardiogram (ăn″ jĭ-ō-kăr′ dĭ-ō-grăm)	angio cardio gram	CF CF S	vessel heart record	An x-ray record of the heart and great vessels that is made visible through the use of a radiopaque contrast medium
angiogram (ăn′ jĭ-ō-grăm)	angio gram	CF S	vessel record	An x-ray record of the blood vessels made visible through the use of an injected radiopaque contrast medium
angiography (ăn″ jĭ-ŏg′ ră-fē)	angio graphy	CF S	vessel recording	The process of making an x-ray record of blood vessels
aortogram (ā-ŏr′ tō-grăm)	aorto gram	CF S	aorta record	An x-ray record of the aorta that is made visible through the use of an injected radiopaque contrast medium
arteriography (ăr″ tē-rĭ-ŏg′ ră-fē)	arterio graphy	CF S	artery recording	The process of making an x-ray record of the arteries
arthrography (ăr-thrŏg′ ră-fē)	arthro graphy	CF S	joint recording	The process of making an x-ray record of a joint
brachytherapy (brăk″ ĭ thĕr′ ă-pē)	brachy therapy	P S	short treatment	Radiation therapy in which the radioactive substance is inserted into a body cavity or organ. The source of radiation is located a short distance from the body area being treated
bronchogram (brŏng′ kō-grăm)	broncho gram	CF S	bronchi record	An x-ray record of the bronchial tree that is made visible through the use of a radiopaque contrast medium
cholangiogram (kō-lăn′ jĭ-ō-grăm)	chol angio gram	R CF S	gall, bile vessel record	An x-ray record of the bile ducts that is made visible through the use of a radiopaque contrast medium
cholecystogram (kō″ lē-sĭs′ tō-grăm)	chole cysto gram	R CF S	gall bladder record	An x-ray record of the gallbladder that is made visible through the use of a radiopaque contrast medium

(Terminology—continued)

Term	Word Parts			Definition
cinematoradio-graphy (sĭn″ ĭ-măt″ ō-rā″ dĭ-ŏg′ ră-fē)	cinemato	CF	motion	The process of making an x-ray record of an organ in motion
	radio	CF	ray	
	graphy	S	recording	
cineradiography (sĭn″ ē-rā″ dē-ŏg′ ră-fē)	cine	R	motion	The process of making a motion picture record of successive x-ray images appearing on a fluoroscopic screen
	radio	CF	ray	
	graphy	S	recording	
cisternography (sĭs″ tĕr-nŏg′ ră-fē)	cisterno	CF	cistern	The process of making an x-ray record of the basal cistern of the brain
	graphy	S	recording	
dosimetrist (dō-sĭm′ ĕt-rĭst)	dosi	CF	a giving	One who specializes in the planning and calculating of radiation dosage
	metr	R	to measure	
	ist	S	one who specializes	
echoencephalo-graphy (ĕk″ ō-ĕn-sĕf″ ă-lŏg′ ră-fē)	echo	CF	echo	The process of using ultrasound to determine the presence of a centrally located mass in the brain
	encephalo	CF	brain	
	graphy	S	recording	
echography (ĕk-ŏg′ ră-fē)	echo	CF	echo	The process of using ultrasound as a diagnostic tool. A record is made of the echo produced when sound waves are reflected back through tissues of different density
	graphy	S	recording	
electrokymogram (ə-lĕk″ trō-kĭ′ mō-grăm)	electro	CF	electricity	An x-ray record of the motion of the heart or other moving structures
	kymo	CF	motion	
	gram	S	record	
fluoroscopy (floo-räs′ kə-pē)	fluoro	CF	fluorescence	The process of examining internal structures by viewing the shadows cast on a fluorescent screen after the x-ray has passed through the body
	scopy	S	to view	
holography (hŏl-ŏg′ ră-fē)	holo	CF	whole	The making of a picture in which the original object appears in three dimensions
	graphy	S	recording	
hysterosalpingo-gram (hĭs″ tĕr-ō-săl-pĭn′ gō-grăm)	hystero	CF	uterus	An x-ray record of the uterus and fallopian tubes that is made visible through the use of a radiopaque contrast medium
	salpingo	CF	fallopian tube	
	gram	S	record	

(Terminology—continued)

Term		Word Parts		Definition
intracavitary (ĭn″ tră-kăv′ ĭt-ă-rē)	intra cavit ary	P R S	within cavity pertaining to	Pertaining to within a cavity
intravenous pyelogram (ĭn″ tră-vē′ nŭs pī′ ĕ-lō-grăm)	intra ven ous pyelo gram	P R S CF S	within vein pertaining to renal pelvis record	An x-ray record of the kidney and renal pelvis that is made visible through the use of an injected radiopaque contrast medium
ionometer (ī ŏn-ō-mē-tĕr)	iono meter	CF S	ion instrument to measure	An instrument used to measure the amount of radiation used by x-rays or radioactive substances
ionotherapy (ī″ ŏn-ō-thĕr′ ă-pē)	iono therapy	CF S	ion treatment	Treatment by introducing ions into the body
iontoradiometer (ī-ŏn″ tō-rā″ dĭ-ŏm′ ĭ-tĕr)	ionto radio meter	CF CF S	ion ray instrument to measure	An instrument used to measure the amount and intensity of x-rays
kilovolt (kĭl′ ō-vōlt)	kilo volt	CF R	one thousand volt	1000 V
kilowatt (kĭl′ ō-wătt)	kilo watt	CF R	one thousand watt	1000 W
lymphangiogram (lĭm-făn″ jē-ō-grăm)	lymph angio gram	R CF S	lymph vessel record	An x-ray record of the lymph vessels that is made visible through the use of radiopaque contrast medium
lymphangiography (lĭm-făn″ jē-ŏg′ ră-fē)	lymph angio graphy	R CF S	lymph vessel recording	The process of making an x-ray record of the lymph vessels
mammography (măm-ŏg′ ră-fē)	mammo graphy	CF S	breast recording	The process of obtaining pictures of the breast through the use of x-rays
milliampere (mĭl″ ĭ-ăm′ pēr)	milli ampere	P R	one-thousandth ampere	0.001 A
millicurie (mĭl″ ĭ-kū′ rē)	milli curie	P R	one-thousandth curie	0.001 Ci
myelogram (mī′ ĕ-lō-grăm)	myelo gram	CF S	spinal cord record	An x-ray record of the spinal cord that is made visible through the use of a radiopaque contrast medium

(Terminology—continued)

Term	Word Parts			Definition
oscilloscope (ŏ-sĭl′ ō-skōp)	oscillo scope	CF S	to swing instrument	An instrument used to record an electrical wave visually on a fluorescent screen of a cathode-ray tube
photofluorogram (fō″ tō-floo′ ĕr-ō-grăm)	photo fluro gram	CF CF S	light fluorescence record	An x-ray record of images seen during fluoroscopic examination
physicist (fĭz′ ĭ-sĭst)	physic ist	R S	nature one who specializes	One who specializes in the science of physics
pneumoence- **phalogram** (nū″ mō-ĕn-sĕf′ ă-lō-grăm)	pneumo encephalo gram	CF CF S	air brain record	An x-ray record of the ventricles and subarachnoid spaces of the brain after the injection of air or gas via a lumbar puncture
radiation (rā-dĭ-ā′ shŭn)	radiat ion	R S	radiant process	The process whereby radiant energy is propagated through space or matter
radioactive (rā″ dĭ-ō-ăk′ tĭv)	radio act ive	CF R S	ray acting nature of	Characterized by emitting radiant energy
radiodermatitis (rā″ dĭ-ō-dur′ mă-tī′ tĭs)	radio dermat itis	CF R S	ray skin inflammation	Inflammation of the skin caused by exposure to x-rays or radioactive substances
radiodiagnosis (rā″ dĭ-ō-dī″ ăg-nō′ sĭs)	radio dia gnosis	CF P S	ray through knowledge	To determine a diagnosis through the use of x-rays
radiogenic (rA″ dĭ-ō-jĕn′ ĭk)	radio genic	CF S	ray formation, to produce	Caused or produced by radioactivity
radiograph (rā′ dĭ-ō-grăf)	radio graph	CF S	ray record	A picture produced on a sensitized film or plate by rays; an x-ray record
radiographer (rā″ dĭ-ŏg′ ră-fĕr)	radio graph er	CF S S	ray record one who	One who is skilled in making x-ray records
radiography (rā″ dĭ-ŏg′ ră-fē)	radio graphy	CF S	ray recording	The process of making an x-ray record

(Terminology—continued)

Term		Word Parts		Definition
radiologist	radio	CF	ray	One who specializes in
(rā″ dĭ-ŏl′ ō-jĭst)	log	R	study of	radiology
	ist	S	one who spcializes	
radiology	radio	CF	ray	The study of x-rays,
(rā″ dĭ-ŏl′ ō-jē)	logy	S	study of	radioactive substances, radioactive isotopes, and ionizing radiation
radiolucent	radio	CF	ray	Property of permitting the
(rā″ dĭ-ō-lū′ sĕnt)	lucent	R	to shine	passage of radiant energy
radionecrosis	radio	CF	ray	Death of tissue caused by
(rā″ dĭ-ō-nē-krō′ sĭs)	necr	R	death	exposure to radiant energy
	osis	S	condition of	
radiopaque	radio	CF	ray	Property of obstructing the
(rā″ dĭ-ō-pāk′)	paque	R	dark	passage of radiant energy
radioscopy	radio	CF	ray	The process of viewing and
(rā″ dĭ-ŏs′ kō-pē)	scopy	S	to view, examine	examining the inner structures of the body through the process of x-rays
radiotherapy	radio	CF	ray	The treatment of disease by
(rā″ dĭ-ō-thĕr′ ă-pē)	therapy	S	treatment	the use of x-rays, radium, and other radioactive substances
roentgenologist	roent	R	roentgen	One who specializes in
(rĕnt″ gĕn-ŏl′ ō-jĭst)	geno	CF	kind	roentgen diagnosis, therapy,
	log	R	study of	or both
	ist	S	one who specializes	
roentgenology	roent	R	roentgen	The study of roentgen rays for
(rĕnt″ gĕn-ŏl′ ō-jē)	geno	CF	kind	diagnostic and therapeutic
	logy	S	study of	purposes
sialography	sialo	CF	salivary	The process of making an
(sī″ ă-lŏg′ ră-fē)	graphy	S	recording	x-ray record of the salivary ducts and glands
sonogram	sono	CF	sound	A record produced by
(sōn′ ō-grăm)	gram	S	record	ultrasonography
teletherapy	tele	R	distant	Radiation therapy in which
(tĕl″ ĕ-thĕr′ ă-pē)	therapy	S	treatment	the radioactive substance is at a distance from the body area being treated

(Terminology—continued)

Term	Word Parts			Definition
thermography (thĕr-mŏg′ ră-fē)	thermo graphy	CF S	heat recording	The process of recording heat patterns of the body's surface; useful in the detection of cancer of the breast
tomography (tō-mŏg′ ră-fē)	tomo graphy	CF S	to cut recording	The process of cutting across and producing images of single tissue planes
ultrasonic (ŭl″ tră-sŏn′ ĭk)	ultra son ic	P R S	beyond sound pertaining to	Pertaining to sounds beyond 20,000 cycles/sec
ultrasonography (ŭl″ tră-sŏn-ŏg′ ră-fē)	ultra sono graphy	P CF S	beyond sound recording	The process of using ultrasound to produce a record of ultrasonic echoes as they strike tissues of different densities
venography (vē-nŏg′ ră-fē)	veno graphy	CF S	vein recording	The process of making an x-ray record of veins
ventriculography (vĕn-trĭk″ ū-lŏg′ ră-fē)	ventriculo graphy	CF S	little belly recording	The process of making an x-ray record of the cerebral ventricles after the introduction of air or other contrast medium
xeroradiography (zē″ rō-rā″ dē-ŏg′ ră-fē)	xero radio graphy	CF CF S	dry ray recording	The process of making an x-ray record by a dry, totally photoelectric process

Vocabulary Words

Vocabulary words are terms that have not been divided into component parts. They are common words or specialized terms associated with the subject of this chapter. These words are provided to enhance your medical vocabulary.

Word	Definition
alopecia (ăl″ ō-pē′ shǐ-ă)	Pertaining to hair loss
alpha ray (ăl′ fə rā)	A ray of positively charged particles of helium moving at a high speed. It is the least penetrating ray and is stopped by skin or a single sheet of paper
ampere (ăm′ pēr)	The unit of strength of electricity
anion (ăn′ ī-ŏn)	An ion that carries a negative charge and is attracted to the positive pole (anode)
anode (ăn′ ōd)	The positive pole of an electrical current
anorexia (ăn″ ō-rĕks′ ĭ-ă)	A condition in which there is a loss of appetite
aplastic anemia (ă-plăs′ tĭk ăn-nē′ mĭ-ă)	A type of anemia in which there is aplasia or destruction of the bone marrow; may be caused by chemotherapeutic agents, x-rays, or other sources of ionizing radiation
artifact (ăr′ tĭ-făkt)	An artificially produced structure or feature
atom (ăd-əm)	The smallest part of an element; consists of a nucleus that contains protons and neutrons and is surrounded by electrons
barium sulfate (bā′ rĭ-ŭm sŭl′ fāt)	A radiopaque barium compound used as a contrast medium in x-ray examination of the digestive tract
beam (bēm)	A ray of light. In radiology and nuclear medicine, a beam is radiant energy emitted by a group of atomic particles traveling a parallel course
beta ray (bā′ tă rā)	A ray of negatively charged electrons moving at a high speed. It penetrates only a few millimeters of body tissue
betatron (bā′ tă-trŏn)	A megavoltage machine used in administering external radiation therapy
bombardment (bŏm-bărd′ mənt)	The process of irradiating an atom
cassette (kă-sĕt′)	A light-proof case or holder for x-ray film

(Vocabulary—continued)

Word	Definition
cathode (kăth′ ōd)	The negative pole of an electrical current
cesium-137 (sē′ zĭ-ŭm)	A radionuclide that is the radioactive substance of choice for the treatment of cervical, uterine, and vaginal cancer
cobalt-60 (kō′ balt)	A radionuclide that serves as the radioactive substance in teletherapy machines. It is also used for implantation (interstitial) in the treatment of some malignancies
collimator (kŏl″ ĭ-madər)	A device on an x-ray machine that makes rays parallel and not diffuse
cone (kōn)	An object on an x-ray or radiation machine that regulates the beam of radiant energy
contrast medium (kōn′ trăst mēd′ ĭ-ŭm)	A radiopaque substance used in certain x-ray procedures to permit visualization of organs or structures
curie (Ci) (kūr′ ē)	A unit of radioactivity
cyclotron (sī′ klō-trŏn)	A megavoltage machine used in administering external radiation therapy
decontamination (dē″ kŏn-tăm″ ĭ-nā′ shŭn)	The process of freeing an object, area, or person of some contaminating substance (bacteria, poisonous gas, or radioactive substances)
diaphanography (dĭ″ ă-făn-ŏg′ ră-fē)	The process of taking infrared photographs of the breast while a white light is being shone through the breast
digital subtraction angiography (dĭj′ ĭ-tăl sŭb-trăk′ shŭn ăn″ jĭ-ŏg′ ră-fē)	A method by which the computer performs instantaneous subtraction of the x-ray images, giving high-quality x-ray images of blood vessels with less x-ray dye
dose (dōs)	The amount of medication or radiation that is to be administered
electron (ē-lĕk′ trŏn)	A charge or unit of negative electricity that revolves around the nucleus of an atom
enema (ĕn′ ē-mă)	The process of introducing a substance or solution into the rectum and colon
energy (ĕn′ ĕr-jē)	The power or capacity to do work

(Vocabulary—continued)

Word	Definition
external radiation (ĕk-stur′ năl rā-dĭ-ā′ shŭn)	The process of administering radiation to the patient via a radiation machine that is located outside the body
film (film)	A thin, cellulose-coated, light-sensitive sheet or slip of material used in taking pictures
film badge (film badj)	A device that is sensitive to ionizing radiation. It is worn by one who is around x-rays to monitor the degree of exposure to beta and gamma rays
fluorescence (floo″ ō-rĕs′ ĕnts)	The property of certain substances to emit light as a result of exposure to and absorption of radiant energy
fractionation (frăk″ shŭn-ā′ shŭn)	The process of delivering a fraction or portion of a dose of radiation over time to minimize untoward radiation effects on normal tissue
gamma ray (găm′ ăh rā)	An electromagnetic wave without mass or electrical charge. It is the most penetrating ray and can pass through the whole body. It can be stopped by lead
Geiger counter (gī′ gĕr kown′ tĕr)	An instrument used to detect, measure, and record ionizing radiation; also called a Geiger-Muller counter
half-life (haf′ līf)	The time required for half of the radioactivity of a substance to be reduced by radioactive decay
implant (ĭm-plănt′)	To place within a body cavity or organ; also means to transfer, to graft, or to insert
in vitro (ĭn vē′ trō)	Within a glass
ion (ī-ən)	An atomic particle consisting of an atom or a group of atoms that carry an electrical charge, either negative or positive
ionization (ī″ ŏn-ĭ-zā′ shŭn)	The process of breaking up molecules into their component parts
ionizing radiation (ī′ ŏn-ī-zĭng rā″ dĭ-ā′ shŭn)	A powerful invisible energy capable of producing ions
iridium-192 (ī-rĭd′ ĭ-ŭm)	A radionuclide used to deliver sealed dosages by internal radiotherapy to certain malignancies
irradiation (ĭ-rā″ dē-ā′ shŭn)	A process of using x-rays, radium rays, ultraviolet rays, gamma rays, or infrared rays in the diagnosis or therapeutic treatment of a patient

(Vocabulary—continued)

Word	Definition
isotope (ī′ sō-tōp)	One of a series of nuclides that are chemically identical yet differ in atomic weight and electrical charge. Radioactive isotopes are composed of unstable atoms, and most are artificially produced. Example: cobalt-60 is a radioactive isotope artificially produced from naturally occurring cobalt-59
lead (lĕd)	A metallic chemical element
linear accelerator (lĭn′ ē-ar ăk-sĕl′ ĕr-ā″ tŏr)	A megavoltage machine used in administering external radiation therapy
megavoltage (mĕg′ ă-vōl″ tĭj)	Pertains to 1,000,000 V
neutron (nū′ trŏn)	An electrically uncharged particle existing in the nuclei of atoms
nuclear magnetic resonance imaging (NMRI) (nū′ klē-ar măg-nĕt′ ĭk rĕz′ ŏ-năns)	A technique that uses radio waves and a magnet. A device emits FM radio waves of a certain frequency that are directed at a specific body area contained within an external magnetic field. After the radio waves are turned off, hydrogen nuclei in the patient emit weak radio waves or microwaves that are analyzed by a computer and transformed into cross-sectional pictures. Also called magnetic resonance imaging (MRI)
orthovoltage (or″ thō-vōl′ tĭj)	Pertains to a voltage range of 140–400 kV. In radiation therapy, it is used in administering low-energy radiation for palliative treatment of cancer
port (pôrt)	In radiation therapy, refers to the skin area of entry for the radiation
proton (prō′ tŏn)	An electrically positive-charged particle existing in the nuclei of atoms
rad (răd)	Refers to the amount of radiation absorbed. The letters stand for **r**adiation **a**bsorbed **d**ose
radionuclide (rā″ dĭ-ō-nū′ klĭd)	A radioactive species of an atomic nucleus identified by its atomic number, mass, and energy state
radiotherapist (rā″ dĭ-ō-thĕr′ ă-pĭst)	One who specializes in the use of radiant energy for therapeutic purposes
radium (rā′ dĭ-ŭm)	A radioactive isotope used in the treatment of certain malignant diseases
roentgen (R) (rĕnt′ gĕn)	The international unit for describing exposure dose of x-ray or γ-radiation

(Vocabulary—continued)

Word	Definition
scan (skăn)	A process of using a moving device or a sweeping beam of radiation to produce images of organs or structures of the body
shield (shēld)	A protective structure used to prevent or reduce the passage of particles or radiation
tagging (tag′ ing)	The process of tracing a radioactive isotope that has become involved in metabolic or chemical actions
volt (V) (vōlt)	The electromotive force or unit of pressure for the flow of electricity
watt (W) (wătt)	The unit of electrical power. One watt is equal to a current of 1 A under 1 V of pressure
x-ray (x′ rā)	An electromagnetic wave of high energy produced by the collision of a beam of electrons with a target in a vacuum tube (x-ray tube)

ABBREVIATIONS

AP	anteroposterior	mCi	millicurie
Ba	barium	MRI	magnetic resonance imaging
BaE	barium enema	Ra	radium
Ci	curie	rad	radiation absorbed dose
CT	computed tomography	NMR	nuclear magnetic resonance
ERT	external radiation therapy	PA	posteroanterior
IRT	internal radiation therapy	PEG	pneumoencephalogram
kV	kilovolt	PET	positron emission
kW	kilowatt		tomography
LL	left lateral	RL	right lateral
mA	milliampere		

Communication Enrichment

This segment is provided for those who wish to enhance their ability to communicate in either English or Spanish.

RELATED TERMS

English	Spanish
x-ray	radiografia (ră-dē-ō-gră-fē-ă)
record	registro (rĕ-*hĭs*-trō)
motion	mocion (mō-sĭ-*ōn*)
electricity	electricidad (ĕ-lĕc-*trĭ*-cĭ-dăd)
measure	medida (mĕ-*dĭ*-dă)
light	ligero; luz (lĭ-*hĕ*-rō; lŭz)
radiant	radiante (ră-dĭ-*ăn*-tĕ)
dark	oscuro (ōs-*cŭ*-rō)
treatment	tratamiento (tră-tă-mĭ-*ĕn*-tō)
ampere	amperio (ăm-*pĕ*-rĭ-ō)
atomic	atomico (ă-*tō*-mĭ-cō)
cassette	cartucho (căr-*tŭ*-chō)
cone	cono (*cō*-nō)
curie	curie (cŭ-*rĕ*)
dose	dosis (*dō*-sĭs)
electron	electrón (ĕ-*lĕc*-trōn)
energy	energia (ĕ-nĕr-*hĭ*-ă)
implant	implantar (ĭm-plăn-*tăr*)
lead	plomo (*plō*-mō)
scan	hojear (ō-hĕ-*ăr*)
shield	escudo (ĕs-*cŭ*-dō)

Learning Exercises

An Overview of Radiology and Nuclear Medicine

Write your answers to the following questions. Do not refer back to the text.

1. Define radiology. _____
   _____

2. Name three characteristics of x-rays.

   a. _____ b. _____

   c. _____

3. Name two dangers of x-rays.

   a. _____ b. _____

4. List five safety precautions designed to prevent unnecessary exposure to x-rays.

   a. _____ b. _____

   c. _____ d. _____

   e. _____

5. Name four diagnostic tools used in diagnostic radiology.

   a. _____ b. _____

   c. _____ d. _____

6. Define radiation therapy. _____
   _____

Word Parts

1. In the spaces provided, write the definition of these prefixes, roots, combining forms, and suffixes. Do not refer to the listings of terminology words. Leave blank those terms you cannot define.
2. After completing as many as you can, refer back to the terminology word listings to check your work. For each word missed or left blank, write the term and its definition several times on the margins of these pages or on a separate sheet of paper.
3. To maximize the learning process, it is to your advantage to do the following exercises as directed. To refer to the terminology listings before completing these exercises invalidates the learning process.

PREFIXES

Give the definitions of the following prefixes:

1. brachy- _____ 2. dia- _____

3. intra- _____ 4. milli- _____

5. ultra- _____

ROOTS AND COMBINING FORMS

Give the definitions of the following roots and combining forms:

1. act _____   2. ampere _____

3. angio _____   4. aorto _____

5. arterio _____   6. arthro _____

7. broncho _____   8. cardio _____

9. cavit _____   10. chol _____

11. chole _____   12. cine _____

13. cinemato _____   14. cisterno _____

15. curie _____   16. cysto _____

17. dermat _____   18. dosi _____

19. echo _____   20. electro _____

21. encephalo _____   22. fluoro _____

23. geno _____   24. holo _____

25. hystero _____   26. iono _____

27. ionto _____   28. kilo _____

29. kymo _____   30. log _____

31. lucent _____   32. lymph _____

33. mammo _____   34. metr _____

35. myelo _____   36. necr _____

37. oscillo _____   38. paque _____

39. photo _____   40. physic _____

41. pneumo _____   42. pyelo _____

43. radiat _____   44. radio _____

45. roent _____   46. salpingo _____

47. sialo _____   48. son _____

49. sono _____   50. tele _____

51. thermo _____   52. tomo _____

53. ven _____   54. veno _____

55. ventriculo _____   56. volt _____

57. watt _____   58. xero _____

SUFFIXES

Give the definitions of the following suffixes:

1. -ary   _____   2. -er   _____

3. -genic   _____   4. -gnosis   _____

5. -gram   _____   6. -graph   _____

7. -graphy   _____   8. -ic   _____

9. -ion   _____   10. -ist   _____

11. -itis   _____   12. -ive   _____

13. -logy   _____   14. -meter   _____

15. -osis   _____   16. -ous   _____

17. -scope   _____   18. -scopy   _____

19. -therapy   _____   _____

Identifying Medical Terms

In the spaces provided, write the medical terms for the following meanings:

1. _____ The process of making an x-ray record of blood vessels

2. _____ The process of making an x-ray record of a joint

3. _____ An x-ray record of the gallbladder that is made visible through the use of a radiopaque contrast medium

4. _____ The process of making an x-ray record of the basal cistern of the brain

5. _____ One who specializes in the planning and calculating of radiation dosage

6. _____ The making of a picture in which the original object appears in three dimensions

7. _____ Pertaining to within a cavity

8. _____ Treatment by introducing ions into the body

9. _____ 1000 V

10. _____ 1000 W

11. _____ The process of obtaining pictures of the breast through the use of x-rays

12. _____ 0.001 Ci

13. _____ One who specializes in the science of physics

14. _____ The process whereby radiant energy is propagated through space or matter

15. _____ Caused or produced by radioactivity

16. _____ One who is skilled in making x-ray records

17. _____ Property of permitting the passage of radiant energy

18. _____ Property of obstructing the passage of radiant energy

19. _____ One who specializes in roentgen diagnosis, therapy, or both

20. _____ A record produced by ultrasonography

Spelling

In the spaces provided, write the correct spelling of these misspelled terms:

1. hystersalpingram _____   2. echgraphy _____

3. lymphangography _____   4. myleogram _____

5. pneumencephalgram _____   6. radiactive _____

7. radigraphy _____   8. silography _____

9. tomgraphy _____   10. vengraphy _____

Review Questions

Matching

Select the appropriate lettered meaning for each numbered line.

_____ 1. alopecia

_____ 2. anorexia

_____ 3. beam

_____ 4. cassette

_____ 5. energy

_____ 6. lead

_____ 7. radium

_____ 8. scan

_____ 9. shield

_____ 10. tagging

a. A protective structure used to prevent or reduce the passage of particles or radiation

b. A radioactive isotope used in the treatment of certain malignant diseases

c. A ray of light

d. Loss of hair

e. Loss of appetite

f. Loss of energy

g. A light-proof case or holder for x-ray film

h. The process of tracing a radioactive isotope that has become involved in metabolic or chemical reactions

i. A process of using a moving device or a sweeping beam of radiation to produce images of organs or structures of the body

j. The power or capacity to do work

k. A metallic chemical element

Abbreviations

Place the correct word, phrase, or abbreviation in the space provided.

_____ 1. anteroposterior

_____ 2. barium

_____ 3. computed tomography

_____ 4. kV

_____ 5. LL

_____ 6. Ra

_____ 7. magnetic resonance imaging

_____ 8. PA

_____ 9. pneumoencephalogram

_____ 10. PET

I

Answer Key

CHAPTER 1

Word Parts

Prefixes

1. without
2. away from
3. against
4. self
5. bad
6. a hundred
7. through
8. different
9. bad
10. small
11. one-thousandth
12. many, much
13. new
14. beside
15. before
16. together
17. three

Roots and Combining Forms

1. stuck to
2. armpit
3. center
4. chemical
5. a shaping
6. formation, produce
7. a thousand
8. large
9. death
10. law
11. rule
12. tumor
13. organ
14. fever

15. heat, fire
16. ray
17. to examine
18. putrefaction
19. hot, heat
20. place
21. cough

Suffixes

1. related to
2. pertaining to
3. pertaining to
4. surgical puncture
5. a key
6. a course
7. shape
8. to flee
9. formation, produce
10. knowledge
11. a step
12. a weight
13. recording
14. condition
15. pertaining to
16. process
17. condition of
18. nature of, quality of
19. liter
20. study of
21. instrument to measure
22. condition of
23. pertaining to
24. disease
25. to carry
26. instrument
27. decay
28. treatment
29. heat
30. condition

Identifying Medical Terms

1. adhesion
2. asepsis
3. axillary
4. chemotherapy
5. heterogeneous
6. malformation
7. microscope
8. multiform
9. neopathy
10. oncology

Spelling

1. antiseptic
2. autonomy
3. centimeter
4. diaphoresis
5. milligram
6. necrosis
7. paracentesis
8. radiology

Matching

1. f	6. k
2. d	7. b
3. j	8. i
4. g	9. c
5. a	10. e

Abbreviations

1. abnormal
2. axillary
3. Bx
4. cardiovascular disease

5. diagnosis-related groups
6. ENT
7. FP
8. GP
9. gynecology
10. pediatrics

CHAPTER 2

Anatomy and Physiology

1. body . . . cells . . . sustain
2. cell membrane
3. protoplasm . . . cytoplasm . . . karyoplasm
4. karyoplasm
5. a. cell reproduction
   b. control over activity within the cell's cytoplasm
6. a. protection
   b. absorption
   c. secretion
   d. excretion
7. connective
8. a. striated (voluntary)
   b. cardiac
   c. smooth (involuntary)
9. a. excitability
   b. conductivity
10. A tissue serving a common purpose
11. A group of organs functioning together for a common purpose
12. a. integumentary
    b. skeletal
    c. muscular
    d. digestive
    e. cardiovascular
    f. blood and lymphatic
    g. respiratory
    h. urinary
    i. endocrine
    j. nervous
    k. reproductive
13. a. above, in an upward direction
    b. in front of, before
    c. toward the back
    d. toward the head
    e. nearest the middle

f. to the side
g. nearest the point of attachment
h. away from the point of attachment
i. the front side
j. the back side
14. midsagittal plane
15. transverse or horizontal
16. coronal or frontal
17. a. thoracic   b. abdominal
    c. pelvic
18. a. cranial   b. spinal

Word Parts

Prefixes

1. both
2. up
3. two
4. color
5. down, away from
6. apart
7. outside
8. within
9. similar, same
10. middle
11. through
12. first
13. one

Roots and Combining Forms

1. fat
2. man
3. life
4. tail
5. cell
6. cell
7. to pour
8. formation, produce
9. tissue
10. water
11. cell's nucleus
12. side
13. disease
14. nature
15. to drink
16. body
17. place
18. a turning
19. body organs

Suffixes

1. pertaining to
2. use, action
3. formation, produce
4. pertaining to
5. process
6. study of
7. form, shape
8. resemble
9. like
10. condition of
11. pertaining to
12. a thing formed, plasma
13. body
14. control, stopping
15. incision

Identifying Medical Terms

1. android
2. bilateral
3. cytology
4. ectomorph
5. karyogenesis
6. somatotrophic
7. unilateral

Spelling

1. adipose
2. caudal
3. cytology
4. diffusion
5. histology
6. mesomorph
7. perfusion
8. pinocytosis
9. somatotrophic
10. unilateral

Matching

1. c	6. i
2. d	7. g
3. e	8. h
4. f	9. j
5. a	10. b

Abbreviations

1. abd
2. anatomy and physiology
3. central nervous system
4. CV
5. GI
6. lateral
7. respiratory
8. endoplasmic reticulum
9. anterior-posterior
10. posterior-anterior

CHAPTER 3

Anatomy and Physiology

1. The skin
2. a. hair
   b. nails
   c. sebaceous glands
   d. sweat glands
3. a. protection
   b. regulation
   c. sensory reception
   d. secretion
4. epidermis . . . dermis
5. a. stratum corneum
   b. stratum lucidum
   c. stratum granulosum
   d. stratum germinativum
6. Keratin
7. Melanin
8. dermis
9. a. papillary layer
   b. reticular layer
10. lunula

Word Parts

Prefixes

1. without, lack of
2. self
3. out
4. upon
5. out
6. excessive
7. under
8. within
9. around
10. below

Roots and Combining Forms

1. a thorn
2. ray
3. gland
4. white
5. cancer
6. heat
7. juice
8. corium
9. skin
10. skin
11. skin
12. skin
13. skin
14. skin
15. red
16. red
17. sweat
18. jaundice
19. tumor
20. horn
21. white
22. study of
23. black
24. black
25. fungus
26. nail
27. nail
28. nail
29. thick
30. a louse
31. wrinkle
32. wrinkle
33. hard
34. oil
35. old
36. hot, heat
37. hair
38. hair
39. nail
40. yellow
41. dry

Suffixes

1. pertaining to
2. pain
3. immature cell, germ cell
4. injection
5. skin
6. excision
7. sensation
8. pencil
9. condition
10. pertaining to
11. process
12. condition of
13. one who specializes
14. inflammation
15. study of
16. softening
17. resemble
18. tumor
19. condition of
20. pertaining to
21. disease
22. skin
23. to eat
24. surgical repair
25. flow, discharge
26. instrument to cut
27. tissue

Identifying Medical Terms

1. actinic dermatitis
2. cutaneous
3. dermatitis
4. dermatology
5. dermatopathy
6. hyperhidrosis
7. hypodermic
8. icteric
9. onychectomy
10. pachyderma
11. thermanesthesia
12. xanthoderma

Spelling

1. causalgia
2. dermomycosis
3. ecchymosis
4. erysipelas
5. hypodermoclysis
6. melanoma
7. onychophagia
8. rhytidectomy
9. scleroderma
10. seborrhea

Matching

1. d   4. h
2. f   5. j
3. e   6. i

7. b   9. a
8. g   10. c

Abbreviations

1. FUO
2. TTS
3. hypodermic
4. I & D
5. SG
6. intradermal
7. T
8. UV
9. foreign body
10. psoralen-ultraviolet-light

Diagnostic and Laboratory Tests

1. c
2. d
3. a
4. b
5. a

CHAPTER 4

Anatomy and Physiology

1. 206
2. a. axial b. appendicular
3. a. flat . . . ribs, scapula,
          parts of
          the pelvic girdle,
          bones of the skull
   b. long . . . tibia, femur,
      humerus, radius
   c. short . . . carpal, tarsal
   d. irregular . . . vertebrae,
                ossicles of
                the ear
   e. sesamoid . . . patella
4. a. shape, support
   b. protection
   c. storage
   d. formation of blood cells
   e. attachment of skeletal
      muscles

f. movement, through
   articulation
5. a. the ends of a developing
      bone
   b. the shaft of a long bone
   c. the membrane that
      forms the covering of
      bones, except at their
      articular surfaces
   d. the dense, hard layer of
      bone tissue
   e. a narrow space or cavity
      throughout the length of
      the diaphysis
   f. a tough connective tis-
      sue membrane lining the
      medullary canal and con-
      taining the bone marrow
   g. the reticular tissue that
      makes up most of the vol-
      ume of bone
6. Numbers of the matching
   answers:
   a. 6   h. 14
   b. 11   i. 1
   c. 4   j. 12
   d. 13   k. 2
   e. 8   l. 3
   f. 10   m. 7
   g. 9   n. 5
7. a. synarthrosis
   b. amphiarthrosis
   c. diarthrosis
8. Abduction
9. the process of moving a
   body part toward the
   midline
10. Circumduction
11. the process of bending a
    body part backward
12. Eversion
13. the process of straightening
    a flexed limb
14. Flexion
15. the process of turning
    inward
16. Pronation
17. the process of moving a
    body part forward
18. Retraction
19. the process of moving a
    body part around a central
    axis

20. Supination

Word Parts

Prefixes

1. without
2. upon, above
3. water
4. between
5. beyond
6. around
7. many, much
8. under, beneath
9. together
10. together

Roots and Combing Forms

1. vinegar cup
2. achilles, heel
3. extremity, point
4. extremity
5. stiffening, crooked
6. joint
7. joint
8. a pouch
9. heel bone
10. heel bone
11. cancer
12. wrist
13. wrist
14. cartilage
15. cartilage
16. little key
17. clavicle
18. tail bone
19. tail bone
20. glue
21. knuckle
22. to bind together
23. rib
24. rib
25. hip
26. hip
27. skull
28. skull
29. finger or toe
30. finger or toe
31. femur
32. fibrous
33. fibula
34. curve

35. humerus
36. ilium
37. ilium
38. ischium
39. a hump
40. lamina (thin plate)
41. bending
42. loin
43. loin
44. lower jawbone
45. jawbone
46. jaw
47. marrow
48. marrow
49. death
50. elbow
51. bone
52. kneecap
53. kneecap
54. disease
55. foot
56. closely knit row
57. a passage
58. pus
59. spine
60. spine
61. radius
62. sacrum
63. flesh
64. shoulder blade
65. hardening
66. curvature
67. curvature
68. spine
69. vertebra
70. sternum
71. sternum
72. tendon
73. tendon
74. tibia
75. elbow
76. elbow
77. vertebra
78. vertebra
79. sword

Suffixes

1. pertaining to
2. pertaining to
3. pain
4. pertaining to
5. pertaining to

6. immature cell, germ cell
7. surgical puncture
8. a breaking
9. binding
10. pain
11. excision
12. swelling
13. formation, produce
14. formation, produce
15. mark, record
16. to write
17. pertaining to
18. inflammation
19. nature of
20. study of
21. softening
22. enlargement, large
23. resemble
24. tumor
25. shoulder
26. condition of
27. disease
28. lack of
29. fixation
30. growth
31. formation
32. surgical repair
33. formation
34. drooping
35. to burst forth
36. suture
37. rupture
38. instrument to cut
39. incision
40. tension

Identifying Medical Terms

1. acroarthritis
2. ankylosis
3. arthrectomy
4. arthritis
5. arthropathy
6. calcaneal
7. carpoptosis
8. chondral
9. chondropathology
10. coccygodynia
11. costal
12. craniectomy
13. dactylic
14. hydrarthrosis

15. intercostal
16. ischialgia; coxalgia
17. lumbar
18. myeloma
19. osteoarthritis
20. osteodynia
21. osteomyelitis or myelitis
22. osteopenia
23. pedal
24. sternalgia
25. xiphoid

Spelling

1. acromion
2. arthredema
3. bursitis
4. chondroblast
5. connective
6. cranioplasty
7. dactylomegaly
8. ischial
9. myelitis
10. osteochondritis
11. osteonecrosis
12. patellar
13. phalangeal
14. rachigraph
15. scoliosis
16. spondylitis
17. symphysis
18. tenonitis
19. ulnocarpal
20. vertebral

Matching

1. i   6. h
2. j   7. g
3. e   8. a
4. c   9. d
5. b   10. f

Abbreviations

1. CDH
2. DJD
3. long leg cast
4. osteoarthritis
5. PEMFs
6. rheumatoid arthritis

7. SPECT
8. thoracic vertebra, first
9. temporomandibular joint
10. Tx

Diagnostic and Laboratory Tests

1. c
2. d
3. c
4. b
5. b

CHAPTER 5

Anatomy and Physiology

1. a. skeletal   b. smooth
   c. cardiac
2. 42
3. a. nutrition b. oxygen
4. a. origin   b. insertion
5. voluntary or striated
6. aponeurosis
7. a. body   b. origin
   c. insertion
8. a. A muscle that counteracts
      the action of another muscle.
   b. A muscle that is primary
      in a given movement.
   c. A muscle that acts with
      another muscle to pro-
      duce movement.
9. involuntary, visceral, or unstriated
10. a. digestive tract
    b. respiratory tract
    c. urinary tract
    d. eye
    e. skin
11. Cardiac
12. a. movement
    b. maintain posture
    c. produce heat

Word Parts

Prefixes

1. lack of
2. away from

3. toward
4. against
5. separation
6. two
7. slow
8. with
9. through
10. difficult
11. into
12. within
13. many
14. with, together
15. three

Roots and Combining Forms

1. agony
2. arm
3. clavicle
4. turmoil
5. neck
6. finger or toe
7. to lead
8. work
9. a band
10. a band
11. a band
12. fiber
13. fiber
14. equal
15. a rind
16. lifter
17. bending
18. breast
19. black
20. to measure
21. muscle
22. muscle
23. muscle
24. muscle
25. nerve
26. nerve
27. disease
28. four
29. to loosen
30. rod
31. to turn
32. flesh
33. flesh
34. hardening
35. to gain
36. convulsive
37. sternum
38. tendon

39. tendon
40. tone, tension
41. twisted
42. to draw
43. will

Suffixes

1. pain
2. pertaining to
3. pertaining to
4. weakness
5. immature cell, germ cell
6. head
7. binding
8. pain
9. excision
10. formation, produce
11. to write, record
12. condition
13. pertaining to
14. process
15. agent
16. inflammation
17. condition
18. motion
19. motion
20. study of
21. destruction
22. softening
23. resemble
24. tumor
25. a doer
26. condition of
27. weakness
28. disease
29. a fence
30. surgical repair
31. stroke, paralysis
32. suture
33. rupture
34. tension, spasm
35. order
36. instrument to cut
37. incision
38. nourishment, development
39. pertaining to

Identifying Medical Terms

1. aponeurorrhaphy
2. atonic
3. bradykinesia
4. dactylospasm

5. dystrophy
6. fascioplasty
7. intramuscular
8. levator
9. myasthenia
10. myogenesis
11. myology
12. myoparesis
13. myoplasty
14. myosarcoma
15. myotenositis
16. myotomy
17. neuromyositis
18. polyplegia
19. tenodesis
20. synergetic
21. triceps

Spelling

1. fascia
2. myokinesis
3. polymyoclonus
4. rhabdomyoma
5. sarcolemma
6. sternocleidomastoid
7. tenotomy
8. torticollis

Matching

1. d   6. a
2. i   7. h
3. g   8. c
4. e   9. b
5. j   10. f

Abbreviations

1. above elbow
2. aspartate transaminase
3. Ca
4. EMG
5. full range of motion
6. musculoskeletal
7. ROM
8. sh
9. total body weight
10. triceps jerk

Diagnostic and Laboratory Tests

1. b
2. d
3. b
4. c
5. a

CHAPTER 6

Anatomy and Physiology

1. a. mouth
   b. pharynx
   c. esophagus
   d. stomach
   e. small intestine
   f. large intestine
2. a. salivary glands
   b. liver
   c. gallbladder
   d. pancreas
3. a. digestion
   b. absorption
   c. elimination
4. A small mass of masticated food ready to be swallowed
5. A series of wave-like muscular contractions that are involuntary
6. Hydrochloric acid and gastric juices
7. duodenum
8. chyme
9. circulatory system
10. cecum, colon, rectum, and the anal canal
11. liver
12. Stores and concentrates bile
13. Produces digestive enzymes
14. a. It plays an important role in metabolism.
    b. It manufactures bile.
    c. It stores iron, vitamins B_{12}, A, D, E, and K
15. small intestine
16. a. parotid c. sublingual
    b. submandibular
17. a. insulin b. glucagon

Word Parts

Prefixes

1. lack of
2. up
3. down
4. difficult
5. above
6. excessive, above
7. deficient, below
8. bad
9. large, great
10. around
11. after
12. backward
13. below

Roots and Combining Forms

1. to suck in
2. gland
3. starch
4. anus
5. appendix
6. appendix
7. gall, bile
8. to cast, throw
9. cheek
10. abdomen, belly
11. lip
12. gall, bile
13. common bile duct
14. colon
15. colon
16. colon
17. colon
18. bladder
19. tooth
20. tooth
21. diverticula
22. duodenum
23. intestine
24. intestine
25. esophagus
26. esophagus
27. stomach
28. stomach
29. gums
30. tongue
31. sweet, sugar
32. blood
33. liver
34. liver
35. hernia

36. ileum
37. ileum
38. lip
39. flank, abdomen
40. to loosen
41. tongue
42. fat
43. study of
44. middle
45. pancreas
46. to digest
47. pharynx
48. meal
49. rectum, anus
50. rectum, anus
51. pylorus, gate keeper
52. rectum
53. saliva
54. sigmoid
55. spleen
56. mouth
57. poison
58. vagus
59. worm

Suffixes

1. pertaining to
2. pertaining to
3. pain
4. pertaining to
5. enzyme
6. hernia
7. injection
8. pain
9. excision
10. vomiting
11. shape
12. formation, produce
13. pertaining to
14. pertaining to
15. process
16. condition of
17. one who specializes
18. inflammation
19. nature of, quality of
20. study of
21. destruction, to separate
22. enlargement, large
23. tumor
24. appetite
25. condition of
26. disease

27. to digest
28. fixation
29. to eat
30. surgical repair
31. suture
32. instrument
33. to view, examine
34. contraction
35. new opening
36. incision
37. pertaining to

Identifying Medical Terms

1. amylase
2. anabolism
3. anorexia
4. appendectomy
5. appendicitis
6. biliary
7. celiac
8. colorrhaphy
9. dysphagia
10. hepatitis
11. herniotomy
12. postprandial
13. proctalgia
14. splenomegaly
15. sigmoidoscope

Spelling

1. biliary
2. colonoscopy
3. enteroclysis
4. gastroenterology
5. hepatotoxin
6. laxative
7. peristalsis
8. sialadenitis
9. vagotomy
10. vermiform

Matching

1.	e	6.	h
2.	f	7.	j
3.	d	8.	a
4.	b	9.	g
5.	i	10.	c

Abbreviations

1. a.c.
2. bowel movement
3. bowel sounds
4. cib
5. GB
6. HAV
7. nasogastric
8. nothing by mouth
9. p.c.
10. TPN

Diagnostic and Laboratory Tests

1. a
2. c
3. d
4. c
5. c

CHAPTER 7

Anatomy and Physiology

1. a. heart   c. veins
   b. arteries   d. capillaries
2. a. endocardium
   b. myocardium
   c. pericardium
3. 300
4. atria . . . interatrial
5. ventricles . . . interventricular
6. a. superior and inferior
      vena cavae
   b. right atrium
   c. tricuspid valve
   d. right ventricle
   e. pulmonary semilunar
      valve
   f. left and right pulmonary
      arteries
   g. lungs
   h. left and right pulmonary
      veins
   i. left atrium
   j. bicuspid or mitral valve
   k. left ventricle
   l. aortic valve
   m. aorta

n. capillaries
7. autonomic nervous system
8. sinoatrial node
9. Purkinje system
10. a. radial . . . on the radial
       side of the wrist
    b. brachial . . . in the
       antecubital space of the
       elbow
    c. carotid . . . in the neck
11. a. the pressure exerted by
       the blood on the walls
       of the vessels
    b. the difference between
       the systolic and diastolic
       readings
12. man's fist . . . 60 to 100
13. 100 and 140 . . . 60 and 90
14. transports blood from the
    right and left ventricles of
    the heart to all body parts
15. transport blood from periph-
    eral tissues to the heart

Word Parts

Prefixes

1. lack of
2. two
3. slow
4. together
5. within
6. within
7. outside
8. excessive, above
9. deficient, below
10. around
11. before
12. half
13. fast
14. three

Roots and Combining Forms

1. vessel
2. to choke, quinsy
3. vessel
4. aorta
5. aorta
6. artery
7. artery
8. artery

9. fatty substance, porridge
10. fatty substance, porridge
11. atrium
12. atrium
13. heart
14. heart
15. heart
16. dark blue
17. to the right
18. to widen
19. electricity
20. a throwing in
21. sweet, sugar
22. blood
23. to hold back
24. motion
25. study of
26. moon
27. thin
28. mitral valve
29. muscle
30. death
31. sour, sharp, acid
32. vein
33. vein
34. sound
35. lung
36. rhythm
37. hardening
38. a curve
39. pulse
40. narrowing
41. chest
42. to draw, to bind
43. contraction
44. pressure
45. clot of blood
46. tone
47. small vessel
48. vessel
49. a carrier
50. vein
51. vein
52. ventricle

Suffixes

1. pertaining to
2. pertaining to
3. pertaining to
4. immature cell, germ cell
5. surgical puncture
6. injection

7. point
8. pain
9. dilatation
10. excision
11. blood condition
12. relating to
13. formation, produce
14. a mark, record
15. to write
16. recording
17. condition
18. pertaining to
19. having a particular quality
20. process
21. condition of
22. one who specializes
23. inflammation
24. nature of, quality of
25. stone
26. study of
27. softening
28. enlargement, large
29. instrument to measure
30. tumor
31. one who
32. condition of
33. disease
34. surgical repair
35. stroke, paralysis
36. prolapse, drooping
37. to pierce
38. suture
39. instrument
40. contraction, spasm
41. contraction
42. instrument to cut
43. incision
44. crushing
45. tissue
46. pertaining to

Identifying Medical Terms

1. angioma
2. angioblast
3. angioplasty
4. angiostenosis
5. arterectomy
6. arteriolith
7. arteriotomy
8. arteritis
9. bicuspid

10. cardiodynia
11. cardiologist
12. cardiomegaly
13. cardiopulmonary
14. constriction
15. embolism
16. phlebitis
17. phlebolith
18. tachycardia
19. vasodilator

Spelling

1. arterectomy
2. atherosclerosis
3. atrioventricular
4. endocarditis
5. extrasystole
6. ischemia
7. myocardial
8. oxygen
9. phlebitis
10. presystolic

Matching

1. d   6. c
2. e   7. a
3. f   8. i
4. g   9. j
5. b   10. h

Abbreviations

1. AMI
2. A-V, AV
3. blood pressure
4. coronary artery disease
5. CC
6. electrocardiogram
7. high-density lipoproteins
8. H & L
9. myocardial infarction
10. tissue plasminogen activator

Diagnostic and Laboratory Tests

1. c   4. c
2. a   5. b
3. b

CHAPTER 8

Anatomy and Physiology

1. a. erythrocytes
   b. thrombocytes
   c. leukocytes
2. transport oxygen and carbon dioxide
3. 5
4. 80–120 days
5. body's main defense against the invasion of pathogens
6. 8000
7. a. neutrophils
   b. eosinophils
   c. basophils
   d. lymphocytes
   e. monocytes
8. plays an important role in the clotting process
9. 200,000–500,000
10. a. A.   b. B   c. AB
    d. O
11. a. It transports proteins and fluids
    b. It protects the body against pathogens
    c. It serves as a pathway for the absorption of fats
12. a. spleen
    b. tonsils
    c. thymus

Word Parts

Prefixes

1. lack of
2. against
3. self
4. through
5. bad
6. excessive
7. deficient
8. one
9. all
10. many
11. before

Roots and Combining Forms

1. gland
2. gland
3. clumping
4. other
5. vessel
6. unequal
7. base
8. lime, calcium
9. smoke
10. destruction
11. clots, to clot
12. flesh, creatine
13. cell
14. cell
15. cell
16. rose-colored
17. red
18. sweet, sugar
19. little grain, granular
20. blood
21. blood
22. blood
23. white
24. white
25. fat
26. study of
27. lymph
28. lymph
29. large
30. neither
31. kernel, nucleus
32. eat, engulf
33. a thing formed, plasma
34. net
35. putrefying
36. whey, serum
37. iron
38. spleen
39. spleen
40. sea
41. clot
42. clot
43. thymus
44. thymus
45. tonsil

Suffixes

1. capable
2. forming
3. immature cell, germ cell
4. body
5. hernia
6. to separate
7. cultivation
8. cell

9. excision
10. blood condition
11. work
12. formation, produce
13. formation, produce
14. protein
15. knowledge
16. condition
17. pertaining to
18. chemical
19. process
20. one who specializes
21. inflammation
22. study of
23. destruction
24. enlargement
25. tumor
26. condition of
27. disease
28. lack of
29. fixation
30. removal
31. attraction
32. attraction
33. fear
34. formation
35. bursting forth
36. bursting forth
37. control, stopping
38. treatment
39. incision

Identifying Medical Terms

1. agglutination
2. allergy
3. antibody
4. anticoagulant
5. antigen
6. antihermorrhagic
7. basocyte
8. coagulable
9. creatinemia
10. eosinophil
11. erythroclastic
12. granulocyte
13. hematologist
14. hemoglobin
15. hyperglycemia
16. hyperlipemia
17. leukocyte
18. lymphostasis
19. mononucleosis

20. prothrombin
21. splenopexy
22. thrombocyte
23. thrombogenic
24. thymitis

Spelling

1. allergy
2. creatinemia
3. dysglycemia
4. erythrocytosis
5. hematocele
6. hematocrit
7. hemorrhage
8. leukemia
9. lymphadenotomy
10. serology

Matching

1. h   6. c
2. d   7. b
3. e   8. a
4. g   9. j
5. f   10. i

Abbreviations

1. AIDS
2. BSI
3. chronic myelogenous leukemia
4. Hb, Hgb
5. hematocrit
6. HIV
7. pneumocystis pneumonia
8. prothrombin time
9. red blood cell (count)
10. RIA

Diagnostic and Laboratory Tests

1. d
2. c
3. c
4. b
5. a

CHAPTER 9

Anatomy and Physiology

1. a. nose   d. trachea
   b. pharynx   e. bronchi
   c. larynx   f. lungs
2. To furnish oxygen for use by individual cells and to take away their gaseous waste product, carbon dioxide
3. The process whereby the lungs are ventilated and oxygen and carbon dioxide are exchanged between the air in the lungs and the blood within capillaries of the alveoli
4. The process whereby oxygen and carbon dioxide are exchanged between the bloodstream and the cells of the body
5. a. Serves as an air passage way
   b. Warms and moistens inhaled air
   c. Its cilia and mucous membrane trap dust, pollen, bacteria, and foreign matter
   d. It contains olfactory receptors that sort out odors
   e. It aids in phonation and the quality of voice
6. a. nasopharynx
   b. oropharynx
   c. laryngopharynx
7. a. Serves as a passageway for air
   b. Serves as a passageway for food
   c. Aids in phonation by changing its shape
8. Acts as a lid to prevent aspiration of food into the trachea
9. A narrow slit at the opening between the true vocal folds
10. The production of vocal sounds

11. Serves as a passageway for air
12. right bronchus ... left bronchus
13. Provides a passageway for air to and from the lungs
14. Cone-shaped, spongy organs of respiration lying on either side of the heart
15. A serous membrane composed of several layers
16. diaphragm
17. mediastinum
18. 3 ... 2
19. alveoli
20. To bring air into intimate contact with blood so that oxygen and carbon dioxide can be exchanged in the alveoli
21. temperature, pulse, respiration, and blood pressure
22. a. The amount of air in a single inspiration or expiration
    b. The amount of air remaining in the lungs after maximal expiration
    c. The volume of air that can be exhaled after a maximal inspiration
23. medulla oblongata ... pons
24. 30 to 80
25. 15 to 20

Word Parts

Prefixes

1. lack of
2. lack of
3. through
4. difficult
5. within
6. good
7. out
8. below, deficient
9. excessive
10. in
11. fast

Roots and Combining Forms

1. air
2. small, hollow air sac
3. coal
4. imperfect
5. bronchi
6. bronchi
7. bronchiole
8. bronchi
9. dust
10. dark blue
11. breathe
12. blood
13. larynx
14. larynx
15. larynx
16. lobe
17. chin
18. fungus
19. nose
20. straight
21. smell
22. oxygen
23. palate
24. breast
25. pharynx
26. voice
27. partition
28. partition
29. speech
30. pleura
31. pleura
32. pleura
33. lung, air
34. lung
35. lung
36. lung
37. pus
38. nose
39. a curve, hollow
40. breath
41. narrowing
42. chest
43. chest
44. almond, tonsil
45. trachea
46. trachea

Suffixes

1. pertaining to
2. pain
3. hernia
4. surgical puncture
5. pain
6. dilation
7. excision
8. a mark, record
9. condition
10. process
11. inflammation
12. instrument to measure
13. condition of
14. disease
15. bearing
16. surgical repair
17. stroke, paralysis
18. breathing
19. to spit
20. bursting forth
21. flow, discharge
22. instrument
23. new opening
24. incision
25. pertaining to

Identifying Medical Terms

1. aeropleura
2. alveolus
3. aphonia
4. bronchiectasis
5. bronchitis
6. bronchoplasty
7. dysphonia
8. eupnea
9. hemoptysis
10. inhalation
11. laryngitis
12. laryngostenosis
13. nasomental
14. pharyngalgia
15. pneumothorax
16. rhinoplasty
17. rhinorrhea
18. sinusitis
19. thoracopathy

Spelling

1. bronchoscope
2. diaphragmatocele
3. expectoration
4. laryngeal
5. orthopnea
6. pleuritis
7. pulmonectomy
8. rhinotomy
9. tachypnea
10. tracheal

Matching

1.	h	6.	b
2.	i	7.	d
3.	k	8.	a
4.	f	9.	e
5.	c	10.	g

Abbreviations

1. AFB
2. cystic fibrosis
3. CXR
4. COLD
5. endotracheal
6. postnasal drip
7. R
8. sudden infant death syndrome
9. SOB
10. tuberculosis

Diagnostic and Laboratory Tests

1. b
2. c
3. c
4. d
5. a

CHAPTER 10

Anatomy and Physiology

1. a. kidneys   c. bladder
   b. ureters   d. urethra
2. Extraction of certain wastes from the bloodstream, conversion of these materials to urine, and transport of the urine from the kidney, via the ureters, to the bladder for elimination
3. a. true capsule
   b. perirenal fat
   c. renal fascia
4. A notch
5. Sac-like collecting portion of the kidney
6. arteries, veins, convoluted tubules, and glomerular capsules
7. inner
8. The structural and functional unit of the kidney
9. renal corpuscle . . . tubule
10. glomerulus and Bowman's capsule
11. To remove the waste products of metabolism from the blood plasma
12. filtration and reabsorption
13. 95 . . . 5
14. 1000 to 1500
15. Narrow, muscular tubes that transport urine from the kidneys to the bladder
16. Muscular, membranous sac that serves as a reservoir for urine
17. Small, triangular area near the base of the bladder
18. Convey urine and semen
19. Convey urine
20. urinary meatus
21. Physical, chemical, and microscopic examination of urine
22. a. yellow to amber
    b. clear
    c. 5.0 to 7.0
    d. 1.015 to 1.025
    e. aromatic
    f. 1000 to 1500 mL/day
23. a. renal
    b. transitional
    c. squamous
24. diabetes mellitus
25. renal disease, acute glomerulonephritis, pyelonephritis

Word Parts

Prefixes

1. not, apart, lack of
2. without
3. against
4. through
5. through
6. difficult, painful
7. within
8. water
9. excessive
10. not
11. scanty
12. beside
13. around
14. excessive

Roots and Combining Forms

1. gland
2. protein
3. bacteria
4. bile
5. calcium
6. colon
7. to hold
8. bladder
9. bladder
10. bladder
11. producing
12. glomerulus, little ball
13. glomerulus, little ball
14. sweet, sugar
15. blood
16. ketone
17. stone
18. study of
19. passage
20. passage
21. to urinate
22. kidney
23. kidney
24. night
25. penis
26. perineum
27. to fold
28. purple
29. pus
30. renal pelvis
31. renal pelvis
32. kidney
33. hardening
34. narrowing
35. mouth
36. trigone
37. urine
38. urinate
39. urea
40. urine
41. ureter
42. ureter
43. urethra
44. urethra
45. urine
46. urine

47. urine
48. urine
49. vagina
50. bladder

Suffixes

1. pertaining to
2. pain
3. pertaining to
4. hernia
5. pain
6. distention
7. dilation
8. excision
9. blood condition
10. a mark, record
11. pertaining to
12. chemical
13. process
14. one who specializes
15. inflammation
16. stone
17. study of
18. destruction, to separate
19. softening
20. enlargement
21. instrument to measure
22. tumor
23. condition of
24. disease
25. fixation
26. to obstruct
27. surgical repair
28. paralysis
29. formation
30. prolapse, drooping
31. bursting forth
32. suture
33. instrument
34. to view, examine
35. condition
36. tension, spasm
37. dripping, trickling
38. new opening
39. instrument to cut
40. incision
41. tension
42. nourishment, development
43. urine

Identifying Medical Terms

1. antidiuretic
2. cystectomy

3. cystitis
4. cystopexy
5. cystorrhaphy
6. dysuria
7. glomerulitis
8. hypercalciuria
9. meatal
10. micturition
11. nephratony
12. nephrolith
13. nephromegaly
14. periurethral
15. pyuria
16. ureteropathy
17. ureterorrhaphy
18. urethralgia
19. urethrospasm
20. urologist

Spelling

1. cystoplasty
2. cystorrhagia
3. enuresis
4. glycosuria
5. hematuria
6. incontinence
7. nephremia
8. nephrocystitis
9. nephromalacia
10. nephroptosis
11. nocturia
12. ureteroplasty
13. urethrophraxis
14. urinalysis
15. urobilin
16. uropoiesis

Matching

1. d   6. g
2. e   7. j
3. b   8. c
4. f   9. h
5. a   10. i

Abbreviations

1. ADH
2. blood urea nitrogen
3. CRF
4. cystoscopic examination
5. genitourinary

6. hemodialysis
7. IVP
8. peritoneal dialysis
9. potential of hydrogen
10. UA

Diagnostic and Laboratory Tests

1. c
2. c
3. b
4. c
5. b

CHAPTER 11

Anatomy and Physiology

1. a. pituitary
   b. pineal
   c. thyroid
   d. parathyroid
   e. islets of Langerhans
   f. adrenals
   g. ovaries
   h. testes
2. a. thymus
   b. placenta during pregnancy
   c. gastrointestinal mucosa
3. It involves the production and regulation of chemical substances (hormones) that play an essential role in maintaining homeostasis
4. A chemical transmitter that is released in small amounts and transported via the bloodstream to a targeted organ or other cells
5. It synthesizes and secretes releasing hormones, releasing factors, release-inhibiting hormones, and release-inhibiting factors
6. Because of its regulatory effects on the other endocrine glands
7. a. growth hormone (GH)
   b. adrenocorticotropin (ACTH)

c. thyroid-stimulating hormone (TSH)

d. follicle-stimulating hormone (FSH)

e. luteinizing hormone (LH)

f. prolactin (PRL)

g. melanocyte-stimulating hormone (MSH)

8. a. antidiuretic hormone (ADH)

   b. oxytocin

9. melatonin and serotonin

10. It plays a vital role in metabolism and regulates the body's metabolic processes.

11. a. thyroxine (T$_4$)

    b. triiodothyronine (T$_3$)

    c. calcitonin

12. serum calcium . . . phosphorus

13. blood sugar

14. glucocorticoids, mineralocorticoids, and the androgens

15. a. Regulates carbohydrate, protein, and fat metabolism

    b. Stimulates output of glucose from the liver

    c. Increases the blood sugar level

    d. Regulates other physiological body processes

    * Optional answers to question 15:

    e. Promotes the transport of amino acids into extracellular tissue

    f. Influences the effectiveness of catecholamines such as dopamine, epinephrine, and norepinephrine

    g. Has an anti-inflammatory effect

    h. Helps the body cope during times of stress

16. a. use of carbohydrates

    b. absorption of glucose

    c. gluconeogenesis

    d. potassium and sodium metabolism

17. Aldosterone

18. A substance or hormone that promotes the development of male characteristics

19. a. dopamine

    b. epinephrine

    c. norepinephrine

20. a. It elevates the systolic blood pressure.

    b. It increases the heart rate and cardiac output.

    c. It increases glycogenolysis, thereby hastening release of glucose from the liver. This action elevates the blood sugar level and provides the body with a spurt of energy.

    * Optional answers to question 20:

    d. It dilates the bronchial tubes.

    e. It dilates the pupils.

21. estrogen and progesterone

22. testosterone

23. a. thymosin

    b. thymopoietin

24. a. gastrin

    b. secretin

    c. pancreozymin-cholecystokinin

    d. enterogastrone

Word Parts

Prefixes

1. toward
2. through
3. within
4. good, normal
5. out, away from
6. out, away from
7. excessive
8. deficient, under
9. all
10. beside
11. before

Roots and Combining Forms

1. acid
2. extremity
3. gland
4. gland
5. cortex

6. flesh
7. cretin
8. to secrete
9. to secrete
10. to secrete
11. small
12. milk
13. old age
14. giant
15. little acorn
16. sweet, sugar
17. seed
18. hairy
19. insulin
20. insulin
21. insulin
22. potassium
23. drowsiness
24. study of
25. mucus
26. eye
27. pine cone
28. pineal body
29. phlegm
30. kidney
31. kidney
32. hardening
33. thymus
34. thymus
35. thyroid, shield
36. thyroid, shield
37. poison
38. nourishment
39. masculine

Suffixes

1. pertaining to
2. pain
3. pertaining to
4. to go
5. excision
6. swelling
7. blood condition
8. formation, produce
9. condition
10. pertaining to
11. condition of
12. one who specializes
13. inflammation
14. study of
15. softening
16. enlargement, large
17. resemble
18. tumor

19. condition of
20. disease
21. fixation
22. growth
23. drooping
24. flow, discharge
25. treatment
26. instrument to cut
27. pertaining to

Identifying Medical Terms

1. adenosis
2. cretinism
3. diabetes
4. endocrinology
5. euthyroid
6. exocrine
7. gigantism
8. glucocorticoid
9. hyperkalemia
10. hypocrinism
11. hypogonadism
12. lethargic
13. pinealoma
14. thymitis

Spelling

1. adenosclerosis
2. cretinism
3. exophthalmic
4. hypothyroidism
5. myxedema
6. pineal
7. pituitary
8. thyroid
9. thyrotome
10. virilism

Matching

1. e   6. i
2. f   7. c
3. b   8. j
4. g   9. d
5. h   10. a

Abbreviations

1. BMR
2. DM

3. fasting blood sugar
4. glucose tolerance tests
5. PBI
6. parathormone
7. radioimmunoassay
8. STH
9. thyroid function studies
10. vasopressin

Diagnostic and Laboratory Tests

1. a
2. c
3. c
4. b
5. c

CHAPTER 12

Anatomy and Physiology

1. a. central b. peripheral
2. Neurons
3. a. Cause contractions in muscles
   b. Cause secretions from glands and organs
   c. Inhibit the actions of glands and organs
4. An axon is a long process reaching from the cell body to the area to be activated.
5. A dendrite resembles the branches of a tree and has short, unsheathed processes that transmit impulses to the cell body.
6. Sensory nerves transmit impulses to the central nervous system.
7. Interneurons
8. a. A single elongated process
   b. A bundle of nerve fibers
   c. Groups of nerve fibers
9. brain . . . spinal cord
10. a. receives impulses
    b. processes information
    c. responds with appropriate action
11. a. dura mater
    b. arachnoid

c. pia mater
12. a. cerebrum
    b. diencephalon
    c. midbrain
    d. cerebellum
    e. pons
    f. medulla oblongata
    g. reticular formation
13. frontal lobe
14. somesthetic area
15. auditory and language
16. vision
17. a. relay center for all sensory impulses
    b. relays motor impulses from the cerebellum to the cortex
18. a. regulator
    b. produce neurosecretions
    c. produces hormones
19. coordination of voluntary movement
20. a. regulate and control breathing
    b. regulate and control swallowing
    c. regulate and control coughing
    d. regulate and control sneezing
    e. regulate and control vomiting
21. a. conduct sensory impulses
    b. conduct motor impulses
    c. reflex center
22. 120 and 150
23. a. olfactory
    b. optic
    c. oculomotor
    d. trochlear
    e. trigeminal
    f. abducens
    g. facial
    h. acoustic
    i. glossopharyngeal
    j. vagus
    k. accessory
    l. hypoglossal
24. a. cervical   c. lumbar
    b. brachial   d. sacral
25. a. controls sweating
    b. controls the secretions of glands
    c. controls arterial blood pressure

d. controls smooth muscle tissue
26. a. sympathetic
    b. parasympathetic

Word Parts

Prefixes

1. lack of
2. lack of
3. star-shaped
4. slow
5. two
6. difficult
7. upon
8. half
9. water
10. excessive
11. below
12. within
13. small
14. little
15. beside
16. beside
17. many
18. fire
19. below
20. above
21. together

Roots and Combining Forms

1. extremity
2. to walk
3. spider
4. imperfect
5. imperfect
6. center
7. head
8. head
9. little brain
10. little brain
11. cerebrum
12. color
13. reservoir, cavity
14. cord
15. skull
16. skull
17. cell
18. tree
19. a disk
20. dura, hard
21. I, self
22. electricity
23. brain
24. brain
25. feeling
26. foramen
27. knot
28. glue
29. blood
30. sleep
31. sleep
32. thin plate
33. lobe
34. study of
35. word
36. large
37. membrane
38. membrane
39. membrane
40. mind
41. memory
42. spinal cord
43. spinal cord
44. muscle
45. nerve
46. nerve
47. nerve
48. papilla
49. to engulf, eat
50. dusky
51. air
52. gray
53. mind
54. mind
55. four
56. spine
57. root
58. root
59. hardening
60. a thorn
61. vertebra
62. body
63. sleep
64. sympathy
65. sympathy
66. tentorium, tent
67. mind, emotion
68. a bore
69. vagus, wandering
70. little belly

Suffixes

1. pertaining to
2. pain
3. pain
4. pertaining to
5. weakness
6. germ cell
7. hernia
8. cell
9. binding
10. excision
11. swelling
12. feeling
13. glue
14. mark, record
15. to write
16. recording
17. condition
18. pertaining to
19. process
20. condition
21. one who specializes
22. inflammation
23. motion
24. motion
25. to talk
26. a sheath, husk
27. diction
28. study of
29. destruction
30. softening
31. madness
32. instrument to measure
33. measurement
34. imitating
35. memory
36. mind
37. tumor
38. eye, vision
39. condition of
40. weakness
41. disease
42. to eat
43. speak
44. fear
45. a wasting
46. formation
47. surgical repair
48. stroke, paralysis
49. action
50. suture
51. strength
52. new opening
53. order
54. instrument to cut
55. incision
56. crushing
57. pertaining to
58. condition

Identifying Medical Terms

1. amnesia
2. analgesia
3. aphagia
4. arachnitis
5. ataxia
6. cephalalgia
7. cerebellar
8. craniectomy
9. dyslexia
10. encephalitis
11. epidural
12. hemiparesis
13. hypnology
14. macrocephalia
15. meningitis
16. meningopathy
17. myelotome
18. neuralgia
19. neuritis
20. neurocyte
21. neurology
22. neuroma
23. neuroplasty
24. neurosis
25. phagomania
26. polyneuritis
27. psychology
28. radiculitis
29. vagotomy
30. ventriculometry

Spelling

1. anesthesia
2. atelomyelia
3. cerebrospinal
4. craniotomy
5. encephalocele
6. meningioma
7. meningomyelocele
8. neuropathy
9. poliomyelitis
10. ventriculogram

Matching

1. g   6. h
2. d   7. j
3. c   8. f
4. b   9. a
5. e   10. i

Abbreviations

1. AD
2. ALS
3. central nervous system
4. cerebral palsy
5. CT
6. HDS
7. intracranial pressure
8. lumbar puncture
9. multiple sclerosis
10. PET

Diagnostic and Laboratory Tests

1. a
2. b
3. c
4. d
5. c

CHAPTER 13

Anatomy and Physiology

1. hearing and equilibrium
2. a. external   c. inner
   b. middle
3. a. auricle
   b. external acoustic meatus
   c. tympanic membrane
4. Auricle
5. a. lubrication
   b. protection
6. a. malleus c. stapes
   b. incus
7. To transmit sound vibrations
8. a. transmitting sound vibrations
   b. equalizing air pressure
   c. control of loud sounds
9. cochlea, vestibule, and the semicircular canals
10. a. cochlear duct
    b. semicircular ducts
    c. utricle and saccule
11. organ of Corti
12. vestibule
13. 8th cranial nerve
14. the position of the head
15. a. endolymph
    b. perilymph

Word Parts

Prefixes

1. within
2. within
3. around

Roots and Combining Forms

1. hearing
2. to hear
3. to hear
4. hearing
5. the ear
6. gall, bile
7. land snail
8. electricity
9. maze
10. maze
11. larynx
12. study of
13. breast
14. fungus
15. drum membrane
16. drum membrane
17. nerve
18. ear
19. ear
20. pharynx
21. voice
22. old
23. pus
24. nose
25. hardening
26. stirrup
27. fat
28. a jingling
29. drum

Suffixes

1. pertaining to
2. pain
3. hearing
4. pain
5. excision
6. a mark, record
7. recording
8. pertaining to
9. one who specializes
10. inflammation
11. stone
12. study of
13. serum, clear fluid
14. instrument to measure

15. measurement
16. form
17. tumor
18. condition of
19. surgical repair
20. flow
21. instrument
22. instrument to cut
23. incision
24. pertaining to
25. pertaining to

Identifying Medical Terms

1. audiologist
2. audiometry
3. auditory
4. endaural
5. labyrinthitis
6. myringoplasty
7. myringotome
8. otodynia
9. otolaryngology
10. otopharyngeal
11. otoscope
12. perilymph
13. stapedectomy
14. tympanectomy
15. tinnitus

Spelling

1. acoustic
2. audiology
3. cholesteatoma
4. electrocochleography
5. labyrinthitis
6. myringoplasty
7. otomycosis
8. otosclerosis
9. tympanic
10. tympanitis

Matching

1. h   6. b
2. e   7. j
3. i   8. c
4. a   9. d
5. g   10. f

Abbreviations

1. AC
2. AD
3. left ear
4. AU
5. ear, nose, throat
6. eyes, ears, nose, throat
7. HD
8. Oto
9. serous otitis media
10. UCHD

Diagnostic and Laboratory Tests

1. a
2. b
3. c
4. d
5. b

CHAPTER 14

Anatomy and Physiology

1. orbit, muscles, eyelids, conjunctiva, and the lacrimal apparatus
2. fatty tissue
3. optic nerve and ophthalmic artery
4. a. support
   b. rotary movement
5. intense light, foreign particles, and impact
6. A mucous membrane that acts as a protective covering for the exposed surface of the eyeball
7. Structures that produce, store, and remove the tears that cleanse and lubricate the eye
8. eyeball, its structures, and the nerve fibers
9. vision
10. optic disk
11. The process of sharpening the focus of light on the retina

12. Answers to the matching question:
   c 1. aqueous humor
   e 2. vitreous humor
   b 3. iris
   a 4. sclera
   f 5. uvea
   d 6. pupil
   h 7. retina
   i 8. rods and cones
   j 9. lens
   g 10. cornea

Word Parts

Prefixes

1. lack of, without
2. two
3. double
4. out
5. in
6. inward
7. beyond
8. within
9. three

Roots and Combining Forms

1. dull
2. disproportionate
3. unequal
4. eyelid
5. eyelid
6. choroid
7. choroid
8. pupil
9. cornea
10. ciliary body
11. ciliary body
12. sac
13. tear
14. tear
15. electricity
16. focus
17. angle
18. iris
19. iris
20. cornea
21. cornea
22. tear
23. study of
24. measure
25. to shut

26. muscle
27. blind
28. eye
29. eye
30. eye
31. eye
32. eye
33. lens
34. lentil, lens
35. light
36. old
37. pupil
38. retina
39. retina
40. sclera
41. point
42. tone
43. turn
44. uvea
45. foreign material
46. dry

Suffixes

1. pertaining to
2. pertaining to
3. pertaining to
4. germ cell
5. binding
6. excision
7. mark, record
8. recording
9. condition
10. pertaining to
11. process
12. condition of
13. one who specializes
14. inflammation
15. study of
16. destruction, to separate
17. softening
18. instrument to measure
19. tumor
20. eye, vision
21. condition of
22. disease
23. fear
24. surgical repair
25. stroke, paralysis
26. prolapse, drooping
27. instrument
28. stretching

Identifying Medical Terms

1. amblyopia
2. bifocal
3. blepharoptosis
4. corneal
5. dacryoma
6. diplopia
7. emmetropia
8. intraocular
9. iridomalacia
10. keratitis
11. keratoplasty
12. lacrimal
13. ocular
14. ophthalmopathy
15. photophobia

Spelling

1. astigmatism
2. cycloplegia
3. iridectomy
4. ophthalmologist
5. phacosclerosis
6. pupillary
7. retinoblastoma
8. scleritis
9. tonometer
10. uveal

Matching

1. e   6. d
2. f   7. g
3. j   8. b
4. h   9. a
5. c   10. i

Abbreviations

1. DVA
2. emmetropia
3. hypermetropia (hyperopia)
4. IOL
5. L & A
6. myopia
7. right eye
8. OS
9. OU
10. exotropia

Diagnostic and Laboratory Tests

1. c
2. b
3. c
4. d
5. d

CHAPTER 15

Anatomy and Physiology

1. a. ovaries
   b. fallopian tubes
   c. uterus
   d. vagina
   e. vulva
   f. breasts
2. To perpetuate the species through sexual or germ cell reproduction
3. a. body   b. isthmus
   c. cervix
4. The bulging surface of the body of the uterus extending from the internal os of the cervix upward above the fallopian tubes
5. a. broad ligaments
   b. round ligaments
   c. uterosacral ligaments
   d. ligaments that attach to the bladder
6. a. peritoneal
   b. endometrium
   c. myometrium
7. a. menstruation
   b. functions as a place for the protection and nourishment of the fetus during pregnancy
   c. uterine wall contracts rhythmically and powerfully to expel the fetus from the uterus
8. a. The process of bending forward of the uterus at its body and neck
   b. The process of bending the body of the uterus

backward at an angle, with the cervix usually unchanged from its normal position

c. The process of turning the fundus forward toward the pubis, with the cervix tilted up toward the sacrum

d. The process of turning the uterus backward, with the cervix pointing forward toward the symphysis pubis

9. uterine tubes or oviducts
10. a. serosa c. mucosa
    b. muscular
11. Finger-like processes that work to propel the discharged ovum into the fallopian tube
12. fertilization
13. a. Serves as a duct for the conveyance of the ovum from the ovary to the uterus
    b. Serve as ducts for the conveyance of spermatozoa from the uterus toward each ovary
14. Almond-shaped organs attached to the uterus by the ovarian ligament
15. a. primary   c. graafian
    b. growing
16. pituitary gland (anterior lobe)
17. a. production of ova
    b. production of hormones
18. musculomembranous . . . vestibule
19. a. female organ of copulation
    b. passageway for discharge of menstruation
    c. passageway for birth of the fetus
20. a. mons pubis
    b. labia major
    c. labia minora
    d. vestibule
    e. clitoris
21. perineum
22. A surgical procedure to pre-

vent tearing of the perineum and to facilitate delivery of the fetus
23. mammary glands
24. areola . . . nipple
25. a. prolactin
    b. insulin
    c. glucocorticoids
26. A thin yellowish secretion containing mainly serum and white blood cells; the "first milk"
27. a. menstruation
    b. proliferation
    c. luteal or secretory
    d. premenstrual or ischemic
28. A condition that effects certain women and may cause distressful symptoms such as nausea, constipation, diarrhea, anorexia, headache, appetite cravings, backache, muscular aches, edema, insomnia, clumsiness, malaise, irritability, indecisiveness, mental confusion, and depression

Word Parts

Prefixes

1. lack of
2. lack of
3. before
4. down
5. together
6. against
7. difficult, painful
8. within
9. good, normal
10. within
11. many
12. new
13. none
14. scanty
15. all
16. beside
17. around
18. after
19. before
20. first
21. false

22. backward
23. three

Roots and Combining Forms

1. to miscarry
2. lamb
3. Bartholin's glands
4. receive
5. cervix
6. a coming together
7. vagina
8. cul-de-sac
9. bladder
10. vulva
11. a bed
12. fibrous tissue
13. belonging to birth
14. female
15. blood
16. hymen
17. womb, uterus
18. womb, uterus
19. study of
20. breast
21. breast
22. month
23. month
24. month
25. womb, uterus
26. uterus
27. muscle
28. birth
29. birth
30. ovum, egg
31. ovary
32. ovary
33. to bear
34. labor
35. cessation
36. pelvis
37. perineum
38. pus
39. rectum
40. tube
41. tube
42. tube
43. birth
44. uterus
45. vagina
46. sexual intercourse
47. turning

Suffixes

1. pertaining to
2. pertaining to
3. hernia
4. surgical puncture
5. pregnancy
6. excision
7. formation, produce
8. recording
9. condition
10. pertaining to
11. process
12. one who specializes
13. inflammation
14. study of
15. measurement
16. tumor
17. condition of
18. surgical repair
19. to burst forth
20. suture
21. flow
22. instrument
23. instrument to cut
24. incision

Identifying Medical Terms

1. abortion
2. amniotome
3. antepartum
4. cervicitis
5. colporrhaphy
6. dysmenorrhea
7. eutocia
8. fibroma
9. gynecology
10. hymenectomy
11. mammoplasty
12. menorrhea
13. neonatal
14. oogenesis
15. postpartum

Spelling

1. amniocentesis
2. bartholinitis
3. dystocia
4. episiotomy
5. hysterotomy
6. menorrhagia

7. oophoritis
8. salpingitis
9. vaginitis
10. venereal

Matching

1. f   6. a
2. j   7. g
3. d   8. h
4. c   9. b
5. e   10. i

Abbreviations

1. abortion
2. AFP
3. abdominal hysterectomy
4. CS; C-section
5. diethylstilbestrol
6. EDC
7. pregnancy one
8. gynecology
9. IUD
10. PID

Diagnostic and Laboratory Tests

1. b
2. c
3. a
4. c
5. d

CHAPTER 16

Anatomy and Physiology

1. a. testes
   b. various ducts
   c. urethra
   d. bulbourethral gland
   e. prostate gland
   f. seminal vesicles
2. a. scrotum   b. penis
3. To provide the sperm cells necessary to fertilize the ovum, thereby perpetuating the species
4. A pouch-like structure located behind the penis

5. corpora cavernosa penis and the corpus spongiosum
6. 15 to 20
7. glans penis
8. The loose skin folds that cover the penis
9. A lubricating fluid
10. a. It is the male organ of copulation
    b. It is the site of the orifice for the elimination of urine and semen from the body.
11. They are two ovoid-shaped organs located in the scrotum. Each testis is about 4 cm long and 2.5 cm wide.
12. Seminiferous tubules
13. a. It is responsible for the development of secondary male characteristics during puberty.
    b. It is essential for normal growth and development of the male accessory sex organs.
    c. It plays a vital role in the erection process of the penis.
    d. It affects the growth of hair on the face.
    e. It affects muscular development and vocal timbre.
14. rete testis
15. A coiled tube lying on the posterior aspect of the testis
16. a. It is a storage site for sperm.
    b. It is a duct for the passage of sperm.
17. ductus deferens or the vas deferens
18. a. ductus deferens
    b. arteries
    c. veins
    d. lymphatic vessels
    e. nerves
19. Production of a slightly alkaline fluid
20. It is about 4 cm wide and weighs about 20 g. It is composed of glandular, connective, and muscular tissues

and lies behind the urinary bladder.
21. Enlargement of the prostate that sometimes occurs in older men
22. bulbourethral . . . Cowper's
23. a. prostatic
    b. membranous
    c. penile
24. It transmits urine and semen out of the body.
25. 20

Word Parts

Prefixes
1. lack of
2. lack of
3. around
4. upon
5. water
6. under
7. scanty
8. beside

Roots and Combining Forms
1. glans
2. to cut
3. hidden
4. bladder
5. testis
6. to pour
7. testicle
8. testicle
9. testicle
10. penis
11. a muzzle
12. prostate
13. prostate
14. a rent (opening)
15. seed
16. seed
17. seed, sperm
18. sperm
19. testicle
20. twisted vein
21. vessel
22. vesicle
23. animal
24. life

Suffixes
1. pain
2. pertaining to
3. immature cell, germ cell
4. hernia
5. to kill
6. excision
7. formation, produce
8. condition
9. process
10. condition of
11. inflammation
12. enlargement
13. condition of
14. fixation
15. surgical repair
16. incision
17. urine

Identifying Medical Terms
1. balanitis
2. epididymectomy
3. orchidectomy
4. orchidoplasty
5. prostatalgia
6. prostatocystitis
7. spermatoblast
8. spermatozoon
9. spermicide
10. testicular

Spelling
1. cryptorchism
2. hypospadias
3. orchidotomy
4. prostatomegaly
5. spermaturia

Matching
1. e   6. i
2. c   7. h
3. f   8. k
4. b   9. a
5. g   10. d

Abbreviations
1. BPH
2. gonorrhea
3. HPV
4. herpes simplex virus-2
5. sexually transmitted diseases
6. TPA
7. transurethral resection
8. urogenital
9. VD
10. WR

Diagnostic and Laboratory Tests
1. c
2. a
3. b
4. c
5. c

CHAPTER 17

An Overview of Cancer
1. a. carcinomas
   b. sarcomas
   c. mixed cancers
2. The process whereby normal cells have a distinct appearance and specialized function
3. The process whereby normal cells lose their specialization and become malignant
4. a. active migration
   b. direct extension
   c. metastasis
5. a. Change in bowel or bladder habits
   b. A sore that does not heal
   c. Unusual bleeding or discharge
   d. Thickening or lump in breast or elsewhere
   e. Indigestion or difficulty in swallowing
   f. Obvious change in a wart or mole
   g. Nagging cough or hoarseness
6. a. surgery
   b. chemotherapy
   c. radiation therapy
   d. immunotherapy

Word Parts

Prefixes

1. up
2. star-shaped
3. excessive
4. new
5. little
6. before

Roots and Combining Forms

1. gland
2. vessel
3. crab
4. cancer
5. cancer
6. cartilage
7. chorion
8. cell
9. tree
10. fiber
11. glue
12. glue
13. blood
14. safe
15. smooth
16. white
17. white
18. fat
19. lymph
20. lymph
21. marrow
22. black
23. membrane
24. mucus
25. fungus
26. marrow
27. muscle
28. kidney
29. kidney
30. nerve
31. tumor
32. bone
33. net
34. retina
35. rod
36. flesh
37. flesh
38. seed
39. mouth
40. monster
41. thymus
42. poison
43. grating
44. dry

Suffixes

1. immature cell
2. blood condition
3. formation
4. produce
5. formation, produce
6. condition
7. pertaining to
8. inflammation
9. tumor
10. pertaining to
11. plate
12. formation
13. a thing formed
14. formation
15. treatment
16. pertaining to

Identifying Medical Terms

1. carcinogen
2. chondrosarcoma
3. glioma
4. hypernephroma
5. leukemia
6. lymphoma
7. melanoma
8. myosarcoma
9. osteogenic sarcoma
10. sarcoma

Spelling

1. anaplasia
2. fibrosarcoma
3. lymphosarcoma
4. myeloma
5. oncogenic
6. seminoma

Matching

1. e   6. f
2. i   7. j
3. d   8. b
4. g   9. h
5. c   10. a

Abbreviations

1. Adeno-CA
2. Bx
3. cancer
4. chemotherapy
5. DNA
6. interleukin-2
7. LAK
8. metastases
9. tumor necrosis factor
10. TNM

CHAPTER 18

An Overview of Radiology and Nuclear Medicine

1. The study of x-rays, radioactive substances, radioactive isotopes, and ionizing radiation
2. a. invisible
   b. cause ionization
   c. excite fluorescence
   *Alternate characteristics to those listed:
   d. travel in a straight line
   e. able to penetrate substances
   f. destroy cells
3. a. Can depress the hematopoietic system, cause leukopenia, leukemia
   b. Can damage the gonads
4. a. wearing a film badge
   b. lead screens
   c. lead-lined room
   d. protective clothing
   e. gonad shield
5. a. computed tomography
   b. magnetic resonance imaging
   c. thermography
   d. scintigraphy
6. Treatment of disease by the use of ionizing radiation

Word Parts

Prefixes

1. short
2. through
3. within
4. one-thousandth
5. beyond

Roots and Combining Forms

1. acting
2. ampere
3. vessel
4. aorta
5. artery
6. joint
7. bronchi
8. heart
9. cavity
10. gall, bile
11. gall
12. motion
13. motion
14. cistern
15. curie
16. bladder
17. skin
18. a giving
19. echo
20. electricity
21. brain
22. fluorescence
23. kind
24. whole
25. uterus
26. ion
27. ion
28. one-thousand
29. motion
30. study of
31. to shine
32. lymph
33. breast
34. to measure
35. spinal cord
36. death
37. to swing
38. dark
39. light
40. nature
41. air
42. renal pelvis
43. radiant
44. ray
45. roentgen
46. fallopian tube
47. salivary
48. sound
49. sound
50. distant
51. heat
52. to cut
53. vein
54. vein
55. little belly
56. volt
57. watt
58. dry

Suffixes

1. pertaining to
2. one who
3. formation, produce
4. knowledge
5. record
6. record
7. recording
8. pertaining to
9. process
10. one who specializes
11. inflammation
12. nature of
13. study of
14. instrument to measure
15. condition of
16. pertaining to
17. instrument
18. to view, examine
19. treatment

Identifying Medical Terms

1. angiography
2. arthrography
3. cholecystogram
4. cisternography
5. dosimetrist
6. holography
7. intracavitary
8. ionotherapy
9. kilovolt
10. kilowatt
11. mammography
12. millicurie
13. physicist
14. radiation
15. radioactive
16. radiographer
17. radiolucent
18. radiopaque
19. roentgenologist
20. sonogram

Spelling

1. hysterosalpingogram
2. echography
3. lymphangiography
4. myelogram
5. pneumoencephalogram
6. radioactive
7. radiography
8. sialography
9. tomography
10. venography

Matching

1. d		6. k	
2. e		7. b	
3. c		8. i	
4. g		9. a	
5. j		10. h	

Abbreviations

1. AP
2. Ba
3. CT
4. kilovolt
5. left lateral
6. radium
7. MRI
8. posteroanterior
9. PEG
10. positron emission tomography

II
APPENDIX
Abbreviations

The process of shortening a word or phrase used in writing is called abbreviation. Abbreviations are the shorthand of the medical field. They are useful in saving time and space and have been recognized as a system of communication between members of the medical team.

Thousands of abbreviations are used in medicine to designate everything from prescriptions to the titles and degrees of health professionals. Typically, abbreviations are used for titles, degrees, licensure, registry, certification, organizations, agencies, associations, departments in hospitals, medications, diseases, lab tests, and specialties in nursing, medicine, and allied health fields. Due to the fast pace of high technology, additional abbreviations are continuously being added to those in common use.

In this section, over 800 abbreviations are listed under the following categories: Common Medical Abbreviations, and Medications and Prescriptions. These selected abbreviations are presented using capital letters without periods except in those cases where lower case letters and periods represent the norm or preferred method.

COMMON MEDICAL ABBREVIATIONS

A	accommodation	ACVD	acute cardiovascular disease	AIH	artificial insemination homologous
	age				
	anterior	AD	right ear (auris dextra)	alb	albumin
A_2	second aortic sound	ADH	antidiuretic hormone	alk	alkaline
AB	abnormal	ADS	antibody deficiency syndrome	alk phos	alkaline phosphatase
	abortion			ALL	acute lymphoblastic leukemia
A/B	acid-base ratio	AF	acid-fast		
abd	abdomen	AFB	acid-fast bacilli	ALS	amyotrophic lateral sclerosis
ABO	blood group	A/G	albumin-globulin ratio		
AC	air conduction	AH	abdominal hysterectomy	AMB	ambulatory
	acromioclavicular	AHD	arteriosclerotic heart disease	AMI	acute myocardial infarction
	alternating current				
ac	acute		autoimmune hemolytic disease	AML	acute myelocytic leukemia
ACH	adrenal cortical hormone	AID	acute infectious disease	ant	anterior
ACIP	Advisory Committee Immunization Practices		artificial insemination donor	A & P	anterior and posterior
		AIDS	acquired immuno-deficiency syndrome		auscultation and percussion
ACTH	adrenocorticotropic hormone			ARD	acute respiratory disease

535

ARF	acute respiratory failure	CMV	cytomegalovirus (herpes virus)	ECT	electroconvulsive therapy
ARM	artificial rupture of the membranes	CO	carbon monoxide	EDC	expected date of confinement
AS	left ear (auris sinistra)	CO_2	carbon dioxide	EEG	electroencephalogram
ASCVD	arteriosclerotic cardio-vascular disease	COLD	chronic obstructive lung disease	EENT	eyes, ears, nose, and throat
AU	both ears (aures unitas)	COPD	chronic obstructive pulmonary disease	EKG	electroencephalogram
AV	atrioventicular	CP	cerebral palsy	EMG	electromyography
ax	axiliary	CPA	carotid phonoangio-graph	EOM	extraocular movement
AZT	Aschheim-Zondek test	CPPB	continuous positive-pressure breathing	EPR	electron paramagnetic resonance
Ba	barium	CPR	cardiopulmonary resuscitation	EPS	extrapyramidal symptoms
BAC	blood alcohol concentration	creat	creatine	ER	emergency room
BaE, BE	barium enema	CRF	chronic renal failure	ERG	electroretinogram
Bld	blood	CS	central supply	ex	excision
BJ	Bence Jones	C & S	culture and sensitivity	exam	examination
BM	bowel movement	CSR	Cheyne-Stokes respira-tion	exp	expiration
BMR	basal metabolic rate		central supply room	F	Fahrenheit
BP, B/P	blood pressure	CT	computerized tomo-graphy	FBS	fasting blood sugar
BPH	benign prostatic hypertrophy	CTZ	chemoreceptor trigger zone	FH	family history
BRP	bathroom privileges			FHR	fetal heart rate
BS	blood sugar	CUC	chronic ulcerative colitis	FHS	fetal heart sound
	bowel sounds	CV	cardiovascular	FME	full mouth extraction
BSP	bromsulphalein	CVA	cardiovascular accident	FP	family practice
BUN	blood urea nitrogen	CVP	central venous pressure	FROM	full range of motion
Bx	biopsy	CXR	chest x-ray	FSH	follicle-stimulating hormone
		cysto	cystoscopy	FT	family therapy
CA	cancer			FUO	fever of unknown origin
Ca	calcium			FX	fracture
CAB	coronary artery bypass	db	decibel		
CAD	computerized assisted design	DC	direct current	GA	gastric analysis
cath	catheter	D & C	dilatation (dilation) and curettage	GB	gallbladder
CBC	complete blood count	D/C	discontinue	GBS	Guillain-Barré syndrome
CBS	chronic brain syndrome	Del	delivery	GC	gonorrhea
CC	chief complaint	diag	diagnosis	GG	gamma globulin
	cardiac cycle	DJD	degenerative joint disease	GH	growth hormone
CCPD	continuous cycle perito-neal dialysis	DM	diabetes mellitus	GI	gastrointestinal
CCU	cardiac care unit	DNA	deoxyribonucleic acid	GP	general practice
CDC	calculated date of con-finement	DOA	dead on arrival	grav 1	pregnancy one (primigravida)
	Center for Disease Control	DOB	date of birth	GS	general surgery
CF	cystic fibrosis	DR, Dr	doctor	GT	glucose tolerance
Ch, Chol	cholesterol	DRGs	diagnosis-related groups	GU	genitourinary
CHF	congestive heart failure	DVA	distance visual acuity	GVH	graft versus host disease
CHO	carbohydrate	Dx	diagnosis	GxT	graded exercise test
cib	food (cibus)			gyn	gynecology
Cl	clinic	EBL	estimated blood loss		
	chlorine	ECG	electrocardiogram	HASHD	hypertensive arterio-sclerotic heart disease
		ECHO	echocardiogram		
		E coli	Escherichia coli		

HB	heart block
Hb, Hgb	hemoglobin
HBP	high blood pressure
HBV	hepatitis B virus
HCT	hematocrit
HDCV	human diploid cell vaccine
HDS	herniated disk syndrome
H & L	heart and lungs
HMD	hyaline membrane disease
HNP	herniated nucleus pulposus
HO	hyperbaric oxygen
H_2O	water
H & P	history and physical
HS	herpes simplex
HSG	hysterosalpingogram
HSV	herpes simplex virus
Ht	height
HV	hospital visit
Hx	history

I	intensity of magnetism
IABP	intra-aortic balloon pump
IASD	interatrial septal defect
ICCU	intensive coronary care unit
ICT	indirect Coombs' test
ict ind	icterus index
ICU	intensive care unit
I & D	incision and drainage
IDS	immunity deficiency state
I/E	inspiratory-expiratory ratio
IEMG	integrated electromyogram
IHD	ischemic heart disease
IMV	intermittent mandatory ventilation
inf	inferior infusion
I & O	intake and output
IOP	intraocular pressure
IP-760	absorbable hemostat made by International Paper Co. and Lederle
IPG	impedance plethysmography
IPPB	intermittent positive-pressure breathing
IQ	intelligence quotient
IUD	intrauterine device

IVCP	inferior vena cava pressure
IVD	intervertebral disk
IVP	intravenous pyelogram
IVSD	interventricular septal defect
IVU	intravenous urogram

JARVIK-7	trademark for pneumatically-driven artificial heart
JRA	juvenile rheumatoid arthritis
jt	joint
JVP	jugular venous pulse

KB	ketone bodies
KCG	kinetocardiogram
KE	kinetic energy
KJ	knee jerk
KUB	kidney, ureter, and bladder
Kv	kilovolt
Kw	kilowatt

L & A	light and accommodation
lab	laboratory
LASER	light amplification by stimulated emission of radiation
lat	lateral
LBBB	left bundle branch block
L & D	labor and delivery
LDD	light-dark discrimination
LE	lupus erythematosus
lg	large
lig	ligament
L K & S	liver, kidney, and spleen
LLL	left lower lobe
LLSB	left lower sternal border
LLQ	left lower quadrant
LMP	last menstrual period
LOM	limitation of motion loss of motion
LP	lumbar puncture
LRDKT	living related donor kidney transplant
LSD	lysergic acid diethylamide
lt	left
LUQ	left upper quadrant

MASER	microwave amplification by stimulated emission of radiation
MBC	maximal breathing capacity
MBD	minimal brain damage
MI	myocardial infarction
MIP	maximal inspiratory pressure
MICU	medical intensive care unit
MND	motor neuron disease
MPJ	metacarpophalangeal joint
MR	mental retardation metabolic rate
MRD	medical record department minimum reacting dose
MS	multiple sclerosis musculoskeletal
MY	myopia

NA	not applicable numerical aperture
NAD	no acute disease
N/C	no complaints
NCV	nerve conduction velocity
NEG	negative
NLP	neuro-linguistic programming
No	number
NPN	nonprotein nitrogen
NPO	nothing by mouth (nulla per os)
NS	not sufficient
NSR	normal sinus rhythm
N & V	nausea and vomiting
NVA	near visual accuity
NVD	nausea, vomiting, and diarrhea neck vein distention

O_2	oxygen
OB	obstetrics
OB-GYN	obstetrics and gynecology
OC	office call
OCG	oral cholecystogram
OD	right eye (oculus dexter)
OIF	oil immersion field

OJ	orange juice	PIP	proximal interphalan-
OL	left eye (oculus laevus)		geal
OM	otitis media	PKU	phenylketonuria
O & P	ova and parasites	PL	light perception
OPD	outpatient department	PLS	primary lateral sclerosis
OPG	oculoplethysmography	PM	physical medicine
OR	operating room		postmortem
OS	left eye (oculus sinister)	PMA	progressive muscular
os	mouth		atrophy
OU	both eyes (oculi unitas)	PMI	point of maximal impulse
		PMP	past menstrual period
	_____	PMR	physical medicine and
			rehabilitation
P	pulse	PMS	premenstrual syndrome
P & A	percussion and ausculta-	PND	postnasal drip
	tion	PO	postoperative
PAC	premature arterial		by mouth (per os)
	contractions	POC	products of conception
PADP	pulmonary artery	PORM	problem-oriented
	diastolic pressure		medical record
PASP	pulmonary artery	pos	positive
	systolic pressure	PP	postpartum
PAP	Papanicolaou smear		postprandial
PAT	paroxysmal atrial tachy-		pulse pressure
	cardia	PPBS	postprandial blood sugar
path	pathology	PPD	purified protein deriva-
PBI	protein-bound iodine		tive (TB skin test)
PBP	progressive bulbar palsy	PPV	positive pressure
PBT₄	protein-bound thyroxine		ventilation
PCV	packed cell volume	PR	peer review
PE	physical examination		peripheral resistance
peds	pediatrics		public relations
PEF	peak expiratory flow		pulse rate
	rate	Pr	presbyopia
PEG	pneumoencephalo-		prism
	graphy	PRC	packed red cells
PERLA	pupils equal, react to	preg	pregnant
	light and accommoda-	preop	preoperative
	tion	prep	prepare
PERRLA	pupils equal, round,	proct	proctology
	regular, react to light	prog	prognosis
	and accommodation	PROM	premature rupture of
PET	preeclamptic toxemia		membranes
PG	pregnant	Pro time	prothrombin time
PGH	pituitary growth	PSP	phenosulfonphthalein
	hormone	PSRO	Professional Standards
PH	past history		Review Organization
	public health	PSS	physiological saline
pH	hydrogen ion concen-		solution
	tration (potential of		progressive systemic
	hydrogen)		sclerosis
PICU	pulmonary intensive	psy,	psychiatry
	care unit	psych	
PID	pelvic inflammatory	PT	paroxysmal tachycardia
	disease		physical therapy
PIF	peak inspiratory flow		

pt	patient
PTB	patellar tendon bearing
PTD	permanent and total
	disability
PTE	parathyroid extract
PU	peptic ulcer
PUD	pulmonary disease
pul	pulmonary
PV	peripheral vascular
	plasma volume
	polycythemia vera
P & V	pyloroplasty and
	vagotomy
PVC	premature ventricular
	contraction
PVD	peripheral vascular
	disease
PVOD	peripheral vascular
	occlusive disease
PVT	paroxysmal ventricular
	tachycardia
pvt	private
PWB	partial weight-bearing
Px	prognosis
	_____
QNS	quantity not sufficient
qt	quiet
	_____
R	rectal
	respiration
Ra	right arm
rad	radiation absorbed dose
RAF	rheumatoid arthritis
	factor
RAI	radioactive iodine
RATₓ	radiation therapy
RBBB	right bundle branch
	block
RBC	red blood cell
	red blood count
RBCV	red blood cell volume
RDA	recommended daily
	allowance
RDS	respiratory distress
	syndrome
rehab	rehabilitation
REM	rapid eye movement
RFS	renal function study
Rh	Rhesus (factor)
Rh neg	Rhesus factor negative
Rh pos	Rhesus factor positive
RHD	rheumatic heart disease

rhm	roentgen (per) hour (at one) meter
RIA	radioimmunoassay
RL	right leg
RLC	residual lung capacity
RLD	related living donor
RLL	right lower lobe
RLQ	right lower quadrant
RMSF	Rocky Mountain spotted fever
RNA	ribonucleic acid
RND	radical neck dissection
ROA	right occipitis anterior
ROM	range of motion rupture of membranes
ROP	right occipitis posterior
ROPS	roll over protection structures
ROS	review of systems
ROT	right occipitus transverse
RPG	retrograde pyelogram
rpm	revolutions per minute
RPO	right posterior oblique
RQ	respiratory quotient
RR	recovery room respiratory rate
RSR	regular sinus rhythm
RT	radiation therapy
rt	right
rt lat	right lateral
rtd	retarded
RU	roentgen unit
RUL	right upper lobe
RUQ	right upper quadrant
RVS	relative value schedule
RW	ragweed
Rx	prescription therapy

———

SA	salicylic acid sinoatrial
S & A	sugar and acetone
SAM	self-administered medication program
SB	stillbirth
SBE	subacute bacterial endocarditis
SCC	squamous cell carcinoma
schiz	schizophrenia
SCID	severe combined immune deficiency
SCUBA	self-contained underwater breathing apparatus

SD	septal defect spontaneous delivery sudden death
SDM	standard deviation of the mean
SDS	sudden death syndrome
sec	second
sed rate	sedimentation rate
seg	segmented neutrophils
SEM	scanning electron microscopy
semi	half
seq	sequela sequestrum
sev	sever severed
SF	scarlet fever spinal fluid
SG	serum globulin skin graft specific gravity
SGOT	serum glutamic-oxaloacetic trans-aminase
SH	serum hepatitis sex hormone
sh	shoulder
SICU	surgical intensive care unit
SID	sudden infant death
SIDS	sudden infant death syndrome
SI Units	International System of Units (Le Système International d'Unités)
SLE	systemic lupus erythematosus
SM	simple mastectomy
sm	small
SMR	submucous resection
SMRR	submucous resection and rhinoplasty
SO	salpingo-oophorectomy
SOB	shortness of breath
SOM	serous otitis media
SOP	standard operating procedure
sp gr	specific gravity
SPBI	serum protein-bound iodine
SPCK	serum creatine phosphokinase
SPE	serum protein electro-phoresis
SPP	suprapubic prostatec-tomy

SR	system review
SS	signs and symptoms soap solution
SSU	sterile supply unit
ST	esotropia
staph	staphylococcus
stat	immediately
STH	somatotropic hormone
STK	streptokinase
ST-MCA	superior temporal—middle cerebral artery anastomosis
strep	streptococcus
STS	serologic test for syphilis
STSG	split thickness skin graft
surg	surgery
SUI	stress urinary incontinence
SVD	spontaneous vaginal delivery
Sx	symptoms

———

T	temperature
T 1/2	half-life
T_3	triiodothyronine
T_4	thyroxine
TA	therapeutic abortion
T & A	tonsillectomy and adenoidectomy
TAH	total abdominal hysterectomy
TAO	thromboangiitis obliterans
TB	tuberculosis
TBD	total body density
TBF	total body fat
TBW	total body weight
TD	total disability
TENS	transcutaneous electrical nerve stimulation
TFS	thyroid function studies
TIA	transient ischemic attack
TKO	to keep open
TLC	tender loving care
TM	temporomandibular
TMJ	temporomandibular joint
Tn	normal intraocular tension
TND	term normal delivery

TPA	*Treponema pallidum* agglutination	ur	urine	VPC	ventricular premature contraction
TPBF	total pulmonary blood flow	URD	upper respiratory disease	VPRC	volume of packed red cells
TPR	temperature, pulse, respiration	URI	upper respiratory infection	VS	vital signs
TDS	Tay-Sach's disease	urol	urology	VSD	ventricular septal defect
TSH	thyroid-stimulating hormone	URQ	upper right quadrant	VT	tidal volume
TSP	total serum protein	US	ultrasonic		
TSS	toxic shock syndrome	UTI	urinary tract infection		———
TUR	transurethral resection	UV	ultraviolet	W	water
TV	tidal volume	UVJ	ureterovesical junction	w	watt
TVH	total vaginal hysterectomy		———	WB	weight-bearing whole blood
TW	tap water	VA	vacuum aspiration visual acuity	WBC	white blood cell white blood count
Tx	traction	VB	viable birth	WDWN	well-developed well-nourished
	———	VC	acuity of color vision vena cava vital capacity	WNL	within normal limits
UC	ulcerative colitis	VCG	vectrocardiogram	WR	Wassermann reaction
U & C	usual and customary	VD	venereal disease	wt	weight
UCD	usual childhood diseases	VDH	valvular disease of the heart		———
UCG	urinary chorionic gonadotropin	VDRL	Venereal Disease Research Laboratory	X	times
UCHD	usual childhood diseases	VG	ventricular gallop	XDP	xeroderma pigmentosum
UE	upper extremity	VH	vaginal hysterectomy	XM	crossmatch
UG	urogenital	VI	volume index	XR	x-ray
UGI	upper gastrointestinal	vin	wine	XT	exotropia
UK	unknown	vit cap	vital capacity		———
UL	upper lobe	VP	venipuncture venous pressure	Yag	yttrium aluminum garnet (laser)
ULQ	upper left quadrant	V & P	vagotomy and pyloroplasty	YOB	year of birth
umb	umbilicus	VBP	ventricular premature beat	yr	year
UN	urea nitrogen				———
UOQ	upper outer quadrant			Z	atomic number zero
UP	uroporphyrin				
UR	upper respiratory				

MEDICATION AND PRESCRIPTION ABBREVIATIONS

$\overline{aa}$	of each	APC	acetylsalicylic acid, phenacetin, caffeine	cap	capsule
ac	before meals (ante cibum)	APC-C	acetylsalicylic acid, phenacetin, caffeine with codeine	caps	capsules
ad lib	as desired (ad libitum) as much as needed			chem	chemotherapy
		aq	water	comp	compound
agit	shake, stir	ASA	acetylsalicylic acid	contra	against
$AgNO_3$	silver nitrate		———	coq	boil
alt dieb	alternating days			CTX	cytoxan
alt hor	alternating hours	BAPS	benzyl alcohol-preserved solutions	DEA	Drug Enforcement Administration
alt noc	alternating nights	bid	two times a day twice daily	dil	dilute
AM	morning			disp	dispense
amp	ampule		———	dist	distill
amt	amount			div	divide
ante	before	$\overline{c}$	with	DMSO	dimethylsulfoxide

dos	doses	KOH	potassium hydroxide	OTC	over the counter (drugs)
DPT	diphtheria pertussis tetanus				
D/S	dextrose and saline	liq	liquid	P	after
DW	distilled water	L/min	liters per minute	PABA	para-aminobenzoic acid
D/W	dextrose in water			p ae	in equal parts (partes aequales)
	————	M	mix	PAM	crystalline penicillin G in 2% aluminum monostearate
elix	elixir	MAO	monoamine oxidase		
emul	emulsion	MAOI	monoamine oxidase inhibitor		
eq	equivalent			PAS	para-aminosalicylic acid
et	and	MED	minimal effective dose	PB	phenobarbital
ext	extract	med	medicine	PBO	placebo
		meds	medicines	PBS	phosphate-buffered saline
	————	meq	milliequivalent		
FDA	Food and Drug Administration	Mg	magnesium	PBZ	pyribenzamine
		$MgSO_4$	magnesium sulfate	pc	after meals (post cibum)
Fe	iron	min	minimal		
fl	fluid	mist	mixture (mistura)	PCN	penicillin
FM	flowmeter	mixt	mixture	PDR	Physicians' Desk Reference
		MLD	minimum lethal dose		
	————	mn	midnight	pen	penicillin
garg	gargle	M & N	morning and night	pent	pentothal
		Mn	manganese	per	through
	————	MO	mineral oil	pil	pill
H	hour	MOM	milk of magnesia	PL	placebo
	hypo	MOPP	nitrogen mustard, oncovin, prednisone, procarbazine	PM	afternoon
(H)	hypodermic			PMI	patient medication instruction
h	hour				
hs	hour of sleep at bedtime	MOPV	monovalent oral poliovirus vaccine	po	by mouth (per os) phone order
H_2O	water	MS	morphine sulfate		
HN_2	nitrogen mustard	MTD	maximum tolerated dose	POMP	prednisone, oncovin, methotrexate, 6-mercaptopurine
hypo	injection under	MTX	methotrexate		
	————		————	pr	per rectum
IDP	initial dose period	Na	sodium	prn	as necessary when needed
IDR	intradermal reaction	ND	new drugs		
IE	immunizing unit (immunitata Einheit)	NDF	new dosage form	PST	penicillin, streptomycin, and tetracycline
		NF	normal flow National Formulary		
IM	intramuscular			pulv	powder
inc	increase	noc	night	PZI	protamine zinc insulin
in d	daily (in die)	noct	at night (nocte)		
inf	infusion	NS	normal saline		————
INH	isoniazid	N/S	normal saline	q	every
inj	inject	NSD	normal single dose	qd	every day (quaque die)
inoc	inoculate			qh	every hour (quaque hora)
IU	immunizing unit		————		
IV	intravenous	O_2	oxygen	q2h	every two hours
	————	OC	oral contraceptive	q3h	every three hours
		OD	overdose	q4h	every four hours
K	potassium	om	every morning (omni mane)	qid	four times a day
KCI	potassium chloride			qm	every morning
KI	potassium iodide	on	every night (omni nocte)	qn	every night
KMnO	potassium permanganate			qod	every other day
		OPV	oral poliovaccine	qs	quantity sufficient

	———	
R	rectal	
Rx	take	
	treatment	
	———	
S, Sig	give the following directions	
$\overline{s}$	without	
sat	saturated	
SC	subcutaneous	
scop	scopolamine	
sig	let it be labeled (sigetur)	
sol	solution	
sos	if it is necessary (si opus sit)	
sp, spir	spirit (spiritus)	
SS	saturated solution	
$\overline{ss}$	one-half	
SSA	salicylsalicylic acid	
SSE	soapsuds enema	
stat	immediately	

std	saturated
STK	streptokinase
STM	streptomycin
STU	skin test unit
subq	subcutaneous
sv	alcoholic spirit (spiritus vini)
syr	syrup
	———
tab	tablet
TAO	triacetyloleandomycin
TAT	tetanus antitoxin
TD	tetanus-diphtheria
TE	tetanus
TEM	triethylenemelamine
tet	tetanus
tid	three times a day
tinct	tincture
TO	telephone order
TOPV	trivalent oral poliovirus vaccine
tr	tincture

troch	troche
tus	cough (tussis)
	———
U	unit
ung	ointment (unguentum)
USP	United States Pharmacopeia
ut dict	as directed (ut dictum)
	———
vag	vagina
ves	bladder
VO	verbal order
vol	volume
	———
wo	without
W/O	water in oil
	———
ZIG	zoster immune globulin

III

Glossary of Component Parts

PREFIXES

a,	no, not, without, lack of, apart	ec,	out, outside, outer	multi,	many, much
ab,	away from	ecto,	outside, outer, out		————
ad,	toward, near, to	em,	in		
ambi,	both	en,	within	neo,	new
an,	no, not, without, lack of	end,	within, inner	nulli,	none
ana,	up	endo,	within, inner		————
ant,	against	ep,	upon, over, above		
ante,	before	epi,	upon, over, above	olig,	little, scanty
anti,	against	eso,	inward	oligo,	little, scanty
apo,	separation	eu,	good, normal		————
astro,	star-shaped	ex,	out, away from		
auto,	self	exo,	out, away from	pan,	all
	————	extra,	outside, beyond	par,	around, beside
			————	para,	beside, alongside, abnormal
bi,	two, double	hemi,	half	per,	through
brachy,	short	hetero,	different	peri,	around
brady,	slow	homeo,	similar, same, likeness	poly,	many, much, excessive
	————	hydr,	water	post,	after, behind
		hydro,	water	pre,	before, in front of
cac,	bad	hyp,	below, deficient	primi,	first
cata,	down	hyper,	above, beyond, excessive	pro,	before, in front of
centi,	a hundred	hypo,	below, under, deficient	proto,	first
chromo,	color		————	pseudo,	false
circum,	around			pyro,	fire
con,	with, together	in,	in, into, not		————
contra,	against	infra,	below		
	————	inter,	between	retro,	backward
		intra,	within		————
de,	down, away from		————		
di(a),	through			semi,	half
dia,	through, between	mal,	bad	sub,	below, under, beneath
dif,	apart, free from, separate	mega,	large, great	supra,	above, beyond
		meso,	middle	sym,	together
dipl,	double	meta,	beyond, over, between, change	syn,	together, with
di(s),	two				————
dys,	bad, difficult, painful	micro,	small	tachy,	fast
	————	milli,	one-thousandth	tri,	three
		mono,	one		————

543

ultra,	beyond	arthro,	joint	cephal,	head
uni,	one	atel,	imperfect	cephalo,	head
		atelo,	imperfect	cept,	receive

ROOTS AND COMBINING FORMS

		ather,	fatty substance, porridge	cere-	
		athero,	fatty substance, porridge	bell,	little brain
		atri,	atrium	cere-	
		atrio,	atrium	bello,	little brain
abort,	to miscarry	audio,	to hear	cerebro,	cerebrum
absorpt,	to suck in	auditor,	hearing	cervic,	cervix
acanth,	a thorn	aur,	the ear	cheil,	lip
aceta-		axill,	armpit	chemo,	chemical
bul,	vinegar cup			chol,	gall, bile
achillo,	Achilles', heel	————		chole,	gall, bile
acid,	acid			chole-	
acoust,	hearing	bacteri,	bacteria	docho,	common bile duct
acr,	extremity, point	balan,	glans	chondr,	cartilage
acro,	extremity	barth-		chondro,	cartilage
act,	acting	olin,	Bartholin's glands	chorio,	chorion
actin,	ray	baso,	base	choroid,	choroid
aden,	gland	bil,	bile	chor-	
adeno,	gland	bili,	gall, bile	oido,	choroid
adhes,	stuck to	bio,	life	chromo,	color
adip,	fat	blephar,	eyelid	chym,	juice
aero,	air	ble-		cine,	motion
agglu-		pharo,	eyelid	cinem-	
tinat,	clumping	bol,	to cast, throw	ato,	motion
agon,	agony	brachi,	arm	cis,	to cut
albin,	white	bronch,	bronchi	cister-	
albumin,	protein	bronchi,	bronchi	no,	reservoir, cavity, cistern
all,	other	bron-		clast,	destruction
alveol,	small, hollow air sac	chiol,	bronchiole	clavicul,	little key
ambly,	dull	broncho,	bronchi	cleido,	clavicle
ambul,	to walk	bucc,	cheek	clon,	turmoil
ametr,	disproportionate	burs,	a pouch	coagul,	clots, to clot
amnio,	lamb			coccyge,	tail bone
ampere,	ampere	————		coccygo,	tail bone
amyl,	starch	calc,	lime, calcium	cochleo,	land snail
andr,	man	calcane,	heel bone	coit,	a coming together
angi,	vessel	cal-		col,	colon
angin,	to choke, quinsy	caneo,	heel bone	colla,	glue
angio,	vessel	calci,	calcium	collis,	neck
aniso,	unequal	cancer,	crab	colo,	colon
ankyl,	stiffening, crooked	capn,	smoke	colon,	colon
ano,	anus	carcin,	cancer	colono,	colon
anthrac,	coal	carcino,	cancer	colpo,	vagina
append,	appendix	card,	heart	condyle,	knuckle
appen-		cardi,	heart	coni,	dust
dic,	appendix	cardio,	heart	connect,	to bind together
aort,	aorta	carp,	wrist	contin-	
aorto,	aorta	carpo,	wrist	ence,	to hold
arachn,	spider	caud,	tail	cor,	pupil
arter,	artery	caus,	heat	cordo,	cord
arteri,	artery	cavit,	cavity	coriat,	corium
arterio,	artery	celi,	abdomen, belly	corne,	cornea
arthr,	joint	centr,	center	cortic,	cortex
		centri,	center		

cost,	rib
costo,	rib
cox,	hip
coxo,	hip
crani,	skull
cranio,	skull
creat,	flesh
creatin,	flesh, creatine
cretin,	cretin
crin,	to secrete
crine,	to secrete
crino,	to secrete
crypt,	hidden
culdo,	cul-de-sac
curie,	curie
cutane,	skin
cyan,	dark blue
cycl,	ciliary body
cyclo,	ciliary body
cyst,	bladder, sac
cysti,	bladder, sac
cysto,	bladder, sac
cyt,	cell
cyth,	cell
cyto,	cell

———

dacry,	tear
dacryo,	tear
dactyl,	finger or toe
dactylo,	finger or toe
dendro,	tree
dent,	tooth
denti,	tooth
derm,	skin
derma,	skin
dermat,	skin
dermato,	skin
dermo,	skin
dextro,	to the right
didym,	testis
dilat,	to widen
disk,	a disc, disk
diverti-culi,	diverticula
dosi,	a giving
duct,	to lead
duoden,	duodenum
dur,	dura, hard
dwarf,	small

———

echo,	echo
ego,	I, self
electro,	electricity

embol,	a throwing in
encep-phal,	brain
ence-phalo,	brain
enchy-ma,	to pour
enter,	intestine
entero,	intestine
eosino,	rose-colored
episio,	vulva, pudenda
erget,	work
erysi,	red
erythro,	red
eso-phage,	esophagus
eso-phago,	esophagus
esthesio,	feeling
eunia,	a bed

———

fasc,	a band
fasci,	a band
fascio,	a band
femor,	femur
fibr,	fibrous tissue, fiber
fibro,	fiber
fibul,	fibula
fluoro,	fluorescence
foc,	focus
fora-mino,	foramen
format,	a shaping
fus,	to pour

———

galacto,	milk
gan-glion,	knot
gastr,	stomach
gastro,	stomach
gen,	formation, produce
gene,	formation, produce
genet,	producing
genital,	belonging to birth
geno,	kind
ger,	old age
gigant,	giant
gingiv,	gums
glandul,	little acorn
gli,	glue
glio,	glue
glomer-ul,	glomerulus, little ball

glomer-ulo,	glomerulus, little ball
glosso,	tongue
gluco,	sweet, sugar
glyc,	sweet, sugar
glyco,	sweet, sugar
glycos,	sweet, sugar
gonad,	seed
gonio,	angle
granulo,	little grain, granular
gryp,	curve
gyneco,	female

———

halat,	breathe
hem,	blood
hemat,	blood
hemato,	blood
hemo,	blood
hepat,	liver
hepato,	liver
hernio,	hernia
hidr,	sweat
hirsut,	hairy
histo,	tissue
holo,	whole
humer,	humerus
hydr,	water
hymen,	hymen
hypn,	sleep
hypno,	sleep
hyster,	womb, uterus
hystero,	womb, uterus

———

icter,	jaundice
ile,	ileum
ileo,	ileum
ili,	ilium
ilio,	ilium
immuno,	safe
insul,	insulin
insulin,	insulin
insu-lino,	insulin
iono,	ion
ionto,	ion
irid,	iris
irido,	iris
isch,	to hold back
ischi,	ischium
iso,	equal

———

kal,	potassium

karyo,	cell's nucleus	meat,	passage	onco,	tumor
kel,	tumor	meato,	passage	onych,	nail
kerat,	horn, cornea	medullo,	marrow	onychi,	nail
kerato,	cornea	melan,	black	onycho,	nail
keton,	ketone	melano,	black	oo,	ovum, egg
kilo,	a thousand	men,	month	oophor,	ovary
kinet,	motion	mening,	membrane	oph-	
kymo,	motion	meninge,	membrane	thalm,	eye
kyph,	a hump	meningi,	membrane	ophthal-	
	————	meningo,	membrane	mo,	eye
		meno,	month	opt,	eye
labi,	lip	ment,	chin, mind	opto,	eye
laby-		mes,	middle	orch,	testicle
rinth,	maze	mester,	month	orchido,	testicle
laby-		metr,	to measure	organ,	organ
rintho,	maze	metr,	womb, uterus	ortho,	straight
lacrim,	tear	metri,	uterus	oscillo,	to swing
lamin,	lamina, thin plate	mic-		osm,	smell
laparo,	flank, abdomen	turit,	to urinate	osteo,	bone
laryng,	larynx	mitr,	mitral valve	oto,	ear
larynge,	larynx	mnes,	memory	ot,	ear
laryngo,	larynx	mucos,	mucus	ovul,	ovary
later,	side	muscul,	muscle	ox,	oxygen
laxat,	to loosen	my,	muscle	oxy,	sour, sharp, acid
leio,	smooth	my,	to shut		————
lemma,	a rind	myc,	fungus		
letharg,	drowsiness	myco,	fungus	pachy,	thick
leuk,	white	myel,	marrow, spinal cord	palato,	palate
leuko,	white	myelo,	marrow, spinal cord	pan-	
levat,	lifter	myo,	muscle	creat,	pancreas
lingu,	tongue	myos,	muscle	papill,	papilla
lip,	fat	myring,	drum, membrane	paque,	dark
lipo,	fat	myringo,	drum, membrane	para,	to bear
litho,	stone	myx,	mucus	partum,	labor
lob,	lobe		————	patell,	kneecap
lobo,	lobe			patella,	kneecap
log,	study of	naso,	nose	path,	disease
logo,	word	nat,	birth	patho,	disease
lord,	bending	nata,	birth	pause,	cessation
lucent,	to shine	necr,	death	pec-	
lumb,	loin	nephr,	kidney	torat,	breast
lumbo,	loin	nephro,	kidney	ped,	foot
lun,	moon	neur,	nerve	pedicul,	a louse
lymph,	lymph	neuri,	nerve	pelvi,	pelvis
lympho,	lymph	neuro,	nerve	pen,	penis
	————	neutro,	neither	penile,	penis
		noct,	night	pept,	to digest
macro,	large	nom,	law	perine,	perineum
mammo,	breast	norm,	rule	perineo,	perineum
mandi-		nucle,	kernel, nucleus	phaco,	lens
bul,	lower jawbone	nyctal,	blind	phago,	to eat, engulf
mano,	thin		————	phak,	lentil, lens
mast,	breast			phalange,	closely knit row
maxill,	jawbone	ocul,	eye	pharyng,	pharynx
maxilla,	jawbone	olecran,	elbow		

phar-	
ynge,	pharynx
pheo,	dusky
phim,	a muzzle
phleb,	vein
phlebo,	vein
phon,	voice
phone,	voice
phono,	sound
photo,	light
phragm,	partition
phrag-	
mato,	partition
phras,	speech
physic,	nature
physio,	nature
pine,	pine cone
pineal,	pineal body
pino,	to drink
pitui-	
tar,	phlegm
plasma,	a thing formed, plasma
pleur,	pleura
pleura,	pleura
pleuro,	pleura
plicat,	to fold
pneumo,	lung, air
pneu-	
mon,	lung
polio,	gray
por,	a passage
porphyr,	purple
prandi,	meal
presby,	old
proct,	rectum, anus
procto,	rectum, anus
prostat,	prostate
prostato,	prostate
psych,	mind
psycho,	mind
pulmo,	lung
pulmon,	lung
pul-	
monar,	lung
pupill,	pupil
py,	pus
pyel,	renal pelvis
pyelo,	renal pelvis
pyo,	pus
pylor,	pylorus, gate keeper
pyret,	fever
pyro,	heat, fire

———

quadri,	four

———

rachi,	spine
rachio,	spine
radi,	radius
radiat,	radiant
radico,	root
radicul,	root
radio,	ray
recto,	rectum
relaxat,	to loosen
ren,	kidney
reno,	kidney
reti-	
culo,	net
retin,	retina
retino,	retina
rhabdo,	rod
rhino,	nose
rhytid,	wrinkle
rhytido,	wrinkle
roent,	roentgen
rotat,	to turn
rrhythm,	rhythm

———

sacr,	sacrum
salping,	tube
sal-	
pingo,	tube
salpinx,	tube, fallopian tube
sarc,	flesh
sarco,	flesh
scapul,	shoulder blade
scler,	hardening, sclera
sclero,	hard
scoli,	curvature
scolio,	curvature
scop,	to examine
sebo,	oil
semin,	seed
senil,	old
sept,	putrefaction
septic,	putrefying
sero,	whey, serum
sert,	to gain
sial,	saliva
sialo,	salivary
sidero,	iron
sig-	
moido,	sigmoid
sino,	a curve
sinus,	a curve, hollow
somat,	body
somato,	body

somn,	sleep
son,	sound
sono,	sound
spadias,	a rent, an opening
spastic,	convulsive
sperm,	seed
spermat,	seed
spermi,	sperm
sphygmo,	pulse
spin,	spine, a thorn
spiro,	breath
splen,	spleen
spleno,	spleen
spondyl,	vertebra
spon-	
dylo,	vertebra
staped,	stirrup
steat,	fat
sten,	narrowing
stern,	sternum
sterno,	sternum
stetho,	chest
stigmat,	point
stom,	mouth
stomat,	mouth
strict,	to draw, to bind
sym-	
path,	sympathy
sym-	
patho,	sympathy
systol,	contraction

———

tele,	distant
tendo,	tendon
teno,	tendon
tenon,	tendon
tenos,	tendon
tens,	pressure
tentori,	tentorium, tent
terat,	monster
testi-	
cul,	testicle
thalass,	sea
thermo,	hot, heat
thoraco,	chest
thorax,	chest
thromb,	clot of blood
thrombo,	clot
thym,	thymus, mind, emotion
thymo,	thymus
thyr,	thyroid, shield
thyro,	thyroid, shield
tibi,	tibia
tinnit,	a jingling

toc,	birth
tomo,	to cut
ton,	tone, tension
tono,	tone
tonsill,	almond, tonsil
topic,	place
topo,	place
torti,	twisted
tox,	poison
toxic,	poison
trache,	trachea
tracheo,	trachea
tract,	to draw
tre-	
phinat,	a bore
trich,	hair
tricho,	hair
trigon,	trigone
trism,	grating
trop,	turn
troph,	a turning
tuss,	cough
tympan,	drum

---

uln,	elbow
ulno,	elbow
ungu,	nail
ur,	urine
ure,	urinate
urea,	urea
uret,	urine
ureter,	ureter
uretero,	ureter
urethr,	urethra
urethro,	urethra
urin,	urine
urinat,	urine
urino,	urine
uro,	urine
uter,	uterus
uve,	uvea

---

vagin,	vagina
vago,	vagus, wandering
varico,	twisted vein
vas,	vessel
vascul,	small vessel
vaso,	vessel
vector,	a carrier
ven,	vein
venere,	sexual intercourse
veni,	vein
veno,	vein

ventri-	
cul,	ventricle
ventri-	
culo,	little belly
vermi,	worm
vers,	turning
vertebr,	vertebra
vertebro,	vertebra
vesic,	bladder
vesicul,	vesicle
viril,	masculine
viscer,	body organs
volt,	volt
volunt,	will

| watt, | watt |

---

xantho,	yellow
xen,	foreign material
xer,	dry
xero,	dry
xiph,	sword

| zoo, | animal |
| zoon, | life |

SUFFIXES

-able,	capable
-ac,	pertaining to
-age,	related to
-al,	pertaining to
-algesia,	pain
-algia,	pain
-ant,	forming
-ar,	pertaining to
-ary,	pertaining to
-ase,	enzyme
-asthenia,	weakness
-ate,	use, action

-betes,	to go
-blast,	immature cell, germ cell
-body,	body

-cele,	hernia
-cen-	
tesis,	surgical puncture
-ceps,	head
-cide,	to kill

-clasia,	a breaking
-clave,	a key
-clysis,	injection
-colon,	colon
-crit,	to separate
-cul-	
ture,	cultivation
-cusis,	hearing
-cuspid,	point
-cyesis,	pregnancy
-cyte,	cell

-derma,	skin
-desis,	binding
-drome,	a course
-dynia,	pain

-ectasia,	distention
-ectasis,	dilatation, dilation, distention
-ectasy,	dilation
-ectomy,	excision
-edema,	swelling
-emesis,	vomiting
-emia,	blood condition
-er,	relating to, one who
-ergy,	work
-esthesia,	feeling

| -form, | shape |
| -fuge, | to flee |

-gen,	formation, produce
-genes,	produce
-genesis,	formation, produce
-genic,	formation, produce
-glia,	glue
-globin,	protein
-gnosis,	knowledge
-grade,	a step
-graft,	pencil
-gram,	a weight, mark, record
-graph,	to write, record
-graphy,	recording

| -hexia, | condition |

| -ia, | condition |
| -ic, | pertaining to |

-ide,	having a particular quality
-in,	chemical, pertaining to
-ine,	pertaining to
-ion,	process
-ism,	condition of
-ist,	one who specializes, agent
-itis,	inflammation
-ity,	condition
-ive,	nature of, quality of

———

| -kinesia, | motion |
| -kinesis, | motion |

———

-lalia,	to talk
-lemma,	a sheath, husk, rind
-lexia,	diction
-liter,	liter
-lith,	stone
-logy,	study of
-lymph,	serum, clear fluid
-lysis,	destruction, to separate

———

-malacia,	softening
-mania,	madness
-megaly,	enlargement, large
-meter,	instrument to measure, measure
-metry,	measurement
-mime-tic,	imitating
-mnesia,	memory
-morph,	form, shape

———

| -noia, | mind |

———

-oid,	resemble, form
-oma,	tumor
-omion,	shoulder
-opia,	eye, vision
-opsia,	eye, vision
-or,	one who, a doer
-orexia,	appetite
-ose,	like
-osis,	condition of
-ous,	pertaining to

———

-paresis,	weakness
-pathy,	disease
-pelas,	skin
-penia,	lack of, deficiency
-pepsia,	to digest
-pexy,	fixation
-phagia,	to eat
-phasia,	speak
-pheresis,	removal
-phil,	attraction
-philia,	attraction
-phobia,	fear
-phore,	bearing
-phoresis,	to carry
-phragm,	a fence
-phraxis,	to obstruct
-phthisis,	a wasting
-physis,	growth
-plakia,	plate
-plasia,	formation
-plasm,	a thing formed, plasma
-plasty,	surgical repair
-plegia,	stroke, paralysis
-pnea,	breathing
-poiesis,	formation
-poietic,	formation
-praxia,	action
-ptosis,	prolapse, drooping
-ptysis,	to spit
-punc-ture,	to pierce

———

-rrhage,	to burst forth, bursting forth
-rrhagia,	to burst forth, bursting forth
-rrhaphy,	suture
-rrhea,	flow, discharge
-rrhexis,	rupture

———

-scope,	instrument
-scopy,	to view, examine
-sepsis,	decay
-sis,	condition
-some,	body
-spasm,	tension, spasm, contraction
-stalsis,	contraction

-stasis,	control, stopping
-staxia,	dripping, trickling
-sthenia,	strength
-stomy,	new opening
-systole,	contraction

———

-tasis,	stretching
-taxia,	order
-therapy,	treatment
-thermy,	heat
-tome,	instrument to cut
-tomy,	incision
-tone,	tension
-tony,	tension
-tripsy,	crushing
-trophy,	nourishment, development

———

-um,	tissue
-uria,	urine
-us,	pertaining to

———

| -y, | condition, pertaining to, process |

Suffixes that mean pertaining to are:
-ac
-al
-ar
-ary
-ic
-in
-ine
-ous
-us
-y

Suffixes that mean condition of are:
-hexia
-ia
-ism
-ity
-osis
-sis
-y

GENERAL INDEX

SPANISH INDEX

Need Extra Help?

Appleton & Lange has the resources to help you *master* medical terminology.

COMPUTERIZED STUDENT SELF-ASSESSMENT

to accompany Jane Rice's *Medical Terminology with Human Anatomy, 3/e.*

A computerized self-assessment is available for Jane Rice's *Medical Terminology with Human Anatomy, 3/e.* This program links each question to a specific page in the text where the answer can be found. After working through the questions, chapter by chapter, a personalized study plan is created based on the learner's performance.

Features!
- 1,500 questions in multiple-choice and fill-in-the-blank format
- Correct answer explained and referenced by page number
- Study plan generated from questions answered incorrectly
- Study plans can be printed out and/or viewed on computer screen
- A superior value at only $19.95 plus $2.95 shipping and handling

3 VOLUME SET OF AUDIO TAPES to accompany Jane Rice's
Medical Terminology with Human Anatomy, 3/e

In order to facilitate learning, these audiotapes are available as an aid to the pronunciation and comprehension of medical terminology. Each term is pronounced, broken into its component parts, the definition of the part is given, and the term pronounced again.

3 Audio Tapes (90 minutes each), ISBN 0-8385-6256-6, A6256-0, $29.95

FREE AUDIO TAPE
Spanish Terms & Tough Terms

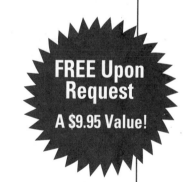

Students may request a free 60-minute audio tape — a compilation of Spanish terms and phrases on one side and those tough terms that need the extra reinforcement on the other. This tape is absolutely free by mailing in the coupon on the reverse side.

Features!
- TOUGH TERMS
  Integumentary System (Ch.3)
  Endocrine System (Ch.11)
  Nervous System (Ch.12)

- SPANISH TERMS
  Terms and phrases pronounced in Spanish, then English, then defined in English.

To order any of these valuable resources, fill out the coupons on the reverse side and mail to the appropriate addresses.

❑ YES! Please send me the **COMPUTERIZED STUDENT SELF-ASSESSMENT**
to accompany Jane Rice's *Medical Terminology with Human Anatomy, 3/e*.

To purchase this interactive learning tool for $19.95 (plus $2.95 shipping and handling), simply call 1-800-748-7734 or clip & mail this coupon to:
Educational Software Concepts, Inc. • P.O. Box 13267 • 660 S. 4th Street • Edwardsville, KS • 66113

Name_____Address _____

City _____State _____ Zip _____

Phone _____

❑ Payment Enclosed   ❑ Bill Me

❑ MasterCard   ❑ Visa   ❑ American Express

Card No. _____ Exp. _____

Signature _____

❑ YES! Please send me the **3 VOLUME SET OF AUDIO TAPES**
(90 minutes each), ISBN 0-8385-6256-6, A6256-0, $29.95

❑ YES! Please send me the ***FREE* SPANISH TERMS AND TOUGH TERMS**
audio tape ($9.95 VALUE!) to accompany Jane Rice's *Medical Terminology with Human Anatomy, 3/e*, ISBN 0-8385-6255-8, A6255-2.

To order, check off the appropriate boxes and mail this valuable coupon to:
Appleton & Lange • Department Rice • 25 Van Zant Street • P.O. Box 5630 • Norwalk, CT • 06856

Name_____Address _____

City _____State _____ Zip _____

Phone _____

School _____Address _____

City _____State _____ Zip _____

Professor_____Name of Course _____

Name of Program _____

❑ Payment Enclosed   ❑ Bill Me

❑ MasterCard   ❑ Visa   ❑ American Express

Card No. _____ Exp. _____

Signature _____

How did you hear about Rice's MEDICAL TERMINOLOGY, 3/e? _____

Are you interested in computerized study tools?_____

NOTE: This free audio tape is available through Appleton & Lange only. Coupon is necessary for fulfillment. No telephone, bookstore, or wholesaler requests will be honored. Limit one per customer.

10/94

RIC-32734-A1(3)

a-, an-	bi-
prefix	prefix
ab-	brachy-
prefix	prefix
ad-	brady-
prefix	prefix
ambi-	cac-, mal-
prefix	prefix
ante-	centi-
prefix	prefix
anti-	con-
prefix	prefix
auto-	contra-
prefix	prefix

two, double

no, not, without, lack of

meaning

meaning

short

away from

meaning

meaning

slow

toward, near, to

meaning

meaning

bad

both

meaning

meaning

a hundred

before

meaning

meaning

with, together

against

meaning

meaning

against

self

meaning

meaning

de-	ep-, epi-
prefix	prefix
dia-	eu-
prefix	prefix
dif-	ex-, exo-
prefix	prefix
dipl-	extra-
prefix	prefix
dys-	hemi-, semi-
prefix	prefix
ec-, ecto-	hetero-
prefix	prefix
end-, endo-	homeo-
prefix	prefix

upon, over, above	down, away from
meaning	meaning

good, normal	through, between
meaning	meaning

out, away from	apart, free from, separate
meaning	meaning

outside, beyond	double
meaning	meaning

half	bad, difficult, painful
meaning	meaning

different	out, outside, outer
meaning	meaning

similar, same	within, inner
meaning	meaning

hydro-	mega-
prefix	prefix
hyper-	meso-
prefix	prefix
hypo-	meta-
prefix	prefix
in-	micro-
prefix	prefix
infra-	milli-
prefix	prefix
inter-	mono-
prefix	prefix
intra-	multi-
prefix	prefix

large, great	water
meaning	meaning
middle	above, beyond, excessive
meaning	meaning
beyond, over, between, change	below, under, deficient
meaning	meaning
small	in, into, not
meaning	meaning
one thousandth	below
meaning	meaning
one	between
meaning	meaning
many, much	within
meaning	meaning

neo-	post-
prefix	prefix
olig-, oligo-	pre-, pro-
prefix	prefix
pan-	pseudo-
prefix	prefix
para-	retro-
prefix	prefix
per-	sub-
prefix	prefix
peri-	supra-
prefix	prefix
poly-	sym-, syn-
prefix	prefix

after, behind

new

meaning

meaning

before, in front of

little, scanty

meaning

meaning

false

all

meaning

meaning

backward

beside, alongside, abnormal

meaning

meaning

below, under, beneath

through

meaning

meaning

above, beyond

around

meaning

meaning

with, together

many, much, excessive

meaning

meaning

tachy-	-blast
prefix	suffix
tri-	-centesis
prefix	suffix
ultra-	-cyte
prefix	suffix
uni-	-ectasis
prefix	suffix
-ac, -al, -ar, -ary, -ic, -in, -ine, -ous, -us, -y	-ectomy
suffix	suffix
-algesia, -algia, -dynia	-emesis
suffix	suffix
-ate	-gen, -genesis, -genic
suffix	suffix

immature cell, germ cell	fast
meaning	meaning
surgical puncture	three
meaning	meaning
cell	beyond
meaning	meaning
dilatation, dilation, distention	one
meaning	meaning
excision	pertaining to
meaning	meaning
vomiting	pain
meaning	meaning
formation, produce	use, action
meaning	meaning

-gram	-megaly
suffix	suffix
-hexia, -ia, -ism, -ity, -osis, -sis, -y	-oma
suffix	suffix
-itis	-pathy
suffix	suffix
-ive	-penia
suffix	suffix
-logy	-plasm
suffix	suffix
-lymph	-plegia
suffix	suffix
-lysis	-ptosis
suffix	suffix

enlargement, large	weight, mark, record
meaning	meaning
tumor	condition of
meaning	meaning
disease	inflammation
meaning	meaning
lack of, deficiency	nature of, quality of
meaning	meaning
a thing formed, plasma	study of
meaning	meaning
stroke, paralysis	serum, clear fluid
meaning	meaning
prolapse, drooping	destruction, to separate
meaning	meaning

-rrhea	-tome
suffix	suffix
-rrhaphy	-tomy
suffix	suffix
-rrhexis	-trophy
suffix	suffix
-scopy	adeno
suffix	combining form
-spasm	arterio
suffix	combining form
-stasis	arthro
suffix	combining form
-staxia	cardio
suffix	combining form

instrument to cut	flow, discharge
meaning	meaning
incision	suture
meaning	meaning
nourishment, development	rupture
meaning	meaning
gland	to view, examine
meaning	meaning
artery	tension, spasm
meaning	meaning
joint	control, stopping
meaning	meaning
heart	dripping, trickling
meaning	meaning

chondro	hepato
combining form	combining form
costo	myo
combining form	combining form
cranio	naso rhino
combining form	combining form
dermato	nephro reno
combining form	combining form
erythro	neuro
combining form	combining form
gastro	patho
combining form	combining form
hemato	thoraco
combining form	combining form

liver	cartilage
meaning	meaning
muscle	rib
meaning	meaning
nose	skull
meaning	meaning
kidney	skin
meaning	meaning
nerve	red
meaning	meaning
disease	stomach
meaning	meaning
chest	blood
meaning	meaning